Hydroxychloroquine and Chloroquine Retinopathy

David J. Browning

Hydroxychloroquine and Chloroquine Retinopathy

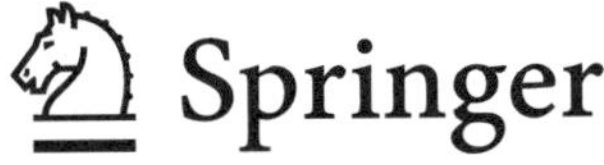 Springer

David J. Browning
Charlotte Eye Ear Nose & Throat Associates
Charlotte, NC, USA

ISBN 978-1-4939-4733-1   ISBN 978-1-4939-0597-3 (eBook)
DOI 10.1007/978-1-4939-0597-3
Springer New York Heidelberg Dordrecht London

Printed on acid-free paper

Springer is part of Springer Science+Business Media (www.springer.com)

To my son, Samuel Judson Browning

Preface

This book provides a single source from which an interested ophthalmologist or optometrist can learn most of what is known in 2014 about the cause, prevention, and detection of hydroxychloroquine and chloroquine retinopathy.

The book is oriented to the needs of the practitioner. In real life, acquisition of ancillary studies is often done at a simpler level than in an academic environment. Whereas avoiding artifacts in ancillary tests is a goal everywhere, the clinician must often make interpretations in spite of them, and real cases are presented in which this has been done.

No monograph can be completely self-contained, but this one aspires to that goal. The intended reader is the ophthalmologist or optometrist who sees patients taking 4-aminoquinolines. Often far removed from their training, these clinicians may not remember the precise meanings of prevalence, odds ratio, pretest probability, sensitivity, epitope, decibels, visual field threshold, and coefficient of variance. Therefore, a refresher is included here. Thus, in addition to the main subject of clinical ophthalmology, the book is a platypus with sections on pathology, physiology, pharmacokinetics, toxicology, and statistics. Along the way, sidebars guide the reader on interesting tangents.

Unfortunately, the literature on 4-aminoquinoline retinopathy is large and dispersed. Even using the Internet, it is difficult to access and synthesize the sources. The aim of this book is to accomplish just that. With this text as your guide, you can become the local expert on this iatrogenic and largely preventable condition.

Nomenclature is important, but confusing. Although the book focuses on chloroquine and hydroxychloroquine, much of it applies to other related drugs (e.g., quinacrine). These drugs were formerly termed antimalarials, as they were first used against malaria. However, their main use currently is in the treatment of autoimmune diseases. Because both chloroquine and hydroxychloroquine are 4-aminoquinolines, a timeless chemical descriptor, this is the preferred usage when writing about both drugs. When only one of the two is referred to, the particular compound is named. When quinacrine is also implied, it is mentioned specifically.

Evidence-based medicine is the benchmark for clinicians in 2014, yet in the field of hydroxychloroquine and chloroquine retinopathy there are no level-1 studies. Instead, we have eminence-based medicine, in the phrase of Graham Hughes, relying on case series and personal experience. In this context, the recognized authorities over the last 50 years were Bernstein and Mackenzie, followed by Easterbrook, and latterly Marmor.

Some have despaired that a higher quality of evidence cannot be achieved. Perhaps the best that can be done is to analyze the literature, identify flaws, and develop a contemporary perspective. Yet the development of a network of ophthalmologists linked by the Internet to a hub with expertise in clinical trials (along the lines of the Diabetic Retinopathy Clinical Research Network) makes one hopeful that questions may eventually be answered in a rigorous manner. In particular, answers are needed to these:

- Why is the perifoveal retina preferentially affected by the toxicity?
- What is the prevalence of 4-aminoquinoline retinopathy?
- What is the relative importance of adjusted daily dose and cumulative dose?
- What are the relative sensitivity and specificity of 10–2 visual fields, multifocal electroretinography, spectral domain optical coherence tomography, and fundus autofluorescence for the detection of 4-aminoquinoline retinopathy?
- Does screening for 4-aminoquinoline retinopathy in properly dosed patients make economic sense?

The field of study is dynamic; some might say volatile. In 1993, 10–2 visual fields were considered optional as screening aids. By 2002, they were recommended in all cases. By 2011, the additional use of multifocal electroretinography, spectral domain optical coherence tomography, and fundus autofluorescence imaging was recommended. By 2013, experts were backing away from these expanded recommendations. The reader can expect even more changes in the future, especially as economic constraints pressure proponents of tests to prove their value.

Elmore Leonard's tenth rule for writing well was to leave out the part that no one reads, which is good advice for writing novels, but not textbooks. For example, a clinician may occasionally want to know how hydroxychloroquine affects the binding of the invariant chain to MHC class II molecules. This, and other recondite facts, are found in this book, which aims to be a resource both for daily practice and for in-depth study.

Finally, although I have attempted to fairly lay out the evidence in support of all sides in controversies surrounding 4-aminoquinoline retinopathy, the facts have led me to a point of view that has not been hidden. The evidence suggests that too many people lose vision from 4-aminoquinoline retinopathy because of insufficient attention paid to dosing. Moreover, the recommendation favoring universal ancillary testing of those taking 4-aminoquinolines seems wasteful, when the emphasis should be on detecting toxic dosing with selective use of tests based on clinically assessed risk. Paracelsus told us 500 years ago, "It is the dose that makes the poison." What follows is an elaboration on the truth of that adage.

Charlotte, NC, USA   David J. Browning

Acknowledgements

Many colleagues helped write this book. Joanna Perey of Springer guided the project from proposal through development and production with professionalism and friendly support. Sara Jarret, Daniel Britt, and Wendy Vetter provided talented assistance in converting sketches into clear figures. Chong Lee was tireless in fact-checking, obtaining references, laying out figures, and completing the tables. Uma Balasubramaniam, Swann Bojaj, Loraine Clark, Donna Jo McClain, Michael McOwen, and Cherish Lynn Watson took the photographs, optical coherence tomographs, and performed the multifocal electroretinograms found in the book. I am thankful every day for their technical skills and caring manner with patients. Clare Browning and Gabriela Ritterspach read chapters critically and identified sections needing rewriting. Will Doak is the best editor an author could have. He clarifies everything his pen touches. I am grateful to all of these talented friends. Any merit the book has is shared with them. Errors that remain are mine.

Contents

Abbreviations

4AQs	4-Aminoquinolines (chloroquine and hydroxychloroquine)
APC	Antigen presenting cell
4AQR	4-Aminoquinoline retinopathy
BM	Bruch's membrane
BRB	Blood–retina barrier
C	Concentration
C_pG ODN	C_pG oligodeoxynucleotide
CD	CD number
CD3	Cluster of differentiation T3 cell co-receptor
CD74 gene	Cluster of differentiation 74 gene
D	Daily dose in mg/kg
DN cells	Double negative cells
DP cells	Double positive cells
EC50	Effective concentration 50 %
ELM	External limiting membrane
FAZ	Foveal avascular zone
GCL	Ganglion cell layer
HLA	Human leukocyte antigen
IFNα	Interferon alpha
Ii	Invariant chain
IκK complex	Inhibitor of kappa B kinase complex
IL	Interleukin
ILM	Internal limiting membrane
INL	Inner nuclear layer
IPL	Inner plexiform layer
IRAK	Interleukin-1 receptor-associated kinase
IS/OS	Inner segment/outer segment
K	Rate constant for elimination
μm	Micrometer
MHC	Major histocompatibility complex
miRNA	MicroRNA
nm	Nanometer
NEMO	Nuclear factor-$\kappa\beta$ essential modifier regulatory subunit
NF-$\kappa\beta$	Nuclear factor-$\kappa\beta$
NFL	Nerve fiber layer
NLRs	Nucleotide-binding and oligomerizing domain-like receptors
OCT	Optical coherence tomography
OPL	Outer plexiform layer
ONL	Outer nuclear layer
PAMP	Pathogen-associated molecular pattern
RA	Rheumatoid arthritis
RCS	Royal College of Surgeons
RPC	Radial peripapillary capillary
RPE	Retinal pigment epithelium
SD-OCT	Spectral domain optical coherence tomography
SLE	Systemic lupus erythematosus
SP cells	Single positive cells
TCR	T cell receptor
TCR–CD3	T cell receptor–cluster of differentiation 3T cell co-receptor complex
TD-OCT	Time domain optical coherence tomography

D.J. Browning, *Hydroxychloroquine and Chloroquine Retinopathy*, DOI 10.1007/978-1-4939-0597-3_1, © Springer Science+Business Media New York 2014

Th cells   Helper T cells
Treg cells   Regulatory T cells
V   Volume of distribution
VEGF   Vascular endothelial growth factor

Concepts and facts in this chapter are drawn from ocular anatomy, physiology, immunology, and pharmacology that are important in understanding the cause, progression, and ways to prevent chloroquine and hydroxychloroquine retinopathy. Because chloroquine and hydroxychloroquine are 4-aminoquinolines (4AQs), the retinopathy that they cause is referred to as 4-aminoquinoline retinopathy (4AQR). It is assumed that the reader has a medical-school background but needs to be refreshed about the relevant topics. Where possible, the particular structures and physiologic steps influenced by 4AQs will be noted. Looking ahead, Chap. 2 reviews the pharmacology of the 4AQs, and Chap. 3 their toxicology and the pathologic ocular changes they can cause. Commonly used abbreviations in this chapter are collected in "Abbreviations" for reference. Each term will be first used in its full form, along with its abbreviation.

1.1 Anatomy and Histology

Histologically, the retina is a multilayered sheet of neuronal, glial, and vascular tissue that lines the inside posterior two-thirds of the eye. It is bounded anteriorly by the vitreous humor and posteriorly by the retinal pigment epithelium (RPE), Bruch's membrane (BM), and choroid. The macula is a circular area of the retina 5.2–5.5 mm in diameter with a center located 17°, or 4.0–5.0 mm temporal, and 0.53–0.8 mm inferior to the center of the optic disc (Fig. 1.1) [1–5]. Of potential significance in 4AQR, the macula receives more total irradiance than the peripheral retina, and the inferior macula receives more irradiance in the blue part of the spectrum (from the sky) than the superior macula [6]. A useful conversion of arc length on the macula to degrees of eccentricity from the fovea is that 1 degree is equivalent to 280 microns, or three first-order retinal vein widths [5]. Among the distinguishing features of the macula are the high

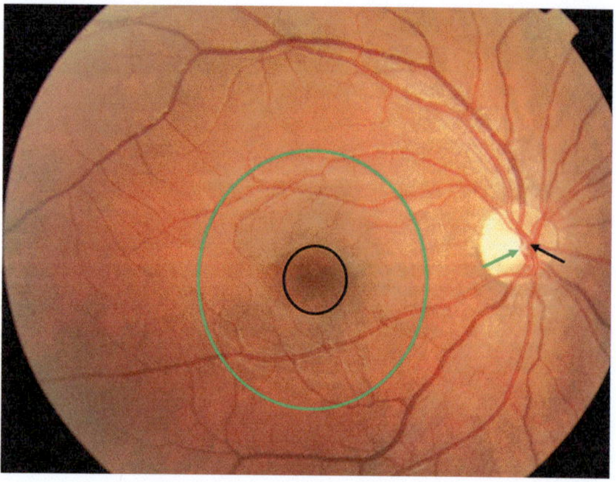

Fig. 1.1 Fundus photograph from a normal eye showing the macula (*green circle*) and fovea (*black circle*). The normal central retinal artery (*black arrow*) is located nasal to the central retinal vein (*green arrow*) in the optic disc. The luteal pigment gives the region encircled in *black* its darker pigmentation relative to the surrounding retina

density of cones, two or more layers of ganglion cells, as well as the presence of the xanthophyll carotenoids lutein and zeaxanthin within photoreceptor axons, bipolar cells, and ganglion cells [1, 3, 7, 8].

Xanthophylls are not synthesized by the body, but must come from the diet [7]. Zeaxanthin is the predominant xanthophyll in the center of the macula with lutein rising in relative concentration in the parafovea [7]. The xanthophylls reduce chromatic aberration, absorb damaging blue light, and protect retinal membranes from photooxidation [7, 9]. The extent of their distribution is similar to the size of the bull's-eye macular lesion in 4AQR and suggests that they may have a role in toxicity. For example, 4AQR in its advanced stages manifests outer retinal atrophy that spares the fovea and is greatest from 2 to 8° eccentric to the fovea [10, 11]. Xanthophylls have their greatest concentrations in the fovea and drop to a lower plateau within 4° of the fovea [9]. The levels are generally nondecreasing once adulthood is reached [7].

The central 1.5 mm circular area of the macula is called the fovea, denoted by a gently curved depression in the retinal surface. Within the fovea is a roughly circular avascular area, the foveal avascular zone (FAZ), approximately 400–500 µm in diameter which contains only cones, present at a density of approximately 125,500–140,000/mm^2 [1, 12].

Deriving the Conversion from Degrees to Micrometers

Without derivation, it has been asserted that $1° \approx 280$ μm [2, 5, 13]. There is pedagogic value in deriving this relationship. Geometrically, an object creates an inverted image which falls upon the concave retina. An image that spans the 5.5 mm curvilinear macula would create a larger image if it were flat on a plane tangent to the posterior pole of the eye. The size of this straightened image can be calculated as follows. The average eye has a diameter of 24.07 mm, creating a radius of 12.035 mm. The angle subtended by a circular segment 5.5 mm in length is (see Fig. 1.2):

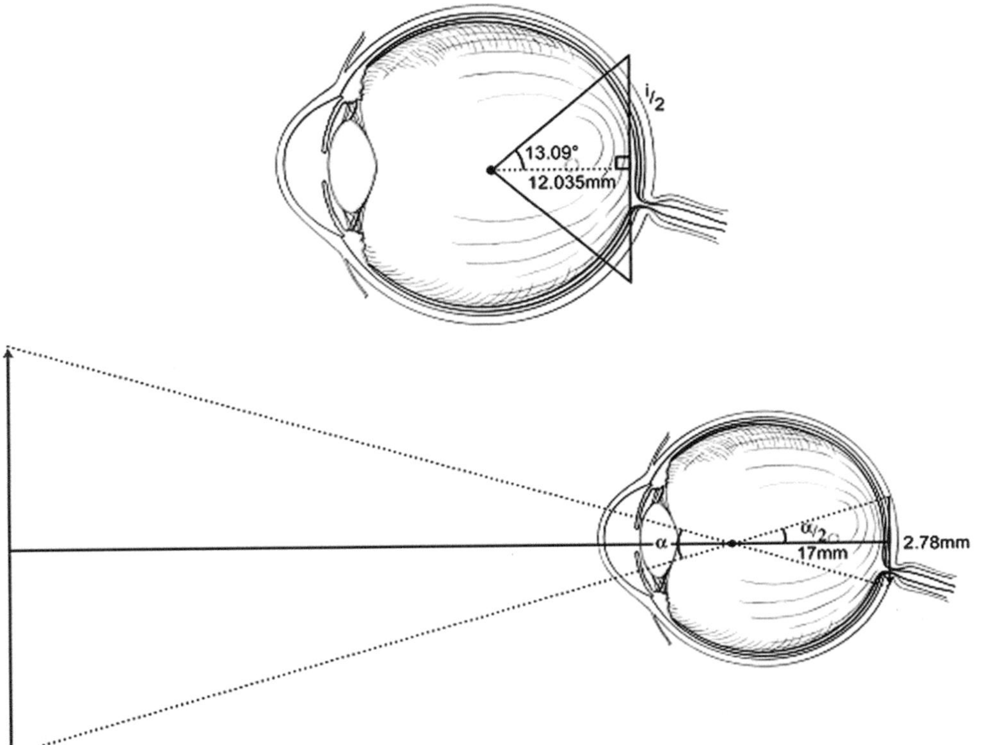

Fig. 1.2 Diagram of schematic eye used in deriving the conversion factor for transforming arc length on the retina to subtended angle

$$360° \,(5.5/\text{circumference of eye}) = 26.18°.$$

One half the straightened image height ($i/2$) can be calculated noting the geometrical relationship:

$$\tan(13.09) = \left(\frac{i}{2}\right)\Big/ 12.035.$$

Solving for i,

$$i = 2 \times 12.035 \times \tan(13.09) = 5.56\,\text{mm},$$

and therefore $i/2 = 2.78$ mm.

The simplified version of the eye is that of a single lens 17 mm in front of the retina (the eye's nodal point). Ray tracing shows the relationship between object and image in Fig. 1.2. One half the angle α subtended by the image from the eye's nodal point can be calculated from the geometrical relationship

$$\tan\left(\frac{\alpha}{2}\right) = 2.78\,/\,17,$$

where

$$\alpha = 2\arctan\left(2.78\,/\,17\right) = 18.57°.$$

The conclusion, then, is that $18.57° = 5.5$ mm, or $1° = 0.296$ mm $= 296$ μm, which is in fair agreement with the published figure.

A cross section through the retina just outside the area centralis shows ten layers (Figs. 1.3 and 1.4). Proceeding from the vitreous to the choroid are the internal limiting membrane (ILM), nerve fiber layer, ganglion cell layer, inner plexiform layer, inner nuclear layer, outer plexiform layer, outer nuclear layer (ONL), external limiting membrane (ELM), rod and cone inner and outer segments, and RPE [14]. In histologic sections the retina is thicker around the disc, where it is 0.56 mm thick, and tapers to 0.18 mm at the equator and 0.11 mm at the ora as the density of all neural elements decreases peripherally [1]. The topography of the macula includes a central thinner zone, the foveal depression, and a thicker paracentral annulus around the fovea where the ganglion cell layer, inner nuclear layer, and outer plexiform layer of Henle are thickest (Fig. 1.4) [1].

In vivo measurements of the thickness of retinal layers can be measured by spectral domain optical coherence tomography (SD-OCT). Table 1.1 shows measurements made for central and pericentral regions in normal human subjects [5]. Macular thicknesses and the thicknesses of intraretinal layers measured with different instruments will differ slightly because of differences in location of the outer retinal boundary line and in the segmentation algorithms used. For example, the Stratus time domain optical coherence tomography (TD-OCT) instrument measures from the ILM to the inner segment/outer segment (IS/OS) junction, the Spectralis SD-OCT between the ILM and the Bruch's membrane–choriocapillaris complex, the Cirrus SD-OCT between the ILM and the photoreceptor outer segment–RPE boundary, and the Optovue SD-OCT between the ILM and the external limit of the RPE [15–17].

The central circular area has a radius of 1.4 mm for the Optovue SD-OCT [5]. For the Cirrus SD-OCT the radius of the central circular zone is 1.0 mm [19]. The pericentral annulus for the Optovue measurements extends from 1.4 to 2.6 mm from the fovea [5]. For the Cirrus measurements the annulus extends from 1.0 to 3.0 mm from the fovea [19].

1.2 Microanatomy of the Retina

The RPE is a monolayer of hexagonal cells external to the photoreceptors (Fig. 1.3). These cells do not divide after embryogenesis. They are multifunctional, pumping ions and water toward the choroid, absorbing photons not involved in phototransduction, protecting the retina from oxidative stress, and participating in the cycling of visual pigments in concert with photoreceptors [6]. The lateral cell membranes of the RPE are connected by zonula occludentes inhibiting the extracellular diffusion of water and ions and constituting the outer blood–retina barrier (BRB) [1].

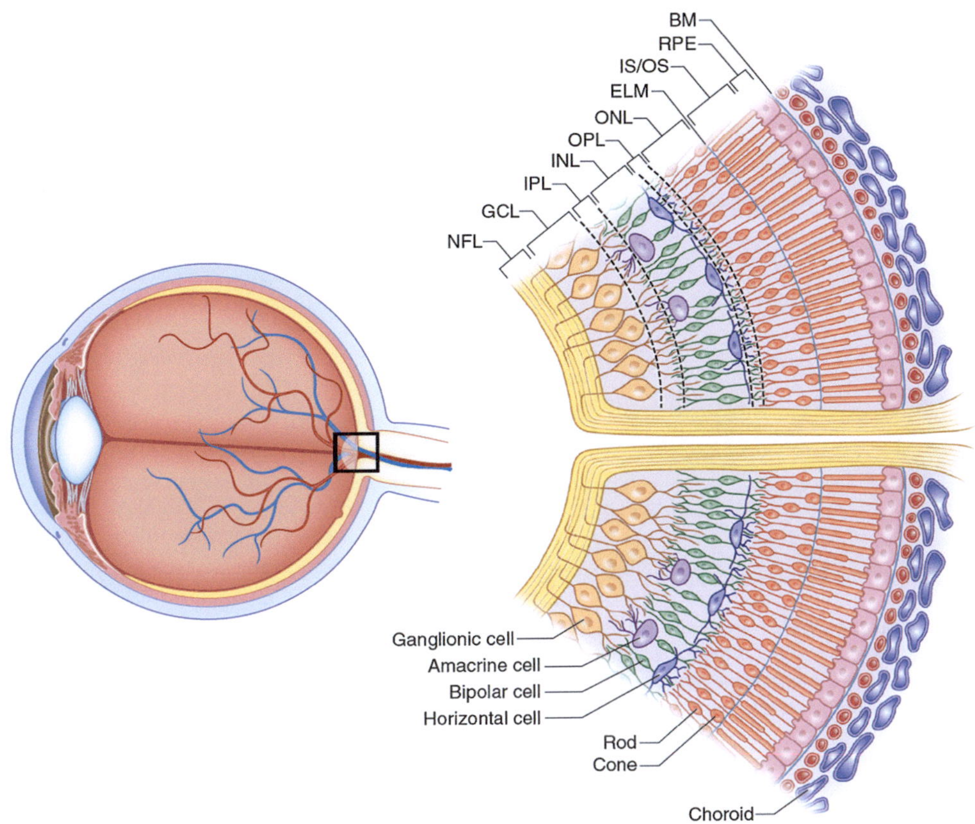

Fig. 1.3 Diagram of the stratified cellular nature of the retina. The axons of the ganglion cells comprise the nerve fiber layer and optic nerve. BM is Bruch's membrane. RPE is the retinal pigment epithelium. IS/OS stands for the inner segment/outer segment of photoreceptors. ELM is the external limiting membrane. ONL is the outer nuclear layer. OPL is the outer plexiform layer. INL is the inner nuclear layer. IPL is the inner plexiform layer. GCL is the ganglion cell layer. NFL is the nerve fiber layer

There are regional variations in RPE biochemistry. Levels of cathepsin D, aryl sulfatase, and acid phosphatase enzyme activity are higher in the macula than in the periphery [6]. Some of these enzymes are inhibited by 4AQs suggesting a potential association with the maculocentric distribution of 4AQR.

The RPE recycles large amounts of photosensitive cell membranes derived from the discs of the photoreceptor outer segments [1]. The apposition of photoreceptor discs to apical RPE plasma membrane triggers a signal for phagocytosis of the discs (Fig. 1.5) [20, 21]. Discs are encompassed by invaginated RPE plasma membrane and the shed discs are internalized into the RPE cell as a phagosome [21–23]. The phagosome moves basally while fusing with lysosomes containing 60 or more hydrolytic enzymes that progressively degrade the discs as well as melanin (Fig. 1.6) [6, 21, 22, 24, 25]. Phagosomes with degraded discs are termed myeloid or myelin bodies. Apposition of RPE to photoreceptor outer segments is essential for disc metabolism. Isolated retinas without apposed RPE do not shed discs, but begin to do so when the retina is reapposed to RPE. Both rods and cones shed discs, but the timing differs by photoreceptor types. Although there are exceptions in certain species, the general pattern is that cones shed their discs with the onset of darkness and rods shed theirs with the onset of light [6]. Melatonin synthesized by the retina primes shedding [24].

In the retina of the rhesus monkey, each RPE cell in the retinal periphery degrades approximately

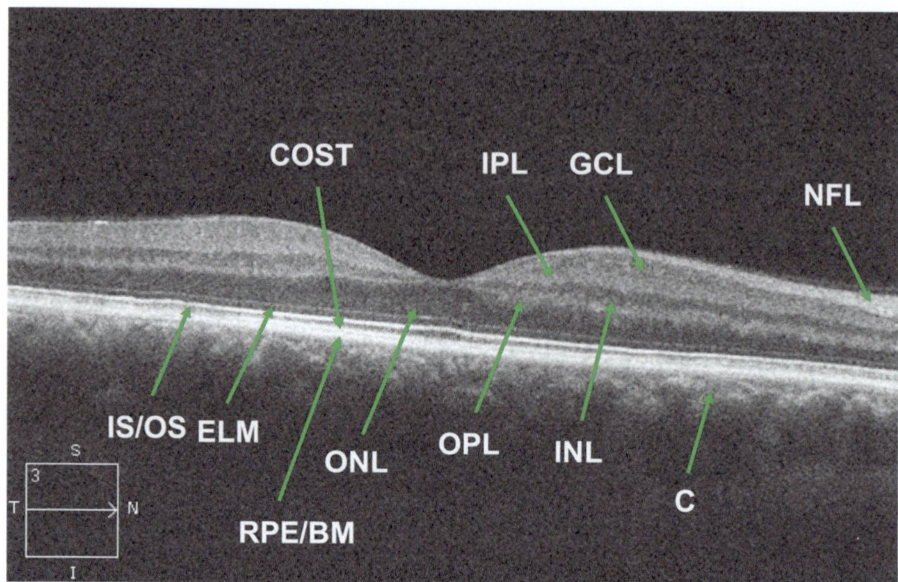

Fig. 1.4 Spectral domain OCT image from a normal right eye depicting the layers of the retina. The vitreous is the black empty space at the top above the retina. The foveal depression is seen in the center. The cones are taller than the rods producing greater separation between the inner segment/outer segment junction and the apical retinal pigment epithelium at the fovea. NFL is the nerve fiber layer. GCL is the ganglion cell layer. IPL is the inner plexiform layer. INL is the inner nuclear layer. OPL is the outer plexiform layer. ONL is the outer nuclear layer. ELM is the external limiting membrane. IS/OS is the inner segment/outer segment junction. COST is the cone outer segment tips. RPE/BM is the retinal pigment epithelium/ Bruch's membrane. C is the choroid. N means nasal. *T* temporal, *S* superior, *I* inferior

Table 1.1 SD-OCT measured thickness of retinal layers in the macula

Retinal layer	Study/instrument/gender	Central circular zone (µM)	Pericentral annulus (µM)
Nerve fiber layer	Pasadikha et al. [5]/Optovue/female	16.93 ± 2.23	37.83 ± 5.25
	Demirkaya et al. [18]/Topcon OCT-1000/both		23.1 ± 1.8
Ganglion cell layer	Demirkaya et al. [18]/Topcon OCT-1000/both		50.6 ± 5.6
Inner plexiform layer	Demirkaya et al. [18]/Topcon OCT-1000/both		40.7 ± 3.3
Ganglion cell layer + inner plexiform layer	Pasadikha et al. [5]/Optovue/female	73.38 ± 8.93	74.26 ± 5.46
Inner nuclear layer	Pasadikha et al. [5]/Optovue/female	29.24 ± 3.16	32.84 ± 2.38
	Demirkaya et al. [18]/Topcon OCT-1000/both		39.6 ± 3.2
Outer plexiform layer	Pasadikha et al. [5]/Optovue/female	32.80 ± 1.94	28.26 ± 1.94
	Demirkaya et al. [18]/Topcon OCT-1000/both	24.4 ± 5.1	29.0 ± 3.5
Outer nuclear layer + photoreceptor inner segment layer	Pasadikha et al. [5]/Optovue/female	90.60 ± 3.23	75.20 ± 3.02
	Demirkaya et al. [18]/Topcon OCT-1000/both	117.0 ± 11.7	95.9 ± 9.3
Photoreceptor outer segment layer	Pasadikha et al. [5]/Optovue/female	33.42 ± 2.75	33.07 ± 3.16
	Demirkaya et al. [18]/Topcon OCT-1000/both	48.6 ± 3.9	42.6 ± 3.6
Retinal pigment epithelium	Demirkaya et al. [18]/Topcon OCT-1000/both	19.2 ± 1.7	18.2 ± 1.9
Total retinal thickness	Pasadikha et al. [5]/Optovue/female	276.38 ± 12.73	281.46 ± 5.69
	Wagner-Schuman et al. [19]/Cirrus/female	253.6 ± 19.3	317.9 ± 13.8
	Grover/Spectralis/female	266.3 ± 21.9	

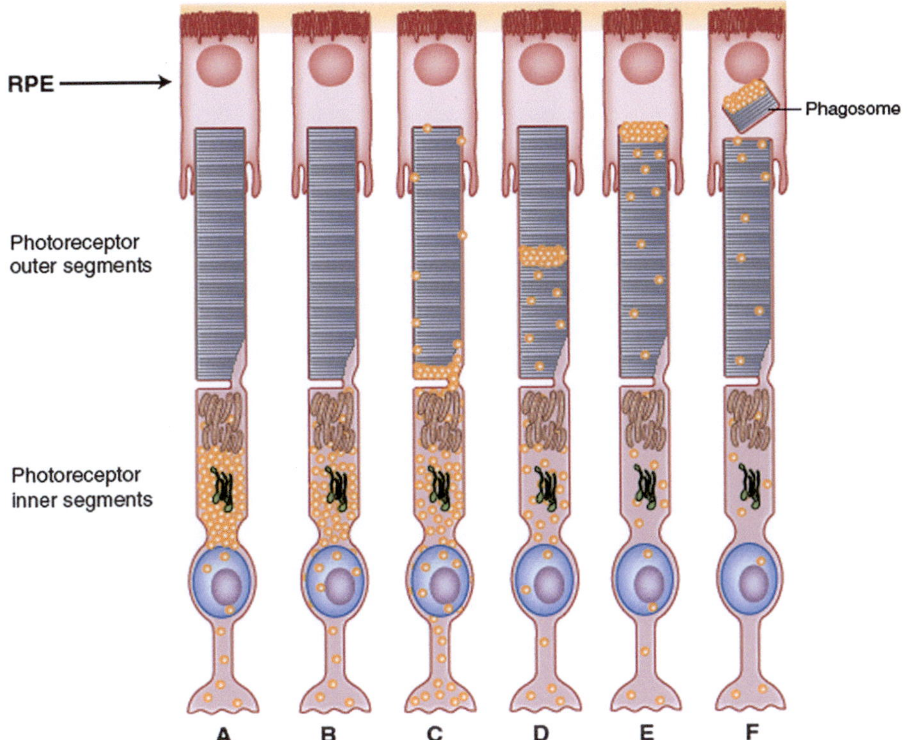

Fig. 1.5 Diagram of rod outer segment disc metabolism. Protein has been radiolabeled (*yellow dots*). The protein is synthesized in the inner segments, is incorporated into a cohort of discs within the photoreceptor outer segments that moves outward, and is phagocytosed by the retinal pigment epithelium when it reaches the apex of the outer segment. Data from Young [26]

4,000 rod outer segment discs per day [24]. The phagocytic load per RPE cell increases with age as RPE cells drop out and fewer remaining cells distribute the burden [6]. Disruption of photoreceptor outer segment recycling by RPE damages the photoreceptors and probably has a role in 4AQR. For example, the photoreceptors prematurely die in the Royal College of Surgeons (RCS) rat, which has a mutation impairing RPE phagocytosis [20, 27].

The product of degradation of photoreceptor outer segments by RPE is lipofuscin, which is contained within lysosomes as undigested residues of oxidatively damaged lipids (Fig. 1.7) [6, 24, 28–31]. Fluorophores within the discs resist full degradation in the RPE lysosomes. Their presence gives lipofuscin its autofluorescence [32]. The RCS rat has decreased levels of RPE lipofuscin because of impaired photoreceptor outer segment phagocytosis [27, 33]. Lipofuscin has its highest concentration in the central retina, where it increases in concentration over a lifetime [28, 34]. It occupies 1 % of the cytoplasmic volume of RPE cells in the first decade of life, but 19 % in the decade 81–90 [28]. In 4AQR, parafoveal hyperautofluorescence is a consequence of the disrupted RPE metabolism of photoreceptor outer segments (Fig. 1.8) [35]. Most investigators consider lipofuscin to be detrimental to cell function, as testified by increased levels in 4AQR, Stargardt disease, age-related macular degeneration, and retinitis pigmentosa (Fig. 1.8) [6, 30, 36]. The toxic component of lipofuscin is A2E, which raises lysosomal pH, inhibits lysosomal degradation of proteins, predisposes RPE cells to blue light-induced apoptosis, and has damaging detergent properties for cell membranes [25, 30, 37–40].

By SD-OCT the average thickness of the RPE layer in a central circle of 1 mm diameter in the

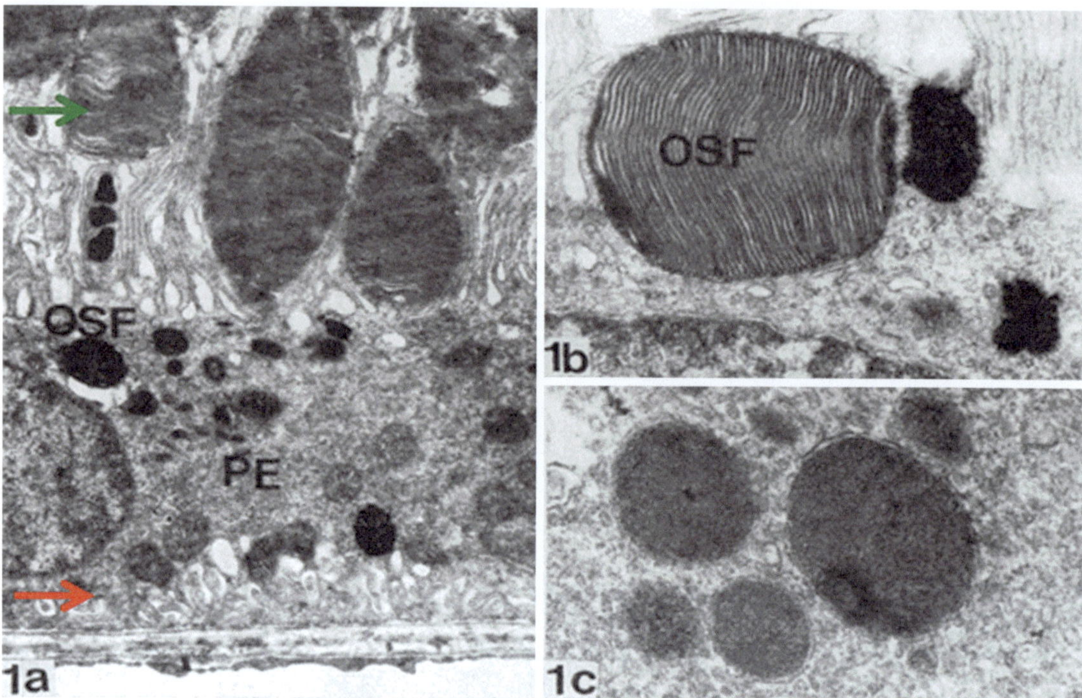

Fig. 1.6 Electron micrograph of retinal pigment epithelial cell (PE) from a rat ingesting photoreceptor outer segments and degrading them through fusion with lysosomes into lysosomal bodies. *1a*: The apical cytoplasm of the retinal pigment epithelium is at the level indicated with the *green arrow* and the basal cytoplasm is at the level of the *red arrow*. OSF: A photoreceptor outer segment fragment that has been phagocytosed by the retinal pigment epithelial cell. *1b*: A more magnified view of a phagocytosed outer segment fragment with the stacked disc structure apparent. *1c*: Lysosomal bodies in which more progressed degradation of the discs than evident in *1b* has resulted in a homogeneous matrix of residual waste material. Reproduced with permission from Drenckhahn and Lullmann-Rauch [41]

macula is 18.3 ± SD 2.4 μm. The RPE in the pericentral annulus of RPE from 1 to 2 mm eccentric to the fovea has similar thickness, but more peripherally the RPE thickness increases. In the annulus from 3 to 6 mm eccentric to the fovea, the average thickness of the RPE is 19.6 ± SD 1.8 μm [18]. The RPE thickness in the central macula increases with age due in part to accumulation of lipofuscin within the cells [18]. Average RPE cell diameter increases with age as some RPE cells die and the remainder spread out to fill in gaps [6]. Toxicologic studies in embryonal chick retina suggest that RPE is more sensitive to chloroquine toxicity than retinal neuronal cells, but the reverse seems to be the case in the primate [42, 43].

Photoreceptors are polarized cells with an outer segment that absorbs quanta of incoming light. The outer segments of photoreceptors are made up of stacks of double membranes derived from a continuously growing and evaginating plasma membrane [24]. Photons of light travel through the translucent inner retina until they strike the photopigment molecules in the stacked discs of the photoreceptor outer segments. The photopigments transduce the light energy in a complex process leading to transmembrane hyperpolarization. The outer segments join the inner segments histologically at the cilium. Outermost in the inner segment is the ellipsoid, a region densely packed with mitochondria for cellular energy production. More vitread to the ellipsoid is the myoid, in which endoplasmic reticulum and golgi apparatus are densely distributed for production of cellular proteins and macromolecules. At the inner terminal of the

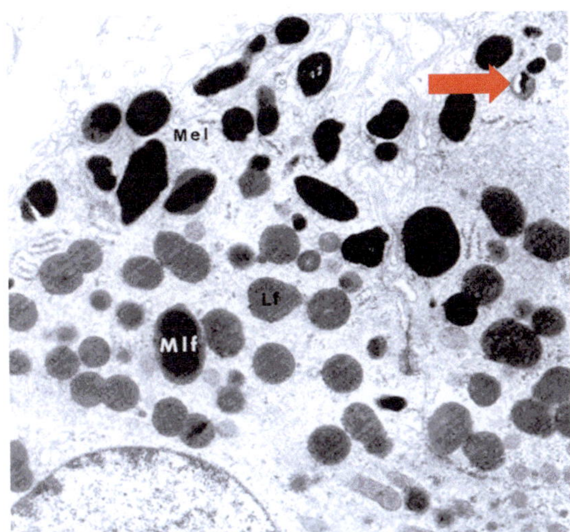

Fig. 1.7 Electron micrograph of the retinal pigment epithelial cell from a 49-year-old person. The *red arrow* indicates a secondary lysosome formed by ingestion of melanin by a primary lysosome. Lysosomal degradation of outer segment discs results in lipofuscin (Lf). Melanolipofuscin (Mlf) is a complex residue resulting from degradation of both disc membranes and melanin by RPE lysosomes. Reproduced with permission from Feeney [22]

photoreceptors is the synaptic terminal with many synaptic vesicles filled with neurotransmitters [24]. The IS/OS junction is a landmark easily seen in normal SD-OCT images (Fig. 1.4). Recent evidence suggests that the IS/OS junction actually represents the band of ellipsoids of adjacent photoreceptor outer segments rather than the band formed by the histologic IS/OS junctions, which is just distal to the band of ellipsoids [44]. Between the outer segments and the RPE is the interphotoreceptor matrix, a complex milieu with signaling molecules, glycoproteins, enzymes, and fatty acids in an extracellular matrix of acid mucopolysaccharides. The third highly reflective line seen in SD-OCT images is termed the cone outer segment tips (COST) (Fig. 1.4) and is thought to correspond to the zone of ensheathment of cone outer segments by apical processes of RPE cells [44]. The fourth highly reflective line arises from the RPE and Bruch's membrane (Fig. 1.4) [44]. All four highly reflective lines in the outer retina can be lost first in the perifovea and later in the central fovea in 4AQR [45, 46].

The retina contains 38.7–125 million rods and 2.2–6.8 million cones [1, 2, 12]. The topographic distribution of rods and cones is illustrated in Fig. 1.9. There is an intuitive relationship of this topographic distribution and the hill of vision as defined by static automated perimetry (Fig.1.10). The density of rods peaks at approximately 150,000/mm [2] in an annular ring around the fovea having a diameter of 3–5 mm, or 10–17° eccentric to the fovea (Fig. 1.9). Although the annular shape of this distribution calls to mind the annular shape of 4AQR, the dimensions do not match. The elliptical annulus of 4AQR has a horizontal and vertical median radius from the

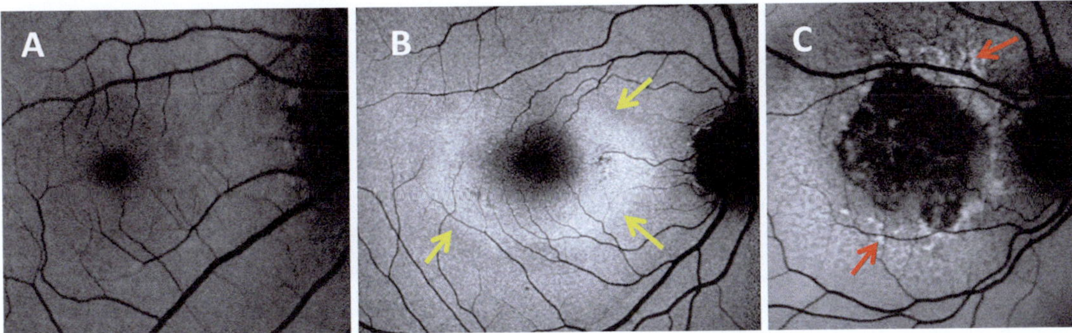

Fig. 1.8 Fundus autofluorescence photography in a normal eye (**a**), an eye with hydroxychloroquine retinopathy (**b**), and age-related macular degeneration with geographic retinal pigment epithelial atrophy (**c**). (**a**) In the normal eye the fovea is hypoautofluorescent compared to the perifovea. (**b**) In this eye with early hydroxychloroquine retinopathy, the perifoveal retinal pigment epithelium has increased lipofuscin, which renders it hyperautofluorescent (*yellow arrows*). (**c**) In this eye with age-related macular degeneration and geographic retinal pigment epithelial atrophy, the area of atrophy is hypoautofluorescent and appears dark. Just outside the border of atrophy are cells with excessive amounts of lipofuscin rendering these patches hyperautofluorescent (*red arrows*)

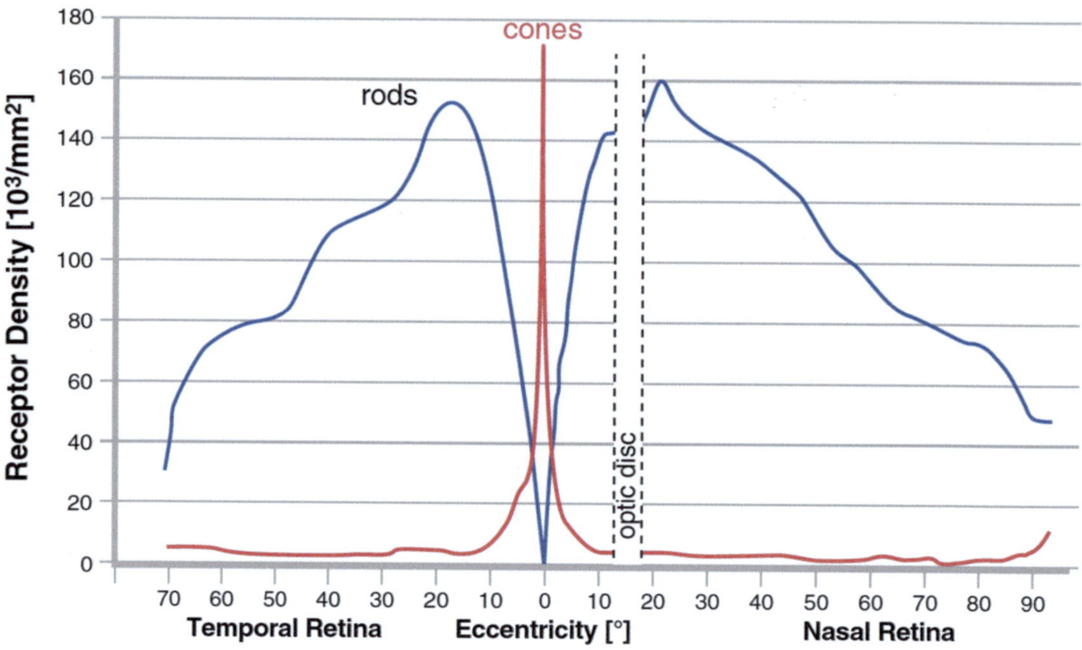

Fig. 1.9 Plot of the density of rods and cones as a function of position relative to the fovea (zero eccentricity) in a sagittal section passing through the fovea and center of the optic nerve. There are no photoreceptors at the location of the optic nerve 15° temporal to the fovea. Note the correspondence to the retinal sensitivity curve (the hill of vision) in Fig. 1.9 (Data from Osterberg [47])

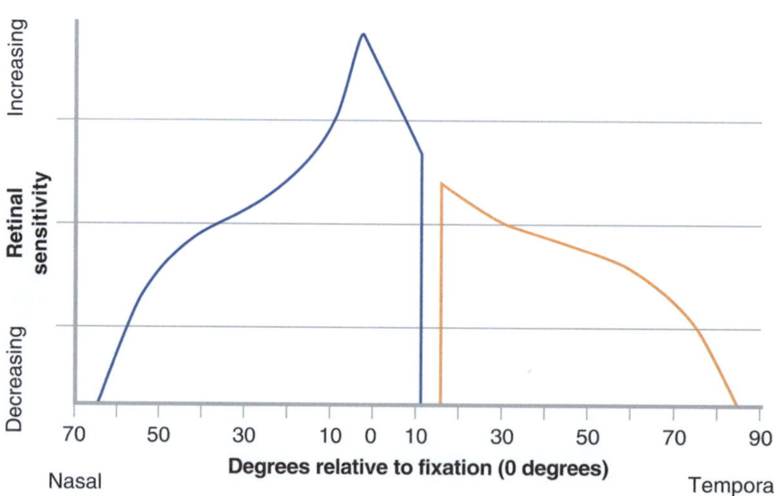

Fig. 1.10 Graph of retinal sensitivity to a light stimulus in static automated perimetry along a sagittal section of the hill of vision passing through the point of fixation and the physiologic blind spot located approximately degrees temporal to fixation. Note the correspondence to the plot of photoreceptor density (Fig. 1.8) relative to location in the retina along a correlative sagittal section. The locus of highest cone density corresponds to the peak sensitivity in the hill of vision. The optic disc, with no photoreceptors, corresponds to the blind spot

fovea of 1.4 and 1.0 mm, respectively (see Chap. 6). The mismatch tends to discount an association of rod density with the pathogenesis of 4AQR. The cone outer segments are taller than the rod outer segments accounting for the subfoveal hump in the IS/OS junction (Fig. 1.4). The length of the outer segments and inner segments together is 58–67 μm in the fovea but 37–40 μm at the equator and beyond [1]. The cones differ from rods in several respects. Their stacked discs are open to the extracellular space. By contrast, in rods the innermost discs are open to the extracellular space, but as the discs move outward with the production of new discs their attachments to the plasma membrane are lost. They become surrounded by plasma membrane and are not bathed in extracellular fluid.

The ONL, comprising the photoreceptor cell bodies, is located just internal to the ELM, a band of zonulae adherens that connect apposed Muller cells and inner segments of photoreceptors (Figs. 1.3 and 1.4) [48, 49]. The ELM is an important landmark seen in SD-OCT images and constitutes a relative diffusion barrier between the interstitium of the inner retina and the subretinal space, as the intercellular space at each zonula adherens narrows to 20 nm [1, 48]. Rods and cones are connected to adjacent Muller cells by zonulae adherens, but are commonly separated from other photoreceptors [1]. The ONL has gentle topographic variation in thickness, from 45 μm nasal to the disc, to 22 μm temporal to the disc, to 50 μm in the perifovea, to 27 μm in the remainder of the peripheral retina [1]. Thinning of the ONL in the perifovea is often seen simultaneously with loss of definition of the IS/OS junction in 4AQR [50, 51].

The outer plexiform layer lies between the inner nuclear layer and ONL and describes a zone of synapses between rod and cone inner segments and the dendrites of horizontal cells (Figs. 1.3 and 1.4). It is characteristically thinner than the inner plexiform layer and may partially impede diffusion of molecules from the inner retinal to outer retinal interstitium. Henle's layer designates the outer plexiform layer adjacent to the fovea where the axons of the rods and the cones turn and travel more parallel with the plane of the retina and away from the fovea [1]. The lengths of individual fibers of Henle are not known for humans, but are longer for the fibers belonging to more centrally located photoreceptors because there is greater distance between these more central photoreceptors and their connecting bipolar cells displaced laterally from the center of the macula [2].

The inner nuclear layer contains the cell bodies of bipolar, horizontal, and amacrine cells (Figs. 1.3 and 1.4) which mediate the initial processing of signals from rods and cones and have receptive fields of varying diameter. The bipolar cells are the most numerous. The cell bodies of the Muller cells are also contained within this layer. Muller cells span the thickness of the retina and are involved in glucose metabolism and ionic and water transport within the retina [1]. Muller cell processes wrap around the axons and dendrites of the intermediate cells of the retina and around capillaries [1]. The inner nuclear layer is a relative bottleneck for the diffusion of macromolecules applied to the vitreal side of the retina [52].

The inner plexiform layer is located between the ganglion and inner nuclear cell layers and ranges in thickness from 18 to 36 μm (Figs. 1.3 and 1.4) [1]. In addition to Muller cell branches and retinal blood vessels, the inner plexiform layer contains synaptic processes of the bipolar, ganglion, and amacrine cells. The bipolar cell axons bring signals from the outer retina to the processing amacrine cells and to the dendrites of the more superficially located ganglion cells. There are at least 25 types of amacrine cells in the human retina, and the lateral span of their dendrites increases with eccentricity from the fovea.

The ganglion cell layer lies between the inner plexiform layer and the nerve fiber layer. In histological sections it varies in thickness from 10 to 20 μm in the nasal retina to 60 to 80 μm in the perifovea (Figs. 1.3 and 1.4) [1]. Measured by SD-OCT, the average thickness of an annulus from 1 to 3 mm from the fovea is 50.6±SD 5.6 μm (Table 1.1). The average thickness of an annulus from 3 to 6 mm from the fovea is 28.5±SD 3.0 μm [18]. This variability in thickness corresponds to the presence of a single lamina of ganglion cells in most of the retina, but 8–10 laminae as the fovea is approached from the optic disc [1].

The average number of ganglion cells in the retina is 1.07 ± 0.4 million [2]. Ganglion cell densities are highest in a horizontally oriented elliptical ring extending from 0.4 to 2.0 mm from the fovea [2]. The size and shape of this area resemble the area of funduscopic damage in 4AQR, which is known to involve ganglion cells at an early stage [43]. The pericentral ganglion cell layer thickness decreases with age, presumably due to attrition of ganglion cells [18]. The ratios of ganglion cells to photoreceptors are 1:100 rods and 1:4 cones, respectively, except in the macula where the ratio of ganglion cells to cones may be as large as 1:2 [2]. This translates physiologically into a smaller receptor field for each ganglion cell in the macula and, therefore, greater acuity. Macular visual field sensitivity correlates with ganglion cell/inner plexiform layer thickness as measured by SD-OCT [53]. The ganglion cells' dendrites extend toward the outer retina and synapse with retinal bipolar and amacrine cells in the inner plexiform layer. The ganglion cell axons are long, making up the retinal nerve fiber layer. They travel within the optic nerve (Fig. 1.3), through the optic chiasm and eventually synapse with cells in the lateral geniculate body. In a primate model of chloroquine toxicity, ganglion cells showed histologic damage earliest [43].

The nerve fiber layer is thickest adjacent to the optic disc where it is 20–30 µm (Figs. 1.3 and 1.4) [1]. The nerve fibers remain unmyelinated until they reach the lamina cribrosa. Muller cell processes interdigitate around the ganglion cell axons which sometimes directly contact their neighbors. The axons assume a generally radial course toward the optic nerve except for those immediately temporal to the macula, which arc above and below the papillomacular bundle that defines the orientation of the horizontal raphe. Since the axons of the papillomacular bundle are the first to develop, they form the center of the optic nerve with axons from the more peripheral retina found more peripherally in the optic nerve. As ganglion cell axons converge toward the optic nerve, the nerve fiber layer thickens. It is absent within the fovea and very thin in the far periphery. Ischemia disrupts physiologic axoplasmic flow and produces both proximal and distal

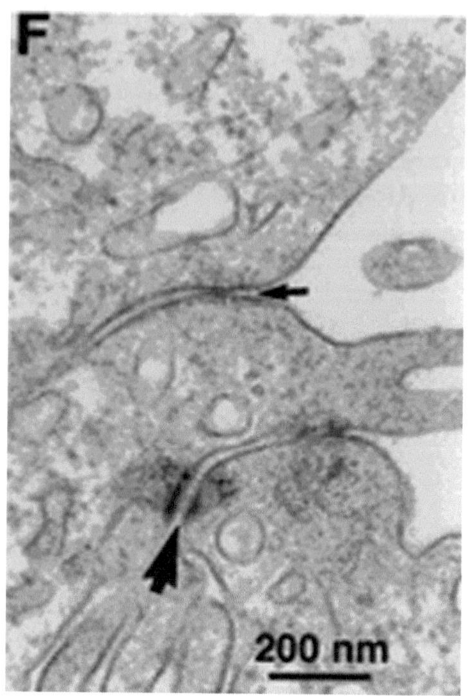

Fig. 1.11 Electron micrograph of a zonule occludens (*smaller arrow*) between cells of the ECV304 cell line. Such junctions between endothelial cells and retinal pigment epithelial cells serve as the basis of the blood–retina barrier. The *larger arrow* denotes a maculae adherens intercellular junction. Reproduced with permission from Penfold et al. [57]

axonal degeneration [54]. The funduscopic correlates of these processes are cotton wool spots and optic disc edema in acute ischemia and the featureless retina lacking nerve fiber layer striations in chronic retinal ischemia [54, 55]. The perifoveal thickness of the combined inner nerve fiber layer–ganglion cell layer as measured by SD-OCT is thinned in patients with hydroxychloroquine retinopathy [5].

The normal BRB is based on tight intercellular junctions between vascular endothelial cells and between retinal pigment epithelial cells. In both sites, the barrier is subsumed by the zonulae occludens (Fig. 1.11). These prevent the easy passage of paracellular ions and hydrophilic small molecules between the neurons of the retina and the vascular system. Amphiphilic substances such as the 4AQs pass through cellular membranes by diffusion and are not impeded by the BRB. The 4AQs in toxic concentrations may degrade the BRB. Vitreous fluorophotometry shows that the BRB is intact in patients taking chloroquine without retinopathy [56]. On the other hand, patients with chloroquine retinopathy have increased permeability of the BRB [56].

The ILM, the sole true basement membrane within the retina, separates the retina from the vitreous. The inner stratum of the ILM is laminated with the basement membrane of the Muller cells. The outer stratum is composed of laminin, proteoglycans, fibronectin, and collagen [16]. The ILM varies in thickness from 2,000 nm over the parafovea to 20 nm over the fovea, since the density of Muller cells decreases in the fovea [17]. Muller cell processes form a continuous but uneven border of attachment with the ILM. The ILM constitutes a barrier for vitreous molecules diffusing toward the retina.

1.3 Vascular Anatomy

The central retinal artery travels through the center of the lamina cribrosa to the optic disc, where it divides into superior and inferior branches that supply the retinal hemispheres. Further equal bifurcations occur downstream as do sidearm branchings of smaller arterioles [58]. Branch retinal arteries lie in the nerve fiber layer or ganglion cell layer, with only the smaller arterioles descending into the inner plexiform layer to supply capillaries [22].

Retinal capillaries reside within various laminae of the inner retina. During normal development, astrocytes in the retina produce vascular endothelial growth factor (VEGF) that induces development of the superficial capillary bed. Later, photoreceptor development in the outer retina causes hypoxia of the inner retina with upregulation of VEGF from the inner nuclear layer and development of the deeper capillary bed within the inner retina [61]. Astrocytes and retinal capillaries colocalize within the retina. Astrocytes and capillaries are absent from the FAZ and in the immediately postoral retina [62].

A superficial network of capillaries called the radial peripapillary capillaries (RPCs) surrounds the optic nerve (Fig. 1.11) [59]. These capillaries lie in the superficial nerve fiber layer and preferentially nourish that layer, but derive from arterioles located deeper at the levels of the outer nerve fiber layer and ganglion cell layer [1]. The RPCs are arranged in parallel rows rather than in the anastomotic net typical of the deeper retinal capillaries. RPCs connect rarely with each other or with deeper retinal capillaries and run parallel to major retinal arteries, rarely crossing them [59].

Besides the RPCs, capillaries of the inner retina assume locations at four depths depending on the thickness of the ganglion cell layer [60]. One lamina of capillaries is present in the nerve fiber layer and ganglion cell layer. Capillaries are regularly found at the outer and inner borders of the inner nuclear layer (which is approximately 40 μm thick); are missing in the inner plexiform layer (approximately 30 μm thick); and are found at the inner or outer boundaries of the ganglion cell layer for the parts where it is approximately 30 μm thick as well as within the ganglion cell layer where it is thicker (50–60 μm in an annulus 0.7–1.8 mm from the fovea) (Fig. 1.12) [60]. The deepest lamina vanishes more proximally in the retinal mid-periphery, the middle lamina vanishes more peripherally, and the most superficial lamina extends almost to the ora serrata which, like the fovea, is bordered by an avascular zone (Fig. 1.13). A capillary-free zone is also found adjacent to retinal arterioles (Fig. 1.14) [1, 62].

Normal retinal capillaries have low permeability, lacking fenestrations and possessing tight intercellular junctions that form the inner BRB impeding passage of water and ions but not 4AQs [21]. The FAZ is approximately 400 μm in diameter [62]. Bordering the FAZ is a single level of capillaries found within the ganglion cell layer (Fig. 1.13). Moving further from the FAZ, the capillary network becomes trilaminar [60]. There is no known relationship of the FAZ to the relatively spared central zone in advanced 4AQR, but its colocalization invites consideration of some pathogenetic linkage.

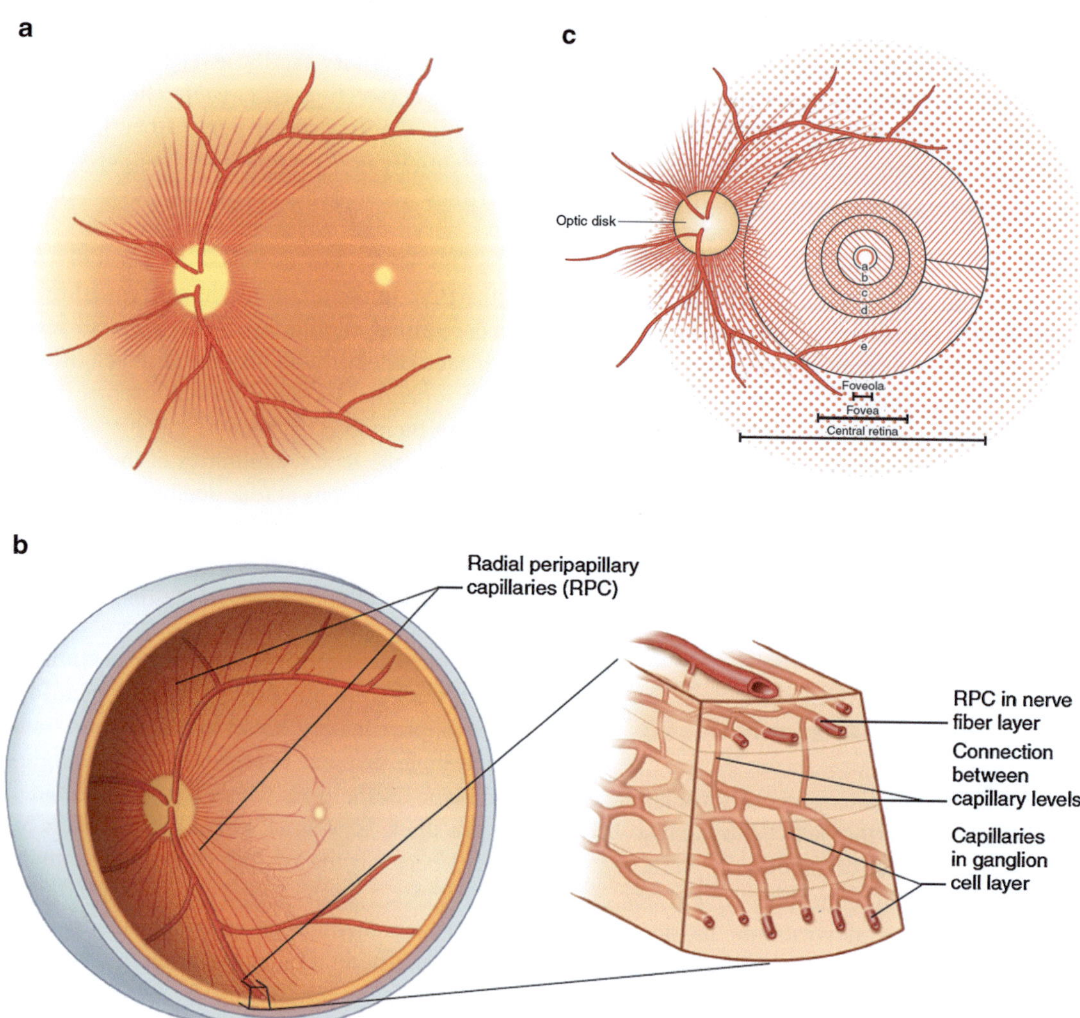

Fig. 1.12 (**a**) Diagram of the distribution of the radial peripapillary capillaries. (**b**) Magnified cutaway diagram showing the sparse anastomoses of the radial peripapillary capillaries with the deeper strata of retinal capillaries. (**c**) Schema of laminar distribution of retinal capillaries. Hatch up and right: Superficial capillaries are at the inner boundary of the inner nuclear layer. Hatch down and right: Capillaries are at the outer boundary of the outer nuclear layer. Cross hatched area: Capillaries are within the ganglion cell layer. Dotted area: Capillaries touch both boundaries of the ganglion cell layer. Data from Henkind [59] and Iwasaki and Inomata [60]

1.4   Immunology

The immune system is composed of the innate response system and the adaptive response system. The innate response system is not antigen specific, shows no immunologic memory, and involves all the immune cells except lymphocytes. That is, it involves the neutrophils, eosinophils, mast cells, basophils, monocytes, macrophages, natural killer cells, and dendritic cells [64]. The adaptive immune system is mediated through lymphocytes, is antigen specific, and manifests immunologic memory [64].

1.4.1   Innate Immunity and Toll-Like Receptors

Innate immunity is mediated through Toll-like receptors (TLRs). TLRs are receptors that bind to evolutionarily conserved molecular structures

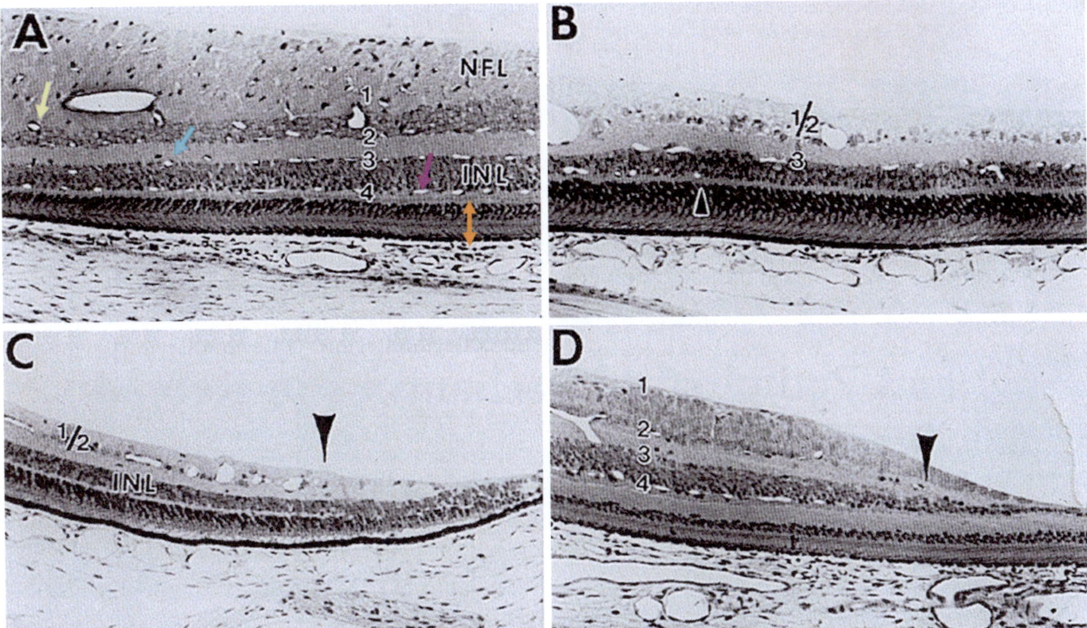

Fig. 1.13 Laminar arrangement of the capillary beds in the primate retina. (**a**) Posterior pole retina with the inner retina labeled 1–4. *1*: Nerve fiber layer (NFL). *2*: Ganglion cell layer. *3*: Inner border of the inner nuclear layer (INL). *4*: Outer border of the inner nuclear layer. The *yellow arrow* denotes a capillary within the deep nerve fiber layer. The *turquoise arrow* denotes a capillary at the inner border of the inner nuclear layer. The *pink arrow* denotes a capillary at the outer border of the inner nuclear layer, which is the deepest level of the inner retina containing capillaries. The *orange double-headed arrow* spans the avascular outer retina comprising the outer plexiform layer, outer nuclear layer, photoreceptor outer segments, and retinal pigment epithelium. (**b**) Sample of the mid-peripheral retina showing the locus of termination of the outermost lamina of capillaries (*arrowhead*). To the right of the *arrowhead*, no capillaries are seen at the outer border of the inner nuclear layer, but capillaries are evident at the inner border of the inner nuclear layer and in the nerve fiber/ganglion cell layer. Slightly more peripherally, the capillary lamina at the inner border of the inner nuclear layer vanishes (not shown). (**c**) The peripheral retina/ora serrata junction showing that the innermost lamina of capillaries vanishes just proximal to the ora serrata. (**d**) Section of the retina from the perifovea (*left side*) to the fovea (*right side*). The foveal avascular zone begins at the *arrowhead*, which denotes the border capillary. Reproduced with permission from Gariano et al. [63]

found in microbes and host cells. These signature molecules are nonspecific to any particular microorganism, but allow discrimination of microbes from the host. The molecules that TLRs recognize are called pathogen-associated molecular patterns (PAMPs). Once a TLR binds to a PAMP an inflammatory cascade is initiated [65]. There are at least 13 TLRs in humans, and more continue to be discovered.

TLRs reside on the surface of cells and intracellularly within endosomes [65, 66]. The cell surface TLRs recognize bacterial and fungal PAMPs whereas the intracellular TLRs recognize viral PAMPs [67]. Related to TLRs are nucleotide-binding and oligomerization domain-like receptors (NOD-like receptors or NLRs) that bind to microbial metabolic products or detritus from cellular damage such as ATP and uric acid [65]. NLRs have a role in inflammatory diseases for which 4AQs may be used as treatment. Binding of ligands to NLRs can activate nuclear factor-κβ (NF-κβ), a step that starts many inflammatory pathways. For example, binding of ligands to NLRP1, NLRP3, and IPAF leads to activation of caspase-1 in inflammasomes, which are multiprotein complexes that are integral to inflammatory reactions [65].

The details of TLR signaling pathways continue to be defined, but an outline is shown in Fig. 1.15. The extracellular domain of a TLR

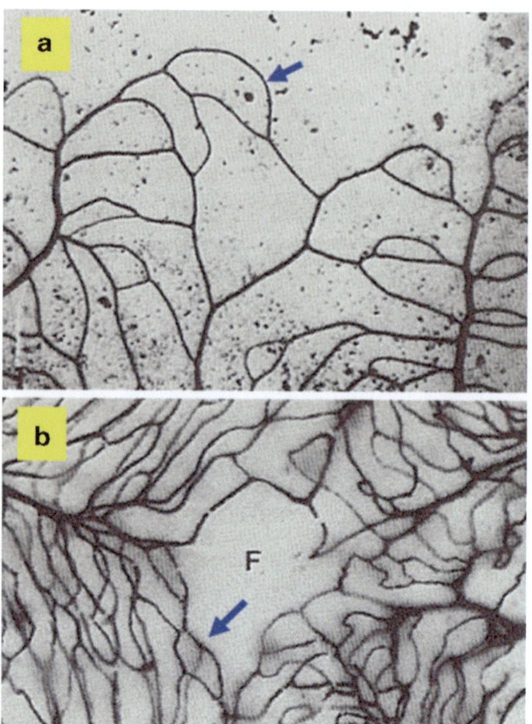

Fig. 1.14 Image of retinal vessels stained for ADPase in the young human. (**a**) Just posterior to the ora serrata the retina is avascular. The *blue arrow* denotes the most peripheral retinal capillary posterior to the ora serrata. (**b**) The center of the macula is avascular (F) and is bordered by the single-layered perifoveal capillary arcade (*blue arrow*). Reproduced with permission from Gariano et al. [63]

binds a ligand which leads to activation of the intracellular domain, the Toll-interleukin-1 resistance domain (TIR). Activation of TIR catalyzes activation of interleukin (IL)-1 receptor-associated kinases-4 and -1 (IRAK4 and IRAK1) and tumor necrosis factor receptor-associated factor 6 (TRAF6). Their activation leads to activation of the inhibitor of kappa B kinase complex (IκκK complex). The IκκK complex contains the NF-κβ essential modifier regulatory subunit (NEMO). NEMO phosphorylates inhibitors of NF-κβ leading to their degradation. The degradation of NF-κβ inhibitors releases NF-κβ for translocation to the cell nucleus, which induces a cascade of pro-inflammatory cytokine production.

There are positive and negative modulators of the TLR signaling pathways. MicroRNAs (miR-NAs) are oligonucleotides that bind to the mRNA of a target gene either increasing or decreasing degradation of the mRNA and causing increases or decreases in translation of the protein encoded by the target gene. For example, miR-146 targets TRAF6 and IRAK1 and reduces the mRNA levels of both of these intermediates in TLR signaling [65]. Ubiquitination is a mechanism regulating the degradation of proteins by the proteasome. Targeted proteins are linked to a chain of ubiquitin molecules by ligation to lysine residues. TRAF6 has ubiquitin ligase activity and can auto-ubiquitinate. Pellino3 is a ubiquitin activating enzyme with ligase activity that promotes ubiquitination of IRAK1. Ubiquitination of TRAF6 and IRAK1 can reduce NF-κβ translocation to the nucleus and downregulate the production of inflammatory cytokines [65].

Intracellular TLRs recognize self-nucleic acid components including immune complexes found in rheumatoid arthritis (RA) and systemic lupus erythematosus (SLE). Normally these self-nucleic acid components would be found extracellularly and would not react with intracellular TLRs, but in antigen processing cells of patients with RA and SLE they are transported intracellularly to endosomal compartments and bind to TLRs [68]. Fcγ receptors on dendritic cells and B cell receptors on the surface of B cells mediate this transportation [68]. The particular nucleic acid motif that interacts with intracellular TLRs is C_pG oligodeoxynucleotide (C_pG ODN). As a result the antigen processing cells are activated to produce interferon α (IFNα) and other cytokines [67, 68]. The endosomal TLRs 3, 7, 8, and 9 seem to be particularly implicated in the pathogenesis of SLE and RA [65, 66, 69]. For example, in a mouse model rheumatoid factor production by activated B cells stimulated by chromatin containing immune complexes requires a signal transmitted by TLR9 [70].

Antimalarial drugs inhibit the function of intracellular TLRs by inhibiting C_pG at nanomolar concentrations that are achieved in clinical use (Fig. 1.14) [68, 71]. Hydroxychloroquine is a TLR7 and TLR9 antagonist [67]. Investigational derivatives of chloroquine such as C_pG-52364 inhibit TLR7, TLR8, and TLR9 and reduce activity of SLE in animal models. The 4AQs are

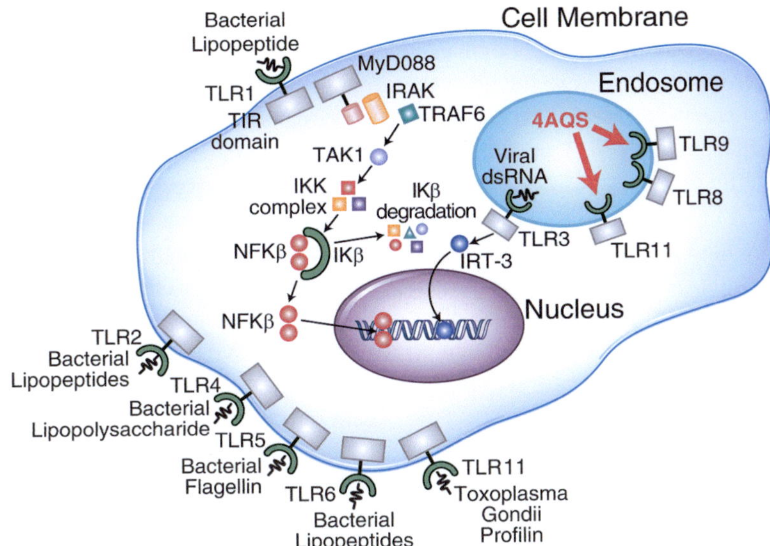

Fig. 1.15 Toll-like receptor-mediated innate immune mechanisms affected by 4-aminoquinolines. Diagram of the activation of Toll-like receptors and effects on gene transcription. Depicted are TLRs exposed to the extracellular space (TLRs 1, 2, 4, 5, 6, and 11), which interact with bacterial and toxoplasmic pathogen-associated molecular patterns (PAMPs), as well as TLRs on endosomal membranes (TLRs 3, 7, 8, and 9), which interact with viral PAMPs and presumably autoimmunity-associated ligands. The diagram shows as an example TLR1 binding a bacterial PAMP that leads to recruitment of a series of proteins including Toll-interleukin-1 resistance domain (TIR), interleukin-1 receptor-associated kinases (IRAK), and tumor necrosis factor receptor-associated factor 6 (TRAF6). Their activation in turn activates the inhibitor of kappa B kinase complex (IκκK complex) which phosphorylates the inhibitor of NF-κβ (Iκβ) leading to its degradation. This releases NF-κβ for translocation to the cell nucleus where it induces a cascade of pro-inflammatory cytokine production via upregulation of transcription of the relevant genes. The sites of action of 4-aminoquinolines (4AQs) are shown by *red block arrows*. In nanomolar concentrations these drugs block TLR7 and 9. Data from Delves et al. [64]

thought to inhibit TLR signaling by raising endosomal pH or by binding to self-DNA epitopes thereby masking them from the TLRs [68]. Short DNA sequences termed immunoregulatory sequences inhibit TLR7 and TLR9, retarding SLE progression in a mouse model of SLE. A different immunoregulatory sequence that blocks TLR7 and TLR9, IMO-3100, inhibited upregulation of TNF-α, IFNα, and IL-17 in human monocyte culture [65]. In a human leukemic T cell line culture, HCQ inhibited T cell receptor (TCR)-mediated increases in cytosolic calcium concentration, but did not affect protein tyrosine phosphorylation, protein kinase phosphorylation, and production of inositol phosphates which are earlier events occurring after TCR–antigen binding [72]. That is, the effects of the 4AQs in TCR signaling appear to be toward the end of the known cascade of steps linking TCR binding to antigen and upregulation of transcription factors NFAT and NF-κB involved in T cell proliferation and differentiation [72].

Genetic polymorphisms of the genes regulating TLR expression have an effect in autoimmune diseases for which chloroquine and hydroxychloroquine are used as treatment. For example, TLR polymorphisms rs10488631, rs2004640, and rs729302 for the TLR protein IRF5 increase susceptibility to SLE [65]. On the other hand, the polymorphism S180L for the TLR protein MAL decreases risk for developing SLE [65].

1.4.2 Adaptive Immunity

A complex sequence of interactions between hematopoietic stem cells and cytokines in the bone marrow produces precursors of the effector cells of the immune system. T-lymphocyte progenitors arising from bone marrow travel to the thymus gland where they interact with thymic hormones and differentiate [64]. T cells that recognize foreign antigenic peptides are positively selected in the thymic cortex and those recognizing self-peptide antigens are negatively selected in the thymic medulla [73]. Thymocyte activity is greatest in the first year of life followed by diminution thereafter at 3 % per year through age 45 and thereafter further diminution at 1 % per year after age 45.

Newly arrived thymocytes express neither CD4 nor CD8 surface markers, nor any TCRs. They are called double negative cells (DN cells). Under the influence of chemokines CCL19 and CCL21 extensive rearrangement of TCR genes follows ultimately leading to expression of a randomly generated TCR on the cell surface as a TCR–CD3 complex, where CD3 is the cluster of differentiation 3T cell co-receptor. Simultaneously, both CD4 and CD8 membrane markers are expressed. At this stage the cells are termed double positive (DP) cells [64]. If the resulting DP cells express on their surface membranes a TCR that fails to recognize self-MHC (major histocompatibility complex) molecules the cells are neglected and undergo apoptosis [64]. If the DP cells express a TCR with low or intermediate affinity for self-MHC molecules, they are saved from apoptosis. If the DP cells express a TCR with high affinity for self-MHC or self-MHC + self-peptide expressed on macrophages or dendritic cells, then they receive a signal resulting in apoptosis, a result termed negative selection [73].

Autoimmune diseases are thought to represent a breakdown of the negative selection pathway. Affected patients fail to express enough self-MHC + self-peptide on thymic epithelial cells to cause avid binding of T cells expressing TCRs for self-peptide antigens. Because these T cells are not deselected, they can later be stimulated by self-antigens and proliferate with pathological consequences [73]. The 4AQs work by raising the pH of lysosomes of antigen presenting cells (APCs) which reduces the expression of self-MHC + self-peptide on their cell surfaces relative to the expression of self-MHC–foreign peptide complexes [73]. The result is that T cells expressing TCRs for self-antigens would be less stimulated and the autoimmune disease would become less active.

After DP cells undergo positive and negative selection in the thymus they exit as single positive (SP) CD4+ or CD8+ cells that recognize epitopes of foreign antigens presented by the individual's MHC molecules. Transcription factors Th-POK, TOX, and GATA-3 favor CD4+ T cell production, whereas transcription factor RUNX3 favors CD8+ T cell development [64]. The SP cells therefore possess either a CD4+ phenotype or a CD8+ phenotype [64, 74]. CD4 and CD8 molecules are co-receptors, along with the TCRs, for MHC–antigen complexes [64].

For both T and B lymphocytes, after traveling from the thymus to the peripheral tissues, the initial exposure to the antigen for which the cell surface receptor is matched results in clonal proliferation of that cell with subsequent differentiation of the progeny into effector cells and memory cells that express receptors for that antigen (Fig. 1.16). This is the primary immune response. A subfraction of the progeny called memory cells are more effective than the naïve lymphocytes at responding to second exposure to the antigen. The subsequent exposure leads to a larger and more rapid proliferation of effector lymphocytes with all the sequelae of immune response [64].

An intricate mechanism links presentation of an antigen and activation of its corresponding T cell. In extrathymic tissues, the first step is binding of a TCR to its paired antigen with TCR cross-linking and activation of the immunoreceptor tyrosine-based activation motif on the cytoplasmic tail of CD3 molecules (Fig. 1.17). A cascade of reactions follows [72]. Tyrosine kinases are activated including p56lck, p59fyn, and ZAP-70 which then phosphorylate multiple intracellular enzymes including phospholipase C (PLC)γ1. Activated PLCγ1 enhances hydrolysis of phosphatidylinositol 4,5-biphosphate (PIP2) to inositol 1,4,5-triphosphate (IP3) and diacylglycerol which cause an increase in cytosolic calcium

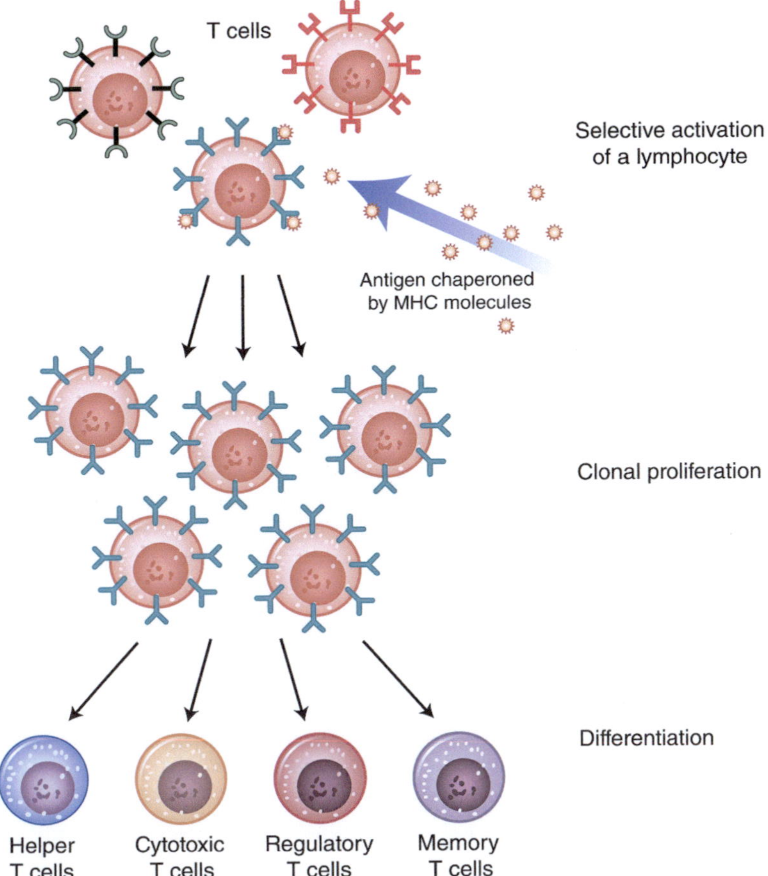

Fig. 1.16 Selective activation, proliferation, and differentiation of a T cell. Naïve T lymphocytes are activated when their T cell receptors bind to antigen presenting cell surface ligands chaperoned by MHC molecules. The activated T cells multiply, and under the governance of a complex mixture of cytokines, differentiate into one of several more specialized types of T cells. Data from Delves et al. [64]

concentration and enhance catalytic activity of protein kinase C (PKC). Higher calcium concentration enhances the activity of calmodulin which binds to calcineurin. Calcineurin regulates nuclear translocation of transcription factors of the nuclear factor of activated T cells family (NFAT) (Fig. 1.17). Subsequently CD69 is upregulated and IL-2 secretion increases [72]. The 4AQs modulate the terminal events in this complex sequence and thereby affect activation of T cells in peripheral tissues [72].

CD8+ T cells are also called cytotoxic T cells and CD4+ T cells are also called helper T cells. Helper T cells (Th) are differentiated into multiple categories of cells. A partial list would include Th1, Th2, regulatory T cells (Treg), and Th17 cells. The cytokines TGF-β, IL-1β, IL-6, IL-21, and IL-23 are involved in the evolution of naïve CD4+ cells into differentiated Th cells [75, 76]. The transcription factors signal-transducer-and-activator-of-transcription-3, retinoic acid receptor-related orphan receptor-γt, and aryl-hydrocarbon-receptor regulate Th17 differentiation [77]. Th1 cells secrete IL-2, IL-γ, and TNF-β. These T cells mediate delayed type hypersensitivity and activation of cytotoxic T cells. Th2 cells secrete IL-4 and facilitate B cell activation [78]. Th17 cells are thought to be involved in the pathogenesis of SLE and RA as an aberrant role in addition to their adaptive role of clearing extracellular Candida and Klebsiella pathogens [76–78]. IL-17, ILs 21–23, and IL-26 are produced by

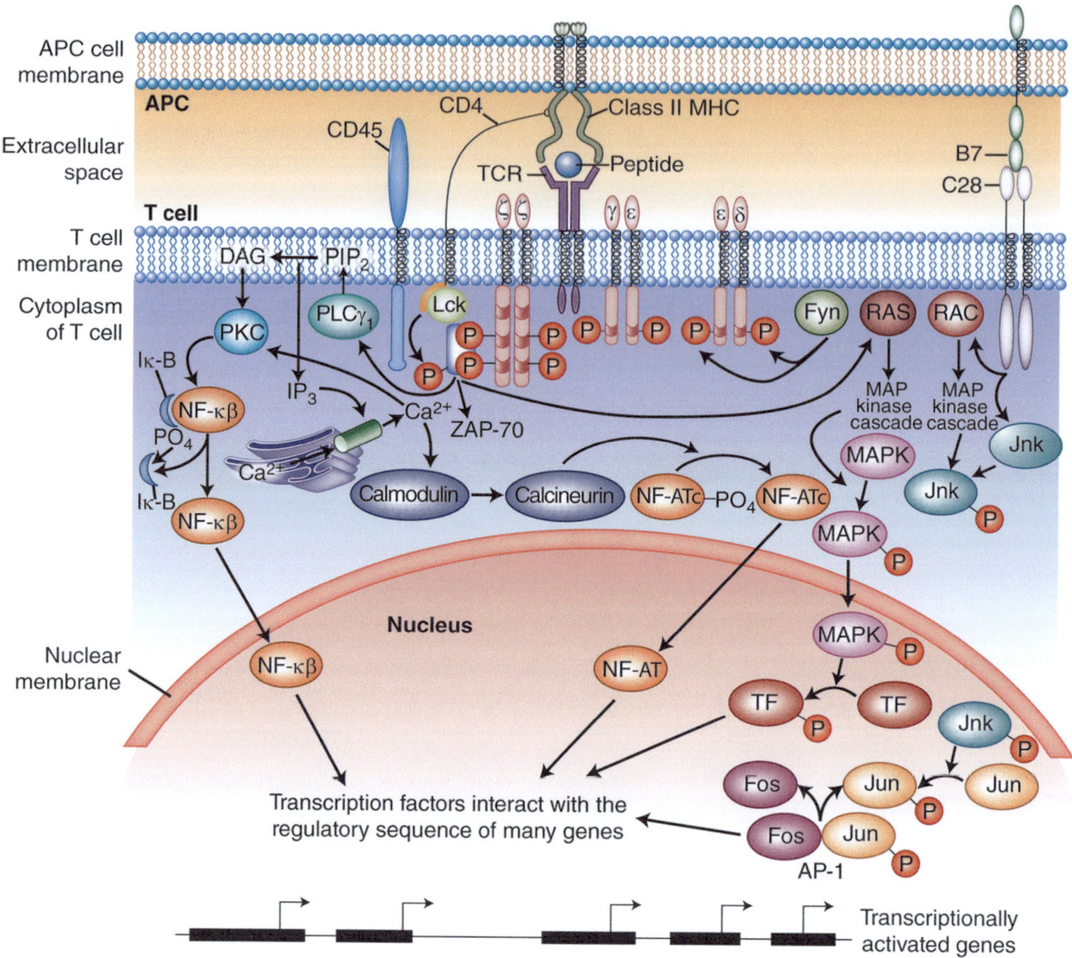

Fig. 1.17 Diagram of the cascade of events involved in T cell activation. The class II MHC molecule–antigen complex activates T cell receptor (TCR) crosslinking on a CD4+ T cell. Multiple T cell tyrosine kinases, including ZAP-70, are activated, which then phosphorylate other intracellular enzymes including phospholipase C (PLC) γ1. Activated PLCγ1 enhances hydrolysis of phosphatidylinositol 4,5-biphosphate (PIP2) to inositol 1,4,5-triphosphate (IP3) and diacylglycerol which effect an increase in cytosolic calcium concentration and enhance catalytic activity of protein kinase C (PKC). Higher calcium concentration enhances the activity of calmodulin which binds to calcineurin which regulates nuclear translocation of transcription factors of the nuclear factor of activated T cells family (NFAT). Other transcription factors (e.g., Fos and Jun) are also involved in regulation of gene expression. Data from Delves et al. [64]

Th17 cells, and these cytokines serve as serum markers that Th17 cells are important in particular diseases [77]. Patients with SLE have increased levels of IL-17 and IL-23 and patients with RA have increased IL-22 [77, 78]. IL-17 is increased in the synovial fluid of patients with RA. IL-17 stimulates increased antibody production by B cells, amplifies inflammatory damage in target organs in SLE, and stimulates osteoclasts in patients with RA [75]. The 4AQs inhibit the production of IL-5, IL-17, IL-22, and TNF-α by peripheral blood mononuclear cells in clinical use and in models using phorbol myristic acid, lipopolysaccharide, and ionomycin as monocyte activators [75, 79–81].

MHC molecules are expressed on the cell surface and serve as platforms for the presentation of antigens to T lymphocytes [82]. In humans,

MHC molecules are also called human leukocyte antigen (HLA) molecules [83]. MHC class I and II molecules work to present antigens to CD8+ T cells and CD4+ T cells, respectively [83, 84]. TCRs for foreign antigens only bind to an antigen when it is presented within the groove of an MHC molecule [64]. MHC molecules are composed of an α and β chain [85]. In MHC class I molecules, α chains vary but β chains do not; they are all β_2 microglobulin. In MHC class II molecules, both the α and β chains vary [86]. The MHC class I molecules are HLA-A, -B, -C, -E, -F, and -G, which are expressed on the surface membranes of almost all nucleated cells [83]. The MHC class II molecules are HLA-DP, -DQ, -DR, -DM, and DO, which are expressed on the surface membranes of macrophages, dendritic cells, and certain B cells [83]. These three types of immune cells are collectively termed professional APCs.

Macrophages phagocytose exogenous proteins and produce smaller foreign peptide nonself antigens [83, 87]. Dendritic cells and B cells are involved in presenting previously processed foreign peptide antigens. All of these professional APCs possess compartments enriched in MHC class II molecules, a characteristic which distinguishes them from nonprofessional APCs. Antigen catabolism and MHC class II molecular maturation occur in communicating compartments of the endosome/lysosome system of APCs [84].

Figure 1.18a is a diagram showing how a CD8+ T lymphocyte is primed by interaction with a foreign antigen synthesized within the cell bearing the MHC class I molecules. In the example shown, a virus has infected a host cell, which expresses class I MHC molecules on its surface membrane. The infected cell synthesizes viral peptides that fit into a pocket formed by the α chain of the class I MHC molecule. The class I MHC molecule–peptide antigen complex is displayed on the surface membrane of the cell. A CD8+ T cell with the corresponding TCR binds to the complex. Costimulatory molecules CD28 (found on the CD8+ T cell), B7 (found on the host APC), and other cytokines released by the APC lead to priming of the CD8+ T cell. A second exposure of the CD8+ T cell to the foreign antigen can trigger the CD8+ T cell to release cytotoxic cytokines and pore-forming molecules that kill the infected cell [88]. In certain circumstances, previously processed foreign antigen may be taken up by APCs and presented with MHC class I molecules on the cell surface to CD8+ T cells, a process termed cross-presentation [84, 89]. Chloroquine increases the CD8+ T cell response to a soluble antigen by decreasing degradation within lysosomes, increasing the cytosolic concentration of antigen, which in turn increases formation of antigen–MHC class I complexes and their expression on surface membranes for interaction with CD8+ T cells [71, 89]. One clinical correlate is that pretreatment with chloroquine of patients receiving hepatitis B vaccination increases the induced antigen-specific CD8+ T cell response [89].

Figure 1.18b illustrates the analogous process for priming of a CD4+ T cell by a professional APC. In the example shown, a macrophage has phagocytosed a bacterial or fungal protein and broken it into smaller antigenic peptides 13–25 amino acids long [87, 90]. The peptide fits in the pocket formed between the α and β chains of the class II MHC molecule [84]. The complex is expressed on the surface membrane of the macrophage [84]. A CD4+ T cell with the appropriate TCR binds to the peptide–class II MHC molecule complex and under the costimulus of B7 protein and various cytokines becomes primed [74]. When CD4+ T cells are primed they can multiply (called clonal expansion) synthesize an array of cytokines, and express costimulatory molecules and cell-adhesion molecules on their surface membranes [88]. Dendritic cells and B cells prime CD4+ T cells in an analogous fashion to macrophages, but present previously processed peptide antigens rather than phagocytosing foreign proteins and digesting them to antigenic peptides.

T cell priming is subject to modulation. For example IL-10 decreases antigen presentation by professional APCs and monoclonal antibodies against B7 can reduce the activation of CD4+ T cells [74]. Chloroquine decreases the catabolism of bacterial proteins into immunogens by macrophages and presentation of bacterial antigens to T

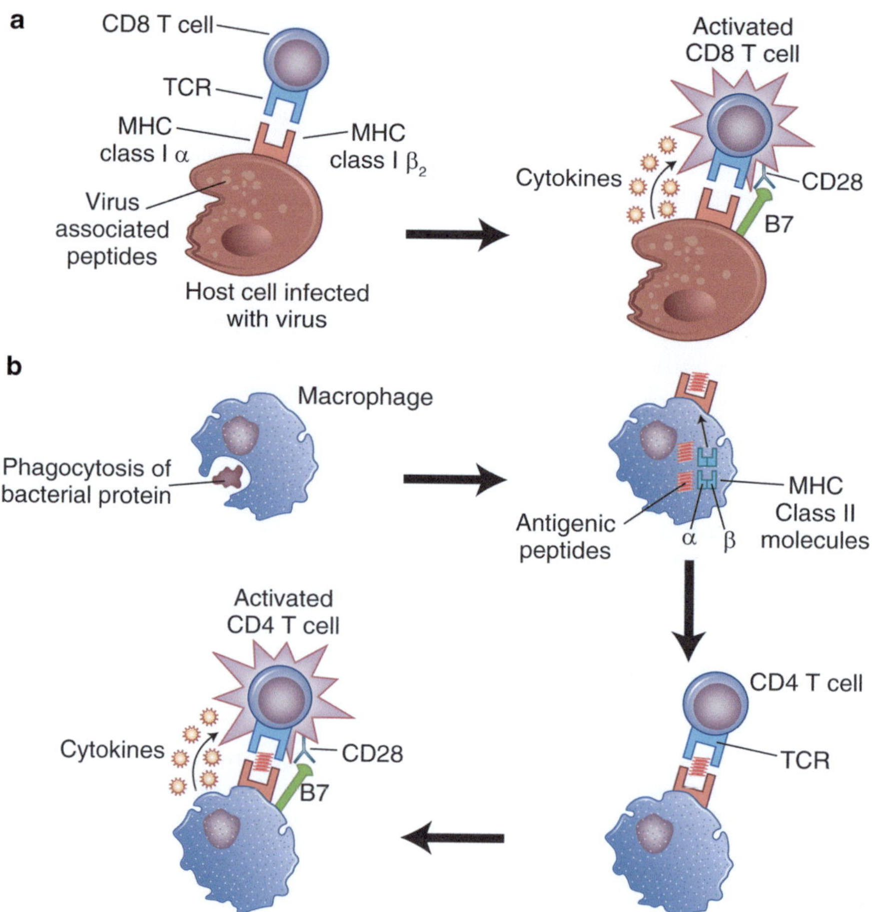

Fig. 1.18 Activation of CD4+ and CD8+ T cells. Priming of CD8+ and CD4+ T cells. (**a**) Diagram of activation of a CD8+ T cell by an MHC class I molecule-bearing host cell that has been infected by a virus. Within the cytoplasm of the infected cell are virally synthesized peptides that fit into the pocket of the α chain of MHC class I molecules. The viral peptide–MHC class I molecule complex is transported and displayed on the cell membrane where it binds to the T cell receptor (TCR) of a CD8+ T cell. This binding, together with costimulation by CD28-B7 molecules and cytokines, leads to priming of the CD8+ T cell and clonal expansion. (**b**) Diagram of activation of a CD4+ T cell by an MHC class II molecule-bearing macrophage that has phagocytosed exogenous bacterial protein. The protein is degraded into foreign antigenic peptides, which are loaded into the groove formed between the α and β chains of the MHC class II molecules stored in organelles within the cytoplasm. The foreign peptide antigen–MHC class II complex is transported to the cell membrane and binds to the TCR of a CD4+ T cell. The combination of receptor binding and costimulation by CD28-B7 molecules and cytokines released by the macrophage results in activation of the CD4 T cell and clonal expansion. Data from Moorthy et al. [88]

lymphocytes, but does not change ingestion of bacteria by macrophages, which tends to implicate an effect of the drug at the level of the lysosome [87].

The work of turning exogenous proteins into antigenic peptides for presentation to CD4+ T cells occurs within the lysosomes of MHC class II APCs [83]. Under conditions of a normal immune response, the MHC class II molecule is dissociated from a chaperone protein called invariant chain (Ii) that is encoded by a nonMHC gene, the cluster of differentiation 74 (CD74) gene [73, 82]. In the place of Ii, the processed antigen binds to the MHC class II molecule and the complex is transported out of the lysosome and on to the cell surface so that the complex is exposed to the extracellular space (Fig. 1.19a) [82, 84, 90, 91]. When the pH inside the lysosome

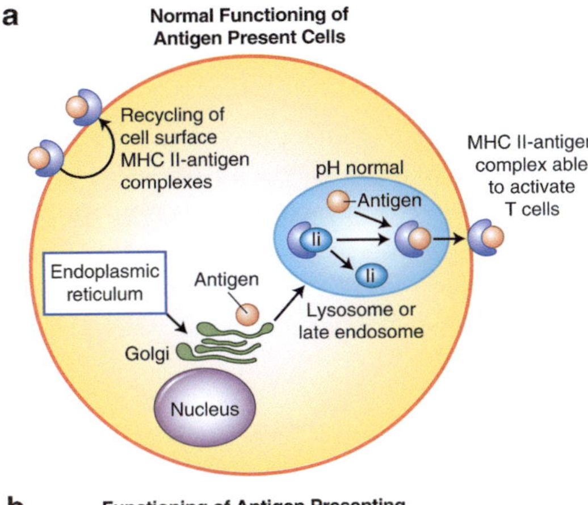

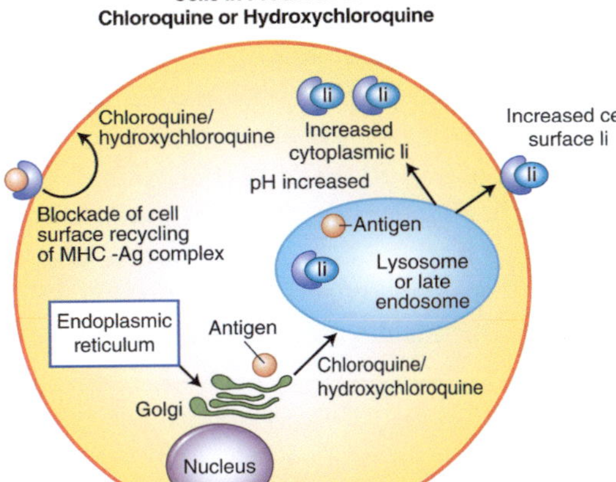

Fig.1.19 Antigen presenting cells and 4-aminoquinolines. Diagram of antigen processing by a professional antigen presenting cell normally (**a**) and in the presence of 4AQs. (**a**) Under normal circumstances the intralysosomally processed antigen displaces the invariant chain Ii from the MHC II molecule and the MHC II–antigen complex is transported to the cell surface membrane. (**b**) In the presence of chloroquine or hydroxychloroquine the invariant chain remains bound to the MHC II molecule and the Ii–MHC II complex is displayed on the cell surface membrane. Less immune activation of T cells matched to the antigen is the result. Data from Schultz and Gilman [74]

is increased, as happens with chloroquine and hydroxychloroquine use, the chaperone protein Ii remains stuck to the MHC class II molecule and this complex is expressed on the cell surface instead of the MHC class II molecule complexed with the processed antigen (Fig. 1.19b) [73, 86, 92, 93]. As a result, the APC less effectively

stimulates the CD4+ cell, and there is a negative influence on the immune response to the antigen [74]. As self-antigens typically have less affinity for MHC class II molecules than foreign antigens, the effect of 4AQs is more marked on autoimmunity than immune responses to exogenous antigens [71]. In this way 4AQs are useful immunomodulators but do not immunosuppress users against infections [94]. Among the many immune-mediated actions of 4AQs, none appear to involve B cells [74]. In summary, by these steps the 4AQs alter MHC II-associated antigen processing [74].

1.5 Pharmacology and Toxicology

1.5.1 Acid–Base Chemistry

The literature on 4AQs frequently refers to concentrations of these drugs in whole blood, plasma, and serum. To be able to compare the articles, one needs to understand the relationships of these types of samples. Whole blood contains erythrocytes, leukocytes, and platelets. Because the 4AQs have higher concentrations within erythrocytes and leukocytes than in the bathing acellular fluid, and because intraindividual variation of hematocrit, leukocyte count, and platelet count is large, the whole blood concentrations of drug will be higher and more variable. Plasma is blood minus the cellular components and is obtained by spinning down a tube of anticoagulated whole blood and removing the supernatant. Serum is obtained from coagulated blood and is therefore deficient in clotting factors, but contains proteins released by platelets during clotting that are not present in plasma [95]. Serum concentrations of metabolites and drugs concentrated in platelets are generally higher than plasma concentrations, although the two concentrations are correlated [95].

The 4AQs are weak bases that undergo ionic trapping within acidic lysosomes and other organelles in the cytosol [96, 97]. The accumulation of 4AQs within lysosomes is termed lysosomotropism [98]. To understand how it works, it may help to review some principles of acid–base chemistry. The relevant reaction is as follows:

$$\text{Acid} \underset{K_2}{\overset{K_1}{\rightleftarrows}} \text{Base} + \text{H}^+$$

where K_1 and K_2 are rate constants for the forward and backward reactions. At equilibrium, $K_1[\text{Acid}] = K_2[\text{Base}] \cdot [\text{H}^+]$. Rearranging,

$[\text{H}^+] = (K_1/K_2) \cdot [\text{Acid}]/[\text{Base}] = K_a \cdot [\text{Acid}]/[\text{Base}]$, where $K_a = K_1/K_2$ is defined as the acid dissociation constant. Taking the negative logarithm to the base 10 of both sides gives

$$\text{pH} = -\log_{10}\left[\text{H}^+\right] = \text{pK}_a + \log_{10}\left(\left[\text{Base}\right]/\left[\text{Acid}\right]\right),$$

which is the Henderson–Hasselbach equation. This equation provides the definition of pK_a. If one notes that at 50 % ionization, [Acid]=[Base], then $\log_{10}[\text{Base}]/[\text{Acid}]=0$ and thus pK_a=pH. In words, the pK_a is the pH at which half the base is protonated [99, p. 19]. In the case of chloroquine there are two basic groups with pK_as of 8.1 and 10.2 [100]. For hydroxychloroquine the pK_as of the two basic groups are 9.8 and 15.6 [101].

The pH of the cytosol and extracellular space is approximately seven, whereas the pH inside a lysosome is approximately four by virtue of an ATPase-dependent proton pump found in the lysosomal membrane [96]. At equilibrium, the ratio of the concentration of monoprotonated 4AQ in the lysosome compared to that in the extralysosomal space is approximately equal to the ratio of the hydrogen ion concentration in the lysosome compared to that in the extracellular space, or $10^{-4}/10^{-7}$, which is 1,000 [98]. Thus, at therapeutic plasma concentrations of 4AQs of approximately 1×10^{-6} M/L, concentrations of 4AQs within lysosomes of 1×10^{-3} M/L can be obtained [98].

1.5.2 Dose–Response Relationships

The half-maximal effective concentration of a drug is a concentration that produces a response halfway between the baseline state and the maximal response. This concept is often termed the effective concentration 50 (EC50) [102]. Similar concepts are the effective dose 50 (ED50), which is the dose at which 50 % of the population will experience the therapeutic effect, and the toxic dose 50 (TD 50), which is the dose at which 50 % of the population will experience a defined toxic effect.

The therapeutic ratio, or index, is a metric designed to express the pharmacologic activity of a drug relative to its toxicity. The concept is typically framed in statistical terms, because of variability across individuals [103, p. 14]. The most common statistic used is the median dose for a therapeutic or toxic effect. Thus,

$$\text{Therapeutic ratio} = \frac{\textit{Median dose to produce toxicity}}{\textit{Median dose to produce therapeutic effect}} = \frac{TD50}{ED50}.$$

From various models of antimalarial activity using mice, rats, chicks, and ducks, hydroxychloroquine has a therapeutic ratio of 2.25–4.5 and chloroquine a therapeutic ratio of 1–2 [104]. Therefore, it is commonly stated that hydroxychloroquine is a safer drug than chloroquine [104], although some disagree because the studies of the two drugs often cannot be directly compared and the results with the two drugs are not greatly different [105].

1.5.3 Pharmacokinetic Relationships

The concentration of a drug in the plasma depends on the dose given, the frequency of dosing, and the kinetics of absorption, redistribution into various compartments in the body, and excretion [106]. For either of the 4AQs, Fig. 1.20 illustrates the various compartments and the

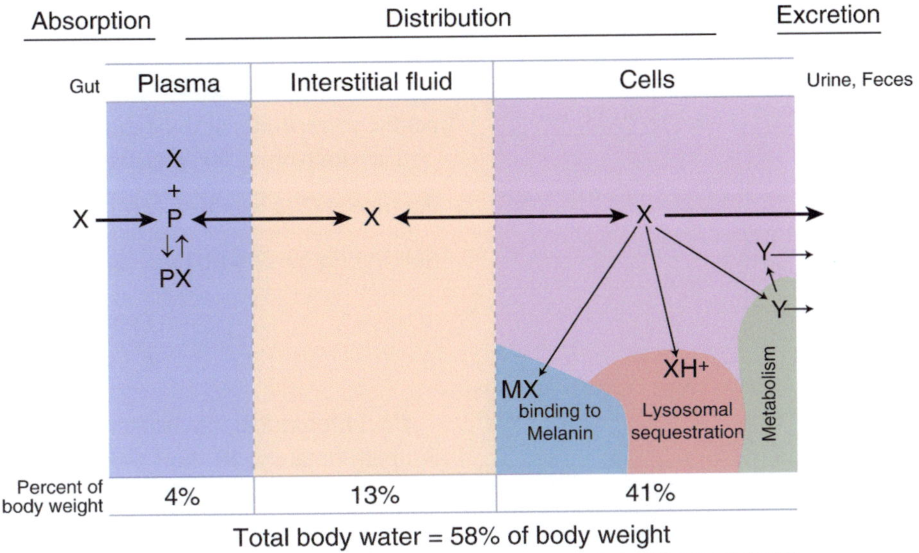

Fig. 1.20 Diagram of the fate of a 4-aminoquinoline (X) from ingestion through excretion. For 4AQs, absorption from the gastrointestinal tract is nearly complete. In plasma the drug is partially bound to protein P. Both 4AQs are amphiphilic and easily pass across cellular membranes, but can be trapped when protonation occurs in intracellular organelles that are acidic, such as lysosomes (XH+) and the Golgi complex. Extensive binding of 4AQs to melanin occurs (MX). In the liver, metabolism converts 4AQs to other compounds (Y) that are excreted and also have their own actions which often mimic those of the parent compound. Data from Goldstein et al. [99, p. 130]

pathways followed by the drug from ingestion through elimination.

The pharmacokinetics of chloroquine and hydroxychloroquine are similar. The 4AQs have complex pharmacokinetic behavior with drug distribution to multiple compartments, including plasma and different peripheral organs that concentrate the drug by different amounts and release it back to the central plasma compartment from which metabolism occurs in the liver and excretion via the feces and urine (see Chap. 2). To be most accurate in modeling drug concentrations over time, therefore, a multicompartmental model fits the situation best (Fig. 1.21a).

There is controversy over which model is best applied—models with two or three compartments or more. Some extremely complex models have been proposed in which the rate of excretion is not constant but instead depends on concentration [107]. These concerns are important in discussing the use of 4AQs to treat malaria acutely, but our interest is in the drugs as they are used to treat autoimmune diseases over months to years and are taken at constant daily doses. In this situation, the processes with short half-times relative to the rate of elimination are unimportant and the modeling becomes simpler [108]. In this situation we can conceive of the situation in terms of a one-compartment model with a large volume of distribution (Fig. 1.21b), V, and an elimination rate constant K_e that is determined by the liver and kidney. The rate of intake of the drug is the daily dose, D, in mg/day.

If we let $X =$ the drug concentration in plasma, the central compartment, then the differential equation that describes the change in concentration with time is

$$\frac{dX}{dt} = \frac{D}{V} - K_e X \qquad (1.1)$$

The solution to this equation (see Box) is

$$X(t) = \frac{D}{K_e V}\left(1 - e^{-K_e t}\right) \qquad (1.2)$$

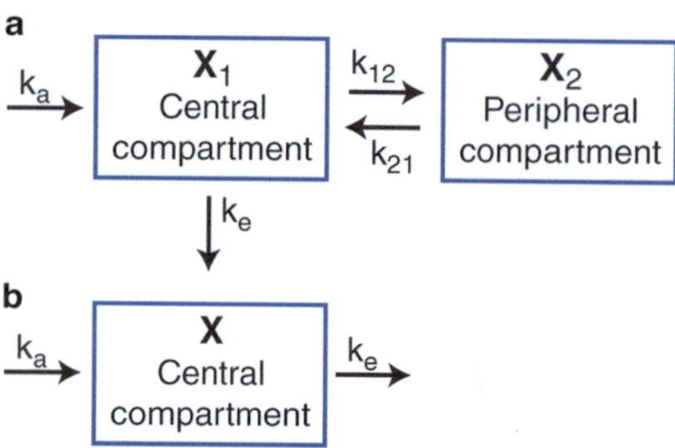

Fig. 1.21 Diagram of compartmental models useful in understanding the pharmacokinetics of 4-aminoquinolines. (**a**) The more realistic model involves the ingestion of drug at a constant rate (K_a), a central compartment (plasma), and a peripheral compartment (all the organs to which the drug distributes). X_1 is the drug concentration in the plasma, X_2 is the drug concentration in the peripheral compartment, K_a equals D/V where D is the daily dose (mg/day), V is the volume of distribution, K_{12} is the rate constant for transfer of drug from the central compartment to the peripheral compartment, K_{21} is the rate constant for transfer of drug from the peripheral compartment to the central compartment, and K_e is the elimination rate constant (partially through the feces and partially through the urine). (**b**) At steady state $K_{12} \cdot X_{12} = K_{21} \cdot X_{21}$. Therefore mass transfer of drug from central to peripheral compartments vanishes, and the model collapses to a simpler one-compartment model as shown

At time $t=0$, $X(0)=0$ and at steady state, when $t = \infty$, $X(\infty) = \dfrac{D}{K_c V}$

We define the steady state plasma concentration of chloroquine as $X_{ss} = X(\infty)$. X_{ss} depends on the daily dose D, the elimination rate constant K_e, and the volume of distribution V. The volume of distribution depends on the size of the individual, which in turn depends on the height and the correlated lean, or ideal, body weight. In a study of hydroxychloroquine, steady state blood concentrations were measured and graphed versus the patients' actual body weights, which differ from ideal body weight due to the variable amount of body fat [109]. Nevertheless, there was a statistically significant relationship as the derivation above predicts (Fig. 1.22). Therefore, it is not surprising that these same variables—daily dose, elimination rate constant (a function of renal and liver function), and ideal body weight—are

recognized as major risk factors in AQR (see Chap. 7). They set the steady state plasma concentration of the AQR, which will be in the subtherapeutic, therapeutic, or toxic range (see below).

The half-time for plasma concentration is the time $t1/2$ at which $X\left(t1/2\right) = \dfrac{1}{2} X_{ss} = \dfrac{D}{2 K_e V}$. Solving Eq. (1.2) with these substitutions yields

$$t1/2 = \frac{0.693}{K_e}. \tag{1.3}$$

For chloroquine, the half-time for elimination is approximately 40 days (see Chap. 2) [110]. When one doses a patient with chloroquine from the beginning with the steady state daily dose, it takes 3–4 months to have a therapeutic effect. If we choose the value 4 months, this equates to three half-times. Figure 1.21 shows a graph of the fraction of steady state drug concentration achieved versus units of time in kt. Three half-times is how long it takes to reach the 87.5th percentile of steady state plasma concentration of drug. Therefore, the delayed onset of therapeutic effect of 4AQs may have to do with pharmacokinetics alone and not to more complicated explanations involving slow translation of drug effect into its therapeutic manifestation via intervening immunologic processes [73, 99]. By beginning therapy with a higher loading dose of drug, onset of therapeutic action may be accelerated [99, p. 323, 106, p. 168].

In the clinical use of the 4AQs, a daily dose is typically ingested at one time. Near total absorption of the ingested dose occurs (see Chap. 2), and the absorption rate constant is so much faster than the elimination rate constant that the time course of plasma concentration of drug over the course of many doses is an asymptotic rise to a steady state concentration as shown in Fig. 1.23. The small fluctuations in plasma concentration caused by daily doses give the plasma concentration curve a sawtooth appearance, but the overall time course in a case with the paired absorption–elimination rate constants that apply to 4AQs resembles that for a constant IV infusion (the smooth curve in Fig. 1.23).

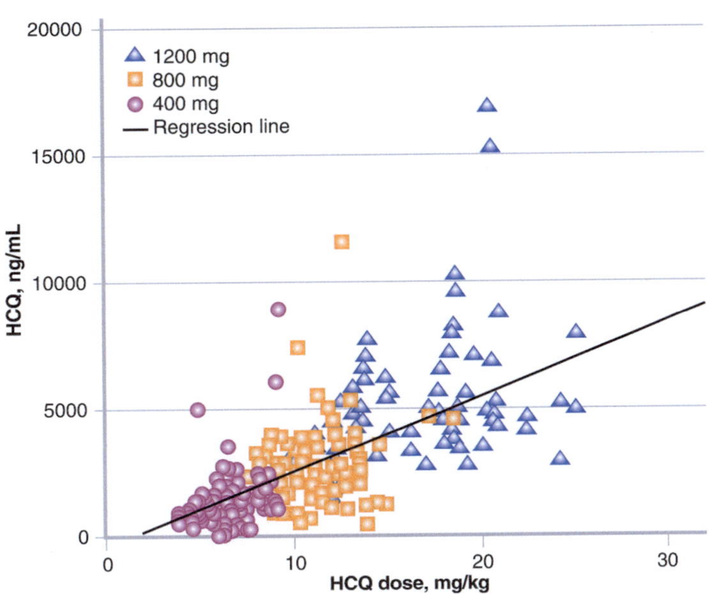

Fig. 1.22 Relationship between the blood concentration of hydroxychloroquine and the hydroxychloroquine daily dose divided by actual body weight in a sample of 123 patients with rheumatoid arthritis. Three doses were used and samples were collected at 5–6 weeks after start of therapy, a time assumed to approximate steady state. Data from Munster et al. [109]

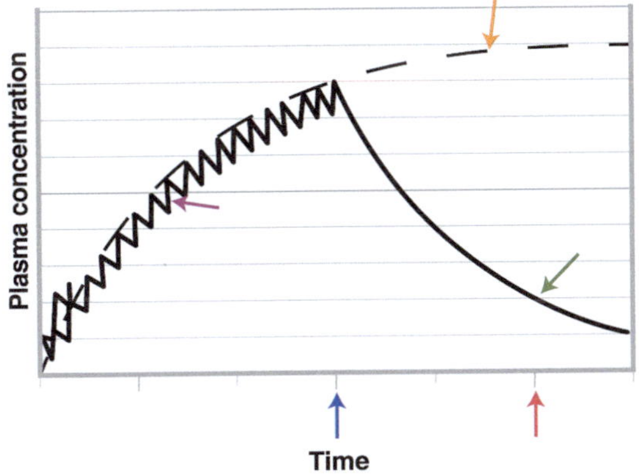

Fig. 1.23 Diagram of plasma concentration of a 4-aminoquinoline given as a daily dose. The sawtooth solid line depicts the actual plasma concentration with small daily fluctuations associated with dosing. The *purple arrow* indicates the size of the increment in plasma concentration caused by a single daily dose. The dotted line is a smoothed curve representing the plasma concentration of an equivalent constant infusion of drug given at a rate of D/V where D is the daily dose and V the volume of distribution. At the *blue arrow*, dosing has stopped and the smooth solid *curve* after this (*green arrow*) shows the elimination of drug that mirrors the rise during dosing. The *orange arrow* shows the plasma concentration that would have been seen had dosing continued. The *red arrow* indicates a time equal to five half-lives, at which point a steady state has been nearly achieved

The plasma concentration of a 4AQ in the context of constant daily dosing shows phase-dependent behavior. In the early phase, the rate of elimination (k_eX) is lower than the rate of drug intake (D/V), because X is near zero. Therefore, at the end of each day and before the next dose, there has occurred an increment in plasma drug concentration (e.g., I_1, I_2, I_3 in Fig. 1.24). On the other hand, as the plasma concentration rises, the rate of elimination, k_eX, increases, and eventually equals the drug intake, D/V. This is the condition for steady state, for which plasma concentration of drug no longer changes.

The steady state can occur at a subtherapeutic concentration, a therapeutic concentration, or a toxic concentration (Fig. 1.24). The steady state concentration depends on the daily dose D and the volume of distribution V, which in turn depends on lean body weight. At a subtherapeutic concentration, the patient probably has no improvement in complaints and the drug dosage may be adjusted upward or the drug discontinued. At therapeutic concentrations, signs and symptoms improve and no toxicity occurs. At toxic concentrations, signs and symptoms are

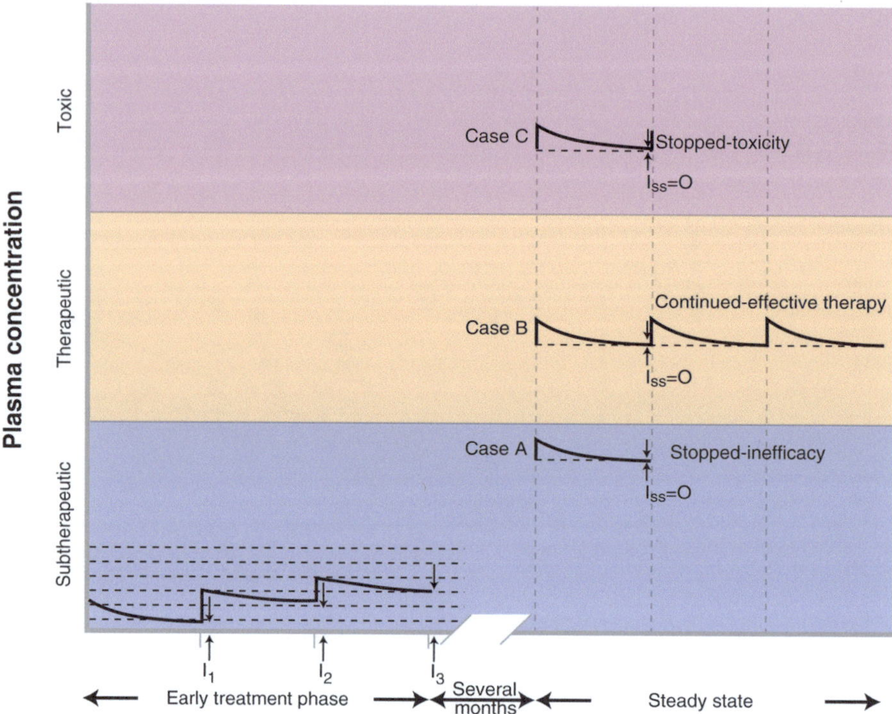

Fig. 1.24 Diagram indicating three clinical scenarios and the associated pharmacokinetic behavior. In the early treatment phase, each dose of drug causes a small increment in plasma concentration (I_1, I_2, $I_3 \neq 0$), because the elimination of drug is nearly zero ($K_e X$ is small because X is nearly 0). At steady state, elimination of drug equals intake ($I_{ss}=0$). Steady state may occur at a subtherapeutic, therapeutic, or toxic plasma concentration (different colored zones). This steady state plasma concentration depends on the daily dose D and the volume of distribution, which depends on ideal body weight (in turn dependent on height)

improved, but retinopathy and other toxic effects eventually develop. The challenge for the ophthalmologist is to determine if the patient falls into this last group, to make changes if possible that place the patient in the therapeutic group, and as a last and least important priority, if the patient falls in the last group, to detect retinopathy at a stage when it can be halted or reversed. A recurring emphasis of this book will be the importance of redirecting clinical attention to the first aim, in contrast to the traditional emphasis in most literature on the last.

Pharmacokinetics of Hydroxychloroquine—Use of Loading Dosing to Achieve Steady State Faster

A randomized clinical trial established that a period of increased dosing with hydroxychloroquine allows a faster onset of clinical response [111]. A 6-week loading dose interval was chosen. The elimination half-life of hydroxychloroquine was assumed to be 40 days [112]. Loading doses with 1,200 mg/day and 800 mg/day were chosen for the intervention groups. The control group was treated as usual with initiation of the maintenance dose of 400 mg/day from day 1. The study designers reported that they expected to reach steady state concentration of the 400 mg/day regimen within 6 weeks for the 1,200 mg/day loading dose group, to reach

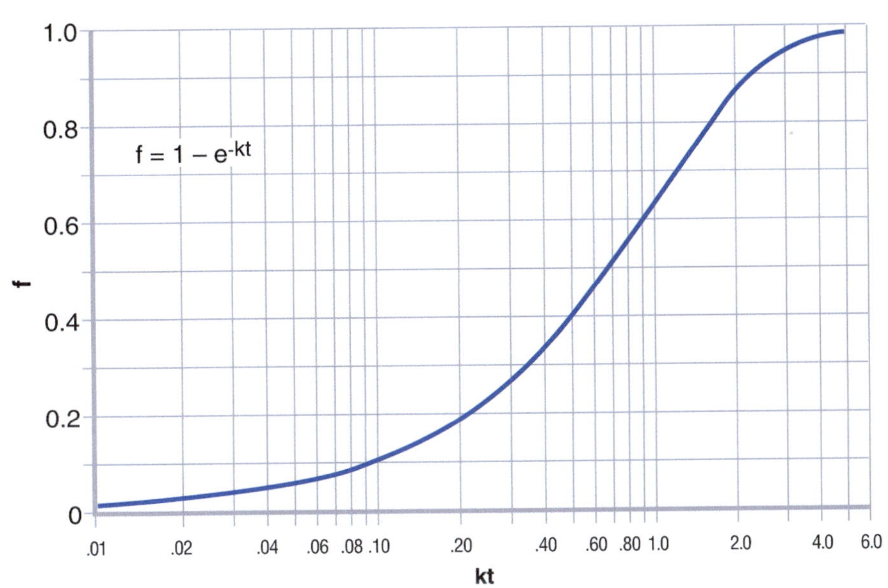

Fig. 1.25 Graph of fractional attainment of steady state plasma concentration (*f*) of a 4-aminoquinoline drug after beginning treatment at a constant daily dose. The abscissa has units of *kt*, where *k* is the elimination rate constant. Because *k* equals $0.693/t_{1/2}$, the actual time to reach a certain percentage of steady state can be determined from known half-times for the 4-aminoquinolines. For chloroquine, $t_{1/2}$ is approximately 40 days; thus, from the graph, >95 % of the steady state concentration is achieved when *kt* equals four. Substituting 0.693/40 days for *k* leads to the conclusion that $t_{>95\%}$ equals 289 days. Data from Goldstein et al. [99, p. 315]

80 % of steady state within 6 weeks for the 800 mg/day loading dose group, and to reach steady state for the 400 mg/day group in 24 weeks [111]. Using the pharmacokinetic principles just discussed, can their projections be confirmed?

For the 400 mg/day group, Eq. (1.3) implies that 24 weeks (or 168 days) would be $(0.693/40) \times 168 = 2.91$ in units of $K_e t$. From Fig. 1.25, at $K_e t = 2.91$, one has reached over 90 % of the steady state concentration, where the steady state concentration is $D/K_e V = 400/K_e V$. For the 800 mg/day group, the steady state concentration is $800/K_e V$. To reach a concentration of 80 % of $400/K_e V$ (i.e., $320/K_e V$), or 40 % of the steady state concentration achieved using 800 mg/day dosing, would require $K_e t = 0.5$ (see Fig. 1.23), or $t = 29$ days, which is approximately 4 weeks, not far off from the authors' claim of 6 weeks. A similar calculation shows a somewhat larger discrepancy regarding the projection to steady state for the 1,200 mg/day loading dose. For that group, the steady state concentration is $1,200/K_e V$. To reach a concentration of $400/K_e V$, or one-third the steady state concentration achieved using 1,200 mg/day dosing, would require $K_e t = 0.4$ (see Fig. 1.25), or $t = 23$ days, which is approximately 55 % of the authors' claim.

1.6   Summary of Key Points

- 4AQ retinopathy is predominantly a maculopathy. The FAZ, the distribution of xanthophylls and retinal pigment epithelial enzymes, and the regional distribution of cones and ganglion cells may affect the maculocentric characteristic of the condition.
- An intimate familiarity with retinal anatomy will improve the clinician's diagnostic skill in examining patients taking 4AQs.
- 4AQ retinopathy follows chronic use of 4AQs in treating autoimmune diseases. The pathogenesis of autoimmune diseases is complex, and the 4AQs act at numerous steps, including:
  - Inhibition of endosomal TLRs TLR7 and TLR9.
  - Inhibition of cytokines IL-3, IL-17, IL-22, and TNF-α produced by mononuclear cells.
  - Inhibition of the terminal steps in T cell activation by self-antigens.
  - Inhibition of antigen processing by professional antigen processing cells.
- The 4AQs are lysosomotropic drugs by virtue of their sequestration in lysosomes which are more acidic than the cytoplasm of the cells containing them.
- The therapeutic ratios of chloroquine and hydroxychloroquine are in the range of 1–2 and 2.25–4.5, respectively. Hydroxychloroquine is a safer drug to use.
- At steady state, the equilibrium concentration of a 4AQ in plasma or whole blood depends on the ideal body weight and the daily dose.
- The elimination half-life of both 4AQs is approximately 40 days, implying that the time to reach steady state is more than 120 days.

References

1. Hogan MJ, Alvarado JA, Weddell JE. Retina. Histology of the human eye: an atlas and textbook. Philadelphia: WB Saunders; 1971. p. 393–522.
2. Curcio CA, Allen KA. Topography of ganglion cells in the human retina. J Comp Neurol. 1990;300:5–25.
3. Gass JDM. Stereoscopic atlas of macular diseases diagnosis and treatment. St Louis: Mosby-Year Book; 1997. p. 1–599.
4. Jonas JB, Nguyen NX, Naumann GO. The retinal nerve fiber layer in normal eyes [Abstract]. Ophthalmology. 1989;96:627–32.
5. Pasadhika S, Fishman GA, Choi D, Shahidi M. Selective thinning of the perifoveal inner retina as an early sign of hydroxychloroquine retinal toxicity. Eye (Lond). 2010;24:756–63.
6. Boulton M. Ageing of the retinal pigment epithelium. Prog Retin Eye Res. 1991;11:125–51.
7. Davies NP, Morland AB. Macular pigments: their characteristics and putative role. Prog Retin Eye Res. 2004;23:533–59.
8. Snodderly DM, Brown PK, Delori FC, Auran JD. The macular pigment. I. Absorbance spectra, localization, and discrimination from other yellow pigments in primate retinas. Invest Ophthalmol Vis Sci. 1984;25:660–74.
9. Snodderly DM, Auran JD, Delori FC. The macular pigment. II. Spatial distribution in primate retinas. Invest Ophthalmol Vis Sci. 1984;25:685.
10. Anderson C, Blaha GR, Marx JL. Humphrey visual field findings in hydroxychloroquine toxicity. Eye (Lond). 2011;25:1535–45.
11. Marmor MF, Chien FY, Johnson MW. Value of red targets and pattern deviation pots in visual field screening for hydroxychloroquine retinopathy. JAMA Ophthalmol. 2013;131:476–80.
12. Jonas JB, Schneider U, Naumann GOH. Count and density of human retinal photoreceptors. Graefes Arch Clin Exp Ophthalmol. 1992;230:505–10.
13. Pasadhika S, Fishman GA. Effects of chronic exposure to hydroxychloroquine or chloroquine on inner retinal structures. Eye (Lond). 2009;24:340–6.
14. William M, Hart J, editors. Adler's physiology of the eye. St. Louis: Mosby; 2003. p. 309–10.
15. Grover S, Murthy RK, Brar VS, Chalam KV. Comparison of retinal thickness in normal eyes using stratus and spectralis optical coherence tomography. Invest Ophthalmol Vis Sci. 2010;51:2644–7.
16. Bentaleb-Machkour Z, Jouffroy E, Rabilloud M, Grange JD, Kodjikian L. Comparison of central macular thickness measured by three OCT models and study of interoperator variability. Scientific World Journal. 2012;2012:1–6.
17. Giani A, Cigada M, Esmaili DD, Salvetti P, Luccarelli S, Marziani E, Luiselli C, Sabella P, Cereda M, Eandi C, Staurenghi G. Artifacts in automatic retinal segmentation using different optical coherence tomography instruments. Retina. 2010;30:607–16.
18. Demirkaya N, van Dijk HW, van Schuppen SM, Abramoff MD, Garvin MK, Sonka M, Schlingemann RO, Verbraak FD. Effect of age on individual retinal layer thickness in normal eyes as measured with spectral-domain optical coherence tomography. Invest Ophthalmol Vis Sci. 2013;54:4934–40.

19. Wagner-Schuman M, Dubis AM, Nordgren RN, Lei Y, Odelll D, Chiao H, Weh E, Fischer W, Sulai Y, Dubra A, Carroll J. Race- and sex-related differences in retinal thickness and foveal pit morphology. Invest Ophthalmol Vis Sci. 2011;52:625–34.

20. Besharse JC, Defoe DM. Role of the retinal pigment epithelium in photoreceptor membrane turnover. In: Marmor MF, Wolfensberger TJ, editors. The retinal pigment epithelium. New York: Oxford University Press; 1998. p. 152–72.

21. Bosch E, Horwitz J, Bok D. Phagocytosis of outer segments by retinal pigment epithelium: phagosome-lysosome interaction. J Histochem Cytochem. 1993;41:253–63.

22. Feeney L. Lipofuscin and melanin of human retinal pigment epithelium. Fluorescence, enzyme cytochemical, and ultrastructural studies. Invest Ophthalmol Vis Sci. 1978;17:583–600.

23. Smith RS, Berson EL. Acute toxic effects of chloroquine on the cat retina: ultrastructural changes. Invest Ophthalmol Vis Sci. 1971;10:237–46.

24. Bok D. Retinal photoreceptor-pigment epithelium interactions. Invest Ophthalmol Vis Sci. 1985;26:1659–94.

25. Holz FG, Schutt F, Kopitz J, Eldred GE, Kruse FE, Volcker HE, Cantz M. Inhibition of lysosomal degradative functions in RPE cells by a retinoid component of lipofuscin. Invest Ophthalmol Vis Sci. 1999;40:737–43.

26. Young RW. Visual cells and the concept of renewal. Invest Ophthalmol Vis Sci. 1976;15:725.

27. Katz ML, Drea CM, Eldred GE, Hess HH, Robison WGJR. Influence of early photoreceptor degeneration on lipofuscin in the retinal pigment epithelium. Exp Eye Res. 1986;43:561–73.

28. Feeney-Burns L, Hilderbrand ES, Eldridge S. Aging human RPE: morphometric analysis of macular, equatorial, and peripheral cells. Invest Ophthalmol Vis Sci. 1984;25:195–200.

29. Cuervo AM, Dice JF. When lysosomes get old. Exp Gerontol. 2000;35:119–31.

30. Radu RA, Han Y, Bui TV, Nusinowitz S, Bok D, Lichter J, Widder K, Travis GH, Mata NL. Reductions in serum vitamin A arrest accumulation of toxic retinal fluorophores: a potential therapy for treatment of lipofuscin-based retinal diseases. Invest Ophthalmol Vis Sci. 2005;46:4393–401.

31. Eldred GE, Lasky MR. Retinal age pigments generated by self-assembling lysosomotropic detergents. Nature. 1993;361:724–6.

32. Sparrow JR, Parish CA, Hashimoto M, Nakanishi K. A2E, a lipofuscin fluorophore, in human retinal pigmented epithelial cells in culture. Invest Ophthalmol Vis Sci. 1999;40:2988–95.

33. Sparrow JR. Lipofuscin of the retinal pigment epithelium. In: Holz FG, Schmitz-Valckenberg S, Spaide RF, Bird AC, editors. Atlas of fundus autofluorescence imaging. Berlin: Springer; 2007. p. 3–16.

34. Kellner U, Renner AB, Tillack H. Fundus autofluorescence and mfERG for early detection of retinal alterations in patients using chloroquine/hydroxychloroquine. Invest Ophthalmol Vis Sci. 2006;47:3531–8.

35. Sundelin SP, Terman A. Different effects of chloroquine and hydroxychloroquine on lysosomal function in cultured retinal pigment epithelial cells. APMIS. 2002;110:481–9.

36. Ben-Shabat S, Parish CA, Vollmer HR, Itagaki Y, Fishkin N, Nakanishi K, Sparrow JR. Biosynthetic studies of A2E, a major fluorophore of retinal pigment epithelial lipofuscin. J Biol Chem. 2002;277:7183–90.

37. Weng J, Mata NL, Azarian SM, Tzekov RT, Birch DG, Travis GH. Insights into the function of rim protein in photoreceptors and etiology of Stargardt's disease from the phenotype in abcr knockout mice. Cell. 1999;98:13–23.

38. De S, Sakmar TP. Interaction of A2E with model membranes. Implications to the pathogenesis of age-related macular degeneration. J Gen Physiol. 2002;120:147–57.

39. Schutt F, Davies S, Kopitz J, Holz FG, Boulton ME. Photodamage to human RPE cells by A2-E, a retinoid component of lipofuscin. Invest Ophthalmol Vis Sci. 2000;41:2303–8.

40. Sparrow JR, Boulton M. RPE lipofuscin and its role in retinal pathobiology. Exp Eye Res. 2005;80:595–606.

41. Drenckhahn D, Lullmann-Rauch R. Drug-induced lipidosis: differential susceptibilities of pigment epithelium and neuroretina toward several amphiphilic cationic drugs. Exp Mol Pathol. 1978;28:360–71.

42. Bruinink A, Zimmermann G, Riesen F. Neurotoxic effects of chloroquine in vitro. Arch Toxicol. 1991;65:480–4.

43. Rosenthal AR, Kolb H, Bergsma D, Huxsoll D, Hopkins JL. Chloroquine retinopathy in the rhesus monkey. Invest Ophthalmol Vis Sci. 1978;17:1158–75.

44. Spaide RF, Curcio CA. Anatomical correlates to the bands seen in the outer retina by optical coherence tomography: literature review and model. Retina. 2011;31:1609–19.

45. Stepien KE, Han DP, Schell J, Godara P, Rha J, Carroll J. Spectral-domain optical coherence tomography and adaptive optics may detect hydroxychloroquine retinal toxicity before symptomatic vision loss. Trans Am Ophthalmol Soc. 2009;107:28–34.

46. Chen E, Brown DM, Benz MS, Fish RH, Wong TP, Kim RY, Major JC. Spectral domain optical coherence tomography as an effective screening test for hydroxychloroquine retinopathy (the "flying saucer" sign). Clin Ophthalmol. 2010;4:1151–8.

47. Osterberg G. Topography of the layer of rods and cones in the human retina. Acta Ophthalmol. 1935;13:6–97.

48. Spitznas M. The fine structure of the so-called outer limiting membrane in the human retina. Graefes Arch Clin Exp Ophthalmol. 1970;180:44–56.

49. Wong IY, Iu LP, Koizumi H, Lai WW. The inner segment/outer segment junction: what have we learnt so far? Curr Opin Ophthalmol. 2012;23:2010–8.

50. Rodriguez-Padilla JA, Hedges III TR, Monson B, Srinivasan V, Wojtkowski M, Reichel E, Duker JS, Schuman JS, Fujimoto JG. High-speed ultra-high-resolution optical coherence tomography findings in hydroxychloroquine retinopathy. Arch Ophthalmol. 2007;125:775–80.

51. Labriola LT, Jeng D, Fawzi AA. Retinal toxicity of systemic medications. Int Ophthalmol Clin. 2012;52: 149–66.

52. Tao Y, Li XX, Jiang YR, Bai XB, Wu BD, Dong JQ. Diffusion of macromolecule through retina after experimental branch retinal vein occlusion and estimate of intraretinal barrier [abstract]. Curr Drug Metab. 2007;8:151–6.

53. Sato S, Hirooka K, Baba T, Tenkumo K, Nitta E, Shiraga F. Correlation between the ganglion cell-inner plexiform layer thickness measured with Cirrus HD-OCT and macular visual field sensitivity measured with microperimetry. Invest Ophthalmol Vis Sci. 2013;54:3046–51.

54. Gomez ML, Mojana F, Bartsch DU, Freeman WR. Imaging of long-term retinal damage after resolved cotton wool spots. Ophthalmology. 2009;116: 2407–14.

55. Mcleod D. Why cotton wool spots should not be regarded as retinal nerve fiber layer infarcts. Br J Ophthalmol. 2005;89:229–37.

56. Raines MF, Bhargava SK, Rosen ES. The blood-retinal barrier in chloroquine retinopathy. Invest Ophthalmol Vis Sci. 1989;30:726–1731.

57. Penfold PL, Wen L, Madigan MC, Gillies MC, King NJC, Provis JM. Triamcinolone acetonide modulates permeability and intercellular adhesion molecule-1 (ICAM-1) expression of the ECV304 cell line: implications for macular degeneration. Clin Exp Immunol. 2000;121:458–65.

58. Singh S, Dass R. The central artery of the retina I. Origin and course. Br J Ophthalmol. 1960;44: 193–212.

59. Henkind P. Radial peripapillary capillaries of the retina. I. Anatomy: human and comparative. Br J Ophthalmol. 1967;51:115–23.

60. Iwasaki M, Inomata H. Relation between superficial capillaries and foveal structures in the human retina. Invest Ophthalmol Vis Sci. 1986;27:1698–705.

61. Stone J, Itin A, Alon T, Pe'er J, Gnessin H, Chan-Ling T, Keshet E. Development of retinal vasculature is mediated by hypoxia-induced vascular endothelial growth factor (VEGF) expression by neuroglia. J Neurosci. 1995;15:4738–47.

62. Gariano RF, Kalina RE, Hendrickson AE. Normal and pathological mechanisms in retinal vascular development. Surv Ophthalmol. 1996;40:481–90.

63. Gariano RF, Iruela-Arispe ML, Hendrickson AE. Vascular development in primate retina: comparison of laminar plexus formation in monkey and human. Invest Ophthalmol Vis Sci. 1994;35:3442–55.

64. Delves PJ, Martin SJ, Burton DR, Roitt IM. Roitt's essential immunology. Oxford: Wiley-Blackwell; 2011.

65. Hennessy EJ, Parker AE, O'Neill LAJ. Targeting toll-like receptors: emerging therapeutics. Rev Drug Discov. 2010;9:293–307.

66. Kyburz D, Brentano F, Gay S. Mode of action of hydroxychloroquine in RA—evidence of an inhibitory effect on toll-like receptor signaling. Nat Clin Pract Rheumatol. 2006;2:458–9.

67. Katz SJ, Russell AS. Re-evaluation of antimalarials in treating rheumatic diseases: re-appreciation and insights into new mechanisms of action. Curr Eye Res. 2011;23:278–81.

68. Wallace DJ, Gudsoorkar VS, Weisman MH, Venuturupalli SR. New insights into mechanisms of therapeutic effects of antimalarial agents in SLE. Nat Rev Rheumatol. 2012;8:522–33.

69. Barrat FJ, Meeker T, Gregorio J, Chan JH, Uematsu S, Akira S, Chang B, Duramad O, Coffman RL. Nucleic acids of mammalian origin can act as endogenous ligands for Toll-like receptors and may promote systemic lupus erythematosus. J Exp Med. 2005;202:1131–9.

70. Leadbetter EA, Rifkin IR, Hohlbaum AM, Beaudette BC, Schlomchik MJ, Marshak-Rothstein A. Chromatin-IgG complexes activate B cells by dual engagement of IgM and Toll-like receptors. Nature. 2002;416:603–7.

71. Kalia S, Dutz JP. New concepts in antimalarial use and mode of action in dermatology. Dermatol Ther. 2007;20:160–74.

72. Goldman FD, Gilman AL, Hollenback C, Kato RM, Premack BA, Rawlings DJ. Hydroxychloroquine inhibits calcium signals in T cells: a new mechanism to explain its immunomodulatory properties. Blood. 2000;95:3460–8.

73. Fox R. Anti-malarial drugs: possible mechanisms of action in autoimmune disease and prospects for drug development. Lupus. 1996;5:S4–S10.

74. Schultz KR, Gilman AL. The lysosomotropic amines, chloroquine and hydroxychloroquine: a potentially novel therapy for graft-versus-host disease. Leuk Lymphoma. 1997;24:201–10.

75. Cruz da Silva J, Mariz HA, da Rocha Jr LF, de Oliveira PSS, Dantas AT, Duarte ALBP, Pitta IDR, Galdino SL, Pitta MGDR. Hydroxychloroquine decreases TH17-related cytokines in systemic lupus erythematosus and rheumatoid arthritis patients. Clinics. 2013;68:766–71.

76. Maddur MS, Miossec P, Kaveri SV, Bayry J. Th 17 cells. Biology, pathogenesis of autoimmune and inflammatory diseases, and therapeutic strategies. Am J. Pathology. 2012;181:8–18.

77. Ferreira da Rocha Jr L, Duarte ALBP, Dantas AT, Mariz HA, Pitta IDR, Galdino SL, Pitta MGDR. Increased serum interleukin 22 in patients with rheumatoid arthritis and correlation with disease activity. J Rheumatol. 2012;39:1320–5.

78. Shah K, Lee WW, Lee SH, Kim SH, Kang SW, Craft J, Kang I. Dysregulated balance of TH17 and Th1 cells in systemic lupus erythematosus. Arthritis Res Ther. 2010;12:R53–63.

79. Weber SM, Levitz SM. Chloroquine Interferes with lipopolysaccharide-induced TNF-α gene expression by a nonlysosomotropic mechanism. J Immunol. 2000;165:1534–40.

80. Wozniacka A, Lesiak A, Narbutt J, McCauliffe DP, Sysa-Jedrzejowska A. Chloroquine treatment influences proinflammatory cytokine levels in systemic lupus erythematosus patients. Lupus. 2006;15:268–75.

81. Karres I, Kremer JP, Dietl I, Steckholzer U, Jochum M, Ertel W. Chloroquine inhibits proinflammatory cytokine release into human whole blood. Am J Physiol. 1998;274:R1058–64.

82. Sant AJ, Miller J. MHC class II antigen processing: biology of invariant chain. Curr Opin Immunol. 1994;6:57–63.

83. Zarbin MA. Recombinant T-cell receptor ligands in the treatment of uveitis. Arch Ophthalmol. 2013;131:399–400.

84. Watts C. Capture and processing of exogenous antigens for presentation on MHC molecules. Annu Rev Immunol. 1997;15:821–50.

85. Nowell J, Quaranta V. Chloroquine affects biosynthesis of Ia Molecules by inhibiting dissociation of invariant chains from α−β dimers in B cells. J Exp Med. 1985;162:1371–6.

86. Loss Jr GE, Sant AJ. Invariant chain retains MHC class II molecules in the endocytic pathway. J Immunol. 1993;150:3187–97.

87. Ziegler HK, Unanue ER. Decrease in macrophage antigen catabolism caused by ammonia and chloroquine is associated with inhibition of antigen presentation to T cells. Proc Natl Acad Sci U S A. 1982;79:175–8.

88. Moorthy RS, Rao PK, Read RW, Van Gelder RN, Vitale AT, Bodaghi B, Parrish CM. Intraocular inflammation and uveitis. San Francisco: American Academy of Ophthalmology; 2012. p. 38–9.

89. Accapezzato D, Visco V, Francavilla V, Molette C, Donato T, et al. Chloroquine enhances human CD8 T cell responses against soluble antigens in vivo. J Exp Med. 2005;202:817–28.

90. Kleijmeer MJ, Ossevoort MS, van Veen CJH, van Hellemond JJ, Neefjes JJ, Kast WM, Melief CIM, Geuze HJ. MHC class II compartments and the kinetics of antigen presentation in activated mouse spleen dendritic cells. J Immunol. 1995;154:5715–24.

91. Maric MA, Taylor MD, Blum JS. Endosomal aspartic proteinases are required for invariant-chain processing. Proc Natl Acad Sci U S A. 1994;91:2171–5.

92. Titus EO. Recent developments in the understanding of the pharmacokinetics and mechanism of action of chloroquine. Ther Drug Monit. 1989;11:369–79.

93. Koch N, Moldenhauer G, Hofmann WJ, Moller P. Rapid intracellular pathway gives rise to cell surface expression of the MHC class II-associated invariant chain (CD74). J Immunol. 1991;147:2643–51.

94. Akhavan PS, Su J, Lou W, Gladman DD, Urowitz MB, Fortin PR. The early protective effect of hydroxychloroquine on the risk of cumulative damage in patients with systemic lupus erythematosus. J Rheumatol. 2013;40:831–41.

95. Yu Z, Kastenmuller G, He Y, Belcredi P, Moller G, Prehn C, Mendes J, et al. Differences between human plasma and serum metabolite profiles. PLoS One. 2011;6:e21230. doi:10.1371/journal.pone.0021230.

96. Kaufmann AM, Krise JP. Lysosomal sequestration of amine-containing drugs: analysis and therapeutic implications. J Pharm Sci. 2007;96:729–46.

97. Oda K, Koriyama Y, Yamada E, Ikehara Y. Effects of weakly basic amines on proteolytic processing and terminal glycosylation of secretory proteins in cultured rat hepatocytes. J Biol Chem. 1986;240:739–45.

98. de Duve C, de Barsy T, Poole B, Trouet A, Tulkens P, Van Hoof F. Lysosomotropic agents. Biochem Pharmacol. 1974;23:2495–531.

99. Goldstein A, Aronow L, Kalman SM. Principles of drug action: the basis of pharmacology. New York: John Wiley and Sons; 2013.

100. Chloroquine. DrugBank: open data drug & drug target database. 2005. http://www.drugbank.ca/drugs/DB00608. Accessed 22 Aug 2013.

101. Hydroxychloroquine. DrugBank: open data drug & drug target database. 2007. http://www.drugbank.ca/drugs/DB01611. Accessed 22 Aug 2013.

102. Ward PA. The chemosuppression of chemotaxis. J Exp Med. 1966;124:209–26.

103. Klaassen CD, Watkins III JB. Casarett and Doull's essentials of toxicology. New York: McGraw Hill; 2010.

104. McChesney EQ, Fitch CD. 4-Aminoquinolines. In: Richards WHG, Peters W, editors. Antimalarial drugs II. Current antimalarials and new drug developments. Berlin: Springer; 1984. p. 3–60.

105. Mackenzie AH. Antimalarial drugs for rheumatoid arthritis. Am J Med. 1983;75:48–58.

106. Shargel L, Wu-Pong S, Yu ABC. Applied biopharmaceutics and pharmacokinetics. New York: McGraw Hill Medical; 2012. p. 153–75.

107. Frisk-Holmberg M, Bergkvist Y, Domeij-Nyberg B, Hellstrom L, Jansson R. Chloroquine serum concentration and side effects: evidence for dose dependent kinetics. Clin Pharmacol Ther. 1979;25:345–50.

108. Miller DR, Fiechtner JJ, Carpenter JR, Brown RR, Stroshane RM, Stecher VJ. Plasma hydroxychloroquine concentrations and efficacy in rheumatoid arthritis. Arthritis Rheum. 1987;30:567–71.

109. Munster T, Gibbs JP, Shen D, Baethge BA, Botstein GR, Caldwell J, Dietz F, Ettlinger R, Golden HE, Lindsley H, et al. Hydroxychloroquine concentration-response relationships in patients with

rheumatoid arthritis. Arthritis Rheum. 2002;46: 1460–9.

110. Rowland M, Tozer TN. Clinical pharmacokinetics and pharmacodynamics. Concepts and applications. Philadelphia: Wolters Kluwer; 2011. p. 579.

111. Furst DE, Lindsley H, Baethge B, Botstein GR, Caldwell J, Dietz F, Ettlinger R, Golden HE, McLaughlin GE, Moreland LW, et al. Dose-loading with hydroxychloroquine improves the rate of response in early, active rheumatoid arthritis. Arthritis Rheum. 1999;42:357–65.

112. Tett S, Cutler D, Day R. Antimalarials in rheumatic diseases. Baillieres Clin Rheumatol. 1990;4: 467–89.

Pharmacology of Chloroquine and Hydroxychloroquine

2

Abbreviations

4AQR	4-Aminoquinoline retinopathy
4AQs	4-Aminoquinolines (chloroquine and hydroxychloroquine)
ABW	Actual body weight
APC	Antigen presenting cell
BCVA	Best corrected visual acuity
C	Chloroquine
C_pG ODN	C_pG oligodeoxynucleotide
CV	Color vision
CYP	Cytochrome P450 enzymes
DFE	Dilated fundus examination
DNA	Deoxyribonucleic acid
ERK	Extracellular signal-regulated kinases
FP	Ferriprotoporphyrin IX
GVF	Goldmann visual fields
HC	Hydroxychloroquine
HIV	Human immunodeficiency virus
HMG-CoA	3-Hydroxy-3-methylglutaryl-coenzyme A reductase
IBW	Ideal body weight
IFN	Interferon
IL	Interleukin
LD_{50}	Lethal dose 50
LDL	Low-density lipoprotein
M	Mole
mRNA	Mitochondrial ribonucleic acid
NG	Not given
RA	Rheumatoid arthritis
RNA	Ribonucleic acid
RPE	Retinal pigment epithelium
SARS	Severe acute respiratory syndrome
SLE	Systemic lupus erythematosus
TLR	Toll-like receptor
TNF	Tumor necrosis factor
TNF-α	Tumor necrosis factor α
V	Volume of distribution

This chapter covers the pharmacology of chloroquine and hydroxychloroquine, which is similar for both drugs [1], but the details are different. For example, both drugs are partially excreted in feces, but the proportions differ slightly—8–10 % for chloroquine and 15–24 % for hydroxychloroquine. Generally, whatever is said in this chapter about one drug can be assumed to apply to the other unless otherwise specified [1, 2]. Because both drugs are derivatives of a 4-aminoquinoline (4AQ) nucleus, they are referred to as 4AQs, and the retinopathy that they can cause is termed 4-aminoquinoline retinopathy (4AQR) [3]. Commonly used abbreviations in this chapter are collected in "Abbreviations" for reference. Each term will be first used in its full form, along with its abbreviation.

2.1 History

In the 1600s, the Jesuits who proselytized Chile discovered from the Incas that the bark of the cinchona tree can cure malaria [4, 5]. Additional medicinal qualities of cinchona bark were described in the 1700s, and the British and Dutch transplanted these trees to Javan plantations in the early 1900s

D.J. Browning, *Hydroxychloroquine and Chloroquine Retinopathy*,
DOI 10.1007/978-1-4939-0597-3_2, © Springer Science+Business Media New York 2014

for the production of quinine. In 1894, Payne described the use of quinine to treat systemic lupus erythematosus (SLE) [6]. Other alkaloids contained in cinchona bark, such as pamaquine, were also successfully used to treat SLE [5].

When the Japanese army occupied Java in World War II, the natural supply of quinine was lost, and synthesis of antimalarials was pursued in the United States [7]. Quinacrine, a 9-aminoacridine compound, was first used, but had the unpleasant side effect of staining the skin and sclera yellow in a manner indistinguishable from icterus [8–10]. The 4AQs, chloroquine and hydroxychloroquine, were found to be effective as antimalarials and did not discolor the skin. Chloroquine was first synthesized in 1934 by Andersag of I.G. Farbenindustrie in a German effort to find drugs better than quinine [11]. The Germans lost interest in the drug when they judged it to be too toxic for use in man, but the Americans restudied the drug and found it to be effective against malaria and sufficiently safe [3, 7, 12]. Hydroxychloroquine was synthesized in 1946 and proposed as a safer alternative to chloroquine in 1955 [13]. Resistance to chloroquine as an antimalarial became a problem in some parts of the world in the 1980s.

In World War II it was observed that servicemen with rashes and inflammatory arthritis who took quinacrine and chloroquine for malaria prophylaxis experienced improvement in their autoimmune conditions [14]. In 1951, Page used quinacrine to treat arthritis and autoimmune dermatologic conditions [15]. Later chloroquine and then hydroxychloroquine were also noted to favorably affect patients with rheumatologic diseases. Over time, both have been widely adopted for these uses. They are commonly used in patients with rheumatoid arthritis (RA), SLE, discoid lupus erythematosus, polymorphous light

eruptions, solar urticaria, recurrent basal cell carcinoma of the skin, porphyrea cutane tarda, antiphospholipid antibody syndrome, and more than 20 other rarer conditions [11, 16–20].

The side effects other than retinopathy of the 4AQs are discussed in Chap. 3. Chapters 4 through 6 cover aspects of retinopathy. The 4AQs and quinacrine can cause retinopathy with the order of frequency chloroquine > hydroxychloroquine >> quinacrine. Chloroquine retinopathy was first described by Hobbs in 1959 [21]. Hydroxychloroquine retinopathy was first described by Braun-Vallon in 1963 [22, 23]. Quinacrine retinopathy is so rare that some have said that it does not exist [5, 24]. Nevertheless, it does, identical in its funduscopic appearance to 4AQR, and was described in 2004 [25].

2.2   Chemistry

The parent molecule for the antimalarials is quinine. Both chloroquine ($C_{18}H_{26}ClN_3$) and hydroxychloroquine ($C_{18}H_{26}ClN_3O$) are alkylated 4-aminoquinolines (4AQs) (Fig. 2.1) [6]. Chloroquine is 7-chloro-4(-4-diethylamino-1-methylbutylamino) quinoline and hydroxychloroquine is its hydroxyl derivative. Chloroquine and hydroxychloroquine have molecular weights of 320 and 336, respectively [26, 27]. Both chloroquine and hydroxychloroquine are amphiphilic weak bases based on two fused aromatic rings having conjugated double bonds, the 4-aminoquinoline nucleus (Fig. 2.1). Both drugs cross cell membranes well [16, 28, 29]. Hydroxychloroquine is more polar, less lipophilic, and has more difficulty diffusing across cell membranes [6, 30, 31]. The 4AQs lack the third benzene ring that is part of the acridine nucleus of quinacrine (Fig. 2.1) [6].

Useful Conversion Factors

In the literature on chloroquine and hydroxychloroquine, some articles express concentrations in μg/mL or ng/mL and others in M/L. The molecular weights of chloroquine and hydroxychloroquine are 320 and 336, respectively; so one mole of chloroquine weighs 320 g and one mole of hydroxychloroquine weighs 336 g. It follows that 1×10^{-6} M of chloroquine and hydroxychloroquine is equivalent to 320 ng/mL (0.320 µg/mL) and 336 ng/mL (0.320 µg/mL), respectively. Conversely, one µg/ml of chloroquine and hydroxychloroquine is equivalent to 3.125×10^{-6} and 2.97×10^{-6} M/L, respectively.

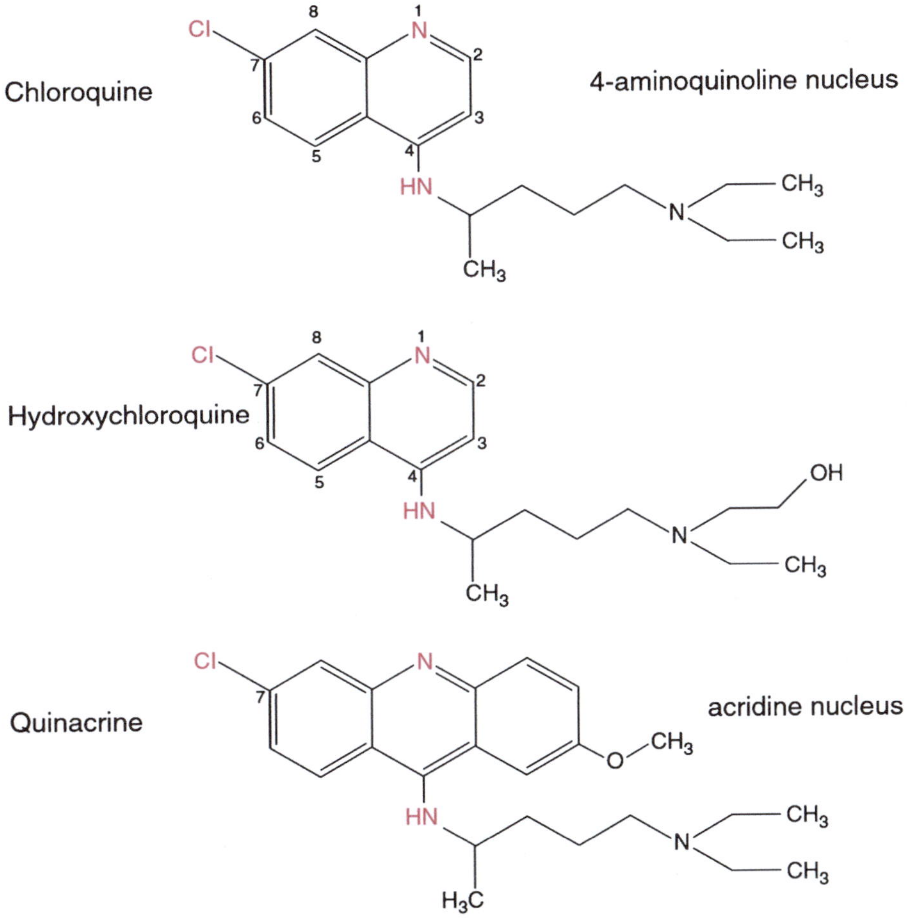

Fig. 2.1 Chloroquine and hydroxychloroquine are 4-aminoquinolines. Quinacrine has a side chain similar to that in chloroquine, but is based on an acridine nucleus

Hydroxychloroquine is more soluble than chloroquine, but both are water-soluble [32]. Chloroquine has two basic groups corresponding to the quinoline-ring nitrogen and the diethyl-amino side-chain nitrogen with ionization constants of 8.1 and 10.2, respectively [33–36]. At a physiologic pH of 7.4, 18 % of chloroquine is monoprotonated but still soluble in lipid and able to traverse cell membranes. However, biprotonated chloroquine, as occurs in a lysosome at a pH of 4–5, is sequestered and prevented from traversing back out to the cytoplasm (see Chap. 1) [34, 37]. Although the amount of free drug present in the plasma is miniscule at the physiologic pH,

Table 2.1 Chemical and brand names of antimalarial drugs

Chemical name	Brand name
Chloroquine phosphate	Aralen, Bemaphate, Chinamine, Delagil, Gontochin, Imagon, Iroquine, Klorokin, Luprochin, Resoquine, Sanoquin, Tanakan, Tresochin, Tochin
Chloroquine diphosphate	Avloclor and Resochin
Chloroquine sulfate	Amokin, Arechin Arthrochin, Artrichin Bemaco, Bemaphate, Bemasulph, Nivaquine, Resoquine
Hydroxychloroquine sulfate	Axenal, Dolquine, Ercoquin, Plaquenil, Polirrheumin, Quensyl
Quinacrine hydrochloride	Acriquine, Atabrine, Atebrin, Chinacrin, Erion, Itaichin, Mepacrine, Palacrin, Metoquine
Amodiaquine dihydrochloride	CAM-AQ1, Camoquinal, Camoquine, Flavoquine, Miaquin,
Quinine sulfate	Qualaquin

Source: Dubois [10]

it is this form of the drug that determines the distribution of the drug between the plasma and the tissues [36]. Induction of acidosis increases the concentration of the drug in the plasma and erythrocytes but does not change drug concentration in the tissues, which have large reservoirs at steady state.

The chemical and brand names of the antimalarial drugs are listed in Table 2.1. Chloroquine diphosphate is the oral form of the drug, and chloroquine hydrochloride is the form used intramuscularly for malaria-induced coma [38]. Neither 4AQ is permitted for routine clinical use in Japan following multiple lawsuits over retinopathy in the 1970s [39]. Hydroxychloroquine is more commonly used in the United States [6]. Chloroquine is rarely used in the United States after multiple lawsuits in the 1960s led Winthrop Laboratories to withdraw the drug's rheumatic indications, but continues to be commonly used in Canada, Mexico, Brazil, Europe, Poland, Turkey, South Africa, and Asia [1, 2, 6, 39–47].

Structure-activity studies of many derivatives of the 4AQs show that halogen substitutions at any position other than seven (Fig. 2.1) reduce pharmacologic activity and toxicity [12]. An aryl rather than an alkyl side chain decreases the therapeutic ratio [12]. Increasing alkyl side-chain length above five carbons decreases the therapeutic ratio and increases toxicity [12].

Chloroquine binds to nucleic acids by electrostatic forces, hydrogen bonds, and van der Waals forces [48]. As a cation at physiologic pH, it binds ionically to melanin, which is a polyanion with many negatively charged carboxyl groups and ortho-semiquinone groups [35, 49–52]. Other binding forces to melanin include van der Waal's forces between the aromatic rings of chloroquine and the indole nuclei of melanin as well as charge transfer complexes in which melanin acts as an electron acceptor [35, 50–54]. The interactions of hydroxychloroquine and melanin parallel those of chloroquine.

Melanin and the 4-Aminoquinolines

Melanin is a name for a family of pigments which are polyanionic polymers formed from the oxidation of tyrosine in cellular vesicles called melanosomes [55]. The term is descriptive, not chemical. Eumelanin is brown or black. Pheomelanin is red or yellow and occurs in red hair [56]. Melanins occur in the retinal pigment epithelium (RPE) of the eye, in the inner ear, and in the substantia nigra of the brain. The highest concentrations are in the eye [55, 56]. The functions of melanin in the eye are to absorb light, preventing scatter, and to protect against free radicals [29, 56]. Although choroidal melanin seems to be synthesized throughout life, melanin in the RPE is synthesized for a brief interval of fetal and perinatal life with little production thereafter [56–58].

The interaction of melanin with 4AQs is complex. Some have written that increased melanin is related to toxicity [55]. Others have denied this or maintained an agnostic viewpoint pending further evidence [29, 54, 56]. Also, the possibility of a protective effect has been raised. The mechanism suggested is that melanin binds the drug and prevents formation of lamellar bodies until its binding capacity is exceeded [19, 51, 56, 59–62]. It has been hypothesized that the extensive binding of 4AQs to melanin produces high local gradients of the drugs that may have importance in identifying cell types that are particularly affected [63]. For example, calculations suggest that the effective concentration of chloroquine in the cytoplasm of the RPE may be in the range of 10^{-5} to 10^{-4} M/L [63]. Chloroquine accumulates in the uveal tract of pigmented animals, but not albino animals, but both types of animals develop 4AQR [64, 65].

Melanin content in the RPE decreases with age [58]. In the first two decades of life, an average of 8 % of cytoplasmic volume is occupied by melanin, but only 3.5 % after age 40 [66]. The decrease is thought to occur by the degradation of melanin, after damage by light or free radicals, into complex granules containing melanolysosomes and melanolypofuscin. The relationship of decreasing melanin and increasing risk of 4AQR with increasing age is intuitive but speculative.

The 4AQs have chiral carbons about which the side chains can be arranged so as to be non-superimposable mirror images of each other [67]. These stereoisomers, called enantiomers, are labeled as R(−) or S(+) forms. Clinically used 4AQs are racemic mixtures with equal amounts of R(−) and S(+) forms [67].

Both enantiomers of chloroquine are equipotent in vitro and in a duck model of malaria. In mice and rats S(+) chloroquine was more potent than R(−) chloroquine, possibly due to stereoselectivity in distribution of drug throughout the body [12, 37, 68, 69].

S(+) chloroquine is more highly bound to plasma proteins than R(−) chloroquine (67 % versus 35 %) [68]. Sequestration of the R(−) enantiomer in ocular tissues is greater than that of the S(+) enantiomer [67]. The toxicity of the S(+) enantiomer is greater than the R(−) enantiomer in mammals [69]. The S(+) enantiomer for both chloroquine and hydroxychloroquine is excreted by the kidneys preferentially compared to the R(−) enantiomer [55, 67, 68]. Because renal failure is associated with 4AQR, it is possible that S(+) chloroquine and S(+) hydroxychloroquine are more toxic in humans than R(−) chloroquine and R(−) hydroxychloroquine, respectively [55].

2.3 Pharmacokinetics and Tissue Distribution of the 4-Aminoquinolines

2.3.1 Absorption

Nearly complete absorption of 4AQs after an oral dose occurs within 2–4 h (Fig. 2.2) [2, 3, 12, 37, 70]. In fasting subjects the absorption of oral chloroquine was 89 ± 16 % and of hydroxychloroquine was 74 ± 13 % [70, 71]. Absorption is relatively unaffected by concomitant ingestion of food. However, intersubject variability of 30–100 % has been reported in extent of absorption, which may explain in part the individual variability of 4AQ effectiveness and toxicity [4, 71, 72].

2.3.2 Distribution and Pharmacokinetics

The pharmacokinetics of chloroquine and hydroxychloroquine are similar [38, 73–75]. However, the explanation is complicated because of their differential sequestration in various

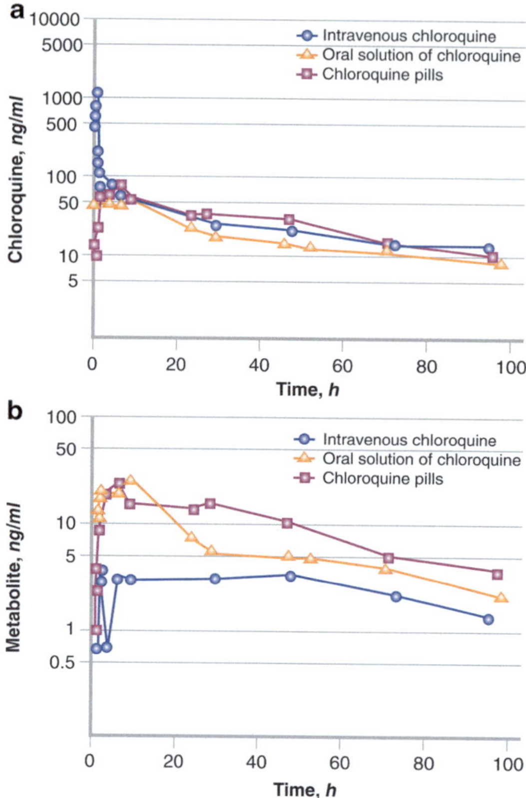

three compartments is considered to be more accurate [37, 75].

The 4AQs have a large volume of distribution (V) due to extensive sequestration of the drugs by tissues. Plasma volumes of distribution up to 65,000 L for chloroquine and 44,257 L for hydroxychloroquine have been reported [71, 75, 77]. Normalized by body mass, reported volumes of distribution for chloroquine have ranged from 204 to 800 L/kg depending on the sensitivity of the method of detecting chloroquine [37]. Drug disposition proceeds in three phases—distribution from blood to tissues, equilibration between blood and tissues, and release from tissues back into blood [19]. These phases have half-lives of 3–8, 40–216 h, and 30–60 days, respectively [13, 37, 70, 75, 78].

The peak plasma concentration after an oral dose of chloroquine is 3–12 h [10, 32, 67]. Thirty-three to 70 % of the drug in plasma is protein-bound [2, 32, 38, 75, 79, 80]. The effects of hypoalbuminemia and altered immunoglobulin composition in patients taking 4AQs are not well understood [80].

The phase of terminal elimination has the greatest importance for the 4AQs as used in autoimmune diseases in which they are given for years and for which steady-state levels are the emphasis. The most commonly quoted median value for the terminal elimination half-life is 40 days [16, 37, 38, 75, 81]. The pharmacokinetics of chloroquine do not differ to a clinically important extent between black and white patients [11, 69, 79]. The average melanin content of a black person is estimated to be 1 g and for a white person is estimated to be 250 mg. This implies that melanin sequestration is not a large factor in systemic pharmacokinetics although the drug continues to elute from melanin at low levels for years after cessation of ingestion [49, 64, 71, 78, 82].

A lower daily dose of chloroquine and hydroxychloroquine leads to a lower plateau concentration in plasma (Fig. 2.3 and Table 2.2). Doses of chloroquine of 3.5–4.0 mg/kg/day based on ideal body weight (IBW) yield serum concentrations of 6 to 9×10^{-7} M/L. Doses of hydroxychloroquine of 6.0–6.5 mg/kg/day based on IBW yield serum concentrations of 1.4 to

Fig. 2.2 Chloroquine bioavailability and elimination in man. A single dose of chloroquine was given intravenously (blue circles), as an oral solution (yellow triangles), or as tablets (purple squares). Panel A shows plasma concentration of chloroquine and panel B chloroquine metabolite. The near superposition of the three curves in panel A is evidence of near-complete absorption of chloroquine from the gastrointestinal tract. Slow elimination is also indicated. Data from Gustafsson [70]

tissues of the body and continuously evolving tests for detection of the drugs in plasma that are increasingly sensitive [37, 75, 76]. As a result, estimates of pharmacokinetic parameters have varied widely over the years [53, 75]. For example, the terminal half-life of chloroquine has been reported variously to be between one and 157 days [53, 70, 75, 76]. In addition, dose-dependent kinetics have been reported by some, while others have claimed that this interpretation arises from artifacts of insensitive detection methods [37, 75–77]. In the 1980s a two-compartment model was thought to best describe the pharmacokinetics of the 4AQs [2]. Now a model with

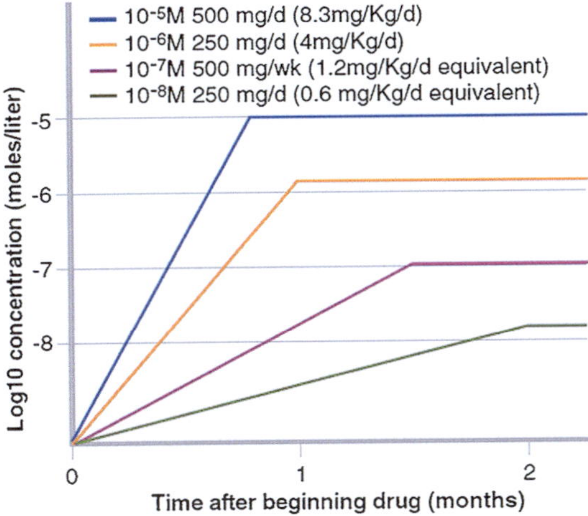

Fig. 2.3 Schematically depicted dependence of final equilibrium plasma concentration and equilibration time on daily dose of chloroquine. The dependence of the final equilibrium concentration on body mass is not shown. However, for a given daily dose the final equilibrium concentration will be lower for a higher body mass. Similar relationships apply to hydroxychloroquine dosing. Data from Mackenzie [2]

1.5×10^{-6} M/L [2]. Daily dosing of chloroquine 250 mg/day produces plasma concentrations at equilibrium of 0.31 to 3.13×10^{-6} M/L depending on body mass [2, 38]. The dependence of time to reach equilibrium levels on daily dosing is schematically represented in Fig. 2.3. Because the half-life to reach a steady-state concentration is not the same for all daily doses, one may conclude that the mechanism of drug elimination is not a first-order process, but rather more complicated with some dependence of the elimination-rate constant on plasma-drug concentration (see Chap. 1) [83, p. 314, [84].

2.3.3 Steady-State Concentration of 4-Aminoquinolines in Various Organs

The concentration of 4AQs in the tissues of the body after ingestion varies. In pigmented rats, the order of concentration of chloroquine after a single dose from greatest to least is uvea > liver > lung > kidney > vitreous > heart > skin > hair > brain > blood > serum [53]. The results are similar in rabbits and humans [11, 82]. Drug binding to melanin explains the differences between pigmented and albino animals [11]. The order of concentration of hydroxychloroquine in various tissues of albino rats is similar, except that concentrations in the albinotic uvea fall to the approximate level of the heart. In pigmented mammals, the eye has the highest concentration due to binding by melanin [74]. Similar results were found after chronic oral administration of chloroquine to albino and pigmented rats (Figs. 2.4 and 2.5) [74].

Limited information from cases of accidental death in persons taking chloroquine and suicides by chloroquine ingestion indicates similar distributions of 4AQs across various tissues in humans [11]. Tissue uptake as a function of dosage is

Table 2.2 Plateau concentrations of 4-aminoquinolines according to daily dosing

Drug/reference	Dosing	Equivalent daily dosing for a subject with IBW of 60 kg (mg/kg/day)	Plateau plasma concentration (M/L)	Plateau blood concentration (M/L)
C [80]	250 mg/week	0.60	10^{-8}	$^{a}5 \times 10^{-8}$
C [80]	500 mg/week	1.19	10^{-7}	$^{a}5 \times 10^{-7}$
C [80]	250 mg/day	4.16	10^{-6}	$^{a}5 \times 10^{-6}$
C [80]	500 mg/day	8.33	10^{-5}	$^{a}5 \times 10^{-5}$
C [69]	310 mg/day	5.17	3.9×10^{-7}	1.95×10^{-6}
HC [175]	224 mg/day	3.73	$^{b}2.5 \times 10^{-7}$	2.0×10^{-6}
HC [71]	155 mg/day	2.58	$^{b}5.88 \times 10^{-7}$	2.94×10^{-6}
HC [71]	310 mg/day	5.17	$^{b}1.18 \times 10^{-8}$	5.88×10^{-6}

In some rows only one plateau concentration was measured, with the other deduced (see *superscripts*). Findings that whole blood concentrations are approximately five times than that of plasma concentrations are denoted by *a*. The finding that plasma concentrations are approximately one-fifth of whole blood concentrations is denoted by *b*

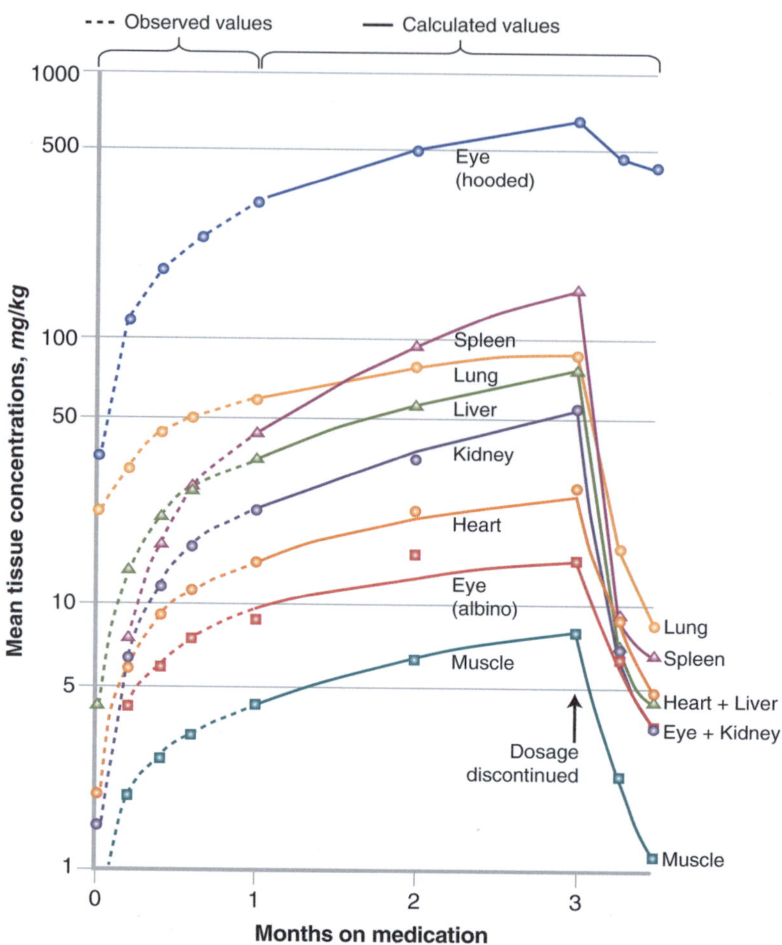

Fig. 2.4 Relative concentration of hydroxychloroquine in various tissues in rats. Tissue levels of hydroxychloroquine in albino rats receiving 40 mg/kg/day of hydroxychloroquine orally by stomach tube, 6 days a week, for 3 months. Groups of four or six animals were sacrificed on days 30, 61, 91, 99, and 106. Results shown project back (mathematically, at intervals) to day 1, as indicated by broken lines. The single curve labeled "Eye (hooded)" refers to pigmented rather than albino rats. The melanin in pigmented tissues sequesters hydroxychloroquine. Data from McChesney EW [74]

nonlinear. In rats, a threefold increase in dosing leads to a 20-fold increase in hydroxychloroquine deposition in liver and spleen [85].

A useful way to understand the differential distribution of 4AQs across various tissues is to consider ratios of concentration in tissues compared to plasma concentration (Table 2.3). The concentration of chloroquine in the liver, spleen, and adrenal gland is 6,000–80,000 times that in plasma, depending on the species chosen for study—whether the species is pigmented or albinotic—and the regimen of drug administration [10, 32, 37]. Within a single organ there are large differences in drug concentration in particular tissues. For example, chloroquine concentrations in the uvea of the rat are 9–32 times that of the retina, which in turn has concentrations six to nine times that of the vitreous [49, 54]. In another example, within skin the 4AQs are more concentrated in the epidermis than the corium with a concentration ratio of 5:1 to 15:1 [86]. The variation reflects sequestration of 4AQs by lysosomes and melanin [37]. Millimolar levels of 4AQs can be found in lysosomes, and melanin can bind a quantity of 4AQs up to 3 % of its weight [37, 87].

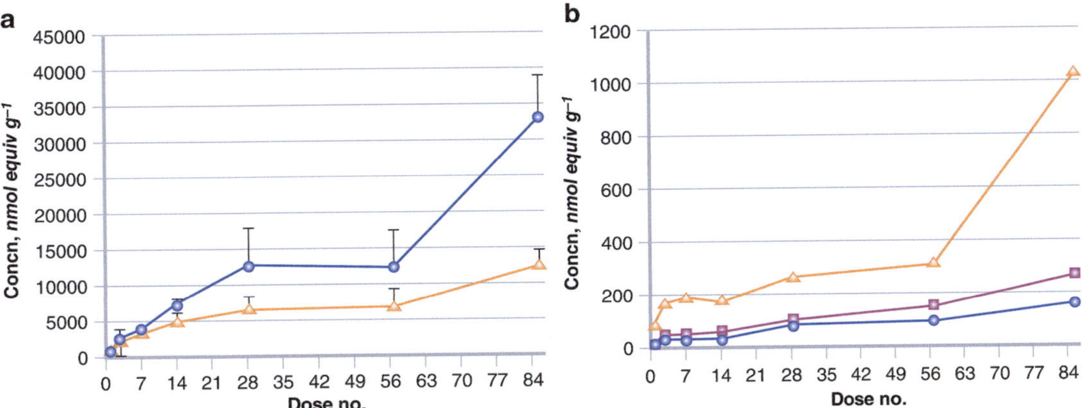

Fig. 2.5 Concentration of chloroquine in ocular tissues of pigmented rats. Panel A—Mean concentration of radioactivity in iris/ciliary body (blue line, circles) and choroid (orange line, triangles) at 24 h after repeated oral administration of ^{14}C-chloroquine at daily doses of 28 mg (0.054 mmol)kg/L under non-fasting conditions in pigmented rats for 84 days. Each value represents the mean ± standard deviation for three rats. Compare the concentrations in iris/ciliary body and choroid to those found in the retina and cornea in panel B. Panel B—Mean concentration of radioactivity in retina (orange line, triangles), cornea (purple line, squares), and vitreous (blue line, circles) after repeated oral administration of ^{14}C-chloroquine at daily doses of 28 mg (0.054 mmol) kg/L under non-fasting conditions in pigmented rats for 84 days. The concentration of chloroquine in the choroid is approximately 12 times higher in the choroid than the retina after the 84th dose. Data from Tanaka [54]

Table 2.3 Relative distribution of chloroquine among tissues

Model	Tissue	Tissue-plasma concentration ratio	Study
Human	Fat, tendon, bone	0.1	Titus [37], McChesney [74]
Albino rat, human	Erythrocytes	1.9–4.0	Berliner [3], Alvan [176], Titus [37, 70]
Albino rat	Whole blood	3.7	Berliner [3]
Albino rat	Brain	4–31	Berliner [3], Titus [37]
Albino rat	Muscle	4–41	Berliner [3], Titus [37]
Human	Skin	6–200	Ramser [87], Tannenbaum [32], Goldman [20]
Albino rat	Heart	150	Berliner [3]
NG	Leukocytes	100–300	Titus [37], Dubois [10]
Albino rat	Kidney	670	Berliner [3]
Albino rat	Lung	640	Berliner [3]
Albino rat	Liver	420	Berliner [3]

In the albino rat model chloroquine 25 mg/kg was given daily for 10 days yielding a mean plasma concentration of 157 g/L [3]. NG means not given

There are clinically unimportant differences in tissue distribution of chloroquine and hydroxychloroquine [78]. For an identical dose of hydroxychloroquine and chloroquine, tissue levels of chloroquine are 2.5 times those of hydroxychloroquine [74]. Tissue-plasma concentration ratios for chloroquine in various albinotic animals range from 28 to 93. For hydroxychloroquine the analogous tissue-plasma concentration ratios range from 33 to 79. In contrast, for both drugs in pigmented animals the tissue-plasma concentration ratios are approximately 1,000–3,000 [11]. The 4AQs remain in human tissues for years. Five years after last ingesting chloroquine, chloroquine and its metabolite have been measured in the urine [85, 88].

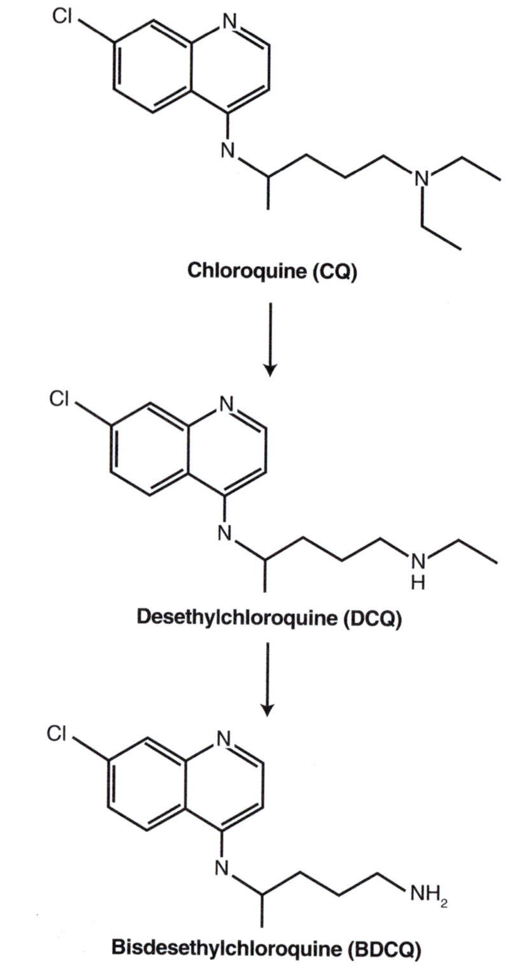

Chloroquine (CQ)

Desethylchloroquine (DCQ)

Bisdesethylchloroquine (BDCQ)

Fig. 2.6 Metabolism of chloroquine by dealkylation. Both metabolites are found in plasma and urine and both have activity similar to the parent compound. Data from Projean [89]

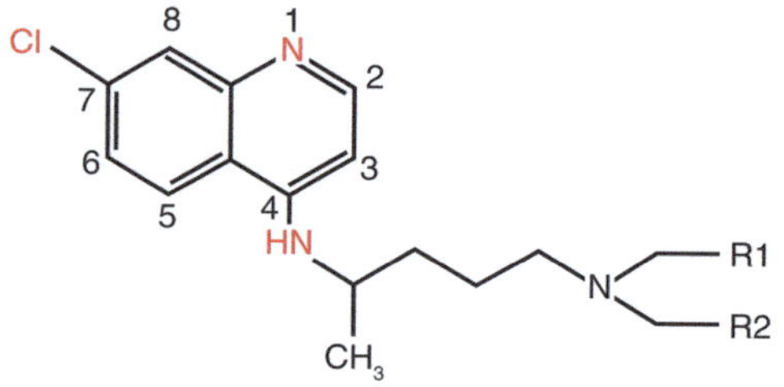

Drug/Metabolite	R1	R2
Chloroquine	$-CH_2CH_3$	$-CH_2CH_3$
Hydroxychloroquine	$-CH_2CH_3$	$-CH_2CHOH$
Desethylchloroquine	$-CH_2CH_3$	$-H$
Desethylhydroxychloroquine	$-H$	$-CH_2CHOH$
Bisdesethylchloroquine	$-H$	$-H$

Fig. 2.7 Chemical structures of the three major metabolites of chloroquine and hydroxychloroquine. Chloroquine has two metabolites, whereas hydroxychloroquine has three

2.3.4 Metabolism

Metabolism of 4AQs is by dealkylation in the liver (Fig. 2.6) [68]. To determine metabolites of chloroquine, carbon-14-labeled chloroquine was administered to monkeys, after which 12 labeled metabolites were detected. The two most important were desethyl chloroquine and bisdesethyl chloroquine, both of which have pharmacologic activity and are thought to be approximately as toxic as the parent compounds [11]. The differential efficacy and toxicity of the metabolites of 4AQs has not been studied, but a suggestion has been made that desethylhydroxychloroquine might have a higher therapeutic ratio than the parent compound hydroxychloroquine [77].

The quinoline ring is resistant to degradation by cytochrome P450 enzymes (CYP) CYP2C8 and CYP3A4, which mediate 80 % of the total metabolism of 4AQs [38, 89–91]. The metabolism of chloroquine and hydroxychloroquine differs only in the number of metabolites produced (Fig. 2.7) [92]. Thirty percent to 79 % of an oral dose of a 4AQ is metabolized and 21–70 % is excreted without metabolism [24, 69, 91, 93].

Desethylchloroquine concentration after a dose of chloroquine reaches 40–48 % of chloroquine concentration. Bisdesethylchloroquine concentration reaches 10–13 % of chloroquine concentration [38, 68, 93, 94]. At steady state the ratio of chloroquine to desethylchloroquine was 7.2 ± 1.88 while the ratio of hydroxychloroquine to desethylhydroxychloroquine was $1.75 \pm .37$ [77].

Inhibition of cytochrome P450 isoenzymes by other drugs and variation across individuals in expression of the isoforms may explain the variation in levels of the two metabolites after ingestion of the same dose of chloroquine or hydroxychloroquine [77, 89]. For example, ketoconazole, an inhibitor of CYP3A4, inhibited the formation of desethylchloroquine by 33 %

Table 2.4   Excretion of 4-aminoquinolines

Fate	Chloroquine (%)	Hydroxychloroquine (%)	References
Excreted unchanged in urine	Range 10–60; median 38	Range 6–60; median 23	Tett [71], Schultz [78], Gustafsson [70], McChesney [11], Berliner [3], Titus [37], Ono [53], McChesney [74], Albert [73]
Excreted as metabolites in urine	Range 7–31; median 18	17	Gustafsson [70], McChesney [11], Titus [37], Ono [53]
Excreted in feces	8–10	24–25	McChesney [11], McChesney [74]
Sloughed off in skin	5	5	Mackenzie [80]
Stored long term in lean tissues	45	45	Mackenzie [80]

and 45 % at concentrations of 1×10^{-6} and 1×10^{-5} M/L, respectively [93]. Cimetidine, another CYP3A4 inhibitor, increased the half-life of an oral dose of chloroquine by 48 % [95]. The elimination half-lives of chloroquine, desethylchloroquine, and bisdesethylchloroquine are all from 20 to 60 days. The half-lives of elimination of the desethyl metabolites of the 4AQs are longer than those of the parent compounds. [77] Chloroquine and metabolites can be found in urine for months after a single oral dose [68].

Caution should be exercised in considering the results of testing in animal models. The results may not translate directly to human metabolism. For example, the dog metabolizes chloroquine by glucuronidation in a manner unlike some other species that leads to a relatively short half-life [11].

2.3.5   Excretion and Storage

4AQs are excreted by the kidney and the liver [96]. For both chloroquine and hydroxychloroquine, approximately 40–60 % is excreted as unchanged or metabolized drug through the kidneys, 8–25 % is excreted in unchanged or changed form in the feces, 5 % is sloughed off through the skin, and 25–45 % is stored long term in lean body tissues (Table 2.4) [3, 11, 37, 38, 53, 73, 74, 80]. Kidney or liver dysfunction decreases excretion of 4AQs and leads to greater drug retention and higher risk of retinopathy [80]. In the anuric patient, compared to subject with normal renal function, the equilibrium level of chloroquine is 70 % higher and for hydroxychloroquine is

25–30 % higher [71]. Declining renal function may be one mechanism by which age becomes a risk factor for retinopathy.

Alkalinization of urine decreases excretion [32]. Acidification of the urine by oral ingestion of ammonium chloride can increase renal excretion 20–80 % [85]. Intramuscular injection of dimercaprol can also increase urinary excretion of chloroquine [85]. Neither of these approaches has been adopted in clinical practice as practical methods to treat chloroquine retinopathy.

2.4   Clinical Uses and Dosing

The 4AQs are commonly used in rheumatologic conditions because they are effective in a high proportion of cases and have fewer side effects than gold, azathioprine, penicillamine, or levamisole [97–100]. The diagnoses for which 4AQs are most prescribed are rheumatoid arthritis (RA) and SLE, which together account for 82–95 % of the cases [23, 101, 102]. An epidemiologic survey, found that 60.1 % of patients with RA and 92.2 % of patients with SLE take hydroxychloroquine at some point in the course of their disease [61].

Antimalarials have a different mechanism of action than other immunomodulating therapies making them useful in combination therapy [42, 103–105]. In RA and SLE it is commonly observed that 60–95 % of patients taking chloroquine have a clinical response measured by subjective improvement, objective responses in laboratory measurements, activities of daily living, and reductions in flares of disease [8, 10, 37, 71, 106–112]. Although initially embraced for patients with milder forms of SLE and RA [10], the recent trend is that 4AQs are being used in a higher proportion of patients with SLE; some have advocated their use in all SLE patients [24, 104]. Many reports pool all patients taking 4AQs together under the assumption that the disease for which the drug is taken is immaterial to the risk of retinopathy [62, 113, 114].

Clinical efficacy may be greater in SLE than in RA [115]. In 15 % of patients the clinical response is dramatic [37]. The erythrocyte sedimentation rate, C-reactive protein, and serum IgG levels typically decrease in patients with autoimmune diseases treated with 4AQs. Occasionally, long-term remission of autoimmune disease is possible with no progression of radiologically documented joint disease [116]. In SLE, use of 4AQs has also improved survival [117]. This may be due to the antiatherogenic and antithrombotic effects of 4AQs as well as their beneficial effects on lipid profile and osteoporosis [103, 104]. When the drugs are stopped, beneficial effects last for several weeks to months, but disease activity generally recurs [116]. There is typically no increase in rates of opportunistic infection. Chloroquine prevents an immunologic response to antigenic proteins requiring digestion, but not the response of T cells to predigested antigenic peptides [118].

Full effects of the 4AQs may take 3–6 months to develop [37, 38, 106, 107, 116, 118–120]. Some have attributed this to a pharmacodynamic mechanism involving an immune process that requires the observed time to develop. However, the effect is predictable based on pharmacokinetics and the time required to saturate lysosomes (see Chap. 1) [83, 94, 121, 122]. The delayed onset of therapeutic effect of the 4AQs after initiation of therapy can be shortened by using a higher loading dose in the first weeks to months at the price of an increased frequency of gastrointestinal side effects [10, 38, 119, 121, 123]. A doubling of the daily dose is common in the first part of a course of rheumatologic therapy [124]. Beginning with the maintenance dose leads to a slower onset of action [121, 123].

Some clinicians give patients a drug holiday during summer as a way of assessing if the drug is still required for control of disease activity [1, 123]. This practice should also reduce the probability of developing 4AQR. Rheumatologists frequently decrease the dosing of 4AQs over time. In one series of 758 patients, 84 % of patients begun on 400 mg/day of hydroxychloroquine had their daily doses reduced over time. This is important, since the most common intervention by ophthalmologists is to suggest dosage reductions, not cessation of 4AQs, in response to concerns of retinopathy [125–127].

Approximately 20–50 % of patients with SLE and 75 % of patients with RA eventually have cessation of the drug by 6–10 years of follow-up, mainly because of inefficacy in the case of RA and because of disease remission in the case of SLE [97, 115, 125, 128, 129]. The rate of discontinuation of 4AQs is highest in the first 2 years. In the case of hydroxychloroquine, by 2 years approximately 34 % of patients with SLE and 54 % of patient with RA will have discontinued the drug [8, 125, 128]. Discontinuation of hydroxychloroquine may be less common in patients treated for SLE than RA. In one series, the overall 5-, 10-, and 15-year discontinuation rates were 20 %, 38 %, and 58 %, respectively [115]. Approximately 5 % of patients stop treatment because of ocular problems such as blurred vision or corneal deposits and 5 % stop because of gastrointestinal complaints, rashes, and other side effects. Rates of stopping 4AQs are dependent on the physician, the patient, and their relationship [97]. Some physicians and patients are more willing than others to tolerate less-than-complete control of disease activity and some degree of side effects [97].

Chloroquine is commonly given in doses of 100–250 mg/day for prophylaxis against malaria [130]. It is given as 1,500 mg over 3 days as a treatment for an acute episode of malaria [131]. The most common doses of chloroquine and hydroxychloroquine in clinical use are 250 and 400 mg/day, respectively, regardless of height or weight of the patient [19, 24, 45, 97, 100, 126]. That is, cumulative doses greater than 100 times that used for prophylaxis or treatment of malaria are administered to patients with autoimmune diseases [11, 100, 115, 130]. Before 1980, dosing of 4AQs was excessive and largely responsible for the greater prevalence of 4AQR reported in this era [10]. For example, in 1978 it was recommended that 400 mg/day of hydroxychloroquine and 250 mg/day of chloroquine were acceptable doses for all adults weighing over 100 lb [10]. The threshold for IBW at which these doses are now recognized to be unacceptable is now recognized to be 135 lb, not 100 lb [32, 127, 132]. More sophisticated regimens seek dosing not greater than 6 mg/kg/day based on actual body weight (ABW) [97] or 6.0–6.5 mg/kg/day based on IBW for hydroxychloroquine [78, 133]. The analogous ceiling for chloroquine is 3.5 mg/kg/day based on IBW. The preferred dosing of 4AQs is based on IBW [80, 114]. If a patient's ABW is less than the IBW based on height, then the ABW should be used to determine dosing [126].

A 250 mg dose of chloroquine phosphate contains 150 mg of chloroquine base [19, 24]. A 200 mg dose of hydroxychloroquine sulfate contains 155 mg of hydroxychloroquine base [1, 19, 24]. The relative potency and toxicity of the two 4AQs is inconsistently portrayed. Some have written that chloroquine is more potent and more toxic than hydroxychloroquine [20, 24, 134], but others have said the reverse. For example, 400 mg of hydroxychloroquine has been assumed to be equivalent to 500 mg of chloroquine [1, 134, 135], yet another report assumes that 400 mg of chloroquine is equivalent to 500 mg of hydroxychloroquine [134]. Other reports state that 400 mg of hydroxychloroquine is equivalent to 250 mg of chloroquine [10, 136].

The best analysis based on multiple forms of administration in different animal models and in human trials is that chloroquine and hydroxychloroquine are equipotent and that chloroquine is approximately twice as toxic [11]. That is, in acute toxicity experiments in animal models, the dose at which 50 % die (LD_{50}) is approximately twice as high with hydroxychloroquine as with chloroquine (see Chap. 3) [11]. Likewise, in subacute and chronic toxicity studies, the tolerated dose for 50 % of animals is approximately twice as high with hydroxychloroquine as with chloro-

quine [11]. Although less rigorous, clinical series in humans suggests the same with a smaller percentage of side effects with hydroxychloroquine compared to chloroquine when the two are given in comparable dosages [137, 138]. Therefore, at the most commonly prescribed daily doses, chloroquine and hydroxychloroquine have been considered equally effective in treating autoimmune diseases with the therapeutic ratio favoring hydroxychloroquine (see Chap. 1).

Reports are inconsistent in the way they report drug concentrations. Plasma, serum, and whole blood concentrations have been used. They are not comparable; plasma concentrations are the lowest, and whole blood concentrations are the greatest. Serum concentrations exceed plasma concentrations because platelets concentrate 4AQs, and upon coagulation of the blood the platelet contents are released into the serum [139]. Plasma levels of chloroquine effective against malaria are 10^{-8} to 10^{-7} M/L [37, 140]. For rheumatological disease higher plasma levels are required—approximately 10^{-6} M/L [34, 37, 71, 89, 140, 141]. Serum concentrations of chloroquine in patients taking chloroquine 250 mg/day for long periods are in the range 6.25×10^{-7} to 1.25×10^{-6} M/L [142]. Therapeutic whole blood concentrations of HC for autoimmune diseases are 8×10^{-7} to 5×10^{-6} M/L, approximately five times higher than plasma concentrations [16, 37, 78, 89]. Using whole blood concentrations is not optimal because 4AQs are preferentially sequestered in erythrocytes and leukocytes which implies that hematocrit and white blood cell count will affect the whole blood concentration in potentially confounding ways. On the other hand, the precision of measurements is higher with whole blood than with plasma, possibly due to the technical difficulty of separating blood cells and platelets from plasma, making whole blood more suited for pharmacokinetic analyses [77].

In a study of patients with rheumatoid arthritis, patients with less morning stiffness and no rheumatoid factor had significantly higher blood concentrations of hydroxychloroquine than patients with more morning stiffness and presence of rheumatoid factor [143]. Other studies have not found a correlation between plasma concentration and clinical response [77, 139, 144]. In patients taking hydroxychloroquine for RA and SLE, daily dosing at 400 mg/day was associated with wide variability in whole blood concentrations [145]. In a study of 143 patients with SLE, those patients with inactive disease had average whole blood concentrations of $3.37 \times 10^{-6} \pm 1.64 \times 10^{-6}$ M/L compared to $2.17 \times 10^{-6} \pm 1.40 \times 10^{-6}$ in those patients with active disease [145]. Higher rates of efficacy can be assured if dosing is calibrated to yield a whole blood concentration of approximately 3.1×10^{-6} M/L [38, 145]. Variability may be due to lack of adherence to therapy or differences in absorption or metabolism of the drugs by individuals. Because of interindividual variability, in certain patients it may not be possible to reach therapeutic concentrations of 4AQs without exceeding daily dose thresholds based on IBW that are considered high risk for causing retinopathy [145]. Patients taking hydroxychloroquine for graft-versus-host disease have higher whole blood concentration targets of 5×10^{-6} to 1.5×10^{-5} M/L. Concerns over retinopathy in these patients are balanced against the more serious nature of their systemic disease. Effective plasma concentrations and effective in vitro concentrations of the drugs are not necessarily closely related, as the drug concentrations may be higher locally due to intracellular organelle sequestration [139, 140]. Other potential confounders include receptor concentrations, the influence of alcohol and smoking, genetic and gender influences, and age [77]. Perhaps because of inconsistency of results, few clinicians measure plasma concentrations of 4AQs to judge adequacy of a trial of drug [24, 139].

One therapeutic strategy used to reduce the risk of retinopathy yet obtain the beneficial disease modifying effects of antimalarial therapy is to combine chloroquine or hydroxychloroquine with quinacrine, which is not a 4-aminoquinoline and is considered to have a lesser risk of causing retinopathy. In practical terms, the patient is begun on hydroxychloroquine 400 mg/day or 6.5 mg/kg/day based on IBW, whichever is lower. After 2 months, if the autoimmune disease has not sufficiently responded, quainacrine 100 mg/day is added. After one additional month if a response has been achieved then the hydroxychloroquine is reduced to 200 mg/day [38]. Although the risk of retinopathy with quinacrine is less than with 4AQs, retinopathy has been associated infrequently with quinacrine [25].

2.5 Pregnancy and Lactation

Antimalarials cross the placenta and can concentrate in the eyes of fetal animals in mice and monkey models [64, 146]. Cord blood concentrations of antimalarials are similar to maternal blood levels [147, 148]. Toxicity in the fetus has not been reported. However, the number of mothers who have taken one of the drugs on a daily basis while pregnant and whose offspring have subsequently been examined for retinopathy has been small and the methods for checking retinopathy insensitive (Table 2.5) [149–151]. A randomized control trial with greater than 400 pregnancies per arm would be required to detect a difference in 5 % in pregnancy loss with alpha error of 0.05 and beta error of 0.8 [152]. Such a study is unlikely to be done, and therefore practice is likely to be guided by evidence of lesser quality. In case–control studies and prospective case series, the rates of spontaneous abortion, fetal death, fetal distress, and congenital malformations have not differed, although the studies have been small with little power to detect small differences in rates [152–154]. Flares of lupus among women who stop 4AQs during pregnancy are more frequent than in women who continue these drugs throughout pregnancy [152, 153]. The general consensus is that mothers using antimalarial drugs during pregnancy need not stop them as they do not appear to affect fetal health [147, 150, 153–156]. Dissenting opinion has been published, but it is based on anecdotal associations of fetal abnormalities in mothers taking 4AQs during pregnancy [8, 32, 71, 157].

Table 2.5   4-Aminoquinoline use in pregnancy and the risk of retinopathy in offspring

Study	Examinations done on offspring	Number of offspring with retinopathy/number of pregnant women taking chloroquine	Number of offspring with retinopathy/number of pregnant women taking hydroxychloroquine
Klinger [149]	BCVA, SLE, DFE, CV, some GVF	0/7	0/14
Motta [150]	Inspect anterior segment, pupillary reaction, DFE		0/35
Parke [156]	Funduscopy	0/4	0/4
Costedoat-Chalumeau [148]	NG		0/11

BCVA best corrected visual acuity, *SLE* slit lamp examination, *CV* color vision, *GVF* Goldmann visual fields, *NG* not given, *DFE* dilated fundus examination

Data on use of antimalarials by lactating mothers is sparse, but small amounts are excreted into breast milk [147, 158]. In a woman given 800 mg of hydroxychloroquine in the course of 48 h, the concentration of drug in breast milk was 9.5×10^{-9} M/L [159]. Doses delivered to breast-feeding infants have been estimated to be 0.06–0.2 mg/kg/day, far less than the threshold of 6.5 mg/kg/day used to regulate pediatric and adult dosing [148, 152].The little evidence available suggests that breastfeeding mothers may continue therapy with hydroxychloroquine and chloroquine [6, 147, 150, 158]. If prescription of a 4AQ is considered during pregnancy, then hydroxychloroquine is preferred over chloroquine because it may be less toxic, because hydroxychloroquine has been used as a treatment for antiphospholipid syndrome, and because hydroxychloroquine is less concentrated in breast milk than chloroquine [38].

2.6   Mechanism of Action

2.6.1   Positive Studies on Mechanism of Action of 4-Aminoquinolines

Mechanisms of action of chloroquine and hydroxychloroquine are thought to be the same [160]. The mechanism that has received the most attention involves lysosomotropism, that is, the property that 4AQs accumulate within lysosomes and other intracellular acidic compartments due to protonation and sequestration of the drug [11, 14, 71, 122, 161]. Uncharged 4AQs readily diffuse into the lysosome, but once protonated at their two basic residues cannot diffuse back out into the cytoplasm [33].

Lysosomes have a pH between four and five maintained by an active transport of protons from the cytosol into the lysosome [38, 122, 162–164]. The cytosol and the extracellular milieu have a pH of approximately 7.4 [122]. Chloroquine is a weak base with $pK_1 = 8.1$ for the amine group at position seven and $pK_2 = 10.1$ for the amine group on the alkyl side chain [52]. Lysosomal concentrations of chloroquine as high as 2×10^{-2} M/L have been measured. [162, 164] The pH of lysosomes exposed to chloroquine increases from the baseline four to six [38, 163]. If the pH gradient is abolished, chloroquine accumulation ceases [164]. Bafilomycin A1, an inhibitor of lysosomal acidification, blocks chloroquine-induced lysosomotropism and toxicity in RPE-19 cell culture [161]. At equilibrium, the ratio of distribution of diacidic bases 4AQs between lysosomes and plasma is given by the ratio (H_L/H_P), [2] where H_L is the hydrogen ion concentration of the lysosome and H_P is the hydrogen ion concentration of the plasma. Thus the ratio of 4AQs between lysosomes and plasma is approximately 160,000. To maintain osmotic balance as chloroquine enters the lysosome, water accompanies it, swelling the organelle [162].

Although lysosomes are a small fraction of intracellular volume, the large gradient of 4AQ suggests the large volumes of distribution empirically measured in pharmacokinetic studies (see Sect. 2.2.3.2) [71]. Besides the sequestration due to diprotonation, there is also binding to acidic polysaccharides and acidic glycolipids found in lysosomal membranes [122].

The inhibition of lysosomal enzymatic function is hypothesized to be the cause of beneficial effects and retinopathy of the 4AQs [29]. Once inside lysosomes, 4AQs inhibit the lysosomal activity of cathepsin B and enzymes involved in degradation of mucopolysaccharides and proteins [33, 71, 118, 165, 166]. Elevation of lysosomal pH by 4AQs inhibits MHC class II-dependent antigen processing and presentation by monocytes [167]. The raised pH increases invariant chain (Ii) dissociation from the MHC class II molecule via decreased activity of aspartyl protease, cathepsin D, and cathepsin B, which cleave Ii from the MHC class II molecule [78]. This decreases antigen binding to the surface of the professional APCs (see Chap. 1). The 4AQs also inhibit lysosomal pinocytosis which inhibits digestion of exogenous proteins into antigenic peptides. With decreased peptide loading into the groove between α and β chains of MHC class II molecules there are fewer peptide-MHC class II complexes for transport to the cell surface and presentation to CD4 T cells (see Chap. 1) [168]. Self-antigens typically have lower affinity for MHC class II molecules than non-self-antigens, thus 4AQs have a preferential inhibitory effect on autoimmunity, and do not impair immunity to exogenous agents [38]. The net effect of 4AQs is dysfunctional protein processing, receptor recycling, protein secretion, reduced production of cytokines and immune mediators, reduced lymphocyte production, and reduced natural killer cell activity [81].

Toxic effects occur when lysosomes exposed to 4AQs accumulate ubiquitinated proteins leading to apoptosis, disruption of autophagy, and oxidative injury [161]. Swollen lysosomes combine with phagosomes containing photoreceptor outer segments to form lamellar inclusion bodies (myeloid or myelin bodies, see Chap. 1) [2, 169].

The increased lysosomal pH inhibits receptor-enzyme dissociation, which may have toxic effects [11]. The sequestered cell membranes and included protein receptors in the myelin bodies are disrupted in their normal recycling which depletes the population of surface membrane receptors without a change in receptor affinity. Disrupted interaction of retinal neuronal and RPE cells with the local environment results in toxicity and eventually morphologic damage [2].

Although lysosomotropic effects have received the most attention, 4AQs affect many other cellular processes, and it can be confusing to tie them together in a comprehensible way. One way to do so is to organize them is by their dependence on concentration. Some authors contend that mechanisms that depend on concentrations higher than 1×10^{-6} M/L in vitro are not relevant to clinical effects. They reason that such concentrations are higher than those expected to be found clinically in the plasma [71, 78, 142, 170]. For example, although hydroxychloroquine at a concentration of 1×10^{-4} M/L affects IL-17 and other cytokine levels produced by the peripheral blood mononuclear cells of patients with RA and SLE in vitro, we are uncertain that this is a physiologic pathway [171]. In another example, significant inhibition of immunoglobulin synthesis and secretion by rat plasma cells in vitro required concentration of 9×10^{-4} M/L chloroquine [172]. These levels of drug are not present in whole blood or plasma, but it is possible that these levels are relevant in intracellular compartments, which are known to have higher concentrations than in plasma [2, 80, 89, 140, 142]. Liver-to-plasma ratios of 200–500 have been recorded in rat models of chloroquine pharmacokinetics (Table 2.3) [89]. In this view, therefore, mechanisms operative at concentrations up to 10^{-4} M may be clinically relevant. Given the persistence of controversy, the coverage here will include mechanisms found at higher concentrations grouped by order of magnitude [37]. Table 2.6 provides a non-exhaustive list of the effects of the 4AQs grouped by concentration dependence.

> **Pharmacologic Tools for Dissecting the Mechanism of Action of 4-Aminoquinolines**
>
> A recurring theme in papers written on the mechanism of action of chloroquine and hydroxy-chloroquine is the use of bafilomycin and ammonium acetate. Ammonium acetate is a cation that crosses cellular membranes easily. It can be used to flatten proton gradients across cell membranes [173]. Bafilomycin is a drug that inhibits the vacuolar proton pump and can decrease the acidification of intracellular vacuoles [173]. It provides a tool for diminishing the uptake of 4AQs by lysosomes and dissecting this mechanism from several candidates.

Table 2.6 Mechanisms of action of 4-aminoquinolines

Mechanism	Concentration range at which relevant (M)
Chloroquine inhibited the interaction of memory B cells but not unprimed B cells specific for foreign antigens [37, 178]	10^{-11} to 10^{-8}
Chloroquine inhibited DNA synthesis and IL-6 secretion by human peripheral blood mononuclear cells stimulated by foreign antigens [173]	10^{-8} to 10^{-7}
1. 4AQs attached to ferriprotoporphyrin IX (FP) to form a toxic complex that increased the membrane permeability of erythrocytes parasitized by malaria protozoans and the protozoans themselves. The erythrocytes and protozoans lost potassium, swelled and were lysed [2, 11, 37, 164, 179, 180]	10^{-7} to 10^{-6}
2. 4AQs inhibited professional APCs from stimulating primed T cells [78, 118]. 4AQs decreased levels of serum IL-1β, IL-2, IL-4, IL-6, IL-17, IL-18, IL-22, IFN-γ, and TNF-α [24, 38, 44, 78, 87, 142, 167, 181]	
3. Chloroquine reduced IL-1β and IL-6 mRNA levels by reducing their stability through a pH dependent mechanism in human monocyte cell culture [182]. Transcription of DNA to RNA was not blocked [182]	
4. Inhibition of TNF-α expression occurred by blocking transcription of DNA into mRNA and not by a mechanism involving sequestration of chloroquine in lysosomes as bafilomycin did not block the effect of chloroquine [183]	
5. In a rat blood-vessel model for assessing prostaglandin inhibition, chloroquine inhibited prostaglandin effects [184]	
6. In patients taking chloroquine for SLE and RA, circulating lymphocytes contained higher numbers of myelin bodies (see Chap. 1) compared to lymphocytes from control patients not taking these drugs and non-rheumatoid control subjects. These were associated with inhibition of lysosomal enzymes cathepsin B_1 and phospholipase A_2 [71, 140, 169, 176, 185, 186]. Chloroquine also inhibited mucopolysaccharidases, alcohol dehydrogenase, and acid phosphodiesterase within lysosomes [166, 187, 188]. Elevation of pH, as would occur in lysosomes exposed to chloroquine, increased the inhibitory potency [185]	
7. Chloroquine inhibited leukotriene release in human lung tissue cell culture that was overcome by arachidonic acid, suggesting inhibition of phospholipase A2 [140]	
8. Chloroquine inhibited the C_pG-oligodeoxynucleotide (C_pG-ODN)-mediated blockade of apoptosis and inhibited IL-6 secretion in a murine B cell lymphoma model [173]	
9. Hydroxychloroquine decreased HIV viral RNA titers [136]	
10. Chloroquine inhibited polypeptide synthesis in rat liver cell free extracts by binding to the polynucleotide and preventing subsequent formation with a polynucleotide-ribosome complex [189]. There was no effect on polypeptide chain initiation or termination [190]	

(continued)

Table 2.6 (continued)

Mechanism	Concentration range at which relevant (M)
1. Chloroquine inhibited chemotaxis of polymorphonuclear leukocytes [71, 191, 192]	10^{-6} to 10^{-5}
2. Chloroquine inhibited production of immunoglobulin secreting cells in response to Staphylococcus aureus by interfering with monocyte secretion of IL-1 in human peripheral mononuclear cells [142]	
3. Chloroquine protected lysosomes against rupture by lysolecithin, progesterone, etiocholanolone, vitamin A, streptolysin S, ultraviolet irradiation, and incubation at neutral pH [193]. 4AQs stabilized lysosomal membranes inhibiting the release of lysosomal enzymes and receptor recycling [168]	
4. Chloroquine inhibited cytokine secretion by mononuclear cells and binding of inositol 1,4,5-triphosphate to its intracellular receptor [173]	
5. 4AQs inhibited activation of toll-like receptors TLR-3, TLR-7, and TLR-9 by raising intralysosomal pH [14, 24, 38, 165, 167, 194–196]	
6. Chloroquine suppressed secretion of catecholamines in bovine adrenal medullary cells by interfering with calcium uptake [197]	
7. Chloroquine caused a decrease in lysosomal β-glucuronidase and arylsulfatase A activity in cultured human fibroblasts [198]	
8. Hydroxychloroquine reduced binding of β2-glycoprotein by antiphospholipid antibodies on phospholipid bilayers [16]	
9. 4AQs increased the activity of HMG-CoA reductase and decreased serum cholesterol and atherosclerosis in SLE [60, 129, 199, 200]	
10. 4AQs reduced serum glucose and incidence of diabetes mellitus in SLE [16, 129, 201, 202]	
11. 4AQs had an antithrombotic effect in SLE [16, 129, 203]. 4 AQs prevented platelet alpha-granule release in vitro [170]. They inhibited release of arachidonic acid from stimulated platelets [14, 24]	
1. Chloroquine inhibited human lymphocyte proliferation stimulated by phytohemagglutinin or conconavalin A [71, 142]. The effect occurred when drug was added early in the culture, but not later, indicating an action involving lysosomes and not via DNA binding [204]	10^{-5} to 10^{-4}
2. Chloroquine inhibited digestion of endocytosed proteins in mouse peritoneal macrophages [205]	
3. Chloroquine inhibited proteolytic conversion of a proform of complement C3 in cultured rat hepatocytes [206]	
4. Chloroquine inhibited phosphorylation of extracellular signal-regulated kinases (ERK) 1 and 2 and mitogen-activated protein kinases [38]	
5. Chloroquine inhibited mitochondrial respiration [12]	
6. Chloroquine inhibited DNA polymerase [71]	
7. Chloroquine competitively inhibited cholinesterase in plasma and human red blood cells [207]	
8. 4AQs inhibited expression on the cell surface of TNF receptors without affecting levels of TNF receptor mRNA in a human histiocytic lymphoma cell line culture and in human peripheral monocytes suggesting inhibition of transport of the receptors from the cytosol to the cell surface [208]	
9. Chloroquine inhibited endotoxin-stimulated TNF-α, IL-1β, and IL-6 from human whole blood and monocytes by an effect on DNA transcription and not a lysosomotropic mechanism [181, 183]	
10. Hydroxychloroquine induced apoptosis in human lymphocytes from normal subjects and synoviocytes taken from RA patients [209, 210]. Chloroquine inhibited extracellular signal-regulated kinase (ERK) in HeLa cells which promoted susceptibility to Fas-mediated apoptosis [211]	
11. Chloroquine blocked DNA repair [212]	

(continued)

Table 2.6 (continued)

Mechanism	Concentration range at which relevant (M)
1. Chloroquine inhibited [124]I-mannose-bovine serum albumin ingestion by inhibiting receptor recycling in rat alveolar macrophages [213]	10^{-4} to 10^{-3}
2. Chloroquine stabilized erythrocyte membranes [34]	
3. Chloroquine inhibited cathepsin B and diamine oxidase enzyme activities and inhibited protein synthesis [11, 14]	
4. Chloroquine attached to double-stranded DNA [173, 214]. Chloroquine attached to single stranded DNA less avidly [173]	
5. Neutrophil phagocytosis was inhibited [192]	
6. Neutrophil oxidative metabolism was inhibited [192]	
7. Proteolytic processing of secretory proteins by hepatocytes was inhibited [206]	
8. Chloroquine inhibited DNA and RNA biosynthesis and was associated with degradation of ribosomes and ribosomal RNA in a bacterial model [215, 216]	
9. Chloroquine raised the pH in the food vacuole of malaria parasites inhibiting the digestion of hemoglobin [71]. Resistant strains of malaria accumulated less chloroquine than those of nonresistant parasites [34]	
10. 4AQs inhibited protein synthesis but not uptake of amino acids in beef RPE cell culture [63].	
1. Chloroquine decreased serum phospholipids concomitant with the appearance of multilamellar myeloid bodies in the RPE, photoreceptors, and ganglion cells in a rat model [60]	Concentrations not reported
2. 4AQs inhibited antigen presentation, chemotaxis, phagocytosis, calcium receptor signaling of T and B cells, and matrix metalloproteinase activity [14]. Chloroquine prevented T cell responses to antigenic proteins but not antigenic peptides implying a mechanism of inhibiting the cleavage of antigenic proteins by macrophages [118]	
3. Hydroxychloroquine increased Fas-mediated apoptosis of synoviocytes [168]	
4. 4AQs inhibited gene expression in T cells in response to immune stimuli [30]	
5. Chloroquine inhibited autophagy in human RPE cells [161]. Inhibition of vacuolar H^+-ATPase by bafilomycin A1 blocked this effect implying that chloroquine acted as a lysosomotropic agent. [161] In a rat pancreas model chloroquine increased the volume of autophagic vacuoles and increased proteolytic lysosomal enzyme activities [217]	
6. Hydroxychloroquine inhibited collagen-induced platelet aggregation and alpha-granule release [16, 170]	
7. Chloroquine inhibited protein synthesis [189]	
8. Chloroquine disrupted the blood-retina barrier as determined by fluorophotometry in patients with retinopathy [218]	
9. Chloroquine inhibited oxidative enzymes found in the ellipsoids of the inner segments of photoreceptors [219]	
10. 4AQs-induced apoptosis of umbilical vascular endothelial cells, peripheral blood lymphocytes, and rheumatoid synoviocytes [87]	
11. Chloroquine decreased retinal glucose-6-phosphate dehydrogenase activity leading to decreased retinal glutathione concentration which increases retinal lipid peroxidation [29]	
12. Chloroquine inhibited low-density lipoprotein uptake or binding to cell surface receptors in human fibroblasts. Degradation of low-density lipoproteins by lysosomes was inhibited [220]. Cholesterol ester formation was stimulated and 3-hydroxy-3-methylglutaryl-coenzyme A activity was inhibited. As a result LDL accumulated within the cell [220]	
13. Chloroquine depleted acid hydrolase receptors on the cell surface and inhibited pinocytosis of acid hydrolases [168]. Secretion of newly synthesized acid hydrolases bearing phosphomannosyl recognition markers was increased [168]	
14. Chloroquine increased nitric oxide synthase activity in endothelial cells [221]	

(continued)

Table 2.6 (continued)

Mechanism	Concentration range at which relevant (M)
15. Chloroquine reduced incorporation of labeled sulfate into cartilage polysaccharide sulfates in a rat model [90]	
16. Chloroquine intercalated between base pairs of DNA as evidenced by the increase in viscosity of DNA exposed to chloroquine [14, 214, 222]	
17. Chloroquine inhibited the mitogenesis in polymorphonuclear leukocytes stimulated by zymosan [192]	
18. Chloroquine inhibited spontaneous and interferon-upregulated natural killer activity in patients with RA [221]	
19. 4AQs interfered with the binding of antiphospholipid antibodies to annexin A5, a potent anticoagulant [24, 81]	
20. 4AQs reduced lipid and triglyceride levels, increased low-density lipoprotein receptor activity, and increased HMG-CoA reductase activity, reducing cardiovascular disease risk [24, 81]. 4AQs decreased the incidence of diabetes and had a hypoglycemic effect, decreased glycosylated hemoglobin levels in patients with diabetes, and improved glucose tolerance in patients with type II diabetes [14, 81, 126]	
21. 4AQs inhibited TLR9-mediated stimulation of perilipin-3 in macrophages [24]	
22. Chloroquine had an antineoplastic effect producing a reduction in the incidence of Burkitt's lymphoma among patients in Tanzania who took the drug for malaria. Chloroquine-induced apoptosis in malignant B cells in patients with chronic lymphocytic leukemia [14]. Hydroxychloroquine had an anti-breast cancer effect. Chloroquine had an anti-colon cancer effect in a mouse model, induced cell death in human A 549 lung cancer cells, and produced better survival in patients with glioblastoma multiforme [14]	
23. 4AQs promoted oxidation of cysteine residues in the peripherin/rds protein leading to disorganization of photoreceptor outer segments and cell death [29]	
24. Chloroquine had a direct depressant effect on smooth muscle of the gut, arteries, trachea, and ciliary body, which might explain the mild ileus and temporary presbyopia that patients often experience after starting the drug [100]	
25. 4AQs inhibit replication of HIV, SARS coronavirus, and influenza [10, 38, 136]	
26. Chloroquine blocked production of IL-1β, IL-6, and TNF-α caused by ultraviolet irradiation of skin of normal subjects but had no effect on expression of these cytokines in unirradiated skin [223]	
27. Chloroquine stimulated nitric oxide production in the kidney and brain with increased vasopressin and natriuresis [224]	
28. Chloroquine enhanced CD8+ T cell responses by APCs against soluble antigens [225]	

4AQ 4-aminoquinoline, *4AQR* 4-aminoquinoline retinopathy, *IL* interleukin, *IFN* interferon, *TNF* tumor necrosis factor, *DNA* deoxyribonucleic acid, *RNA* ribonucleic acid, *SLE* systemic lupus erythematosus, *RA* rheumatoid arthritis, *RPE* retinal pigment epithelium, *HIV* human immunodeficiency virus, *TLR* toll-like receptor, *HMG-CoA* 3-hydroxy-3-methylglutaryl-coenzyme A reductase, *mRNA* mitochondrial ribonucleic acid, *LDL* low-density lipoprotein, *SARS* severe acute respiratory syndrome, *APC* antigen presenting cell

2.6.2 Negative Studies on Mechanism of Action of 4-Aminoquinolines

A number of studies have excluded mechanisms by which 4AQs produce effects. Hydroxychloroquine does not inhibit cyclo-oxygenases or decrease prostaglandin production [94]. Binding of 4AQs to DNA is not thought to be a clinically important mechanism; mefloquine does not bind to DNA, yet is an effective antimalarial drug [164]. The beneficial effects of 4AQs on polymorphous light eruptions are not due to a light-screening effect as they did not act as a physical barrier to the passage of ultraviolet radiation [86]. Chloroquine did not affect mitochondrial respiration and oxidative phosphorylation in mouse-liver homogenates or rat-liver mitochondria [90]. Neither did it affect adenosine triphosphate activity of cow visual pigment extracts [174]. Chloroquine did not affect the internalization of oligonucleotides via acidified vesicles [173].

2.6.3 Drug Interactions

Proton pump inhibitors such as omeprazole may inhibit the accumulation of 4AQs in lysosomes by decreasing the pH of these organelles. A potentially antagonizing effect of such drugs on the immunomodulating effects of 4AQs has been hypothesized [175]. Drugs that inhibit CYP3A4 such as ketoconazole and cimetidine can increase plasma levels of 4AQs [93, 95].

2.7 Summary of Key Points

- The pharmacology of chloroquine and hydroxychloroquine is similar.
- The molecular weights of chloroquine and hydroxychloroquine are 320 and 336, respectively.
- Chloroquine and hydroxychloroquine are alkylated 4AQs that are water soluble, weak, amphiphilic bases that readily cross cell membranes.
- Melanin can bind 3 % of its weight in 4AQs, but whether this protects against, exacerbates, or has no effect on the risk of retinopathy is unknown.
- The 4AQs are lysosomotropic by virtue of protonation and trapping inside acidic lysosomes.
- Absorption of 4AQs is nearly complete with a peak plasma concentration at 3–12 h after an oral dose, a volume of distribution greater than 40,000 L, and a terminal elimination half-life of approximately 40 days.
- Equilibrium plasma concentrations depend on daily dose and IBW.

- With chronic ingestion of 4AQs in non-albinotic mammals, the tissue concentration of drug is highest in the uvea and RPE with a concentration 10,000 times that of plasma. In albinotic mammals, uveal drug concentrations approximate that of the heart. The 4AQs are lipophobic with concentrations in fat that are one-tenth that of plasma.
- The major metabolites of 4AQs are the desethyl and bisdesethyl derivatives of the parent drugs. The metabolites are pharmacologically active. CYP2C3 and CYP3A4 are responsible for 80 % of the metabolism of 4AQs.
- Forty to 60 % of 4AQs is excreted by the kidneys, 8–25 % is excreted in the feces, 5 % is sloughed off with the skin, and 25–45 % is stored in lean tissues.
- Renal and hepatic insufficiency leads to higher plasma concentrations for a given daily dose and raise the risk of toxicity.
- The clinical effects of 4AQs take 3–6 months to develop when no loading doses are used. The time course follows the pharmacokinetics to steady-state concentrations.
- Four hundred milligram per day of hydroxychloroquine and 250 mg/day of chloroquine are acceptable if the lesser of a patient's IBW and ABW is 135 lb or more.
- Hydroxychloroquine and chloroquine are equipotent but chloroquine is more toxic; thus the therapeutic ratio is higher for hydroxychloroquine.
- Whole blood concentrations of 4AQs are approximately five times the plasma concentrations, are more precise, and are favored for pharmacokinetic measurements.
- A clinically therapeutic concentration of a 4AQ is greater than 3×10^{-6} M/L.
- 4AQs should not be stopped during pregnancy and lactation.
- There are more than 20 actions of 4AQs. The lysosomotropic mechanisms are the most important clinically. Because of these effects, the 4AQs have a dichotomous effect on T cells. They inhibit CD4 T cell stimulation but promote CD8 T cell stimulation. The combined effect is a beneficial action in autoimmunity without a penalty of increased opportunistic infections.

References

1. Bunch TW, O'Duffy JD. Disease modifying drugs for progressive rheumatoid arthritis. Mayo Clin Proc. 1980;55:161–79.
2. Mackenzie AH. Pharmacologic actions of 4-aminoquinoline compounds. Am J Med. 1983;75:1–7.
3. Berliner RW, Earle Jr DP, Taggart JV, Zubrod CG, Welch WJ, Conan NJ, Bauman E, Scudder ST, Shannon JA. Studies on the chemotherapy of the human malarias. VI. The physiological disposition, antimalarial activity, and toxicity of several derivatives of 4-aminoquinoline. J Clin Invest. 1948;27:98–107.
4. Bothwell B, Furst DE. Hydroxychloroquine. In: Day RO, Furst DE, editors. Antirheumatic therapy: actions and outcomes. Basel: Piet L.C.M. van Riel and Barry Bresnihan; 2005. p. 81–92.
5. Wallace DJ. Antimalarials-the 'real' advance in lupus. Lupus. 2001;10:385–7.
6. Rynes RI, Parke AL. Introduction to symposium on antimalarial therapy and lupus. Lupus. 1993;2:S1.
7. Wallace DJ. The history of antimalarials. Lupus. 1996;5:S2–3.
8. Rynes RI. Antimalarial drugs in the treatment of rheumatological diseases. Br J Rheumatol. 1997;36:799–805.
9. Hobbs HE, Calnan CD. Visual disturbances with antimalarial drugs, with particular reference to chloroquine keratopathy. Arch Dermatol. 1959;80:557–63.
10. Dubois EL. Antimalarials in the management of discoid and systemic lupus erythematosus. Semin Arthritis Rheum. 1978;8:33–51.
11. McChesney EQ, Fitch CD. 4-Aminoquinolines. In: Peters W, Richards WHG, editors. Antimalarial drugs II. Current antimalarials and new drug developments. Berlin: Springer; 1984. p. 3–60.
12. Thompson PE, Webel LM. Antimalarial agents: chemistry and pharmacology. New York: Academic Press; 1972. p. 150–96.
13. Tzekov R. Ocular toxicity due to chloroquine and hydroxychloroquine: electrophysiological and visual function correlates. Doc Ophthalmol. 2005;110:111–20.
14. Ben-Zvi I, Kivity S, Langevitz P. Hydroxychloroquine: from malaria to autoimmunity. Clin Rev Allergy Immunol. 2012;42:145–53.
15. Lozier JR, Friedlander MH. Complications of antimalarial therapy. Int Ophthalmol Clin. 1989;29:172–8.
16. Rand JH, Wu XX, Quinn AS, Chen PP, Hathcock JJ, Taatjes DJ. Hydroxychloroquine directly reduces the binding of antiphospholipid antibody-beta2-glycoprotein I complexes to phospholipid bilayers. Blood. 2008;112:1687–95.
17. Pillsbury DM, Jacobson C. Treatment of chronic discoid lupus erythematosus with chloroquine (Aralen). JAMA. 1954;154:1330–3.
18. The Canadian Hydroxychloroquine Study Group. A randomized study of the effect of withdrawing hydroxychloroquine sulfate in systemic lupus erythematosus. New Engl J Med. 1991;324:150–4.
19. Banks CN. Melanin: blackguard or red herring? Another look at chloroquine retinopathy. Aust N Z Ophthalmol. 1987;15:365–70.
20. Goldman L, Preston RH. Reactions to chloroquine observed during the treatment of various dermatologic disorders. Am J Trop Med Hyg. 1957;6:654–7.
21. Hobbs HE, Sorsby A, Freedman A. Retinopathy following chloroquine therapy. Lancet. 1959;2:478–80.
22. Bernstein H. Ocular safety of hydroxychloroquine sulfate (Plaquenil). South Med J. 1992;85:274–9.
23. Shearer RV, Dubois EL. Ocular changes induced by long-term hydroxychloroquine (Plaquenil) therapy. Am J Ophthalmol. 1967;64:245–52.
24. Wallace DJ, Gudsoorkar VS, Weisman MH, Venuturupalli SR. New insights into mechanisms of therapeutic effects of antimalarial agents in SLE. Nat Rev Rheumatol. 2012;8:522–33.
25. Browning DJ. Bull's-eye maculopathy associated with quinacrine therapy for malaria. Am J Ophthalmol. 2004;137:577–9.
26. Chloroquine. DrugBank: open data drug & drug target database. 2005. http://www.drugbank.ca/drugs/DB00608. Accessed 22 Aug 2013.
27. Hydroxychloroquine. DrugBank: open data drug & drug target database. 2007. http://www.drugbank.ca/drugs/DB01611. Accessed 22 Aug 2013.
28. Potts AM. The reaction of uveal pigment in vitro with polycyclic compounds. Invest Ophthalmol. 1964;3:405–16.
29. Toler SM. Oxidative stress plays an important role in the pathogenesis of drug-induced retinopathy. Exp Biol Med. 2004;229:607–15.
30. Sundelin SP, Terman A. Different effects of chloroquine and hydroxychloroquine on lysosomal function in cultured retinal pigment epithelial cells. APMIS. 2002;110:481–9.
31. Ferrari V, Cutler DJ. Kinetics and thermodynamics of chloroquine and hydroxychloroquine transport across the human erythrocyte membrane. Biochem Pharmacol. 1991;41:23–30.
32. Tanenbaum L, Tuffanelli DL. Antimalarial agents: chloroquine, hydroxychloroquine, and quinacrine. Arch Dermatol. 1980;116:587–91.
33. Wibo M, Poole B. Protein degradation in cultured cells. II. The uptake of chloroquine by rat fibroblasts and the inhibition of cellular protein degradation and cathepsin B1. J Cell Biol. 1974;63:430–40.
34. Homewood CA, Warhurst DC, Peters W, Baggaley VC. Lysosomes, pH, and anti-malarial action of chloroquine. Nature. 1972;235:50–2.
35. Stepien KB, Wilczok T. Studies of the mechanism of chloroquine binding to synthetic dopa-melanin. Biochem Pharmacol. 1982;31:3359–65.

36. Jailer JW, Zubrod CG, Rosenfeld M, Shannon JA. Effect of acidosis and anoxia on the concentration of quinacrine and chloroquine in blood. J Pharmacol Exp Ther. 1948;92:345–51.

37. Titus EO. Recent developments in the understanding of the pharmacokinetics and mechanism of action of chloroquine. Ther Drug Monit. 1989;11:369–79.

38. Kalia S, Dutz JP. New concepts in antimalarial use and mode of action in dermatology. Dermatol Ther. 2007;20:160–74.

39. Kishimoto M, Deshpande GA, Yokogawa N, Buyon JP, Okada M. Use of hydroxychloroquine in Japan. J Rheumatol. 2012;39:1296–7.

40. Araiza-Casillas R, Cardenas F, Morales Y, Cardiel MH. Factors associated with chloroquine-induced retinopathy in rheumatic diseases. Lupus. 2004;13: 119–24.

41. Easterbrook M. The ocular safety of hydroxychloroquine. Semin Arthritis Rheum. 1993;23:62–7.

42. Meinao IM, Sato EI, Andrade LEC, Ferraz MB, Atra E. Controlled trial with chloroquine diphosphate in systemic lupus erythematosus. Lupus. 1996;5: 237–41.

43. Akman F, Cerman E, Yenice O, Kazokoglu H. Two cases with chloroquine and hydroxychloroquine maculopathy. Marmara Med J. 2011;24:68–72.

44. Wozniacka A, Lesiak A, Narbutt J, McCauliffe DP, Sysa-Jedrzejowska A. Chloroquine treatment influences proinflammatory cytokine levels in systemic lupus erythematosus patients. Lupus. 2006;15: 268–75.

45. Bartel PR, Roux P, Robinson E, Anderson IF, Brighton SW, Van der Hoven HJ, Becker PJ. Visual function and long-term chloroquine treatment. S Afr Med J. 1994;84:32–4.

46. Missner S, Kellner U. Comparison of different screening methods for chloroquine/hydroxychloroquine retinopathy: multifocal electroretinography, color vision, perimetry, ophthalmoscopy, and fluorescein angiography. Graefes Arch Clin Exp Ophthalmol. 2012;250:319–25.

47. Easterbrook M. Ocular effects and safety of antimalarial agents. Am J Med. 1988;85:23–9.

48. Parker FS, Irvin JL. The interaction of chloroquine with nucleic acids and nucleoproteins. J Biol Chem. 1952;199:897–909.

49. Tanaka M, Ono C, Yamada M. Absorption, distribution and excretion of 14C-levofloxacin after single oral administration in albino and pigmented rats: binding characteristics of levofloxacin-related radioactivity to melanin in vivo. J Pharm Pharmacol. 2004;56:463–9.

50. Tjalve H, Nilsson M, Larsson B. Studies on the binding of chlorpromazine and chloroquine to melanin in vivo. Biochem Pharmacol. 1981;30:1845–7.

51. Larsson BS. Interaction between chemicals and melanin. Pigment Cell Res. 1993;6:127–44.

52. Larsson B, Tjalve H. Studies on the mechanism of drug-binding to melanin. Biochem Pharmacol. 1979;28:1181–7.

53. Ono C, Yamada M, Tanaka M. Absorption, distribution and excretion of 14C-chloroquine after single oral administration in albino and pigmented rats: binding characteristics of chloroquine-related radioactivity to melanin in-vivo. J Pharm Pharmacol. 2003;55:1647–54.

54. Tanaka M, Takashina H, Tsutsumi S. Comparative assessment of ocular tissue distribution of drug-related radioactivity after chronic oral administration of C14-levofloxacin and C14-chloroquine in pigmented rats. J Pharm Pharmacol. 2004;56: 977–83.

55. Salazar-Bookaman MM, Wainer I, Patil PN. Relevance of drug-melanin interactions to ocular pharmacology and toxicology. J Ocul Pharmacol. 1994;10:217–39.

56. Leblanc B, Jezequei S, Davies T, Hanton G, Taradach C. Binding of drugs to eye melanin is not predictive of ocular toxicity. Regul Toxicol Pharmacol. 1998;28:124–32.

57. Feeney L. Lipofuscin and melanin of human retinal pigment epithelium. Fluorescence, enzyme cytochemical, and ultrastructural studies. Invest Ophthalmol Vis Sci. 1978;17:583–600.

58. Boulton M. Ageing of the retinal pigment epithelium. Prog Retin Eye Res. 1991;11:125–51.

59. Ivanina TA, Zueva MV, Lebedeva MN, Bogoslovsky AI, Bunin AJ. Ultrastructural alterations in rat and cat retina and pigment epithelium induced by chloroquine. Graefes Arch Clin Exp Ophthalmol. 1983;220:32–8.

60. Gaafar KM, Abdel-Khalek LR, El-Sayed NK, Ramadan GA. Lipidemic effect as a manifestation of chloroquine retinotoxicity. Arzneimittelforschung. 1995;45:1231–5.

61. Wolfe F, Marmor MF. Rates and predictors of hydroxychloroquine retinal toxicity in patients with rheumatoid arthritis and systemic lupus erythematosus. Arthritis Care Res. 2010;62:775–84.

62. Marmor MF. Comparison of screening procedures in hydroxychloroquine toxicity. Arch Ophthalmol. 2012;130:461–9.

63. Gonasun LM, Potts AM. In vitro inhibition of protein synthesis in the retinal pigment epithelium by chloroquine. Invest Ophthalmol Vis Sci. 1974;13: 107–15.

64. Mason CG. Ocular accumulation and toxicity of certain systemically administered drugs. J Toxicol Environ Health. 1977;2:977–95.

65. Kasuya Y, Miyata H, Watanabe M. Toxicological studies on the chloroquine-melanin affinity in vivo and in vitro in relation to chloroquine retinopathy. J Toxicol Stud. 1976;1:32–8.

66. Feeney-Burns L, Hilderbrand ES, Eldridge S. Aging human RPE: morphometric analysis of macular, equatorial, and peripheral cells. Invest Ophthalmol Vis Sci. 1984;25:195–200.

67. Iredale J, Fieger H, Wainer IW. Determination of the stereoisomers of hydroxychloroquine and its major metabolites in plasma and urine following a single

oral administration of racemic hydroxychloroquine. Semin Arthritis Rheum. 1993;23:74–81.

68. Ducharme J, Farinotti R. Clinical pharmacokinetics and metabolism of chloroquine. Focus on recent advancements. Clin Pharmacokinet. 1996;31:257–74.

69. Rollo IM. Drugs used in the chemotherapy of malaria. In: Goodman LS, Gilman A, editors. The pharmacological basis of therapeutics. New York: Macmillan; 1975. p. 1045–68.

70. Gustafsson LL, Walker O, Alvan G, Beermann B, Estevez F, Gleisner L, Lindstrom B, Sjoqvist F. Disposition of chloroquine in man after single intravenous and oral doses. Br J Clin Pharmacol. 1983;15:471–9.

71. Tett S, Cutler D, Day R. Antimalarials in rheumatic diseases. Baillieres Clin Rheumatol. 1990;4:467–89.

72. Laaksonen AL, Koskiahde V, Juva K. Dosage of antimalarial drugs for children with juvenile rheumatoid arthritis and systemic lupus erythematosus. A clinical study with determination of serum concentrations of chloroquine and hydroxychloroquine. Scand J Rheumatol. 1974;3:103–8.

73. Albert DA, Debois LKL, Lu KF. Antimalarial ocular toxicity, a critical appraisal. J Clin Rheumatol. 1998;4:57–62.

74. McChesney EW. Animal toxicity and pharmacokinetics of hydroxychloroquine sulfate. Am J Med. 1983;75:11–8.

75. Tett SE, Cutler DJ, Day RO, Brown KF. A dose-ranging study of the pharmacokinetics of hydroxychloroquine following intravenous administration to healthy volunteers. Br J Clin Pharmacol. 1988;26:303–13.

76. Tett SE, Cutler DJ. Apparent dose-dependence of chloroquine pharmacokinetics due to limited assay sensitivity and short sampling times. Eur J Clin Pharmacol. 1987;31:729–31.

77. Munster T, Gibbs JP, Shen D, Baethge BA, Botstein GR, Caldwell J, Dietz F, Ettlinger R, Golden HE, Lindsley H, et al. Hydroxychloroquine concentration-response relationships in patients with rheumatoid arthritis. Arthritis Rheum. 2002;46:1460–9.

78. Schultz KR, Gilman AL. The lysosomotropic amines, chloroquine and hydroxychloroquine: a potentially novel therapy for graft-versus-host disease. Leuk Lymphoma. 1997;24:201–10.

79. Buchanan N, Can der Walt LA. The binding of chloroquine to normal and kwashiorkor serum. Am J Trop Med Hyg. 1977;26:1025–7.

80. Mackenzie AH. Dose refinements in long-term therapy of rheumatoid arthritis with antimalarials. Am J Med. 1983;75:40–5.

81. Katz SJ, Russell AS. Re-evaluation of antimalarials in treating rheumatic diseases: re-appreciation and insights into new mechanisms of action. Curr Eye Res. 2011;23:278–81.

82. Lawwill T, Appleton B, Altstatt L. Chloroquine accumulation in human eyes. Am J Ophthalmol. 1968;65:530–2.

83. Goldstein A, Aronow L, Kalman SM. Principles of drug action: the basis of pharmacology. New York: Wiley; 2013.

84. Rowland M, Tozer TN. Clinical pharmacokinetics and pharmacodynamics. Concepts and applications. Philadelphia: Wolters Kluwer; 2011. p. 579.

85. Rubin M, Bernstein H, Zvaifler NJ. Studies on the pharmacology of chloroquine. Recommendations for the treatment of chloroquine retinopathy. Arch Ophthalmol. 1963;70:474–81.

86. Shaffer B, Cahn MM, Levy EJ. Absorption of antimalarial drugs in human skin: spectroscopic and chemical analysis in epidermis and corium. J Invest Dermatol. 1958;30:341–5.

87. Ramser B, Kokot A, Metze D, Weib N, Luger TA, Bohm M. Hydroxychloroquine modulates metabolic activity and proliferation and induces autophagic cell death of human dermal fibroblasts. J Invest Dermatol. 2009;129:2419–26.

88. Smith B, O'Grady F. Experimental chloroquine myopathy. J Neurol Neurosurg Psychiatry. 1966;29:255–8.

89. Projean D, Baune B, Farinotti R, Flinois JP, Beaune P, Taburet AM, Ducharme J. In vitro metabolism of chloroquine: Identification of CYP2cb, CYP3A4, and CYP2D6 as the main isoforms catalyzing *N*-desethylchloroquine formation. Am Soc Pharmacol Exp Ther. 2003;31:748–54.

90. Whitehouse MW, Bostrom H. Biochemical properties of anti-inflammatory drugs-VI. The effects of chloroquine (Resochin) and some of their potential metabolites on cartilage metabolism and oxidative phosphorylation. Biochem Pharmacol. 1965;14:1173–84.

91. Kuroda K. Detection and distribution of chloroquine metabolites in human tissues. J Pharmacol Exp Ther. 1962;137:156–61.

92. Estes ML, Ewing-Wilson D, Chou SM, Mitsumoto H, Hanson M, Shirey E, Ratliff NM. Chloroquine neuromyotoxicity. Clinical and pathological perspective. Am J Med. 1987;82:447–55.

93. Kim KA, Park JY, Lee SJ, Lim S. Cytochrome P450 2C8 and CYP3A4/5 are involved in chloroquine metabolism in human liver microsomes. Arch Pharm Res. 2003;26:631–7.

94. Ben-Chetrit E, Tischel R, Hinz B, Levy M. The effects of colchicine and hydroxychloroquine on the cyclo-oxygenases COX-1 and COX-2. Rheumatol Int. 2005;25:332–5.

95. Ette E, Brown-Awala EA, Essien EE. Chloroquine elimination in humans: effect of low-dose cimetidine. J Clin Pharmacol. 1987;27:813–6.

96. Bernstein HN. Ocular safety of hydroxychloroquine. Ann Ophthalmol. 1991;23:292–6.

97. Runge LA. Risk/benefit analysis of hydroxychloroquine sulfate treatment in rheumatoid arthritis. Am J Med. 1983;75:52–6.

98. Terrell III WL, Haik KG, Haik Jr GM. Hydroxychloroquine sulfate and retinopathy. South Med J. 1988;81:1327–8.

99. Dwosh IL, Stein HB, Urowitz MB, Smythe HA, Hunter T, Ogryzlo MA. Azathioprine in early rheumatoid arthritis. Comparison with gold and chloroquine. Arthritis Rheum. 1977;20:685–92.

100. Mackenzie AH. An appraisal of chloroquine. Arthritis Rheum. 1970;13:280–91.

101. Tobin DR, Krohel G, Rynes RI. Hydroxychloroquine-seven-year experience. Arch Ophthalmol. 1982;100:81–3.

102. Henkind P, Rothfield NF. Ocular abnormalities in patients treated with synthetic antimalarial drugs. New Engl J Med. 1963;269:434–9.

103. Molad Y, Gorshtein A, Wysenbeek AJ, Guedj D, Weinberger A, Amit-Vazina M. Protective effect of hydroxychloroquine in systemic lupus erythematosus. Prospective long-term study of an Israeli cohort. Lupus. 2002;11:356–61.

104. Akhavan PS, Su J, Lou W, Gladman DD, Urowitz MB, Fortin PR. The early protective effect of hydroxychloroquine on the risk of cumulative damage in patients with systemic lupus erythematosus. J Rheumatol. 2013;40:831–41.

105. Scull E. Chloroquine and hydroxychloroquine therapy in rheumatoid arthritis. Arthritis Rheum. 1962; 5:30–6.

106. Bagnall AW. The value of chloroquine in rheumatoid disease. A four year study of continuous therapy. Can Med Assoc J. 1957;77:182–94.

107. Adams EM, Yocum DE, Bell CL. Hydroxychloroquine in the treatment of rheumatoid arthritis. Am J Med. 1983;75:321–6.

108. Haydu GG. Rheumatoid arthritis therapy: a rationale and the use of chloroquine diphosphate. Am J Med Sci. 1953;225:71–5.

109. The Canadian Hydroxychloroquine Study Group, Tsakonas E, Joseph L, Esdaile JM, Choquette D, et al. A long-term study of hydroxychloroquine withdrawal on exacerbations in systemic lupus erythematosus. Lupus. 1998;7:80–5.

110. Clark P, Cases E, Tugwell R, Medina C, Gheno C, Tenorio G, Orozco JA. Hydroxychloroquine compared with placebo in rheumatoid arthritis. Ann Intern Med. 1993;119:1067–71.

111. Maksymowych W, Russell AS. Antimalarials in rheumatology: efficacy and safety. Semin Arthritis Rheum. 1987;16:206–21.

112. Freedman A. Chloroquine and rheumatoid arthritis. A short-term controlled trial. Ann Rheum Dis. 1956;15:251–7.

113. Rynes RI. Ophthalmologic safety of long-term hydroxychloroquine sulfate treatment. Am J Med. 1983;75:35–9.

114. Browning DJ. Hydroxychloroquine and chloroquine retinopathy: screening for drug toxicity. Am J Ophthalmol. 2002;133:649–56.

115. Wang C, Fortin PR, Li Y, Panaritis T, Gans M, Esdaile JM. Discontinuation of antimalarial drugs in systemic lupus erythematosus. J Rheumatol. 1999; 26:808–15.

116. Paulus HE. An overview of benefit/risk of disease modifying treatment of rheumatoid arthritis as of today. Ann Rheum Dis. 1982;41:26–9.

117. Alarcon GS, McGwin G, Bertoli AM, Fessler BJ, Calvo-Alen J, Bastian HM, Vila LM, Reveille JD. Effect of hydroxychloroquine on the survival of patients with systemic lupus erythematosus: data from LUMINA, multiethnic US cohort (LUMINA L). Ann Rheum Dis. 2007;66:1168–72.

118. Fox R. Anti-malarial drugs: possible mechanisms of action in autoimmune disease and prospects for drug development. Lupus. 1996;5:S4–10.

119. Abarientos C, Sperber K, Shapiro DL, Aronow WS, Chao CP, Ash JY. Hydroxychloroquine in systemic lupus erythematosus and rheumatoid arthritis and its safety in pregnancy. Expert Opin Drug Saf. 2011;10:705–14.

120. American College of Rheumatology Ad Hoc Committee on Clinical Guidelines. Guidelines for the management of rheumatoid arthritis. Arthritis Rheum. 1996;39:713–22.

121. Furst DE, Lindsley H, Baethge B, Botstein GR, Caldwell J, Dietz F, Ettlinger R, Golden HE, McLaughlin GE, Moreland LW, et al. Dose-loading with hydroxychloroquine improves the rate of response in early, active rheumatoid arthritis. Arthritis Rheum. 1999;42:357–65.

122. Kaufmann AM, Krise JP. Lysosomal sequestration of amine-containing drugs: analysis and therapeutic implications. J Pharm Sci. 2007;96:729–46.

123. Elman A, Gullberg R, Nillson E, Rendahl I, Wachtmeister L. Choroquine retinopathy in patients with rheumatoid arthritis. Scand J Rheumatol. 1976;5:161–6.

124. Percival SPB, Behrman J. Ophthalmological safety of chloroquine. Br J Ophthalmol. 1969;53:101–9.

125. Grierson DJ. Hydroxychloroquine and visual screening in a rheumatology outpatient clinic. Ann Rheum Dis. 1997;56:188–90.

126. Browning DJ. Impact of the revised American Academy of Ophthalmology guidelines regarding hydroxychloroquine screening on actual practice. Am J Ophthalmol. 2013;155:418–28.

127. Browning DJ. Reply to impact of the revised American Academy of Ophthalmology guidelines regarding hydroxychloroquine screening on actual practice. Am J Ophthalmol. 2013;156:410–1.

128. Morand EF, McCloud PI, Littlejohn GO. Continuation of long term treatment with hydroxychloroquine in systemic lupus erythematosus and rheumatoid arthritis. Ann Rheum Dis. 1992;51:1318–21.

129. Petri M. Hydroxychloroquine use in the Baltimore Lupus Cohort: effects on lipids, glucose and thrombosis. Lupus. 1996;5:S16–22.

130. Bruce-Chwatt LJ. Chloroquine blindness? Lancet. 1968;2:1039.

131. Reed H, Campbell AA. Central scotomata following chloroquine therapy. Can Med Assoc J. 1962;86: 176–8.

132. Easterbrook M. Clinical characteristics of hydroxychloroquine retinopathy. Evid Based ophthalmol. 2011;12:132–3.

133. Mavrikakis I, Sfikakis PP, Mavrikakis E, Rougas K, Nikolaou A, Kostopoulos C, Mavrikakis M. The incidence of irreversible retinal toxicity in patients treated with hydroxychloroquine—a reappraisal. Ophthalmology. 2003;110:1321–6.

134. Arden GB, Kolb H. Antimalarial therapy and early retinal changes in patients with rheumatoid arthritis. Br Med J. 1966;1:270–3.

135. Finbloom DS, Silver K, Newsome DA, Gunkel R. Comparison of hydroxychloroquine and chloroquine use and the development of retinal toxicity. J Rheumatol. 1985;12:692–4.

136. Savarino A, Trani LD, Donateli I, Cauda R, Cassone A. New insights into the antiviral effects of chloroquine. Reflection React. 2006;6:67–8.

137. Carr RE, Henkind P, Rothfield N, Siegel IM. Ocular toxicity of antimalarial drugs-long-term follow-up. Am J Ophthalmol. 1968;66:738–44.

138. Percival SPB, Meanock I. Chloroquine: ophthalmological safety and clinical assessment in rheumatoid arthritis. Br Med J. 1968;3:579–84.

139. Miller DR, Fiechtner JJ, Carpenter JR, Brown RR, Stroshane RM, Stecher VJ. Plasma hydroxychloroquine concentrations and efficacy in rheumatoid arthritis. Arthritis Rheum. 1987;30:567–71.

140. Kench JG, Seale JP, Temple DM, Tennant C. The effects of non-steroidal inhibitors of phospholipase A2 on leukotriene and histamine release from human and guinea-pig lung. Prostaglandins. 1985;30: 199–208.

141. Frisk-Holmberg M, Bergqvist Y. Chloroquine disposition in man. Br J Clin Pharmacol. 1982;14: 624P–6.

142. Salmeron G, Lipsky PE. Immunosuppressive potential of antimalarials. Am J Med. 1983;75:19–24.

143. Tett SE, Day RO, Cutler DJ. Concentration-effect relationship of hydroxychloroquine in rheumatoid arthritis—a cross sectional study. J Rheumatol. 1993;20:1874–9.

144. Wollheim FA, Hanson A, Laurell CB. Chloroquine treatment in rheumatoid arthritis. Scand J Rheumatol. 1978;7:171–6.

145. Costedoat-Chalumeau N, Amoura Z, Hulot JS, Hummoud HA, Aymard G, Cacoub P, Frances C, Wechsler B, et al. Low blood concentration of hydroxychloroquine is a marker for and predictor of disease exacerbations in patients with systemic lupus erythematosus. Arthritis Rheum. 2006;65: 3284–90.

146. Ullberg S, Lindquist NG, Sjostrand SE. Accumulation of chorio-retinotoxic drugs in the foetal eye. Nature. 1970;227:1257–8.

147. Cimaz R, Brucato A, Meregalli E, Muscara M, Sergi P. Electroretinograms of children born to mothers treated with hydroxychloroquine during pregnancy and breast-feeding: comment on the article by Costedoat-Chalumeau et al. Arthritis Rheum. 2004;50:3056–7.

148. Costedoat-Chalumeau N, Amoura Z, Aymard G, Hong DLT, Wechsler B, et al. Evidence of transplacental passage of hydroxychloroquine in humans. Arthritis Rheum. 2002;46:1123–4.

149. Klinger G, Morad Y, Westall CA, Laskin C, Spitzer KA, Koren G, Buncic RJ. Ocular toxicity and antenatal exposure to chloroquine or hydroxychloroquine for rheumatic diseases. Lancet. 2001;358: 813–4.

150. Motta M, Tincani A, Faden D, Zinzini E, Chirico G. Antimalarial agents in pregnancy. Lancet. 2002;359: 524–5.

151. Parke A, West B. Hydroxychloroquine in pregnant patients with systemic lupus erythematosus. J Clin Rheumatol. 1996;23:1715–8.

152. Clowse MEB, Magder L, Witter F, Petri M. Hydroxychloroquine in lupus pregnancy. Arthritis Rheum. 2006;54:3640–7.

153. Khamashta MA, Buchanan NMM, Hughes GRV. The use of hydroxychloroquine in lupus pregnancy: the British experience. Lupus. 1996;5:S65–6.

154. Costedoat-Chalumeau N, Amoura Z, Duhaut P, Huong DLT, Sebbough D, Wechsler B, et al. Safety of hydroxychloroquine in pregnant patients with connective tissue disease: a study of one hundred thirty-three cases compared with a control group. Arthritis Rheum. 2003;48:3207–11.

155. Borden MB, Parke AL. Antimalarial drugs in systemic lupus erythematosus: use in pregnancy. Drug Saf. 2001;24:1055–83.

156. Parke A. Antimalarial drugs and pregnancy. Am J Med. 1988;85:30–3.

157. Hart CW, Naunton RF. The ototoxicity of chloroquine phosphate. Arch Otolaryngol. 1964;80: 407–12.

158. Costedoat-Chalumeau N, Amoura Z, Sebbough D, Piette JC. Reply. Arthritis Rheum. 2004;50:3057–8.

159. Ostensen M, Brown ND, Chiang PK, Aarbakke J. Hydroxychloroquine in human breast milk. Eur J Clin Pharmacol. 1985;28:357.

160. Yam JCS, Kwok AKH. Ocular toxicity of hydroxychloroquine. Hong Kong Med J. 2006;12:294–304.

161. Yoon YH, Cho KS, Hwang JJ, et al. Induction of lysosomal dilatation, arrested autophagy, and cell death by chloroquine in cultured ARPE-19 cells. Invest Ophthalmol Vis Sci. 2010;51:6030–7.

162. de Duve C, de Barsy T, Poole B, Trouet A, Tulkens P, Van Hoof F. Lysosomotropic agents. Biochem Pharmacol. 1974;23:2495–531.

163. Ohkuma S, Poole B. Fluorescence probe measurement of the intralysosomal pH in living cells and the perturbation of pH by various agents. Proc Natl Acad Sci U S A. 1978;75:3327–33.

164. Ginsburg H, Geary TG. Current concepts and new ideas on the mechanism of action of quinoline-containing antimalarials. Biochem Pharmacol. 1987;36:1567–76.

165. Kyburz D, Brentano F, Gay S. Mode of action of hydroxychloroquine in RA—evidence of an inhibitory effect on toll-like receptor signaling. Nat Clin Pract Rheumatol. 2006;2:458–9.

166. Stauber WT, Hedge AM, Trout JJ, Schottelius BA. Inhibition of lysosomal function in red and white skeletal muscles by chloroquine. Exp Neurol. 1981;71:295–306.

167. Lafyatis R, York M, Marshak-Rothstein A. Antimalarial agents: closing the gate on toll-like receptors? Arthritis Rheum. 2006;54:3068–70.

168. Gonzalez-Noriega A, Grubb JH, Talkad V, Sly WS. Chloroquine inhibits lysosomal enzyme pinocytosis and enhances lysosomal enzyme secretion by impairing receptor recycling. J Cell Biol. 1980;85:839–52.

169. Jones CJP, Salisbury RS, Jayson MIV. The presence of abnormal lysosomes in lumphocytes and neutrophils during chloroquine therapy: a quantitative ultrastructural study. Ann Rheum Dis. 1984;43:710–5.

170. Prowse C, Pepper D, Dawes J. Prevention of the platelet alpha-granule release reaction by membrane-active drugs. Thromb Res. 1982;25:219–27.

171. Cruz da Silva J, Mariz HA, da Rocha Jr LF, de Oliveira PSS, Dantas AT, Duarte ALBP, Pitta IDR, Galdino SL, Pitta MGDR. Hydroxychloroquine decreases TH17-related cytokines in systemic lupus erythematosus and rheumatoid arthritis patients. Clinics. 2013;68:766–71.

172. Antoine JC, Gould B, Jovanne C, Maurice M, Feldman G. Ammonium chloride, methylamine and chloroquine reversibly inhibit antibody secretion by plasma cells. Biol Cell. 1985;55:41–54.

173. Macfarlane DE, Manzel L. Antagonism of immunostimulatory CpG-oligodeoxynucleotides by quinacrine, chloroquine, and structurally related compounds. J Immunol. 1998;160:1122–31.

174. McConnell DG, Wachtel J, Havener WH. Observations on experimental chloroquine retinopathy. Arch Ophthalmol. 1964;71:552–3.

175. Namazi MR. The potential negative impact of proton pump inhibitors on the immunopharmacologic effects of chloroquinere and hydroxychloroquine. Lupus. 2009;18:104–5.

176. Bondeson J, Sundler R. Antimalarial drugs inhibit phospholipase A2 activation and induction of interleukin 1 beta and tumor necrosis factor alpha in macrophages: implications for their mode of action in rheumatoid arthritis. Gen Pharmacol. 1998;30:357–66.

177. Alvan G. Determination of chloroquine and its desethyl metabolite in plasma, red blood cells and urine by liquid chromotography. J Chromatogr. 1982;229:241–7.

178. Sanders VM, Uhr JW, Vitetta ES. Antigen-specific memory and virgin B cells differ in their requirements for conjugation to T cells. Cell Immunol. 1987;104:419–25.

179. Macomber PB, Sprinz H. Morphological effects of chloroquine on Plasmodium berghei in mice. Nature. 1967;214:937–9.

180. Martin RE, Marchetti RV, Cowen AI, Howitt SM, Broer SV, Kirk K. Chloroquine transport via the malaria parasite's chloroquine resistance transporter. Science. 2009;325:1680–2.

181. Karres I, Kremer JP, Dietl I, Steckholzer U, Jochum M, Ertel W. Chloroquine inhibits proinflammatory cytokine release into human whole blood. Am J Physiol. 1998;274:R1058–64.

182. Jang CH, Choi JH, Byun MS, Jue DM. Chloroquine inhibits production of TNF-alpha, IL-1 beta, and IL-6 from lipopolysaccharide-stimulated human monocytes/macrophages by different modes. Rheumatology. 2006;45:703–10.

183. Weber SM, Levitz SM. Chloroquine interferes with lipopolysaccharide-induced TNF-α gene expression by a nonlysosomotropic mechanism. J Immunol. 2000;165:1534–40.

184. Manku MS, Horrobin DF. Chloroquine, quinine, procaine, quinidine, tricyclic antidepressants, and methylxanthines as prostaglandin agonists and antagonists. Lancet. 1976;20:1115–7.

185. Loffler BM, Bohn E, Hesse B, Kunze H. Effects of antimalarial drugs on phospholipase A and lysophospholipase activities in plasma membrane, mitochondrial, microsomal and cytosolic subcellular fractions of rat liver. Biochim Biophys Acta. 1985;835:448–55.

186. Matsuzawa Y, Hostetler KY. Effects of chloroquine and 4,4′-bis (diethylaminoethoxy)á, â-diethyldiphenylethane on the incorporation of [3H]glycerol into the phospholipids of rat liver lysosomes and other subcellular fractions, in vivo. Biochim Biophys Acta. 1980;620:592–602.

187. Trout JJ, Stauber WT, Schottelius BA. Increased autophagy in chloroquine treated tonic and phasic muscles: an alternative view. Tissue Cell. 1982;13:393–401.

188. Fiddick R, Heath H. Inhibition of alcohol dehydrogenase by chloroquine. Nature. 1967;213:628–9.

189. Roskoski Jr R, Jaskunas SR. Chloroquine and primaquine inhibition of rat liver cell-free polynucleotide-dependent polypeptide synthesis. Biochem Pharmacol. 1972;21:391–9.

190. Lefler CF, Lilja HS, Holbrook Jr DJ. Inhibition of aminoacylation and polypeptide synthesis by chloroquine and primaquine in rat liver in vitro. Biochem Pharmacol. 1973;22:715–28.

191. Ward PA. The chemosuppression of chemotaxis. J Exp Med. 1966;124:209–26.

192. Labro MT, Babin-Chevaye C. Effects of amodiaquine, chloroquine, and mefloquine on human polymorphonuclear neutrophil function in vitro. Antimicrob Agents Chemother. 1988;32:1124–30.

193. Weissmann G. Lysosomes (concluded). New Engl J Med. 1965;273:1143–9.

194. Brentano F, Schorr O, Gay RE, Gay S, Kyburz D. RNA released from necrotic synovial fluid cells activates rheumatoid arthritis synovial fibroblasts via Toll-like receptor 3. Arthritis Rheum. 2005;52:2656–65.

195. Leadbetter EA, Rifkin IR, Hohlbaum AM, Beaudette BC, Schlomchik MJ, Marshak-Rothstein A. Chromatin-IgG complexes activate B cells by dual engagement of IgM and Toll-like receptors. Nature. 2002;416:603–7.

196. Tehrani R, Ostrowski RA, Hariman R, Jay WM. Ocular toxicity of hydroxychloroquine. Semin Ophthalmol. 2008;23:201–9.

197. Wada A, Sakurai S, Kobayashi H, Yanagihara N, Izumi F. Suppression by phospholipase A2 inhibitors of secretion of catecholamines from isolated adrenal medullary cells by suppression of cellular calcium uptake. Biochem Pharmacol. 1983;32:1175–8.

198. Wiesmann EN, DiDonato S, Herschkowitz NN. Effect of chloroquine on cultured fibroblasts: release of lysosomal hydrolases and inhibition of their uptake. Biochem Biophys Res Commun. 1975;66:1338–43.

199. Roman MJ, Shanker BA, Davis A, Lockshin MD, Sammaritano L, Simantov R, Crow MK, et al. Prevalence and correlates of accelerated atherosclerosis in systemic lupus erythematosus. N Engl J Med. 2003;349:2299–406.

200. Wallace DJ, Metzger AL, Stecher VJ, Turnbull BA, Kern PA. Cholesterol-lowering effect of hydroxychloroquine in patients with rheumatic disease: reversal of deleterious effects of steroids on lipids. Am J Med. 1990;89:322–6.

201. Wasko MCM, Hubert HB, Lingala VB, Elliott JR, Luggen ME, Fries JF, Ward MM. Hydroxychloroquine and risk of diabetes in patients with rheumatoid arthritis. JAMA. 2007;298:187–93.

202. Kitridou R, Rees RG, Smith MJ, Peiris A, Kissebah AH. Effect of chloroquine on insulin and glucose homeostasis in normal subjects and patients with non-insulin dependent diabetes mellitus. Br Med J. 1987;294:900–1.

203. Ruiz-Irastorza G, Egurbide MV, Pijoan JI, Garmendia M, Villar I, Martinez-Berriotxoa A, Erdozain JG, Aguirre C. Effects of antimalarials on thrombosis and survival in patients with systemic lupus erythematosus. Lupus. 2006;15:577–83.

204. Hurvitz D, Hirschhorn K. Suppression of in vitro lymphocyte responses by chloroquine. N Engl J Med. 1965;273:23–6.

205. Ohkuma S, Chudzik J, Poole B. The effects of basic substances and acidic ionophores on the digestion of exogenous and endogenous proteins in mouse peritoneal macrophages. J Cell Biol. 1986;102:959–66.

206. Oda K, Koriyama Y, Yamada E, Ikehara Y. Effects of weakly basic amines on proteolytic processing and terminal glycosylation of secretory proteins in cultured rat hepatocytes. J Biol Chem. 1986;240:739–45.

207. Wright CI, Sabine JC. Cholinesterases of human erythrocytes and plasma and their inhibition by antimalarial drugs. J Pharmacol Exp Ther. 1948;93:230–9.

208. Jeong JY, Choi JW, Jeon KI, Jue DM. Chloroquine decreases cell-surface expression of tumour necrosis factor receptors in human histiocytic U-937 cells. Immunology. 2002;105:83–91.

209. Meng XW, Feller JM, Ziegler JB, Pittman SM, Ireland CM. Induction of apoptosis in peripheral blood lymphocytes following treatment in vitro with hydroxychloroquine. Arthritis Rheum. 1997;40:927–35.

210. Kim WU, Yoo SA, Min SY, Park SH, Koh HS, Song SW, Cho CS. Hydroxychloroquine potentiates Fas-mediated apoptosis of rheumatoid synoviocytes. Clin Exp Immunol. 2006;144:503–11.

211. Weber SM, Chen JM, Levitz SM. Inhibition of mitogen-activated protein kinase signaling by chloroquine. J Immunol. 2002;168:5303–9.

212. Ghigo D, Aldieri E, Todde R, Costamagna C, Garbarino G, Pescarmona G, Bosia A. Chloroquine stimulates nitric oxide synthesis in murine, porcine, and human endothelial cells. J Clin Invest. 1998;102:595–605.

213. Tietze C, Schlesinger P, Stahl P. Chloroquine and ammonium ion inhibit receptor-mediated endocystosis of mannose-glyconjugates by macrophages: apparent inhibition of receptor recycling. Biochem Biophys Res Commun. 1980;93:1–8.

214. Allison JL, O'Brien RL, Hahn FE. DNA: reaction with chloroquine. Science. 1965;149:1111–3.

215. Ciak J, Hahn FE. Chloroquine: mode of action. Science. 1966;151:347–9.

216. O'Brien RL, Olenick JG, Hahn FE. Reactions of quinine, chloroquine, and quinacrine with DNA and their effects on the DNA and RNA polymerase reactions. Proc Natl Acad Sci USA. 1966;55:1511–7.

217. Yucel-Lindberg T, Jansson H, Glaumann H. Proteolysis in isolated autophagic vacuoles from the rat pancreas. Effects of chloroquine administration. Virchows Arch B Cell Pathol. 1991;61:141–5.

218. Raines MF, Bhargava SK, Rosen ES. The blood-retinal barrier in chloroquine retinopathy. Invest Ophthalmol Vis Sci. 1989;30:1726–31.

219. Weisinger HS, Pesudovs K, Collin HB. Management of patients undergoing hydroxychloroquine (Plaquenil) therapy. Clin Exp Optom. 2000;83:32–6.

220. Goldstein JL, Brunschede GY, Brown MS. Inhibition of the proteolytic degradation of low density lipoprotein in human fibroblasts by chloroquine, concanavalin A, and Triton WR 1339. J Biol Chem. 1975;250:7854–62.

221. Ausiello CM, Barbieri P, Spagnoli GC, Ciompi ML, Gasciani CU. In vivo effects of chloroquine treatment on spontaneous and interferon-induced natural killer activities in rheumatoid arthritis patients. Clin Exp Rheumatol. 1986;4:255–9.

222. O'Brien RL, Allison JL, Hahn FE. Evidence for intercalation of chloroquine into DNA. Biochim Biophys Acta. 1966;129:622–4.

223. Wozniacka A, Lesiak A, Boncela J, Smolarczyk K, McCauliffe DP, Sysa-Jedrzejowska A. The influence of antimalarial treatment on IL-1beta, IL-6 and TNF-alpha mRNA expression on UVB-irradiated skin in systemic lupus erythematosus. Br J Dermatol. 2008;159:1124–30.

224. Ahmed MH, Ashton N, Balment RJ. The effect of chloroquine on renal function and vasopressin secretion: a nitric oxide-dependent effect. J Pharmacol Exp Ther. 2003;304:156–61.

225. Accapezzato D, Visco V, Francavilla V, Molette C, Donato T, et al. Chloroquine enhances human CD8 T cell responses against soluble antigens in vivo. J Exp Med. 2005;202:817–28.

3

Toxicology of Hydroxychloroquine and Chloroquine and the Pathology of the Retinopathy They Cause

Abbreviations

ABW	Actual body weight
4AQs	4-Aminoquinolines (chloroquine and hydroxychloroquine)
4AQR	4-Aminoquinoline retinopathy
A2E	*N*-retinylidene-*N*-retinylethanolamine
C	Chloroquine
C-tubes	Curvilinear tubules
d	Day
ED50	Effective dose 50
EOG	Electrooculogram
ERG	Electroretinogram
GCL	Ganglion cell layer
g	Gram
HC	Hydroxychloroquine
IBW	Ideal body weight
IM	Intramuscular
INL	Inner nuclear layer
IP	Intraperitoneal
IPL	Inner plexiform layer
IV	Intravenous
kg	Kilogram
L	Liter
LD50	Lethal dose 50
M	Mole
MCB	Membranous cytoplasmic body
mfERG	Multifocal electroretinography
mg	Milligram
μM	Micromoles/L
nm	Nanometer
NSAID	Nonsteroidal anti-inflammatory drug
PR	Photoreceptor
RA	Rheumatoid arthritis
RPE	Retinal pigment epithelium
TD50	Toxic dose 50

The 4-aminoquinolines (4AQs) are thought to be universally toxic under the proper circumstances, although there may be individual genetic factors that modulate risk [1, 2]. That is, the toxic effects on the retina are not idiosyncratic and can be reproducibly observed if a high enough dose of these drugs is given for a long enough period [1]. This is true in animal models and in clinical studies in humans. There is a gradation of toxicity, however, so that clinical retinopathy occurs in a small subset of patients if appropriate dosing by ideal body weight (IBW) is observed [3]. This chapter covers the toxicology of the 4AQs and their histopathologic effects. The remainder of the book is devoted to 4-aminoquinoline retinopathy (4AQR), beginning with its many definitions in Chap. 4, following with epidemiology in Chap. 5, and natural history in Chap. 6. Commonly used abbreviations are collected in "Abbreviations" for reference. Each term will be first used in its full form, along with its abbreviation.

Although the 4AQs are derived from quinine, their toxicities differ from the parent compound. Acute quinine toxicity is characterized by a macular cherry-red spot, electroretinogram (ERG) changes including a reduced b-wave, and a depressed electrooculogram (EOG) Arden ratio [4]. Acutely the retinal vessels have normal caliber [4, 5]. Later optic atrophy develops with

D.J. Browning, *Hydroxychloroquine and Chloroquine Retinopathy*,
DOI 10.1007/978-1-4939-0597-3_3, © Springer Science+Business Media New York 2014

narrowed arterioles and pigmentary changes in the retina [4, 5]. A bull's-eye maculopathy does not develop, in contrast to 4AQR.

The toxicity of chloroquine and hydroxychloroquine is directly related to the 4AQ nucleus, modulated by various side-chain substitutions. Halogen substitutions at any position other than seven (see Chap. 2, Fig. 2.1) reduce pharmacologic activity and toxicity [6]. An aryl rather than an alkyl side chain decreases the therapeutic ratio [6]. Increasing alkyl side-chain length above five carbons decreases the therapeutic ratio and increases toxicity [6]. The 8-aminoquinolines primaquine and quinocide lack the 4AQ nucleus and cause no retinopathy [7]. Quinacrine is not a 4AQ, but rather a derivative of an acridine nucleus (see Chap. 2, Fig. 2.1). For years it was thought not to cause retinopathy [8]; in fact, it had been suggested as a substitute for patients who had discontinuation of 4AQs over concerns regarding retinopathy [8]. Unfortunately quinacrine retinopathy has been reported more recently characterized by a bull's-eye macular lesion indistinguishable from that of 4AQR [9, 10]. However, the prevalence of retinopathy in quinacrine users is much lower [9]. It is probably unwise to place a patient with 4AQR on quinacrine, although this action has been suggested when the mechanism of action of antimalarials is desired with a lesser risk of retinopathy [11].

3.1 Toxic Concentrations

Toxicity has been studied in several different ways, including dose–response curves for lethality in animal models and dose–response curves for frequency of side effects in clinical studies. In a retinal pigment epithelium (RPE)-19 cell culture model of chloroquine toxicity, no toxicity was present at a concentration of 10 micromolar (μM), 100 % toxicity occurred at 250 μM, and the mean dose at which 50 % of cells were killed (lethal dose 50, LD_{50}) was 120 μM [12]. In an intravenous-dosing model in mice, the LD_{50} for chloroquine was 25 mg/kg and was 45 mg/kg for hydroxychloroquine [13]. This order of toxicity is also seen in an intravenous-dosing model in dogs.

It is not seen in rabbits, in which the two drugs reach LD_{50} at similar doses [13]. From cases of suicide, the lethal dose of chloroquine in the adult human is estimated to be 2.5–6 g and 0.75–1 g in a child [14–16]. The lethal dose of hydroxychloroquine is less well established than that of chloroquine, but based on data from animal models it is estimated to be 2–3 times that of chloroquine [15]. One patient survived ingestion of 5.8 g with a plasma level of 1.8×10^{-5} M/L [13]. Death from 4AQ poisoning occurs after hypotension, apnea, and convulsions. The toxicity may be reversible if life support is provided [14].

In clinical practice, the frequency of side effects depends on serum and blood concentrations. In adults, none were noted for serum concentrations of chloroquine below 4.5×10^{-7}–1.25×10^{-6} M/L but occurred in 80–89 % of patients at serum concentrations above 2.5×10^{-6} M/L [15, 17, 18]. The incidence of gastrointestinal side effects in weeks 1–3 of therapy was related to hydroxychloroquine concentration in the blood in one study. The frequency ranged from less than 10% of patients with blood concentrations below 2.2×10^{-6} M/L to 30 % of patients with concentrations of 4.5×10^{-6} M/L and above [19]. In children, side effects were not noted for chloroquine concentrations below 8.75×10^{-7} M/L or for hydroxychloroquine concentrations below 1.40×10^{-6} M/L [20]. A maximum safe serum concentration has been estimated to be 8.75×10^{-7} M/L for chloroquine and 1.4×10^{-6} M/L for hydroxychloroquine [15].

Although it has been stated that the side effects of the 4AQs depend on the serum concentration and not on the cumulative dose [21], such a view does not account for the evidence supporting cumulative dose as a risk factor for retinopathy (see Chap. 7). Retinopathy and other forms of toxicity depend strongly on drug concentration, and hence daily dose; it is rarely seen in patients taking 4AQs for malaria prophylaxis in which dosing is much less than in patients taking the drugs for chronic autoimmune diseases [22, 23].

Plasma concentrations of 4AQs are rarely measured in clinical practice, but abundant information has been collected for daily dosage, a crude surrogate rendered cruder when used in the

Table 3.1 Suggested thresholds at which the risk of retinopathy increases

Drug	Daily dose (mg/kg)	Study
Chloroquine	3.0 (IBW)/day	Marmor et al. [24, 25], Schwartz et al. [26], Missner and Kellner [27], Fung et al. [28], Labriola et al. [29]
	3.5–4.0	Ehrenfeld et al. [30]
	<3.74 (ABW)/day	Mackenzie [31]
	3.85	Fleck et al. [32]
	4.0 (IBW)/day	Cox and Paterson [33], Mackenzie [31], Laaksonen et al. [20], Elman et al. [34]
	4.0 is "too high"	Easterbrook [35]
	4.0 (ABW)/day	Scherbel [36], Sundelin and Terman [37], Elman et al. [34]
	5.35 (IBW)/day	Mackenzie [31]
Hydroxychloroquine	5.0–7.0	Laaksonen et al. [20]
	6.0	Scherbel [36]
	6.15	Fleck et al. [32]
	6.0–6.5	Ehrenfeld et al. [30]
	6.5 (IBW)/day	Marmor et al. [24, 25], Schwartz and Mieler [26], Sundelin and Terman [37], Missner and Kellner [27], Michaelides et al. [38], Browning [39], Levy et al. [40], Mavrikakis et al. [41], Cox et al. [33], Fung et al. [28], Lai et al. [42], Albert et al. [43], Labriola [29], Mackenzie [44]
	7.7 (ABW)/day	Mackenzie [31]

ABW actual body weight, *IBW* is ideal body weight

absence of information on IBW (see Chap. 7). Based on numerous retrospective case series, the current best estimates for dose thresholds at which risk of toxicity increases are 3 and 6.5 mg/kg/day based on IBW (Table 3.1). These thresholds are not optimal dosages, but ceilings above which dosing should not exceed [14]. The similar concept of threshold cumulative dose is analogous to the threshold concentration or adjusted daily dose at which risk of toxicity increases. Unlike the case of adjusted daily dose, there is no clear consensus about what the inflection point might be (see Chap. 7).

3.2 Mechanism of Toxicity

The mechanism of toxicity of the 4AQs is unknown, but the 4AQ nucleus is considered to be the critical factor causing toxicity. Potential mechanisms of toxicity include all the known mechanisms of action of the drug (see Chap. 2) carried to excess [13, 45–47]. In a model using RPE-19 cultured cells, chloroquine inhibited protein degradation within autophagic vacuoles, leading to accumulation of ubiquitinated proteins that might be toxic [12]. Banks has noted that intravitreal chloroquine damages photoreceptors but systemically administered chloroquine spares photoreceptors and instead preferentially damages ganglion cells followed by the RPE [48, 49]. From this observation, he hypothesized that the RPE detoxifies photoreceptors with accumulation of some by-products until a critical threshold is reached, at which point the RPE is destroyed [7]. Mechanisms of toxicity related to melanin binding have been discounted as have mechanisms of therapeutic effects (see Chap. 2). For example, 4AQR occurs in albino animal models [50]. In fact, binding to melanin may be protective rather than harmful [24].

The retinal toxicity of 4AQs may be derived from the toxic effects of metabolic by-products from photopigment recycling. Lipofuscin is an accumulation of breakdown products of visual pigments within the RPE. Lipofuscin's main component is *N*-retinylidene-*N*-retinylethanolamine (A2E) with lesser amounts of isoA2E, all-trans-retinal dimer phosphatidylethanolamine, and all-trans-retinal dimer-E. A2E is photooxidized to peroxy-A2E, furano-A2E, and epoxides [51, 52]. These endoperoxides are potentially cytotoxic and may cause RPE damage and atrophy [51, 53, 54]. Chloroquine and hydroxychloroquine may potentiate the toxic effects by forming complexes with polar lipids, rendering these lipids indigestible and leading to excessive intralysosomal storage of the complexes [47]. These ideas are sketchy, and none has been developed into a testable hypothesis.

The maculocentric nature of 4AQR has prompted speculation of a role for light energy or the distribution of cones or rods (see Chap. 1) [24]. Short-wavelength (blue) light is more damaging to retinal neurons than longer-wavelength light. The blue light of the sky originates in the superior visual field and is focused on the inferior macula, the location of the earliest funduscopically visible damage in 4AQR. Thus, one possible mechanism of 4AQ toxicity is to unmask the susceptibility of the macula, and especially the inferior hemimacula, to the damaging effects of blue light. The relative resistance to 4AQ toxicity of the fovea compared to the perifovea has not been explained [55].

3.3 Nonretinal Ocular Toxicity

The 4AQs have nonretinal ocular toxic effects. Corneal deposits occur frequently with chloroquine use, infrequently with hydroxychloroquine use, and are reversible when the drug is discontinued. They do not spontaneously resolve as long as drug is continued [8, 14, 34, 56–67]. Rates of keratopathy reported in various series are shown in Table 3.2. The weighted mean estimates for chloroquine and hydroxychloroquine are 78 % and 2 %, respectively. The provenance of the deposits is debated. Some claim that they are salts of 4AQs, whereas others say that they are lipid deposits [68, 69]. The deposits may appear as punctate dots in the corneal subepithelium and Bowman's layer as a fine powder-like stippling. They may also appear as a vortex figure similar to amiodarone keratopathy, with the highest concentration below the pupil (Fig. 3.1) [60, 61, 65, 70, 71]. Sometimes these changes are best

Table 3.2 Rates of 4-aminoquinoline keratopathy in various case series

Study	Drug	N	Percentage with keratopathy
Hobbs et al. [73]	C	28	79
Percival and Behrman [74]	C	198	37.9
Hobbs et al. [65]	C	165	33.3
Henkind and Rothfield [60]	C	45	73.3
Araiza-Casillas et al. [75]	C	78	50
Easterbrook [67, 68]	C	~1,500	90
Marks and Power [76]	C	222	15
Weighted mean rate	C	2,014	78
Henkind and Rothfield [60]	HC	6	16.6
Grierson [63]	HC	758	0.9
Mantyjarvi [77]	HC	63	1.6
Elder and Rahman [78]	HC	262	0.4
Easterbrook [67, 68]	HC	~500	5
Weighted mean rate	HC	1,589	2

C is chloroquine, *HC* is hydroxychloroquine

seen on retroillumination and are easier to see in a patient with dilated pupils [35, 57, 72]. They can occur within 3 weeks of starting the drug, and are related to the daily dosage ingested [60, 65]. Their frequency is dose related. Twenty-eight percent of patients taking hydroxychloroquine at doses of greater than 800 mg/day had corneal verticillata, whereas at doses of 400 mg/day fewer than 5 % of patients did [8, 68]. They usually disappear within 6–8 weeks after stopping the drug, but can occasionally persist up to 2 years [58, 68].

Reports are inconsistent as to whether keratopathy is a risk factor for retinopathy. Presence of keratopathy was a risk factor for retinopathy in one series [75]. In others, presence of corneal deposits did not imply higher risk of retinopathy, and cases of retinopathy have developed in patients who never had keratopathy [34, 65, 79]. Few cases with retinopathy develop keratopathy. For example, none of the 16 cases with retinopathy in Michaelides' series had corneal changes, nor any of the author's series of cases of 4AQR [38].

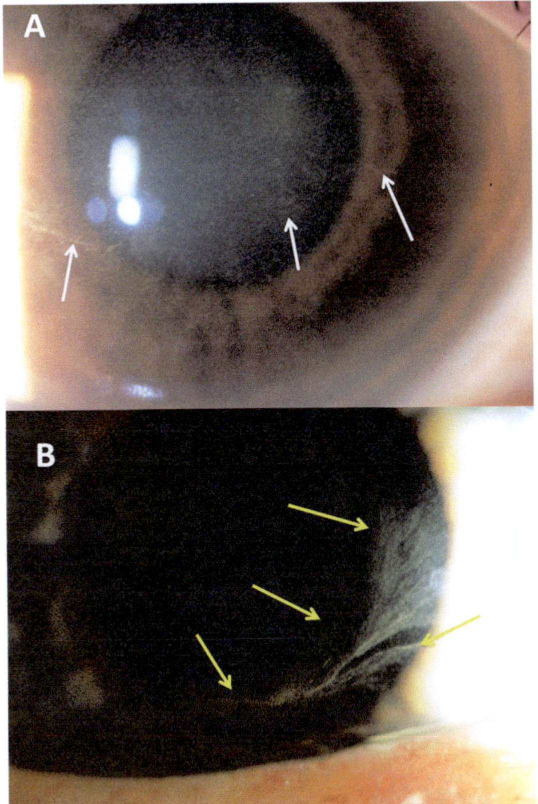

Fig. 3.1 This 52-year-old woman with rheumatoid arthritis was placed on hydroxychloroquine 400 mg/day for 6 months before being examined. Her slit lamp examination showed bilateral verticellate keratopathy (*white arrows*, panel **a**). She was not taking amiodarone or other drugs that are known to cause corneal deposits besides hydroxychloroquine. She was 5 ft 1 in. tall and weighed 211 lb. Her IBW was 127 lb. Thus her adjusted daily dose was 6.93 mg/kg/day—a toxic dose. She was advised that she had hydroxychloroquine deposits in her corneas that might go away with revision of her dosage to a nontoxic level. (**b**) For comparison, a typical example of a patient with amiodarone keratopathy is shown (*yellow arrows*)

Keratopathy does not occur more commonly in one autoimmune disease than another, and is not gender or age dependent [65]. Some authors state that presence of keratopathy implies overdosage and a need to reduce dosing [20, 72, 75]. Easterbrook states that this is not the case for chloroquine, but if prominent in a patient taking hydroxychloroquine it should raise the issue for more thorough investigation [68]. Corneal deposits without retinopathy are not an indication to stop 4AQs [76, 80].

Chloroquine corneal deposits are associated with symptoms of halos around lights in approximately 1 % of patients, but some observers report higher percentages [56, 65, 68]. Easterbrook has never seen a symptomatic case of hydroxychloroquine corneal deposits, nor has the author [68]. Visual acuity is not reduced in the presence of keratopathy. Decreased corneal sensitivity in association with keratopathy has been noted [59, 74]. Decreased corneal sensitivity has been reported to occur in 51.7 % of patients taking 4AQs compared to less than 10 % in a control group of nonrheumatic subjects not taking 4AQs [60]. This corneal effect need not be related to the presence of corneal deposits and typically is bilateral [60].

Cataracts have occasionally been listed as associations with 4AQ toxicity, but the relative high frequency of these in older patients makes such a link difficult to support [81, 82]. Difficulty with accommodation is common with the use of 4AQs, but often subsides over time, and is less of a problem with hydroxychloroquine than chloroquine [81–83]. Diplopia has occasionally been reported with the use of 4AQs [82]. Abducens palsy and optic atrophy have been occasionally associated with chloroquine ingestion [71]. Whitening of hair and eyelashes has been reported in 1.8 % of patients [60, 84].

3.4 Relative Toxicity of Chloroquine and Hydroxychloroquine

In animal models, the preponderance of the evidence suggests that hydroxychloroquine is less toxic than chloroquine on a weight basis (Table 3.3) [6]. For example, in rats given equal doses of hydroxychloroquine and chloroquine, growth rates have slowed more (evidence of toxicity) in the rats receiving chloroquine [85].

The literature on toxicity in humans is inconsistent on the issue of differential toxicity of the antimalarial drugs. Although no scientifically valid studies have been done, it is the common clinical impression that chloroquine at 250 mg/day is more toxic than hydroxychloroquine

Table 3.3 Relative toxicity of 4-aminoquinolines

Animal model (Reference)	Mode of administration	Toxicity index chloroquine	Toxicity index hydroxychloroquine	Toxicity ratio of chloroquine to hydroxychloroquine
Mouse [6]	Acute IV	$LD_{50}=40$ mg/kg	$LD_{50}=74$ mg/kg	1.85
	Acute IP	$LD_{50}=73-125$ mg/kg	$LD_{50}=300$ mg/kg	2.4–4.1
	Acute oral	$LD_{50}=250-1,000$ mg/kg	$LD_{50}=1,000$ mg/kg	1–4
Dog [6]	Acute IM	Maximal tolerated dose = 6 mg/kg	Maximal tolerated dose = 25 mg/kg	4.2
	Chronic oral	Maximal tolerated dose = 12 mg/kg/day × 28 weeks	Maximal tolerated dose = 32 mg/kg/day × 13 weeks	2.7

IV intravenous, *IP* is intraperitoneal, *IM* is intramuscular, *LD50* is lethal dose 50

at 400 mg/day [33, 38, 43, 75, 86–93]. At these doses, the rate of adverse effects observed in clinical practice is approximately half as much with hydroxychloroquine [15, 93]. Other circumstantial evidence to support the view includes the fact that 30 cases of chloroquine retinopathy appeared in the UK over a 30 year span, but only five cases of hydroxychloroquine retinopathy did [33]. The numbers of patients exposed to the two drugs were not known, but hydroxychloroquine usage was estimated to be more than one-sixth the rate of usage of chloroquine [33]. The rate of side effects increases more rapidly as dose increases with chloroquine than with hydroxychloroquine (Fig. 3.2) [20]. In RPE cell culture, hydroxychloroquine was a less potent enhancer of lipofuscinogenesis than chloroquine. The inhibition of lysosomal enzymes was less with hydroxychloroquine [37]. In some patients unable to tolerate chloroquine because of side effects, hydroxychloroquine may be tolerated [92]. The reverse is rarely the case [92]. One hypothesis advanced for the differential toxicity is that the hydroxyl group present in hydroxychloroquine but not in chloroquine gives the former less ability to penetrate the blood–retinal barrier [94, 95]. In addition, chloroquine but not hydroxychloroquine has been documented to cause breakdown of the blood–retina barrier, although if hydroxychloroquine were tested, it might also show this effect [95].

A way to quantitate the relative toxicity of drugs involves the concept of the therapeutic ratio (see Chap. 1). The therapeutic ratio is the ratio of the toxic dose in half of the population

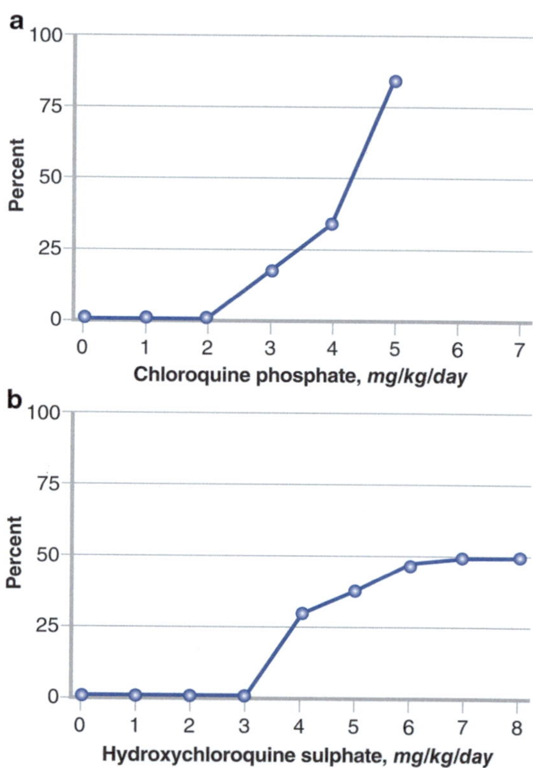

Fig. 3.2 Frequency of complications in percent related to dose of chloroquine (**a**) and hydroxychloroquine (**b**) in mg/kg/day of actual body weight. Data from Laaksonen [20]

(TD50) to the minimum dose effective in half of the population (ED50). Some have estimated that hydroxychloroquine is 50–80 % as effective as chloroquine [88, 96]. Estimates of the relative toxicity of hydroxychloroquine compared to chloroquine range from 33 to 60 % in humans and animal models [13, 14, 50, 88, 97, 98]. This can be reframed quantitatively using the concept of therapeutic ratio. Assume the ED50 of chloroquine (C) is one. If hydroxychloroquine (HC) is two-thirds as effective as chloroquine, then $ED50_{HC} = 0.67ED50_C$. If hydroxychloroquine is one-half as toxic, then $TD50_{HC} = .50TD50_C$. Therefore, the therapeutic ratio of HC is $TD50_{HC}/ED50_{HC} = .67TD50_C/.5ED50_C = 1.33(TD50_C/ED50_C)$. That is, the therapeutic ratio of hydroxychloroquine is 1.33 times that of chloroquine. A higher therapeutic ratio implies greater safety.

The therapeutic ratio may depend on the particular toxicity being discussed. For retinopathy, conclusions about the relative toxicity of 4AQs are inconsistent. Finbloom and colleagues reported that of 31 patients taking chloroquine with a mean dose of 329 mg/day, 6 developed retinopathy [91]. By comparison, none of the 66 patients taking hydroxychloroquine at a mean dose of 280 mg/day developed retinopathy. On the basis of this experience, he concluded that chloroquine was a more toxic drug. However, it should be considered that the mean dose of chloroquine in this series would be high for most patients based on IBW, whereas the mean dose of hydroxychloroquine would not be high for most people. That is, the conclusion of different relative toxicity cannot convincingly be made based on this evidence. Mackenzie assumed that an average therapeutic daily dosage of chloroquine was 4.0 mg/kg/day based on actual body weight (ABW) and of hydroxychloroquine was 6.5 mg/kg/day. His data in patients with retinopathy indicated an average daily dose of 5.11 and 7.77 mg/kg/day based on ABW for chloroquine and hydroxychloroquine, respectively. From these data, the therapeutic ratio was calculated to be 1.27 and 1.20 for chloroquine and hydroxychloroquine, respectively. Looked at in this way, the relative toxicity of the two compounds with respect to retinopathy was approximately equal. The worse clinical experience with chloroquine may reflect the fact that the smallest pill size for chloroquine is 78 % of a toxic dose for a person with an IBW of 60 kg, but the smallest pill size for hydroxychloroquine (200 mg) is 40 % of a toxic dose for hydroxychloroquine in a person of this IBW. Others have agreed that there is no convincing evidence of differential toxicity of the

4AQs [31, 39, 80, 99, 100]. A more nuanced view is that differential toxicity is present at doses above 4 mg/kg/day but that no differential toxicity exists at lower doses [20]. Synthesizing both animal and human data, the weight of the imperfect evidence supports the concept that chloroquine is more toxic than hydroxychloroquine. That is, the therapeutic ratio for hydroxychloroquine is higher.

3.5 Nonocular Toxicity of Chloroquine and Hydroxychloroquine

As might be expected for a biologic toxin, retinopathy is not the only manifestation of chloroquine and hydroxychloroquine toxicity. In a pigmented rabbit model of chloroquine toxicity, serum hypo- and dysproteinemia developed with decreases in serum albumin and alpha 1 and 2 globulin fractions and increases in beta and gamma globulin fractions [101]. Serum amino acid profiles changed with disappearance of tyrosine; decrease in taurine, aspartine, glutamine, tryptophan, and arginine; and increases in serine, alanine, GABA, and ornithine [101].

Most information in humans regarding the toxic side effects of the 4AQs relative to other drugs used for rheumatologic diseases comes from observational studies which are limited by confounding, variable thresholds for diagnosing side effects and different follow-up times [102, 103]. For example, if nonsteroidal anti-inflammatory drugs (NSAIDs), gold, penicillamine, and cyclophosphamide are given for rheumatological disease of different severity, then the prevalence of side effects may reflect the differences in disease severity and not the drugs used. In one study, increasing follow-up from 5 to 15 years doubled the rate of reported side effects leading to drug stoppage [102]. Prospective studies with standardized definitions of side effects yield more reliable data than retrospective observational studies. In one prospective study of patients with early rheumatoid arthritis (RA) randomized to NSAIDs, hydroxychloroquine, gold, or methotrexate, total side effects and those severe enough to cause discontinuation of drug were found in the following order: gold (65 and 30 %)>methotrexate (64 and 11 %)>hydroxychloroquine (49 and 8 %)>NSAIDS (34 % and not given) [104]. In prospective, double-blind studies, the key statistic to consider is the differential frequency of side effects between patients taking 4AQs. For example, in one such study side effects were noted in 40 % of patients in the control group, but 62.5 % of patients taking chloroquine [105].

As with ocular side effects, nonocular side effects are less frequent with hydroxychloroquine (9–17 %) than chloroquine (16–19 %) at usual clinical doses [45, 83, 102, 103]. Approximately 6–10 % of patients who begin to take chloroquine and 5–17 % of patients who begin to take hydroxychloroquine are unable to continue taking the drugs because of side effects [78, 102, 106–108]. Many of the side effects resolve spontaneously if the drug is continued, if the daily dose is divided, or if nocturnal dosing is used [103]. Because the side effects occur at similar rates in patients taking a placebo, it is difficult in some cases to tie them to the ingestion of the 4AQ [15]. The most common nonocular side effect of both 4AQs is gastrointestinal upset accompanied by cramps, nausea, and loss of weight, which has been noted in 6–12 % [75, 88, 92, 102, 106, 109, 110]. Depigmentation of hair can be noted, and can resolve spontaneously even if the drug is continued [70, 83, 84, 92, 110, 111]. Other tissues not exposed to light, such as the palate, can also become depigmented [14, 83]. Ototoxicity, neuropathy, and myopathy have been described [112, 113]. Cutaneous allergy develops in 1–3 % and may include rash or symptoms of itching, hives, and exfoliation [14, 70, 92, 106, 110]. Occasionally patients taking chloroquine develop a blue-gray discoloration of the tibia, face, and palate attributed to increased melanin and hemosiderin production [83, 99]. Psoriasis may be exacerbated [114]. Mild ileus can occur [14]. Rarely, bronchospasm has been reported [114]. Reduced amplitude of the T wave in the electrocardiogram without cardiovascular symptoms has been reported [115]. Although it is rare, leukopenia, lymphopenia, thrombocytopenia, aplastic anemia, and hemolysis have been observed [114].

Skeletal and cardiac myopathy has been described in chloroquine users [36, 116]. Chloroquine myopathy often occurs in concert with chloroquine retinopathy [117, 118]. In one report, 55 % of patients with chloroquine myopathy had concomitant retinopathy [117]. Lower limbs tend to be affected more severely than upper limbs [117]. Cases have generally occurred in patients taking 500 mg/day or more of chloroquine for at least 1 year [119]. The cumulative doses of chloroquine consumed in reported cases have ranged from 45 to 100 g. Once patients stop the chloroquine, they tend to improve, regaining strength [120–122]. In a cell culture model of chloroquine myopathy, characteristic changes of toxicity occur at concentrations of 2.5×10^{-5} M/L [123]. It has been hypothesized, but not demonstrated, that similar mechanisms are responsible for chloroquine retinopathy and myopathy [123]. Chloroquine ototoxicity has also been described [124]. Less documented, and somewhat in doubt, is chloroquine peripheral neuropathy [125].

3.6 Pathology of 4-Aminoquinoline Retinopathy and Nonocular Cytopathy

The pathology of 4AQ toxicity has been studied in a number of experimental animal models and in rare human material from documented cases of clinical retinopathy and other cytopathies. The majority of studies concern chloroquine, but as there is no evidence that the mechanisms or pathologic changes differ by drug, the results for both 4AQs will be covered together.

3.6.1 Cell Culture and Animal Models

In animal models, differences in pathologic effects of chloroquine have been reported depending on the species studied. In the rat model, published results are inconsistent regarding which retinal

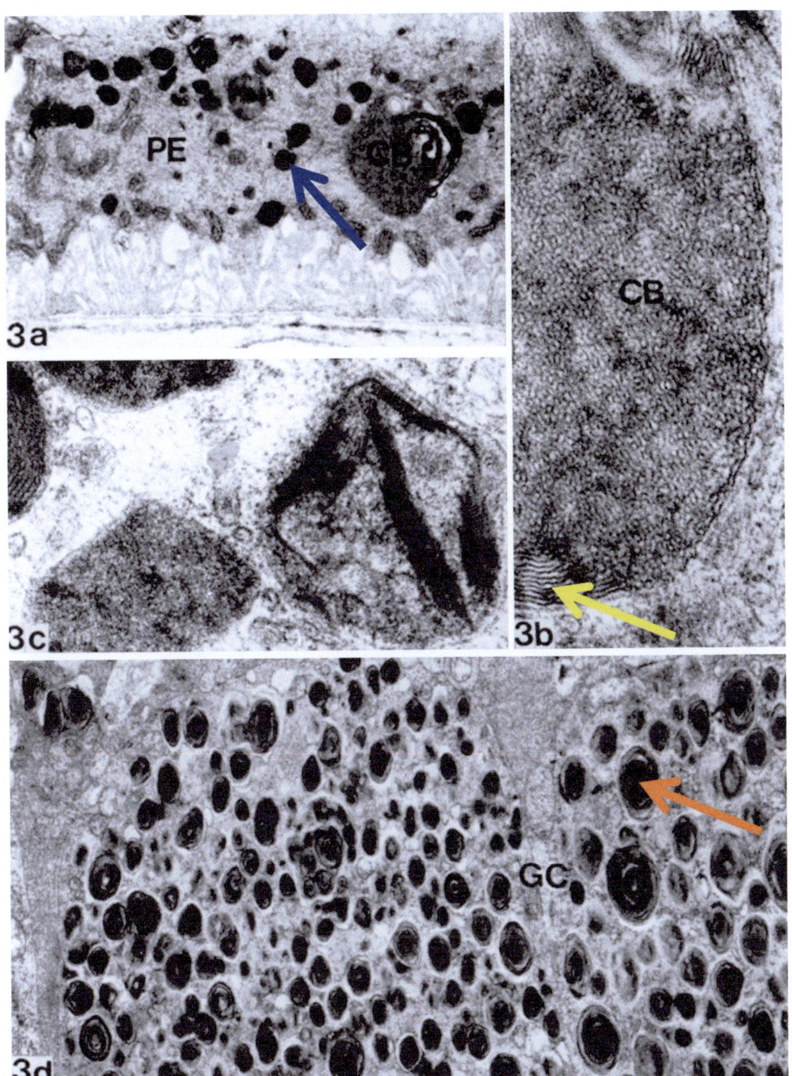

Fig. 3.3 Electron micrograph of a rat exposed to chloroquine 75 mg/kg for 16 weeks. (**a**) The retinal pigment epithelial cell (PE) contains a crystalloid body (CB), which is presumed to represent a lysosomal structure distended with indigestible membranous lipid debris, and numerous other lysosomes (*blue arrow*) that resemble those of control animals. (**b**) A higher magnification view of a crystalloid body. A nidus of residual disc material remains (*yellow arrow*) but most has been digested to a homogenous matrix. (**c**) Higher magnification view of enlarged RPE lysosomes containing some linear and concentric bands of indigestible membranous material. (**d**) A myriad of multilamellated lysosomal inclusions (*orange arrow*) in ganglion cells. Reproduced with permission from Drenckhahn [127]

cells are most sensitive to toxicity. In one report, the earliest damage occurred in the ganglion cell and inner plexiform layer (IPL), later involving photoreceptors (Fig. 3.3) [126, 127]. In another, there was concomitant damage to ganglion cells, RPE, and photoreceptors [128]. Rats with chloroquine retinopathy show an increase in lysosomal-associated organelles as well as immunoreactivity to amyloid precursor protein, amyloid β protein, apolipoprotein E, ubiquitin, and cathepsin D that colocalizes with the damaged ganglion cells [126, 129]. Spiral membranes develop in photoreceptors and inner nuclear layer (INL) cells of albino rats a few days after ganglion cell damage is noted [49]. Multilamellated bodies occur internal to the external limiting membrane of photoreceptors [127]. At the same time, an increased number of lysosomes and close packed membranes are noted in the apical cytoplasm of RPE cells [49]. These were fewer than the inclusions found in the ganglion cells [127]. Autophagic

granules developed in cones but not rods in a rat model of chloroquine retinopathy, suggesting a preferential damaging effect of chloroquine on cones [129]. Pathologic changes are seen in both albino and pigmented rat models, implying that binding of chloroquine to melanin is not critical in the pathophysiology of the toxicity [22].

Pathological Synonyms

Although many authors report lamellar lipid-based structures in pathological studies of 4AQR and other cytopathies associated with 4AQ toxicity, they use different terms for the same structures. Depending on the report, one may encounter the terms membranous cytoplasmic bodies (MCBs), lamelliform bodies, myeloid bodies, myelin bodies, lamellar inclusions, curvilinear cytoplasmic bodies, and curvilinear tubules. These probably all refer to the same thing. In this chapter, the terms used by the authors have been retained.

Pathological results may depend on the dose and route of drug administered in the same animal model [130]. In a mouse model of chloroquine retinopathy in which chloroquine was administered enterally in drinking water at 1.2 mg/mL for 6 months, damage was found only in ganglion cells [131]. In a pigmented mouse model in which 10 mg/kg of chloroquine was administered intraperitoneally for 62 days there was destruction of photoreceptors (PRs), IPL, RPE, and Muller cells. In this study, MCBs accumulated in cells of the inner retina [130].

In both pigmented and albino rat models of chloroquine toxicity, the number and size of lysosomes in bipolar and ganglion cells have increased [132]. This was not the case with the RPE. The rats developed MCBs in the cytoplasm of bipolar cells, ganglion cells, and Muller cells, but not photoreceptors [22, 132]. Dog, cat, and mouse models of chloroquine toxicity also developed MCBs occurring as early as 3 days after beginning drug ingestion [132]. The MCBs are thought to represent lipids and phospholipids inappropriately accumulated because of decreased activity of degradative enzymes contained in lysosomes [112]. There is some controversy regarding whether myeloid bodies and

phagosomes containing lamellar inclusions are the same or not [133].

In a cat model in which toxic doses of chloroquine were administered orally for 50–250 days, the RPE was thickened with increased acid mucopolysaccharide accumulation [134]. Subsequently, photoreceptor atrophy was noted. Retinopathy progressed even if the drug was stopped at the first sign of retinal pigmentation clinically [134]. In a different cat model in which intravitreal chloroquine was injected, all retinal layers were lost over areas of the retina without melanin, suggesting a protective effect of melanin [49]. In yet another cat model in which 0.5 mg of chloroquine was injected intravitreally, the earliest changes were lamellar cytoplasmic inclusions within ganglion cells and shortened photoreceptor outer segments that were disoriented relative to the underlying RPE [133]. Subsequently, similar lamellar inclusions formed in the RPE whether or not the photoreceptors overlay pigmented or nonpigmented pigment epithelium [133].

In a pigmented rabbit model of chloroquine retinopathy, the earliest histopathologic changes occurred in photoreceptors and RPE, with later changes occurring in the inner retina [101].

The photoreceptor outer segment discs lost their regular structure and mitochondria were swollen in photoreceptors and Muller cells [101].

In a rhesus monkey model of chloroquine retinopathy, the choroid, RPE, ciliary body, and iris showed preferential accumulation of drug compared to the optic nerve, lens, and cornea [48]. The common denominator among the tissues with higher chloroquine concentration was the presence of melanin which binds avidly to the drug [48]. The site of greatest histologic damage in the rhesus model was the perifoveal retina [48]. Initially the ganglion cells are damaged, and later the photoreceptors and RPE [48, 129]. Within 3 months, ganglion cells accumulated MCBs (elsewhere and in other models termed myeloid bodies, or curvilinear cytoplasmic bodies). Subsequently, the ganglion cells developed vacuolated cytoplasm and shrank. After 1 year of toxic chloroquine intake the photoreceptor layer began to degenerate with pyknosis of photoreceptor outer nuclei. After 2 years the RPE began to atrophy. During this time, there were no clinical fundus changes and the ERG was unchanged [48].

The sequence of changes was the same when a lower dose with slower onset of toxicity was used. After retinal damage was manifest, choroidal damage developed in which MCBs formed [48]. Although the ganglion cells are affected first, the photoreceptors are more severely affected because of the more severe dysfunction of lysosomes [48]. The correlation between these histopathologic observations in a primate and the selective thinning of the ganglion cell layer (GCL) and IPL complex in humans exposed to hydroxychloroquine without otherwise observable retinopathy is compelling evidence that this may be the earliest site of toxicity within the retina [135, 136, 137].

Proportions of abnormalities differ by model too. In the rhesus monkey model, myeloid bodies were a more prominent component of the histopathology, whereas swollen mitochondria and disorganized photoreceptor outer segments dominated in the rabbit model [48, 101]. In a bovine RPE model, chloroquine raised the pH of RPE cells and induced increased accumulation of rod outer segments within RPE lysosomes [129].

There are no anatomic features of the perifoveal RPE that have been hypothesized to explain the particular susceptibility of this zone to toxicity [138]. However, the greater number of ganglion cells in the affected zone and the greater concentration of luteal pigment are correlations that might warrant further study.

Hypotheses for the Sequential Changes of 4-Aminoquinoline Retinopathy

The maculocentricity of 4AQR, its horizontally elliptical shape, typical dimensions (see Chap. 6), tendency to begin inferiorly, and annular characteristic have led to speculations about relevant factors, including

1. Xanthophyll distribution [139]
2. Foveal avascular zone border
3. Ganglion cell distribution [140]
4. Effects of age on GCL thickness [140]
5. Regional distribution of lipofuscin
6. Asymmetrical exposure of the perifovea to blue light
7. Distribution of rods and cones (see Chap. 1)

No testable hypothesis tying any of these factors to a pathophysiological pathway has yet been advanced.

3.7   Human Pathology

A pathological study of an eye from a patient exposed to chloroquine without clinically recognized retinopathy showed cytoplasmic inclusions most prominently in the ganglion cells, with lesser accumulations in IPL, INL, and RPE. Minimal PR loss was found [141].

The cornea of a 58-year-old woman who was treated with chloroquine 750 mg/day for 1 year followed by 250 mg/day for 5 years is shown in Fig. 3.4. Her eyes were examined pathologically when she died of an accident 1 year after chloroquine was discontinued due to retinopathy. The basal layer of the corneal epithelium had swollen, pale staining cytoplasm. The nuclei were enlarged and vesicular.

In human cases of chloroquine retinopathy, destruction of rods and cones has been described with migration of pigment-laden macrophages into the outer retina (Fig. 3.5) [141, 143–146]. The outer nuclear layer was destroyed in two cases [144, 146]. In one case reported, the photoreceptors of the fovea centralis were relatively spared [144]. The anterior segment and choroid are normal in one case, but in a case with typical chloroquine keratopathy there were hyperplastic basal epithelial cells with large leptochromatic nuclei [144, 146]. Retinal vessels, ganglion cells, and the INL were normal to light microscopy [144]. Electron microscopic studies showed MCBs and short curvilinear tubules (C-tubes) that were hypothesized to be remnants of smooth endoplasmic reticulum captured at different phases of autophagy. MCBs and C-tubes were distributed

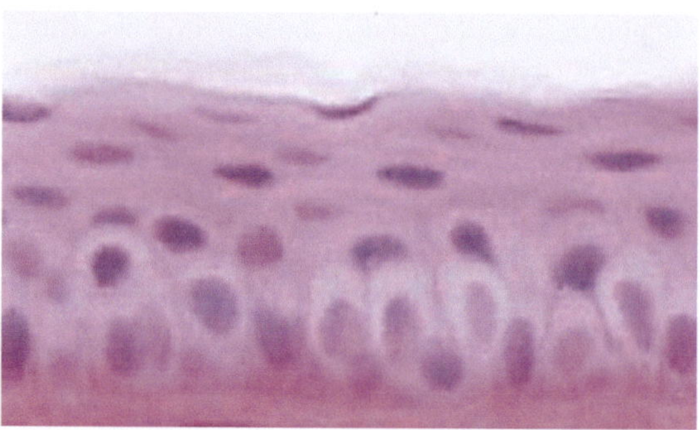

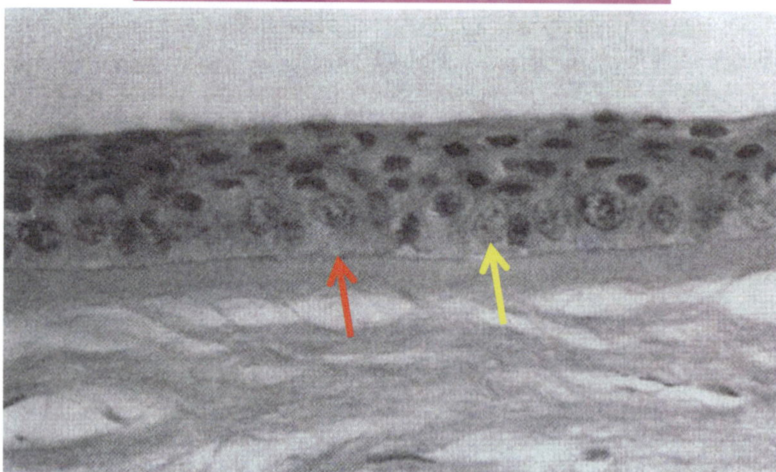

Fig. 3.4 Corneal epithelial changes in a patient with both chloroquine keratopathy and retinopathy. The *top panel* shows a normal control cornea. The *bottom panel* shows the cornea from the patient with keratopathy. The *red arrow* indicates the swollen, pale staining cytoplasm. The *yellow arrow* indicates the vesicular nuclear changes. Reproduced with permission from Lloyd [142]

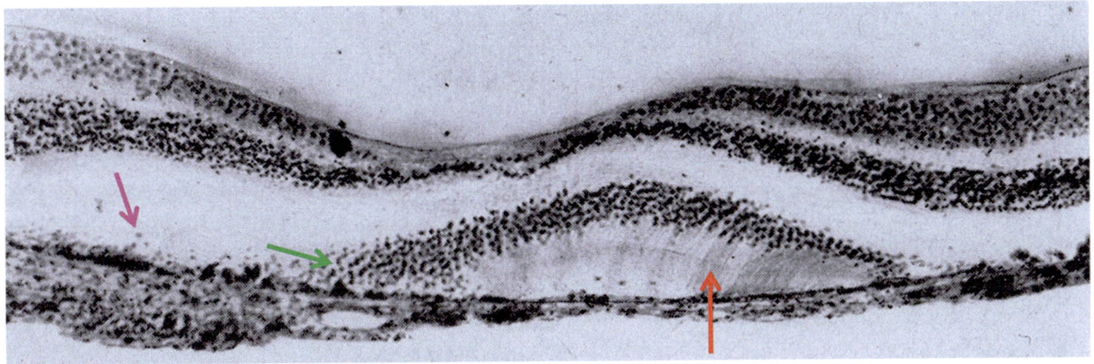

Fig. 3.5 Histopathology of advanced chloroquine retinopathy. This patient was noted to have a bull's-eye maculopathy. The foveal photoreceptors were spared (*red arrow*), but the perifoveal photoreceptors were destroyed. The outer nuclear layer was maintained centrally but was destroyed more peripherally than the border of loss of photoreceptors (*green arrow*). Pigment migration into the outer plexiform layer (*pink arrow*) was noted. Reprinted with permission from Bernstein [143]

widely throughout the retina, but were densest in the GCL [141]. In the RPE, C-tubes but not MCBs were found [141]. C-tubes were seen in the smooth muscle cells of the ciliary muscle and in the striated muscle of the recti [141]. Similar changes have been seen in cardiac muscle of patients with hydroxychloroquine and chloroquine cardiomyopathy [147]. At least with respect to cardiac tissue, follow-up biopsies after cessation of chloroquine ingestion suggest the potential for tissue recovery. After 7 months without chloroquine ingestion, a follow-up biopsy showed that a lower percentage of myocytes were affected [147].

Chloroquine myopathy and cardiomyopathy are similar and show similar changes to those seen in 4AQR. Affected muscle cells show vacuolar degeneration with myelin figures thought to be derived from lysosomes [111]. Mitochondrial changes include an increase in electron density by electron microscopy and distortion of cristae [111]. In histopathological investigations, chloroquine skeletal myopathy features autophagic vacuoles that are filled with periodic acid–Schiff-staining material thought to be glycogen [117, 121, 148]. These vacuoles are 80 nm to 2 μm in diameter [120].

Chloroquine inhibits hexokinase, an enzyme mediating glycogen metabolism [117]. Mitochondrial vacuolization with sequestration of glycogen has also been described (Fig. 3.6). It is thought that the glycogen derives from cytoplasmic autophagy because there is no plasma glycogen due to the existence of plasma amylase [148]. The material within autophagic vacuoles undergoes further degradation, resulting in double-layered membranes that form curvilinear myeloid bodies identical to those seen in retinopathy and in Batten's disease [118–120, 123, 149]. This material is autofluorescent, stains with Sudan black B and is considered to be composed of phospholipids derived from sarcoplasmic reticulum, especially phosphatidyl choline, phosphatidyl ethanolamine, phosphatidyl inositol, and bis-(monoacyl-glycero)-phosphate [118, 121, 150]. It is hypothesized that this material is responsible for the increased fundus autofluorescence seen in chloroquine and hydroxychloroquine retinopathy [151]. Myeloid bodies can be seen in muscle biopsies taken years after the cessation of chloroquine in a patient with myopathy, and a certain amount seems compatible with normal muscle function [118]. Red muscle fibers (type 1, or tonic) are preferentially affected compared to white muscle fibers (type 2, or phasic), perhaps due to binding of chloroquine to myohemoglobin that is found in increased concentrations in red muscle fibers compared to white fibers [119, 120, 125, 150].

Aside from myocytes and retinal cells, myelin bodies have been described in a mouse

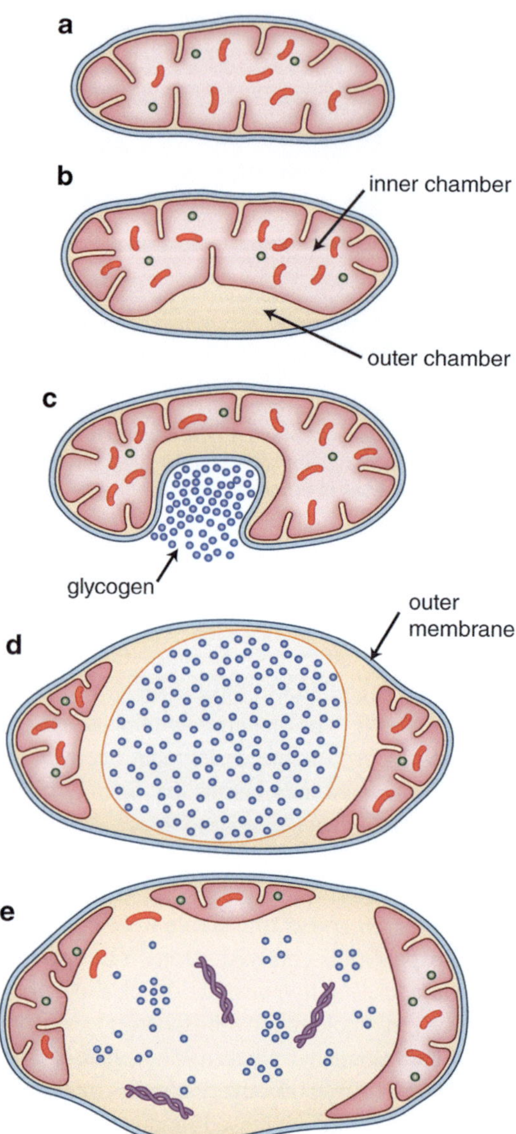

Fig. 3.6 Hypothesized effects of chloroquine in toxic concentrations on a mitochondrion. (**a**) Normal mitochondrion. (**b**) Separation of inner and outer mitochondrial membranes. Two spaces are defined, an inner chamber and an outer chamber. (**c**) Invagination of glycogen-containing cytoplasm. (**d**) Glycogen-containing cytoplasm surrounded by the pinched-off outer mitochondrial membrane contained within the outer chamber. (**e**) Breakdown of the outer mitochondrial membrane surrounding the glycogen vacuole with release of glycogen into the outer chamber. Data from Mastaglia [120]

macrophage cell culture model of chloroquine toxicity [123]. In cell culture models, development of autophagic vacuoles is dose dependent and reversible [150]. The autophagic vacuoles also have increased acid phosphatase activity [119]. In a chicken model, chloroquine was associated with development of lamelliform structures in the cardiac sarcoplam and subsequent vacuolar myopathy [152]. In a pig model of chloroquine toxicity, membranous and granular cytoplasmic inclusions were induced in neurons, striated myocytes, as well as endothelial and epithelial cells [83]. In a rat model of chloroquine toxicity, myocytes developed vacuolization and myeloid bodies [83].

3.8 Summary of Key Points

- Toxicity of 4AQs is predictable and dose dependent. It is not idiosyncratic. There is no evidence that the toxicologic and pathologic changes induced by chloroquine and hydroxychloroquine differ.
- There may be individual factors for susceptibility, such as a genetic profile.
- Toxicity is related to the 4AQ nucleus with structure–toxicity relationships related to the side chains of the nucleus.
- Blood concentrations of 4AQs less than 2.2×10^{-6} M/L are associated with a risk of side effects less than 10 %.
- A daily dose of chloroquine of 3 mg/kg based on IBW is associated with a low risk of retinopathy or other toxicity.
- A daily dose of hydroxychloroquine of 6.5 mg/kg based on IBW is associated with a very low risk of retinopathy or other toxicity.
- The most important mechanism of retinopathy and other cytopathies is impaired lysosomal degradation of phospholipids, although many other pathways may contribute.
- Keratopathy is approximately 40 times as prevalent with chloroquine as hydroxychloroquine and does not imply an increased risk of retinopathy or a need to stop the drug.
- Chloroquine is approximately twice as toxic as hydroxychloroquine on a weight basis.
- More than ten nonocular side effects of 4AQs have been reported. Of these, gastrointestinal upset is the most common, occurring in approximately 12 % of persons who take these drugs.

- The pathology of 4AQR in animal models is notable for the accumulation of myeloid bodies in multiple types of cells. The sequence of pathological changes depends on the animal model used. In primates, myeloid bodies occur first in perifoveal ganglion cells, followed by photoreceptors and RPE. Perifoveal photoreceptors and RPE cells are eventually lost, with retention of foveal layers until the most advanced stage of retinopathy.
- The pathology of 4AQ myopathy resembles 4AQR in the presence of myeloid bodies. In addition, vacuolization of mitochondria is prominent.

References

1. Carr RE, Henkind P, Rothfield N, Siegel IM. Ocular toxicity of antimalarial drugs-long-term follow-up. Am J Ophthalmol. 1968;66:738–44.
2. Shroyer NF, Lewis RA, Lupski JR. Analysis of the ABCR (ABCA4) gene in 4-aminoquinoline retinopathy: Is retinal toxicity by chloroquine and hydroxychloroquine related to Stargardt disease? Am J Ophthalmol. 2001;131:761–6.
3. Jones SK. Ocular toxicity and hydroxychloroquine: guidelines for screening. Br J Dermatol. 1999; 140:3–7.
4. Bacon P, Spalton DJ, Smith SE. Blindness from quinine toxicity. Br J Ophthalmol. 1988;72:219–24.
5. Canning CR, Hague S. Ocular quinine toxicity. Br J Ophthalmol. 1988;72:23–6.
6. Thompson PE, Webel LM. 4-Aminoquinolines. Antimalarial agents. 1972;150–196.
7. Banks CN. Melanin: blackguard or red herring? Another look at chloroquine retinopathy. Aust N Z J Ophthalmol. 1987;15:365–70.
8. Shearer RV, Dubois EL. Ocular changes induced by long-term hydroxychloroquine (Plaquenil) therapy. Am J Ophthalmol. 1967;64:245–52.
9. Browning DJ. Bull's-eye maculopathy associated with quinacrine therapy for malaria. Am J Ophthalmol. 2004;137:577–9.
10. Rothfield N. Efficacy of antimalarials in systemic lupus erythematosus. Am J Med. 1988;85:53–6.
11. Wallace DJ, Gudsoorkar VS, Weisman MH, Venuturupalli SR. New insights into mechanisms of therapeutic effects of antimalarial agents in SLE. Nat Rev Rheumatol. 2012;8:522–33.
12. Yoon YH, Cho KS, Hwang JJ, et al. Induction of lysosomal dilatation, arrested autophagy, and cell death by chloroquine in cultured ARPE-19 cells. Invest Ophthalmol Vis Sci. 2010;51:6030–7.
13. McChesney EQ, Fitch CD. 4-Aminoquinolines. In: Peters W, Richards WHG, editors. Antimalarial drugs II. Current antimalarials and new drug developments. Berlin: Springer; 1984. p. 3–60.
14. Mackenzie AH. An appraisal of chloroquine. Arthritis Rheum. 1970;13:280–91.
15. Tett S, Cutler D, Day R. Antimalarials in rheumatic diseases. Baillieres Clin Rheumatol. 1990;4:467–89.
16. Cann HM, Verhulst HL. Fatal acute chloroquine poisoning in children. Pediatrics. 1961;27:95–102.
17. Titus EO. Recent developments in the understanding of the pharmacokinetics and mechanism of action of chloroquine. Ther Drug Monit. 1989;11:369–79.
18. Frisk-Holmberg M, Bergkvist Y, Domeij-Nyberg B, Hellstrom L, Jansson R. Chloroquine serum concentration and side effects: evidence for dose dependent kinetics. Clin Pharmacol Ther. 1979;25:345–50.
19. Munster T, Gibbs JP, Shen D, Baethge BA, Botstein GR, Caldwell J, Dietz F, Ettlinger R, Golden HE, Lindsley H, et al. Hydroxychloroquine concentration-response relationships in patients with rheumatoid arthritis. Arthritis Rheum. 2002;46:1460–9.
20. Laaksonen AL, Koskiahde V, Juva K. Dosage of antimalarial drugs for children with juvenile rheumatoid arthritis and systemic lupus erythematosus. A clinical study with determination of serum concentrations of chloroquine and hydroxychloroquine. Scand J Rheumatol. 1974;3:103–8.
21. Frisk-Holmberg M, Bergqvist Y. Chloroquine disposition in man. Br J Clin Pharmacol. 1982;14: 624P–6.
22. Abraham R, Hendy RJ. Irreversible lysosomal damage induced by chloroquine in the retinae of pigmented and albino rats. Exp Mol Pathol. 1970;12: 185–200.
23. Bruce-Chwatt LJ. Chloroquine blindness? Lancet. 1968;2:1039.
24. Marmor MF, Carr RE, Easterbrook M, et al. Recommendations on screening for chloroquine and hydroxychloroquine retinopathy. Ophthalmology. 2002;109:1377–82.
25. Marmor MF. New American Academy of Ophthalmology recommendations on screening for hydroxychloroquine retinopathy. Arthritis Rheum. 2003;48:1764–70.
26. Schwartz SG, Mieler WF. Retinal and choroidal manifestations of systemic medications. In: Arevalo JF, editor. Retinal and choroidal manifestations of selected systemic diseases. New York: Springer; 2013. p. 479–92.
27. Missner S, Kellner U. Comparison of different screening methods for chloroquine/ hydroxychloroquine retinopathy: multifocal electroretinography, color vision, perimetry, ophthalmoscopy, and fluorescein angiography. Graefes Arch Clin Exp Ophthalmol. 2012;250:319–25.
28. Fung AE, Samy CN, Rosenfeld PJ. Optical coherence tomography findings in hydroxychloroquine and chloroquine-associated maculopathy. Retinal Cases Brief Rep. 2007;1:128–30.
29. Labriola LT, Jeng D, Fawzi AA. Retinal toxicity of systemic medications. Int Ophthalmol Clin. 2012;52:149–66.

30. Ehrenfeld M, Nesher R, Merin S. Delayed-onset chloroquine retinopathy. Br J Ophthalmol. 1986;70:281–3.

31. Mackenzie AH. Dose refinements in long-term therapy of rheumatoid arthritis with antimalarials. Am J Med. 1983;75:40–5.

32. Fleck BW, Bell AL, Mitchell JD, Thomson BJ, Hurst NP, Nuki G. Screening for antimalarial maculopathy in rheumatology clinics. Br Med J. 1985;291:782–5.

33. Cox NH, Paterson WD. Ocular toxicity of antimalarials in dermatology: a survey of current practice. Br J Dermatol. 1994;131:878–82.

34. Elman A, Gullberg R, Nillson E, Rendahl I, Wachtmeister L. Chloroquine retinopathy in patients with rheumatoid arthritis. Scand J Rheumatol. 1975;5:161–6.

35. Easterbrook M. Ocular effects and safety of antimalarial agents. Am J Med. 1988;85:23–9.

36. Scherbel AL. Use of synthetic antimalarial drugs and other agents for rheumatoid arthritis: historic and therapeutic perspectives. Am J Med. 1983;75:1–4.

37. Sundelin SP, Terman A. Different effects of chloroquine and hydroxychloroquine on lysosomal function in cultured retinal pigment epithelial cells. APMIS. 2002;110:481–9.

38. Michaelides M, Stover NB, Francis PJ, Weleber RG. Retinal toxicity associated with hydroxychloroquine and chloroquine: risk factors, screening, and progression despite cessation of therapy. Arch Ophthalmol. 2011;129:30–9.

39. Browning DJ. Hydroxychloroquine and chloroquine retinopathy: screening for drug toxicity. Am J Ophthalmol. 2002;133:649–56.

40. Levy GD, Munz SJ, Paschal J, Cohen HB, Prince KJ, Peterson T. Incidence of hydroxychloroquine retinopathy in 1,207 patients in a large multicenter outpatient practice. Arthritis Rheum. 1997;40:1482–6.

41. Mavrikakis I, Sfikakis PP, Mavrikakis E, Rougas K, Nikolaou A, Kostopoulos C, Mavrikakis M. The incidence of irreversible retinal toxicity in patients treated with hydroxychloroquine—a reappraisal. Ophthalmology. 2003;110:1321–6.

42. Lai TYY, Chan WM, Li H, Lai RYK, Lam DSC. Multifocal electroretinographic changes in patients receiving hydroxychloroquine therapy. Am J Ophthalmol. 2005;140:794–807.

43. Albert DA, Debois LKL, Lu KF. Antimalarial ocular toxicity, a critical appraisal. J Clin Rheumatol. 1998;4:57–62.

44. Mackenzie AH. Antimalarial drugs for rheumatoid arthritis. Am J Med. 1983;75:48–58.

45. Maksymowych W, Russell AS. Antimalarials in rheumatology: efficacy and safety. Semin Arthritis Rheum. 1987;16:206–21.

46. Leblanc B, Jezequei S, Davies T, Hanton G, Taradach C. Binding of drugs to eye melanin is not predictive of ocular toxicity. Regul Toxicol Pharmacol. 1998;28:124–32.

47. Duncker G, Bredehorn T. Chloroquine-induced lipidosis in the rat retina: functional and morphological changes after withdrawal of the drug. Graefes Arch Clin Exp Ophthalmol. 1996;234:378–81.

48. Rosenthal AR, Kolb H, Bergsma D, Huxsoll D, Hopkins JL. Chloroquine retinopathy in the rhesus monkey. Invest Ophthalmol Vis Sci. 1978;17:1158–75.

49. Ivanina TA, Zueva MV, Lebedeva MN, Bogoslovsky AI, Bunin AJ. Ultrastructural alterations in rat and cat retina and pigment epithelium induced by chloroquine. Graefes Arch Clin Exp Ophthalmol. 1983;220:32–8.

50. Mcchesney EW. Animal toxicity and pharmacokinetics of hydroxychloroquine sulfate. Am J Med. 1983;75:11–8.

51. Sparrow JR. Lipofuscin of the retinal pigment epithelium. In: Holz FG, Schmitz-Valckenberg S, Spaide RF, Bird AC, editors. Atlas of fundus autofluorescence imaging. Berlin: Springer; 2007. p. 3–16.

52. Dillon J, Wang Z, Avalle LB, Gaillard ER. The photochemical oxidation of A2E results in the formation of a 5, 8, 6', 8'-bis-furanoid oxide. Exp Eye Res. 2004;79:537–42.

53. Jang CH, Choi JH, Byun MS, Jue DM. Chloroquine inhibits production of TNF-alpha, IL-1 beta, and IL-6 from lipopolysaccharide-stimulated human monocytes/ macrophages by different modes. Rheumatology. 2006;45:703–10.

54. Eldred GE, Lasky MR. Retinal age pigments generated by self-assembling lysosomotropic detergents. Nature. 1993;361:724–6.

55. Mititelu M, Wong BJ, Brenner M, Bryar PJ, Jampol LM, Fawzi AA. Progression of hydroxychloroquine toxic effects after drug therapy cessation. New evidence from multimodal imaging. Arch Ophthalmol. 2013;131:1187–97.

56. Zeller RW, Deering D. Corneal complication of chloroquine (Aralen) Phosphate therapy. JAMA. 1958;168:2263–4.

57. Calkins LL. Corneal epithelial changes occurring during chloroquine (Aralen) therapy. AMA Arch Ophthalmol. 1958;60:981–8.

58. Hobbs HE, Calnan CD. Visual disturbances with antimalarial drugs, with particular reference to chloroquine keratopathy. AMA Arch Dermatol. 1959;80:557–63.

59. Mason CG. Ocular accumulation and toxicity of certain systemically administered drugs. J Toxicol Environ Health. 1977;2:977–95.

60. Henkind P, Rothfield NF. Ocular abnormalities in patients treated with synthetic antimalarial drugs. New Engl J Med. 1963;269:434–9.

61. Hobbs HE, Calnan CD. The ocular complications of chloroquine therapy. Lancet. 1958;1:1207–9.

62. Graniewski-Wijnands HS, Van Lith GHM, Vijfvinkel-Bruinenga S. Ophthalmological examination of

patients taking chloroquine. Doc Ophthalmol. 1979; 48:231–4.

63. Grierson DJ. Hydroxychloroquine and visual screening in a rheumatology outpatient clinic. Ann Rheum Dis. 1997;56:188–90.

64. Yam JCS, Kwok AKH. Ocular toxicity of hydroxychloroquine. Hong Kong Med J. 2006;12:294–304.

65. Hobbs HE, Eadie SP, Somerville F. Ocular lesions after treatment with chloroquine. Br J Ophthalmol. 1961;45:284–97.

66. Smith JL. Ocular complications of rheumatic fever and rheumatoid arthritis. Am J Ophthalmol. 1957;43:575–82.

67. Easterbrook M. Is corneal deposition of antimalarial any indication of retinal toxicity? Can J Ophthalmol. 1990;25:249–51.

68. Easterbrook M. The ocular safety of hydroxychloroquine. Semin Arthritis Rheum. 1993;23:62–7.

69. Weise EE, Yannuzzi LA. Ring maculopathies mimicking chloroquine retinopathy. Am J Ophthalmol. 1974;78:204–10.

70. Reed H, Campbell AA. Central scotomata following chloroquine therapy. Can Med Assoc J. 1962;86:176–8.

71. Scherbel AL, Mackenzie AH, Nousek JE, Atdjian M. Ocular lesions in rheumatoid arthritis and related disorders with particular reference to retinopathy—a study of 741 patients treated with and without chloroquine drugs. New Engl J Med. 1965;273:360–6.

72. Easterbrook M. Screening for antimalarial toxicity. Can J Ophthalmol. 1993;28:51–2.

73. Hobbs HE, Sorsby A, Freedman A. Retinopathy following chloroquine therapy. Lancet. 1959;2:478.

74. Percival SPB, Behrman J. Ophthalmological safety of chloroquine. Br J Ophthalmol. 1969;53:101–9.

75. Araiza-Casillas R, Cardenas F, Morales Y, Cardiel MH. Factors associated with chloroquine-induced retinopathy in rheumatic diseases. Lupus. 2004;13:119–24.

76. Marks JS, Power BJ. Is chloroquine obsolete in treatment of rheumatic disease? Lancet. 1979;1:371–3.

77. Mantyjarvi M. Hydroxychloroquine treatment and the eye. Scand J Rheumatol. 1985;14:171–4.

78. Elder M, Rahman AMA. Early paracentral visual field loss in patients taking hydroxychloroquine. Arch Ophthalmol. 2006;124:1729–33.

79. Teoh SC B, Lim J, Koh A, Lim T, Fu E. Abnormalities on the multifocal electroretinogram may precede clinical signs of hydroxychloroquine retinotoxicity. Eye (Lond). 2006;20:129–32.

80. Bunch TW, O'Duffy JD. Disease modifying drugs for progressive rheumatoid arthritis. Mayo Clin Proc. 1980;55:161–79.

81. Bernstein HN. Ophthalmologic considerations and testing in patients receiving long-term antimalarial therapy. Am J Med. 1983;75:25–34.

82. Lozier JR, Friedlander MH. Complications of antimalarial therapy. Int Ophthalmol Clin. 1989;29:172–8.

83. Dubois EL. Antimalarials in the management of discoid and systemic lupus erythematosus. Semin Arthritis Rheum. 1978;8:33–51.

84. Fuld H. Retinopathy following chloroquine therapy. Lancet. 1959;2:617–8.

85. Mcchesney EW, Banks Jr WF, Sullivan DJ. Metabolism of chloroquine and hydroxychloroquine in albino and pigmented rats. Toxicol Appl Pharm. 1965;7:627–36.

86. Easterbrook M. An ophthalmological view on the efficacy and safety of chloroquine versus hydroxychloroquine. J Rheumatol. 1999;26:1866–7.

87. Block JA. Hydroxychloroquine and retinal safety. Lancet. 1998;351:771.

88. Rynes RI. Antimalarial drugs in the treatment of rheumatological diseases. Br J Rheumatol. 1997;36:799–805.

89. Rynes R. Ophthalmologic considerations in using antimalarials in the United States. Lupus. 1996;5:S73–4.

90. Spalton DJ. Retinopathy and antimalarial drugs-the British experience. Lupus. 1996;5:S70–2.

91. Finbloom DS, Silver K, Newsome DA, Gunkel R. Comparison of hydroxychloroquine and chloroquine use and the development of retinal toxicity. J Rheumatol. 1985;12:692–4.

92. Goldman L, Preston RH. Reactions to chloroquine observed during the treatment of various dermatologic disorders. Am J Trop Med Hyg. 1957;6:654–7.

93. Bothwell B, Furst DE. Hydroxychloroquine. In: Day RO, Furst DE, editors. Antirheumatic therapy: actions and outcomes. Basel: Piet L.C.M. van Riel and Barry Bresnihan; 2005. p. 81–92.

94. Raines MF, Bhargava SK, Rosen ES. The blood-retinal barrier in chloroquine retinopathy. Invest Ophthalmol Vis Sci. 1989;30:1726–31.

95. Blomquist PH. Screening for hydroxychloroquine toxicity. Comp Ophthalmol Update. 2000;1:245–50.

96. Arden GB, Kolb H. Antimalarial therapy and early retinal changes in patients with rheumatoid arthritis. Br Med J. 1966;1:270–3.

97. Tzekov R. Ocular toxicity due to chloroquine and hydroxychloroquine: electrophysiological and visual function correlates. Doc Ophthalmol. 2005;110:111–20.

98. Schultz KR, Gilman AL. The lysosomotropic amines, chloroquine and hydroxychloroquine: a potentially novel therapy for graft-versus-host disease. Leuk Lymphoma. 1997;24:201–10.

99. Tanenbaum L, Tuffanelli DL. Antimalarial agents: chloroquine, hydroxychloroquine, and quinacrine. Arch Dermatol. 1980;116:587–91.

100. Rynes RI. Ophthalmologic safety of long-term hydroxychloroquine sulfate treatment. Am J Med. 1983;75:35–9.

101. el-Sayed NK, Abdel-Khalek LR, Gaafar KM, Hanafy LK. Profiles of serum proteins and free amino acids associated with chloroquine retinopathy. Acta Ophthalmol Scand. 1998;76:422–30.

102. Wang C, Fortin PR, Li Y, Panaritis T, Gans M, Esdaile JM. Discontinuation of antimalarial drugs in systemic lupus erythematosus. J Rheumatol. 1999;26:808–15.

103. Petri M. Hydroxychloroquine use in the Baltimore Lupus Cohort: effects on lipids, glucose and thrombosis. Lupus. 1996;5:S16–22.

104. van Jaarsveld CHM, Jahangier ZN, Jacobs JWG, Blaauw AAM, van Albada-Kuipers GA, ter Borg EJ, Brus HLM, Schenk Y, van der Veen MJ, Bijlsma JWJ, Rheumatic Research Foundation. Toxicity of anti-rheumatic drugs in a randomized clinical trial of early rheumatoid arthritis. Rheumatology. 2000;39:1374–82.

105. Freedman A, Steinberg VL. Chloroquine in rheumatoid arthritis. A double blindfold trial of treatment for one year. Ann Rheum Dis. 1960;19:243–50.

106. Runge LA. Risk/benefit analysis of hydroxychloroquine sulfate treatment in rheumatoid arthritis. Am J Med. 1983;75:52–6.

107. Scull E. Chloroquine and hydroxychloroquine therapy in rheumatoid arthritis. Arthritis Rheum. 1962;5:30–6.

108. Morand EF, McCloud PI, Littlejohn GO. Continuation of long term treatment with hydroxychloroquine in systemic lupus erythematosus and rheumatoid arthritis. Ann Rheum Dis. 1992;51:1318–21.

109. Wilson W. Retinopathy following chloroquine therapy. Br J Ophthalmol. 1961;45:756–8.

110. Percival SPB, Meanock I. Chloroquine: ophthalmological safety and clinical assessment in rheumatoid arthritis. Br Med J. 1968;3:579–84.

111. Hughes JT, Esiri M, Oxbury JM, Whitty CWM. Chloroquine myopathy. Q J Med. 1971;40:85–93.

112. Estes ML, Ewing-Wilson D, Chou SM, Mitsumoto H, Hanson M, Shirey E, Ratliff NM. Chloroquine neuromyotoxicity: clinical and pathological perspective. Am J Med. 1987;82:447–55.

113. Seckin U, Ozoran K, Ikinciogullari A, Borman P, Bostan EE. Hydroxychloroquine ototoxicity in a patient with rheumatoid arthritis. Rheumatol Int. 2000;19:203–4.

114. Ben-Zvi I, Kivity S, Langevitz P. Hydroxychloroquine: from malaria to autoimmunity. Clin Rev Allergy Immunol. 2012;42:145–53.

115. Rollo IM. Drugs used in the chemotherapy of malaria. In: Goodman LS, Gilman A, editors. The pharmacological basis of therapeutics. New York: Macmillan; 1975. p. 1045–68.

116. Aguayo AJ, Hudgson P. Observations on the short-term effects of chloroquine on skeletal muscle; an experimental study in the rabbit. J Neurol Sci. 1970;11:301–25.

117. Eadie MJ, Ferrier TM. Chloroquine myopathy. J Neurol Neurosurg Psychiatry. 1966;29:331–7.

118. Neville HE, Maundry-Sewry CA, McDougall J, Sewell JR, Dubowitz V. Chloroquine-induced cytosomes with curvilinear profiles in muscle. Muscle Nerve. 1979;2:376–81.

119. Macdonald RD, Engel AG. Experimental chloroquine myopathy. J Neuropathol Exp Neurol. 1970;29:479–99.

120. Mastaglia FL, Papadimitriou JM, Dawkins RL, Beveridge B. Vacuolar myopathy associated with chloroquine, lupus erythematosus and thymoma; report of a case with unusual mitochondrial changes and lipid accumulation in muscle. J Neurol Sci. 1977;34:315–28.

121. Rewcastle NB, Humphrey JG. Vacuolar myopathy; clinical, histochemical, and microscopic study. Arch Neurol. 1965;12:570–82.

122. Begg TB, Simpson JA. Chloroquine neuromyopathy. Br Med J. 1964;1:770.

123. Fedorko ME, Hirsch JG, Cohn ZA. Autophagic vacuoles produced in vitro; I. Studies on cultured macrophages exposed to chloroquine. J Cell Biol. 1968;38:377–91.

124. Hart CW, Naunton RF. The ototoxicity of chloroquine phosphate. Arch Otolaryngol. 1964;80:407–12.

125. Smith B, O'Grady F. Experimental chloroquine myopathy. J Neurol Neurosurg Psychiat. 1966;29:255–8.

126. Yoshida T, Fukatsu R, Tsuzuki K, Aizawa Y, Hayashi Y, Sasaki N, Takamuru Y, Fujii N, Takahata N. Amyloid precursor protein, A beta and amyloid-associated proteins involved in chloroquine retinopathy in rats—immunopathological studies. Brain Res. 1997;764:283–8.

127. Drenckhahn D, Lullmann-Rauch R. Drug-induced lipidosis: differential susceptibilities of pigment epithelium and neuroretina toward several amphiphilic cationic drugs. Exp Mol Pathol. 1978;28:360–71.

128. Gaafar KM, Abdel-Khalek LR, el-Sayed NK, Ramadan GA. Lipidemic effect as a manifestation of chloroquine retinotoxicity. Arzneimittelforschung. 1995;45:1231–5.

129. Mahon GJ, Anderson HR, Gardiner TA, McFarlane S, Archer DB, Stitt AW. Chloroquine causes lysosomal dysfunction in neural retina and RPE: implications for retinopathy. Curr Eye Res. 2004;28:277–84.

130. Gaynes BI, Torczynski E, Varro Z, Grostern R, Perlman J. Retinal toxicity of chloroquine hydrochloride administered by intraperitoneal injection. J Appl Toxicol. 2008;28:895–900.

131. Hallberg A, Naeser P, Andersson A. Effects of long-term chloroquine exposure on the phospholipid metabolism of the retina and pigment epithelium of the mouse. Acta Ophthalmol Scand. 1990;68:125–30.

132. Gregory MH, Rutty DA, Wood RD. Differences in the retinotoxic action of chloroquine and phenothiazine derivatives. J Pathol. 1970;102:139–50.

133. Smith RS, Berson EL. Acute toxic effects of chloroquine on the cat retina: ultrastructural changes. Invest Ophthalmol Vis Sci. 1971;10:237–46.

134. Meier-Ruge W. Experimental investigation of the morphogenesis of chloroquine retinopathy. Arch Ophthalmol. 1965;73:540–4.

135. Bonanomi MT, Dantas NC, Medeiros FA. Retinal nerve fiber layer thickness measurements in patients using chloroquine. Clin Experiment Ophthalmol. 2006;34:130–6.

136. Pasadhika S, Fishman GA, Choi D, Shahidi M. Selective thinning of the perifoveal inner retina as an early sign of hydroxychloroquine retinal toxicity. Eye (Lond). 2010;24:756–63.

137. Pasadhika S, Fishman GA. Effects of chronic exposure to hydroxychloroquine or chloroquine on inner retinal structures. Eye (Lond). 2009;24:340–6.

138. Wolfe F, Marmor MF. Rates and predictors of hydroxychloroquine retinal toxicity in patients with rheumatoid arthritis and systemic lupus erythematosus. Arthritis Care Res. 2010;62:775–84.

139. Davies NP, Morland AB. Macular pigments: their characteristics and putative role. Prog Retin Eye Res. 2004;23:533–59.

140. Demirkaya N, van Dijk HW, van Schuppen SM, Abramoff MD, Garvin MK, Sonka M, Schlingemann RO, Verbraak FD. Effect of age on individual retinal layer thickness in normal eyes as measured with spectral-domain optical coherence tomography. Invest Ophthalmol Vis Sci. 2013;54:4934–40.

141. Ramsey MS, Fine BS. Chloroquine toxicity in the human eye-histopathologic observations by electron microscopy. Am J Ophthalmol. 1972;73:229–35.

142. Lloyd LA, Hiltz JW. Ocular complications of chloroquine therapy. Can Med Assoc J. 1965;92:508–13.

143. Bernstein HN, Ginsberg J. The pathology of chloroquine retinopathy. Arch Ophthalmol. 1964;71:238–45.

144. Wetterholm DH, Winter FC. Histopathology of chloroquine retinal toxicity. Arch Ophthalmol. 1964;71:82–7.

145. Bernstein H, Zvaifler N, Rubin M, Mansour AM. The ocular deposition of chloroquine. Invest Ophthalmol Vis Sci. 1963;2:384–92.

146. Bailey LA, Hiltz JW. Ocular complications of chloroquine therapy. Can Med Assoc J. 1965;6:508–13.

147. Ratliff NB, Estes ML, Myles JL, Shirey EK, McMahon JT. Medial intelligence-diagnosis of chloroquine cardiomyopathy by endomyocardial biopsy. New Engl J Med. 1987;316:191–3.

148. Stauber WT, Hedge AM, Trout JJ, Schottelius BA. Inhibition of lysosomal function in red and white skeletal muscles by chloroquine. Exp Neurol. 1981;71:295–306.

149. Schmalbruch H. The early changes in experimental myopathy induced by chloroquine and chlorphentermine. J Neuropathol Exp Neurol. 1980;39:65–81.

150. Trout JJ, Stauber WT, Schottelius BA. Increased autophagy in chloroquine treated tonic and phasic muscles: an alternative view. Tissue Cell. 1982;13:393–401.

151. Kellner U, Renner AB, Tillack H. Fundus autofluorescence and mfERG for early detection of retinal alterations in patients using chloroquine/hydroxychloroquine. Invest Ophthalmol Vis Sci. 2006;47:3531–8.

152. Fischer VW. Evolution of a chloroquine-induced cardiomyopathy in the chicken. Exp Mol Pathol. 1976;25:242–52.

Definitions of Hydroxychloroquine and Chloroquine Retinopathy

4

Abbreviations

4AQ	4-Aminoquinoline (chloroquine or hydroxychloroquine)
4AQR	4-Aminoquinoline retinopathy
FA	Fluorescein angiography
HC	Hydroxychloroquine
mfERG	Multifocal electroretinogram
RPE	Retinal pigment epithelium
SAP	Standard automated perimetry
SD-OCT	Spectral domain optical coherence tomography

This chapter covers the definitions of retinopathy encountered in the literature on chloroquine and hydroxychloroquine (HC) retinopathy. The name 4-aminoquinoline (4AQ) will be used to refer to both chloroquine and hydroxychloroquine. The definitions of 4-aminoquinoline retinopathy (4AQR) apply to both drugs [1]. Commonly used abbreviations in this chapter are collected in "Abbreviations" for reference. Each term will be first used in its full form, along with its abbreviation.

Confusion arises from the number and variety of definitions for hydroxychloroquine and chloroquine retinopathy [2–5]. An example has to do with whether an abnormality on an ancillary test is the same as toxicity and whether toxicity is the same as retinopathy. It has been stated that an abnormality on multifocal electroretinography or other electrodiagnostic tests is different from toxicity [6, 7]. An abnormality, in this understanding, might represent a pharmacologic effect of the drug. However, because all toxic effects of drugs are pharmacologic effects (i.e., harmful ones), the distinction amounts to a tautology. The effects of hydroxychloroquine on the multifocal electroretinogram (mfERG) are not desirable. Therefore, they represent toxicity. The clinically important issue is not the semantic one, but rather reversibility [7]. Whether one calls an effect pharmacologic, toxic, or retinopathic, what matters is whether it goes away if the drug is stopped. Because we do not know at the time the mfERG is obtained whether it is reversible or not, it is difficult to see how such a distinction is useful.

Lack of agreement on the definition of various stages of chloroquine and hydroxychloroquine retinopathy makes it difficult to compare results across series [8]. For example, Henkind and colleagues could not compare their color vision results to those of Okun because of variability in case severity between the two series [8, 9]. Rates of retinopathy can vary more than tenfold depending on how inclusive or exclusive the definitions of retinopathy are (see Chap. 5) [10]. For example, using a definition of retinopathy based entirely on the mfERG, Lyons and Severn concluded that 37 of 131 eyes (28 %) of patients taking hydroxychloroquine had retinopathy [11]. Using a definition based on cessation of 4AQs after consideration of the totality of the evidence, including mfERG, Browning found that 2 of 183 patients (1.1 %) had retinopathy [12]. Even when

D.J. Browning, *Hydroxychloroquine and Chloroquine Retinopathy*,
DOI 10.1007/978-1-4939-0597-3_4, © Springer Science+Business Media New York 2014

clinicians agree on a definition, the variability in interpretation of findings upon which the definitions of retinopathy are based implies frequent disagreements over whether a particular case has retinopathy or not [5, 13, 14].

In general, there are three stages of 4AQR (see Chap. 6). The term premaculopathy implies that a functional change has occurred but no morphologic change (Fig. 4.1a, b). Reversibility is part of the definition. However, premaculopathy is a fuzzy concept and difficult to apply reproducibly. If one stipulates a morphologic criterion as part of the definition of retinopathy, then one has probably failed in the attempt to detect reversible effects. There is scant evidence that morphologic

changes on spectral domain optical coherence tomography (SD-OCT), fundus photography, or fluorescein angiography (FA) resolve [15]. The advantage of morphologic criteria is that they are more reproducible than functional definitions. The price paid—irreversibility of the change in most cases—may be acceptable in setting the definition if progression can be averted when more advanced changes than purely functional ones have occurred.

Early retinopathy is more advanced than premaculopathy, but means different things to different investigators [16, 17]. Fundus changes can be present, but no bull's-eye lesion (Fig. 4.1c) [3, 9, 18]. Many patients with definite early toxicity

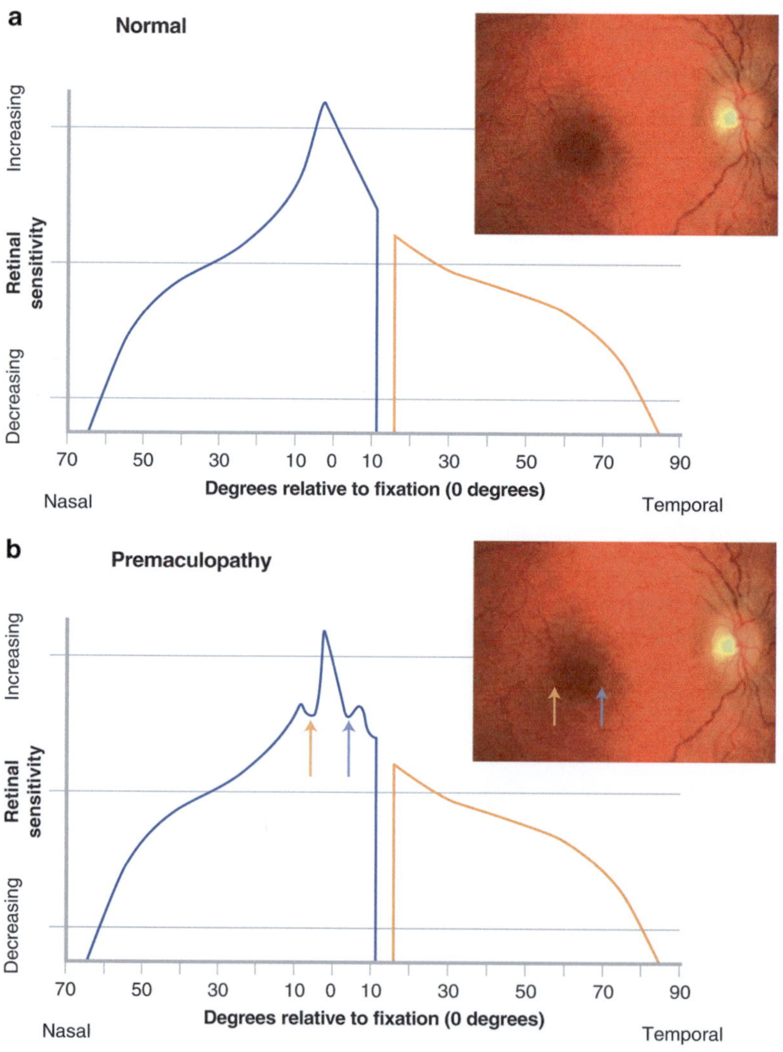

Fig. 4.1 (continued)

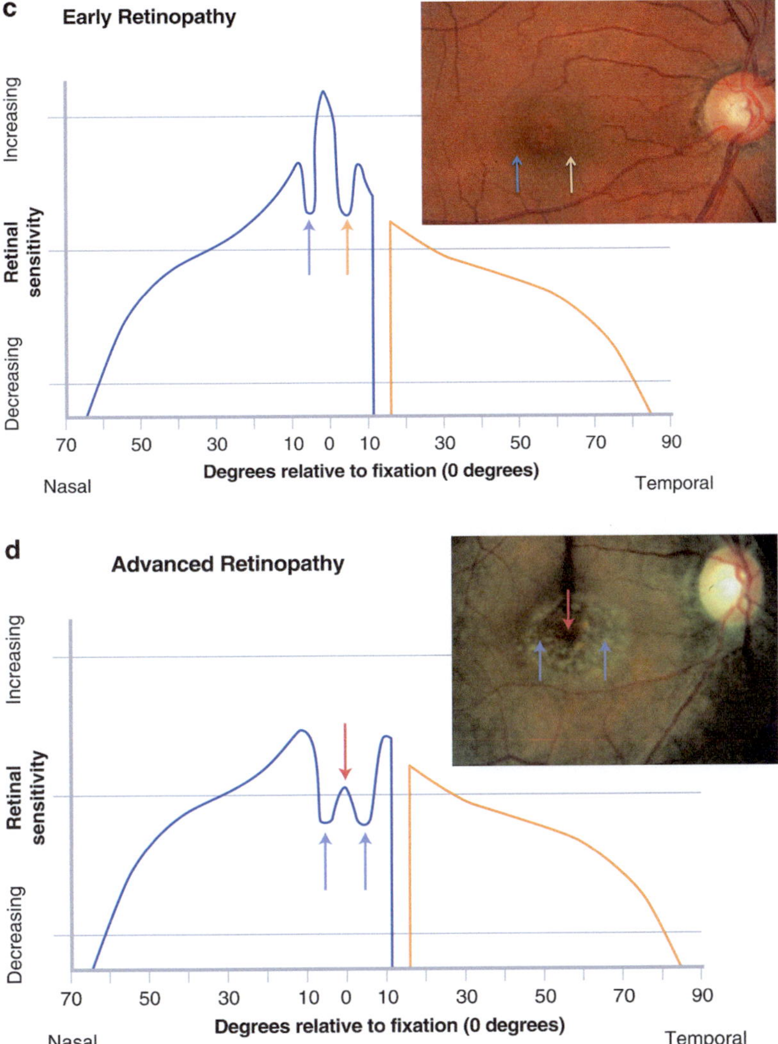

Fig. 4.1 Fundus photographs and diagrams of retinal sensitivity to standardized automated perimetry corresponding to common definitions for the three stages of 4-aminoquinoline retinopathy. (**a**) Depiction of the normal retina. The macular appearance is normal and the hill of vision has the normal configuration with highest sensitivity at the fovea and gradually decreasing sensitivity with increasing eccentricity from the fovea. (**b**) Depiction of premaculopathy. The macular appearance is normal in this case, but it can also show mild mottling. There is a functional abnormality, with decreased retinal sensitivity corresponding to perifoveal locations (relative paracentral scotoma). The relative paracentral scotoma is reversible in some but not all cases. (**c**) Depiction of early maculopathy. The macular appearance is abnormal in this case with mottling of the retinal pigment epithelium, but it can also be normal. There is a more pronounced functional abnormality with a more pronounced decrease in perifoveal retinal sensitivity (deeper paracentral scotoma). The fundus pigmentary change and paracentral scotoma are irreversible, but have a low probability of progressing if drug is stopped at this stage. (**d**) Depiction of advanced retinopathy. The macula has a bull's-eye abnormality that is irreversible. The foveal sensitivity is decreased (relative central scotoma) and the perifoveal retinal sensitivity is even less than in early retinopathy (deeper paracentral scotoma). Even with cessation of drug, at this stage there is a clinically important but poorly defined probability that progressive funduscopic and perimetric worsening will occur over time

have normal fundi [19–22]. Other patients have no visual field abnormalities but have macular pigment stippling [23]. Some authors require that there be visual field scotomata, but do not allow fundus abnormalities [22]. Some authors describe patients in this group as having color vision problems but no visual field defects [17]. Patients often do not have symptoms at this stage, but many do and some authors require symptoms as part of their definition of early retinopathy [18, 24, 25]. Although some have said that early fundus changes are reversible in up to 50 % of such cases [26], skepticism is appropriate as there has not been photographic documentation to analyze [27]. Patients with early retinopathy may have mfERG abnormalities with or without visual field abnormalities [17].

The classically recognized bull's-eye lesion of 4AQR signifies advanced retinopathy that never reverts to normal (Fig. 4.1d) [11, 28–32]. The presence of a bull's-eye lesion is accompanied by an annular scotoma and usually by symptoms. Patients at this stage will have more severe mfERG abnormalities [17]. Although a bull's-eye maculopathy is the hallmark of advanced 4AQR, it is not specific [33].

Table 4.1 compares definitions of chloroquine and hydroxychloroquine retinopathy across published studies. It is apparent that these papers are not addressing retinopathy at the same stage, and thus can only be compared with reservations. Some only consider cases with advanced retinopathy [15, 34]. Others are addressing patients with early retinopathy [35]. Some consider retinopathy to include all stages of toxicity, from functional, and reversible stages, to full-fledged, funduscopic changes with no hope of visual function recovery.

Dubious Cases in the Literature

As a result of the inconsistency of definitions of chloroquine and hydroxychloroquine retinopathy, there are many cases in the literature for which the diagnosis may be reasonably suspected to be incorrect. For example, a case was reported in which a dense central scotoma and 20/120 visual acuity developed with no funduscopic change visible in a patient who had taken no more than 250 mg/d of chloroquine for 1 year, yielding a cumulative dose of 91 g [50]. Another case report has been questioned as representing macular edema rather than HC retinopathy [41]. In another case, the published photographs and visual fields do not appear to be consistent with the diagnosis of chloroquine retinopathy [51].

In other areas of ophthalmology, progress has been slowed by inconsistency in terminology. Examples include uveitis, white dot syndromes, and macular telangiectasia (the MacTel Project) [52, 53]. Once international working groups standardized definitions, more sharply defined questions were made possible and understanding was enhanced. The field of 4AQR needs a similar venture.

4.1   Summary of Key Points

- There are no standardized definitions of 4AQR.
- It is difficult to compare different studies because they use different definitions.
- In broad terms, premaculopathy is a stage of retinopathy with functional but no morphologic changes. It is associated with a higher probability of reversibility if the drug is stopped.
- Early maculopathy is a more advanced stage with a higher probability of irreversibility and a higher proportion of cases with some pigmentary macular changes, but no bull's-eye lesion.
- Advanced retinopathy implies a bull's-eye lesion, an annular or (in the most advanced cases) central scotoma, and uniform irreversibility.
- An international working group to standardize definitions would help.

Table 4.1 Definitions of 4-aminoquinoline retinopathy

Year	Study/stage of retinopathy	Perimetric characteristic	mfERG	SD-OCT	Funduscopy	FA	Other criteria	Number of elements
1968	Carr [36]/NS	None	None	None	Pigmentary abnormality	None	None	1
1971	Marks [23]/NS	None	None	None	Pigmentary abnormality	None	None	1
1985	Easterbrook [37, 38]/NS	Bilateral reproducible visual field defects by two different techniques (e.g., Amsler grid and 10-2 VF with white II targets)	None	None	None	None	None	1
1985	Finbloom [39]/NS	Elevated cone threshold with Goldman-Weeks adaptometer and a <1° red light	None	None	Pigmentary abnormality	None	Color vision abnormality, total dose >100 g	3
1987	Johnson [40]/NS	On 10-2 VF testing with red test object, two or more adjacent points of 5 dB loss or a single point of 10 dB loss	None	None	None	None	None	1
1992	Bernstein [41]/NS	Persistent central or pericentral scotoma to suprathreshold white stimuli	None	None	Bull's-eye lesion qualifies even if no VF done	None	>9 months if daily dose >400 mg/d	3
1993	Easterbrook [2]/NS	Bilateral Amsler grid defects confirmed on perimetry	None	None	None	None	None	1
2000	Neubauer [16]/mild	No reproducible defects on Amsler grid or 10-2 visual field testing	None	None	Pigmentary abnormality	None	None	1

(continued)

Table 4.1 (continued)

Year	Study/stage of retinopathy	Perimetric characteristic	mfERG	SD-OCT	Funduscopy	FA	Other criteria	Number of elements
2000	Neubauer [16]/ advanced	Reproducible, bilateral visual field defects	None	None	Typical bull's-eye macular change and	None	None	2
2003	Mavrikakis [42]/NS	Two or more adjacent defects of 0.8–1.2 log units or one defect of 1.4–1.8 log units in an area of a previous scotoma	None	None	None	None	None	1
2004	Maturi [35]/NS	None	Any abnormality of mfERG—by hexagon or by ring, either amplitude or implicit time	None	None	None	None	1
2004	Araiza-Casillas [34]/NS	Scotoma at 10°	None	None	Pigmentary abnormality	Window defects	None	3
2006	Elder [43]/NS	Paracentral VF defects on 2 10-2 VFs separated by 2 months	None	None	None	None	None	1
2007	Shinjo [25]/NS	None	None	None	Pigmentary abnormality	None	Ocular symptoms	2
2007	Lyons [44]/NS	None	R1/R2>2.6	None	None	None	None	1
2007	Ruther [45]/NS	None	Abnormal mfERG	None	Pigmentary abnormality	None	None	2
2008	Hanna [3]/NS	Persistent paracentral scotoma to threshold white perimetry	None	None	None	None	None	1

2009	Lyons [11]/NS	None	Any of the following: 1. R1 amplitude less than the age-specific lower 99 % limit of normal 2. R1/R2 > 2.64 3. R1/R3 > 4.51 4. R1/R4 > 6.87 5. R1/R5 > age-specific 99 % upper limit of normal	none	none	none	None	1
2010	Bergholz [1]/NS	Reproducible, bilateral paracentral scotoma on SAP	Reproducible bilateral decrease in paracentral amplitude; if equivocal, then at least 2 of the VA, VF, or fundus criteria	None	1. No AMD 2. Either bull's-eye or peripheral pigmentary atrophy	None	Decreased BCVA if other causes except 4AQR ruled out	3
2010	Wolfe [28]/NS	Bull's-eye scotoma if no fundus picture	None	None	Bull's-eye maculopathy	None	None	1
2011	Anderson [46]/NS	Paracentral VF defects on ≥2 SAP tests (10-2 or 30-2)	None	None	None	None	None	1
2011	Michaelides [19], Chen [47]/NS	None	None	None	None	None	Cessation of drug based on totality of evidence	?
2011	Kellner [17]/early	None	Abnormal mfERG	None	Pigmentary abnormality	None	Abnormal color vision	3
2011	Kellner [17]/more advanced	Normal Goldmann VF	Abnormal mfERG	None	Mild bull's-eye maculopathy	None	Abnormal color vision	3

(continued)

Table 4.1 (continued)

Year	Study/stage of retinopathy	Perimetric characteristic	mfERG	SD-OCT	Funduscopy	FA	Other criteria	Number of elements
2011	Kellner [17]/severe retinopathy	Paracentral and mid-peripheral Goldmann VF abnormalities	Abnormal mfERG	None	Severe bull's-eye maculopathy	None	Abnormal color vision	4
2012	Missner [48]/NS	None	Either ring amplitude less than the lower 95 % confidence limit for normals or the ring implicit times greater than the 95 % confidence limit for normals	None	None	None	None	1
2012	Adam [49]/NS	Abnormal 10-2 VF[a]	None	Confirmatory finding on SD-OCT or funduscopy	Confirmatory finding on SD-OCT or funduscopy	None	None	2
2013	Browning [12]/NS	Reproducible paracentral scotomata on 10-2 VF testing	R1/R2 > 2.6	Loss of perifoveal inner segment/outer segment junction or RPE layer	None	None	None	1
2013	Mititelu [15]	None	None	None	Macular RPE changes typically in a concentric fashion around the fovea	None	None	1

[a]In this case, abnormal was undefined. NS means not specified. SD-OCT is spectral domain optical coherence tomography. mfERG is multifocal electroretinogram. VF is visual field. RPE is retinal pigment epithelium. R1, R2, etc. is the averaged amplitude of signals from the ring of hexagons centered on the fovea in the multifocal electroretinogram. SAP is standard automated perimetry

References

1. Bergholz R, Schroeter J, Ruther K. Evaluation of risk factors for retinal damage due to chloroquine and hydroxychloroquine. Br J Ophthalmol. 2010;94: 1637–42.
2. Easterbrook M. Long-term course of antimalarial maculopathy after cessation of treatment. Can J Ophthalmol. 1992;27:237–9.
3. Hanna B, Holdeman NR, Tang RA, Schiffman JS. Retinal toxicity secondary to Plaquenil therapy. Optometry. 2008;79:90–4.
4. Maksymowych W, Russell AS. Antimalarials in rheumatology: efficacy and safety. Semin Arthritis Rheum. 1987;16:206–21.
5. Dubois EL. Antimalarials in the management of discoid and systemic lupus erythematosus. Semin Arthritis Rheum. 1978;8:33–51.
6. Marmor MF. The dilemma of hydroxychloroquine screening: new information from the multifocal ERG. Am J Ophthalmol. 2005;140:894–5.
7. Morsman CDG, Livesey SJ, Richards IM, Jessop JD, Mills PV. Screening for hydroxychloroquine retinal toxicity: is it necessary? Eye. 1990;4:572–6.
8. Henkind P, Carr RE, Siegel IM. Early chloroquine retinopathy: clinical and functional findings. Arch Ophthalmol. 1964;71:157–65.
9. Okun E, Gouras P, Bernstein H, von Sallmann L. Chloroquine retinopathy-A report of eight cases with ERG and Dark-Adaptation findings. Arch Ophthalmol. 1963;63:93–105.
10. Browning DJ. Reply to Impact of the revised American Academy of Ophthalmology guidelines regarding hydroxychloroquine screening on actual practice. Am J Ophthalmol. 2013;156:410–1.
11. Lyons JS, Severns ML. Using multifocal ERG ring ratios to detect and follow Plaquenil retinal toxicity: a review. Doc Ophthalmol. 2009;118:29–36.
12. Browning DJ. Impact of the revised American academy of ophthalmology guidelines regarding hydroxychloroquine screening on actual practice. Am J Ophthalmol. 2013;155:418–28.
13. Marmor MF. Efficient and effective screening for hydroxychloroquine toxicity. Am J Ophthalmol. 2013;155:413–4.
14. Jones SK. Ocular toxicity and hydroxychloroquine: guidelines for screening. Br J Dermatol. 1999;140: 3–7.
15. Mititelu M, Wong BJ, Brenner M, Bryar PJ, Jampol LM, Fawzi AA. Progression of hydroxychloroquine toxic effects after drug therapy cessation. New evidence from multimodal imaging. Arch Ophthalmol. 2013;131:1187–97.
16. Neubauer AS, Samari-Kermani K, Schaller U, Welge-Luben U, Rudolph G, Berninger T. Detecting chloroquine retinopathy: electro-oculogram versus color vision. Br J Ophthalmol. 2003;87:902–8.
17. Kellner U, Kraus H, Foerster MH. Multifocal ERG in chloroquine retinopathy: regional variance in retinal dysfunction. Graefes Arch Clin Exp Ophthalmol. 2000;238:94–7.
18. Angi M, Romano V, Valldeperas X, Romano F, Romano M. Macular sensitivity changes for detection of chloroquine toxicity in asymptomatic patient. Int Ophthalmol. 2010;30:195–7.
19. Michaelides M, Stover NB, Francis PJ, Weleber RG. Retinal toxicity associated with hydroxychloroquine and chloroquine: risk factors, screening, and progression despite cessation of therapy. Arch Ophthalmol. 2011;129:30–9.
20. Rosenthal AR, Kolb H, Bergsma D, Huxsoll D, Hopkins JL. Chloroquine retinopathy in the rhesus monkey. Invest Ophthalmol Vis Sci. 1978;17: 1158–75.
21. Kobak S, Deveci H. Retinopathy due to antimalarial drugs in patients with connective tissue diseases: are they so innocent? A single center retrospective study. Int J Rheum Dis. 2010;13:e11–5.
22. Sataline LR, Farmer H. Medical Intelligence-Impaired vision after prolonged chloroquine therapy. N Engl J Med. 1962;266:346–7.
23. Marks JS, Power BJ. Is chloroquine obsolete in treatment of rheumatic disease? Lancet. 1979;1:371–3.
24. Mills PV, Beck M, Power BJ. Assessment of the retinal toxicity of hydroxychloroquine. Trans Ophthalmol Soc U K. 1981;101:109–13.
25. Shinjo SK, Junior OOM, Tizziani VAP, Morita C, Kochen JAL, Takahashi WY, Laurindo IMM. Chloroquine-induced bull's eye maculopathy in rheumatoid arthritis: related to disease duration? Clin Rheumatol. 2007;26:1248–53.
26. Banks CN. Melanin: blackguard or red herring? Another look at chloroquine retinopathy. Aust N Z J Ophthalmol. 1987;15:365–70.
27. Rynes RI. Ophthalmologic safety of long-term hydroxychloroquine sulfate treatment. Am J Med. 1983;75:35–9.
28. Wolfe F, Marmor MF. Rates and predictors of hydroxychloroquine retinal toxicity in patients with rheumatoid arthritis and systemic lupus erythematosus. Arthritis Care Res. 2010;62:775–84.
29. Shearer RV, Dubois EL. Ocular changes induced by long-term hydroxychloroquine (Plaquenil) therapy. Am J Ophthalmol. 1967;64:245–52.
30. Yam JCS, Kwok AKH. Ocular toxicity of hydroxychloroquine. Hong Kong Med J. 2006;12:294–304.
31. Warner AE. Early hydroxychloroquine macular toxicity. Arthritis Rheum. 2001;44:1959–61.
32. Graniewski-Wijnands HS, Van Lith GHM, Vijfvinkel-Bruinenga S. Ophthalmological examination of patients taking chloroquine. Doc Ophthalmol. 1979; 48:231–4.
33. Weise EE, Yannuzzi LA. Ring maculopathies mimicking chloroquine retinopathy. Am J Ophthalmol. 1974;78:204–10.
34. Araiza-Casillas R, Cardenas F, Morales Y, Cardiel MH. Factors associated with chloroquine-induced retinopathy in rheumatic diseases. Lupus. 2004;13: 119–24.

35. Maturi RK, Yu M, Weleber RG. Multifocal electro-retinographic evaluation of long-term hydroxychloroquine users. Arch Ophthalmol. 2004;122:973–81.

36. Carr RE, Henkind P, Rothfield N, Siegel IM. Ocular toxicity of antimalarial drugs-long-term follow-up. Am J Ophthalmol. 1968;66:738–44.

37. Easterbrook M. The ocular safety of hydroxychloroquine. Semin Arthritis Rheum. 1993;23:62–7.

38. Easterbrook M. Ocular effects and safety of antimalarial agents. Am J Med. 1988;85:23–9.

39. Finbloom DS, Silver K, Newsome DA, Gunkel R. Comparison of hydroxychloroquine and chloroquine use and the development of retinal toxicity. J Rheumatol. 1985;12:692–4.

40. Johnson MW, Vine AK. Hydroxychloroquine therapy in massive total doses without retinal toxicity. Am J Ophthalmol. 1987;104:139–44.

41. Bernstein H. Ocular safety of hydroxychloroquine sulfate (Plaquenil). South Med J. 1992;85:274–9.

42. Mavrikakis I, Sfikakis PP, Mavrikakis E, Rougas K, Nikolaou A, Kostopoulos C, Mavrikakis M. The incidence of irreversible retinal toxicity in patients treated with hydroxychloroquine—a reappraisal. Ophthalmology. 2003;110:1321–6.

43. Elder M, Rahman AMA. Early paracentral visual field loss in patients taking hydroxychloroquine. Arch Ophthalmol. 2006;124:1729–33.

44. Lyons JS, Severns ML. Detection of early hydroxychloroquine retinal toxicity enhanced by ring ratio analysis of multifocal electroretinography. Am J Ophthalmol. 2007;143:801–9.

45. Ruther K, Foerster J, Berndt S, Schroeter J. Chloroquine/hydroxychloroquine: variability of retinotoxic cumulative doses. Ophthalmologe. 2007;104:875–80.

46. Anderson C, Blaha GR, Marx JL. Humphrey visual field findings in hydroxychloroquine toxicity. Eye. 2011;25:1535–45.

47. Chen E, Brown DM, Benz MS, Fish RH, Wong TP, Kim RY, Major JC. Spectral domain optical coherence tomography as an effective screening test for hydroxychloroquine retinopathy (the "flying saucer" sign). Clin Ophthalmol. 2010;4:1151–8.

48. Missner S, Kellner U. Comparison of different screening methods for chloroquine/hydroxychloroquine retinopathy: multifocal electroretinography, color vision, perimetry, ophthalmoscopy, and fluorescein angiography. Graefes Arch Clin Exp Ophthalmol. 2012;250:319–25.

49. Adam MK, Covert DJ, Stepien KE, Han DP. Quantitative assessment of the 103 hexagon multifocal electroretinogram in detection of hydroxychloroquine retinal toxicity. Br J Ophthalmol. 2012;96:723–9.

50. Reed H, Campbell AA. Central scotomata following chloroquine therapy. Can Med Assoc J. 1962;86:176–8.

51. Bernstein HN, Ginsberg J. The pathology of chloroquine retinopathy. Arch Ophthalmol. 1964;71:238–45.

52. Jabs DA, Nussenblatt RB, Rosenbaum JT, Standardization of Uveitis Nomenclature (SUN) Working Group. Standardization of uveitis nomenclature for reporting clinical data. Results of the First International Workshop. Am J Ophthalmol. 2005;140:509–16.

53. Clemons TE, Gillies MC, Chew EY, Bird AC, Peto T, Figueroa M, Harrington MW, The Mac Tel Research Group. The National Eye Institute visual function questionnaire in the Macular Telangiectasia (MacTel) project. Invest Ophthalmol Vis Sci. 2008;49:4340–6.

Epidemiology of Hydroxychloroquine and Chloroquine Retinopathy

5

Abbreviations

4AQR	4-Aminoquinoline retinopathy
4AQs	4-Aminoquinolines (chloroquine and hydroxychloroquine)
ABW	Actual body weight
AG	Amsler grid
C	Chloroquine
CE	Clinical examination
CT	Cone thresholds
CV	Color vision testing
DA	Dark adaptation test
EOG	Electrooculogram
ERG	Electroretinogram
FP	Fundus photography
HC	Hydroxychloroquine
IBW	Ideal body weight
KVF	Kinetic visual field testing
LPT	Light photo stress test
NG	Not given
RA	Rheumatoid arthritis
RPE	Retinal pigment epithelium
SAP	Static automated perimetry
SLE	Systemic lupus erythematosus
TS	Tangent screen testing
VA	Visual acuity

A theme in this book so far has been that chloroquine and hydroxychloroquine are similar in pharmacology, toxicology, and pathologic effects. In considering the epidemiology of the retinopathies caused by antimalarial drugs, the situation is different. Chloroquine retinopathy is so much more prevalent than hydroxychloroquine retinopathy that avoidance of chloroquine has been advised and the use of hydroxychloroquine has been recommended [1, 2]. Although the difference in prevalence has been attributed to greater toxicity of chloroquine, it may be simply a fluke related to the fact that the usual daily dose for chloroquine, 250 mg, represents a higher dose relative to the mean ideal body weight (IBW) of the target population than does the usual daily dose for hydroxychloroquine, 400 mg [3]. To appreciate the significance of this, consider that the average height of a woman in the USA is 64 inches, with a corresponding IBW of 140 pounds (63.6 kg) using the National Heart Lung and Blood Institute table. This average woman taking one 250 mg tablet of chloroquine per day would be taking a dose of 3.9 mg/kg/day, or 112 % of the toxic threshold of 3.5 mg/kg/day. On the other hand, an average woman taking 400 mg of hydroxychloroquine would be taking a dose of 6.3 mg/kg/day, or 97 % of the toxic threshold of 6.5 mg/kg/day.

Of the epidemiologic concepts reviewed here, the prevalence is the most important, because this is the initial estimate of the probability of the presence of retinopathy in a given patient seen for screening [4, 5]. Other factors, such as height and history of renal disease, will inform the clinician's thoughts and modify the initial probability that the clinician settles on before performing any ancillary testing, but the prevalence is the starting point. Unfortunately, the precision of published estimates of prevalence is poor, and the methodologies

D.J. Browning, *Hydroxychloroquine and Chloroquine Retinopathy*,
DOI 10.1007/978-1-4939-0597-3_5, © Springer Science+Business Media New York 2014

flawed. A review of epidemiologic principles will be worthwhile to understand the gaps in our knowledge more clearly.

When both hydroxchloroquine and chloroquine are under discussion, they will be termed 4-aminoquinolines (4AQs) and their retinopathies will be termed 4-aminoquinoline retinopathy (4AQR). Commonly used abbreviations in this chapter are collected in "Abbreviations" for reference. Each term will be first used in its full form, along with its abbreviation.

5.1 Demographics of Patients Taking 4-Aminoquinolines

More women than men take 4AQs because the prevalence of rheumatoid arthritis (RA) and systemic lupus erythematosus (SLE) is higher in women than men [6]. In most series, the proportion of females among cases of retinopathy is 80 % or greater [7–9]. The weighted average percentage of patients who are female is 83 % (Table 5.1). Moreover, the demographic characteristics of patients who take 4AQs are consistent across countries from which case series have been reported [10, 11].

By pooling studies and weighting the reported statistics by sample size, the weighted median age of patients is 54 years. The age distribution of patients taking hydroxychloroquine has been estimated in the literature (Fig. 5.1 and Table 5.2). The ages of treated patients range from 10 to 100 with a peak in the decade 51 to 60.

The list of diseases for which patients take 4AQs is long, but the most common diagnoses are SLE and rheumatoid arthritis (RA). Table 5.3 shows selected data from the literature on this issue. The weighted mean percentages of patients taking 4AQs for RA, SLE, and other autoimmune diseases are 62 %, 29 %, and 9 %, respectively.

5.2 Prevalence and Incidence

The concepts of prevalence and incidence are commonly confused and the terms interchanged [38–40]. The most common error is that authors

Table 5.1 Gender and age of case series of patients taking 4-aminoquinolines

Study	N	Percentage female	Median age
Elder [12]	262	79	55
Almony [13]	68	94	43[a]
Mavrikakis [14]	526	83	46
Tobin [15]	65	61	51
Wolfe [16]	3,995	86	62
Shearer [17]	94	90	36
Rynes [18]	99	77	50
Mantyjarvi [19]	63	65	55[b]
Levy [20]	1,476	83	47[a]
Bergholz [21]	51	90	54
Heravian [22]	86	93	N/A[c]
Bonanomi [23]	34	79	42.2[a]
Neubauer [4]	93	71	50.8[a]
Percival [24]	198	77	NG
Fleck [25]	39	77	52.5[a]
Tanga [26]	48	75	51.4[a]
Bartel [27]	64	77	NG
Bray [28]	437	73	48[a]
Bailey [29]	45	56	NG
Spalton	77	99	37.2[a]
Kabok [30]	85	96	28.5[a]
Wang [31]	156	87	34[a]
Wasko [32]	1,808	80	53.7[a]
Weighted median	9,869[d]/9,476[e]	*83*	*54*

NG is not given

[a]Is mean, not median

[b]Indicates that ages were reported in decades, and that the midpoint of the median decade chosen as the median

[c]Means "not applicable" because these authors restricted inclusion to patients age 20–50

[d]Is the total number of patients for calculating the weighted median percentage female

[e]Is total number of patients for calculating the weighted median age

write about incidence (which implies a number of cases among susceptible individuals **over** a certain interval of time) when they mean prevalence (a certain number of cases among susceptible individuals **at** a given time) [39, 40]. The definitions follow.

- *Prevalence*—The number of cases of the disease divided by the population at one time, expressed as a percentage [41]. A prevalence study is sometimes called a cross-sectional study [42].

- *Incidence*—The number of new cases that arise during a span of time divided by the population at risk but disease-free at the beginning of that time [41]. The time span is specified as in 5-year incidence.

There are fewer studies of the incidence of 4AQR because an incidence study requires two identical examinations using standardized techniques for detection at two separate times.

There is little controversy that more cases of chloroquine retinopathy than hydroxychloroquine retinopathy have occurred [43, 44]. In 2011, Easterbrook had personally cared for 217 cases of 4AQR, with 200 of them attributable to chloroquine [45]. As a result of the higher prevalence of chloroquine retinopathy and perceived higher risk, prescription of chloroquine has almost vanished in the USA and Japan, although it continues to be widely used in Europe, Mexico, Brazil, Turkey, and China [21, 46–49].

The situation is different with hydroxychloroquine. It has been estimated that more than one million persons have taken hydroxychloroquine, yet the number of cases of retinopathy was reported to be less than 47 in 2006 [50, 51]. There is skepticism that hydroxychloroquine retinopathy occurs often enough to be a public health problem [52–54].

To rationally discuss the issue, good data on prevalence of retinopathy are needed. Yet in 1998, Albert and colleagues wrote "There is no epidemiologically sound study that determines the frequency of ocular toxicity in patients treated with antimalarials; therefore, the incidence, prevalence, and risk of toxicity cannot be determined accurately" [55]. In 2014, this statement remains true. To determine the prevalence and incidence of hydroxychloroquine and chloroquine retinopathy would require a population-based study that could be replicated by others: using standardized examinations, prospective follow-up, and pre-specified definitions of hydroxychloroquine and chloroquine retinopathy [41]. It is unlikely that a proper study will ever be done, because the resources required are probably not justified relative to the importance of the information gained, especially in the context of other, more pressing, health care needs. This is part of the reason that screening has intentionally not been recommended in the UK [52, 56–58]. The possible benefit seemed incommensurate with the expense to the panel convened to develop national policy.

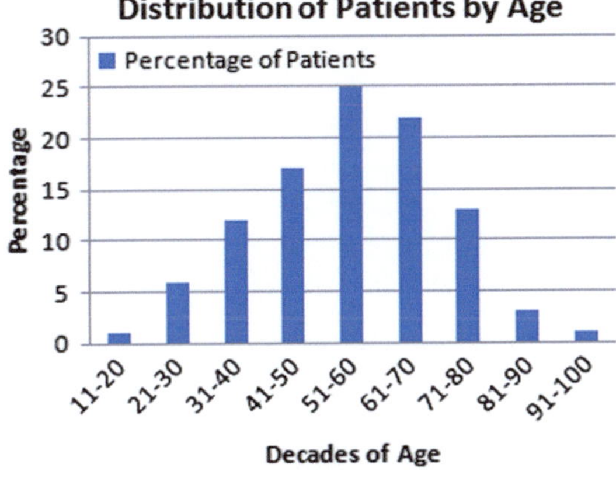

Fig. 5.1 Age distribution of patients taking hydroxychloroquine

Table 5.2 Distribution of ages of patients taking 4-aminoquinolines

Study	N	Decades of age								
		11–20	21–30	31–40	41–50	51–60	61–70	71–80	81–90	91–100
Grierson [33]	841	1	9	16	21	29	18	6	0	0
Elder [12]	275	4	22	37	49	50	46	56	10	1
Author's data	1,010	11	29	85	140	245	268	163	58	11
Pooled number of patients	2,126	23	127	258	365	539	465	269	68	12
Pooled percentage of patients	*100*	*1.1*	*6.0*	*12.1*	*17.2*	*25.4*	*21.9*	*12.7*	*3.2*	*0.6*

N is the number of patients in the study

Table 5.3 Diseases for which patients take 4-aminoquinolines

Study	N	Drug	SLE (%)	RA (%)	Other (%)
Bonanomi [23]	34	C	59	41	0
Mavrikakis [14]	400	HC	40	60	0
Bray [28]	43	Both	22	69	9
Bailey [29]	45	C	16	76	8
Finbloom [34]	110	Both	64	24	12
Kobak [30]	85	Both	14	45	41
Neubauer [4]	93	C	39	40	21
Voipio [35]	121	C	55	28	17
Marks [36]	222	C	9	91	0
Scherbel [37]	408	C	12	78	10
Weighted mean	1,561	Both	29	62	9

SLE is systemic lupus erythematosus. RA is rheumatoid arthritis. C is chloroquine. HC is hydroxychloroquine

In the absence of population-based prevalence estimates, we are left with estimates from observational, retrospective studies and small prospective studies. The prevalences of retinopathy reported from these limited studies for various subsets of patients vary from none to 40 % [3, 13, 14, 16, 17, 20, 35, 43, 47, 50, 58–64]. This uselessly wide range of estimates arises from the different definitions of retinopathy used by different authors (see Chap. 4), different detection methods, differences in risk factor profiles among samples of patients, different stages of retinopathy studied, failure to report cases, publication bias, failure to detect retinopathy by the screening physicians, multiply-counting the same patients with 4AQR over different publications covering the same samples, and failure of patients taking the drugs to comply with screening [21, 43, 58, 65].

Estimates of prevalence depend on sample size. For example, one group reported the prevalence of retinopathy at their center in serial publications over time. As their sample size increased, the reported prevalence decreased from 3.4 to 0.5 %. In this cohort, the sample size at the time of the first report was only 58, but the follow-up report was 400 [14]. Small samples give unreliable point estimates of prevalence.

The risk factors for 4AQR are the drug used (chloroqine or hydroxychloroquine), daily dose adjusted for IBW, cumulative dose (and its surrogate duration of use), age, renal or liver dysfunction, and pre-existing maculopathy (see Chap. 7). Therefore, it is expected that epidemiologic indices of risk would vary in patient samples having different characteristics. The most important variable affecting prevalence is the proportion of patients properly dosed according to IBW. In patients taking doses of hydroxychloroquine less than 6.5 mg/kg/day the prevalence of retinopathy has been estimated to be from 0 to 0.5 % [14, 20, 51, 54, 66–68]. Hydroxychloroquine toxicity at the recommended daily dose adjusted for IBW does occur but is so rare that the only documentation is in the form of isolated case reports [40, 69–72]. At this low rate the concept of prevalence becomes meaningless because the numerator is so small and the denominator so large. For example, Levy and colleagues found no cases of retinopathy in the subgroup of patients taking a nontoxic dose (N not reported) out of a larger sample of 1,207 patients taking hydroxychloroquine within the Kaiser Permanente health care system in California [20]. Mavrikakis found two cases out of 360 patients taking nontoxic daily doses [73]. Perhaps because of this, the index that has been reported more often in the literature has been the total number of cases of hydroxychloroquine retinopathy that have been published. This number was four in 1999 [72] and 47 in 2005 [74]. It follows that a program emphasizing proper dosing of 4AQs based on IBW would be expected to reduce the rate of 4AQR in a cost-effective manner.

The prevalence of chloroquine retinopathy based on daily dosing adjusted for IBW or, if that is not available, for actual body weight (ABW) is less well defined. In one series of patients with chloroquine retinopathy, 7.4 % of those patients with chloroquine retinopathy were dosed at less than 3 mg/kg of ABW/d, but 40 % were taking 3–4 mg/kg (ABW)/d [72]. Different series having different rates of overdosing by weight will be expected to show different prevalences of retinopathy. Although good estimates of prevalence of chloroquine retinopathy are lacking, the available data show that the prevalence is higher than that of hydroxychloroquine retinopathy.

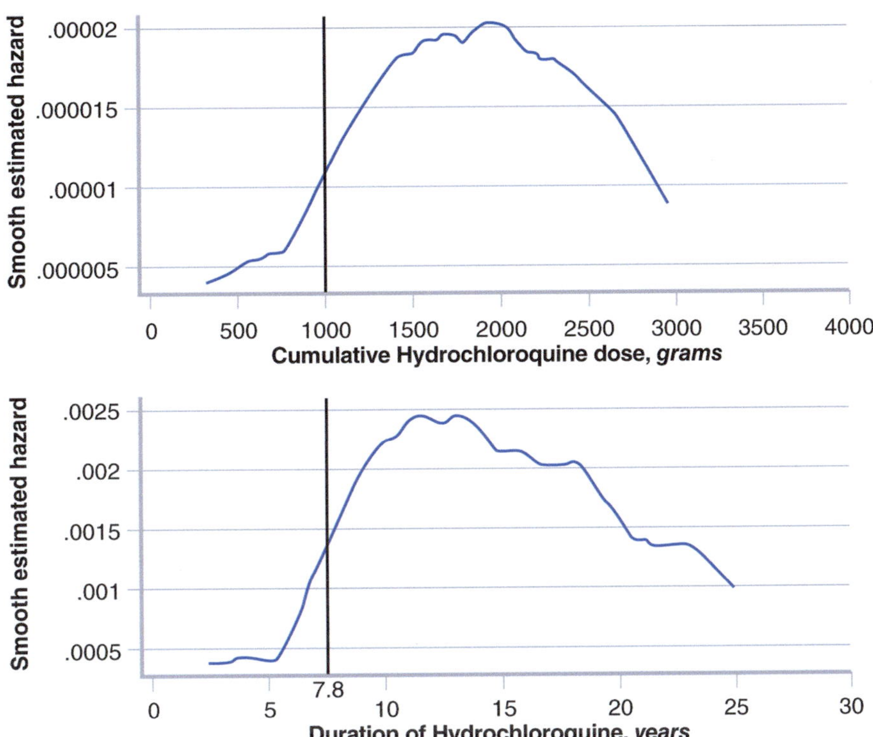

Fig. 5.2 Estimated hazard functions for hydroxychloroquine therapy as a function of cumulative dosage (*top panel*) and duration of therapy (*bottom panel*) based on modeling. In this study the vertical line indicates a cumulative dosage of 1,000 g in the *top panel* and the duration of therapy corresponding to the mean daily dosage of hydroxychloroquine (344 mg) in the *lower panel*, as observed in the study of 3,995 patients with systemic lupus erythematosus or rheumatoid arthritis who took hydroxychloroquine. Data from Wolfe [16]

Prevalence of 4AQR would also be expected to depend on cumulative dose or its surrogate, duration of therapy. The prevalence has not been examined in this way. A related epidemiologic index, the hazard function, has been modeled as a function of these variables [16]. The hazard function gives the rate of occurrence of 4AQR at a given value of the cumulative dose or duration of therapy subject to the condition that the 4AQR has not yet occurred. Wolfe and colleagues found that the hazard function for retinopathy increased for cumulative doses of hydroxychloroquine between 750 and 1,500 g or durations of use from 5 to 10 years (Fig. 5.2) [16].

Referral bias is a problem in estimating prevalence of 4AQR. One would expect to see a higher prevalence in patients seen in a retina referral clinic than in a rheumatology clinic, which in turn would be expected to be higher than in a population-based surveillance study of patients taking 4AQs. Table 5.4 lists the common sources of patients studied. Lastly, a problem tending to inflate estimates of prevalence is the occurrence of the same case in multiple publications, which can be difficult to track [37].

Given the list of obstacles preventing reliable assessment of prevalence, it is not surprising that inconsistent statistics have been published. A small sample of published prevalences among certain subsets of patients follows. A word of caution: some or all of the following observations cannot be accepted to be true generally because of the flaws mentioned.

- 50 % of patients taking more than 600 g of chloroquine developed retinopathy [39].
- 90 % of patients of age 60 or greater who have taken more than 600 g of chloroquine developed retinopathy [39].

Table 5.4 Sources of patients in studies estimating prevalence of 4-aminoquinoline retinopathy

Source of patients	Studies
Retina clinic referrals	Michaelides [65], Marmor [7]
Electrophysiology laboratory referrals	Farrell [75], Maturi [76]
General ophthalmology clinic referrals	Browning [77], Kellner [78], Elder [12],Grierson [33],Mititelu [40]
Rheumatology clinic patients	Almony [13], Mavrikakis [14], Tobin [15], Shearer [17], Rynes [79], Wallace [2], Morand [80], Bailey [29], Spalton [63], Finbloom [34], Kobak [30], Wang [31], Petri [81], Wasko [32], Percival [82], Marks [36]
Patients receiving hydroxychloroquine prescriptions at a health maintenance organization	Levy [20]
Patients in a National Rheumatology Registry willing to complete a 28 page questionnaire	Wolfe [16]

- 0.002 % of patients taking less than 6.5 mg/kg/day (not stated with respect to actual or IBW) of hydroxychloroquine for less than 5 years developed retinopathy [50, 83].
- No patients taking hydroxychloroquine at less than 6.5 mg/kg/day based on IBW for less than 6 years and who had normal renal and liver function developed retinopathy [84].
- Of patients with lupus taking chloroquine or hydroxychloroquine, the prevalences of retinopathy were 10 % and 3 %, respectively [2].

In the absence of sound data on prevalence, Table 5.5 shows a nonexhaustive list of the methodologically flawed estimates arising from prospective and retrospective case series, and surveys.

The most influential epidemiologic study of 4AQR was that of Wolfe and Marmor [16]. It asserted that the prevalence of retinopathy increases for patients taking hydroxychloroquine for more than 5 years. Moreover, it downplayed the importance of daily dose as a risk factor for retinopathy, despite lacking information regarding dosing for 39.3 % of the patients in the sample.

Table 5.5 Methodologically flawed estimates of prevalence of chloroquine and hydroxychloroquine retinopathy

Drug	Study/design/year	Screening tests used	N	Prevalence (%)
C	Kobak [30]	CE, SAP	85	24.7
C	Bailey [29]	KVF, CE	45	15
C	Nebbioso [85]	NG	NG	7.4
C	Wallace [2]	NG	NG	10
C	Finbloom [34]	CE, CV, CT	31	19
C	Elman [86]	VA, KVF, CV, ERG	270	0.37
C	Mackenzie [87]	NG	NG	0.1
C	Hobbs [88]	CE	170	2.9
C	Shinjo [47]	CE	607	4.4
C	Fuld [61]	CE	100	1.0
C	Henkind [38]	CE	48	17.7
C	Butler [89]	CE	82	2.4[a]
C	Percival [82]	CE, TS, FP, CV	272	4.0
C	Marks [36]	CE	222	10
C	Shearer[b] [17]	CE, VA, VF, CV, FA	81	14
C(83 %)[c]	Neubauer [4]	CE, CV, EOG, AG	93	40.8 Mild, 4.3 advanced
C(58 %)[c]	Bernstein[d] [5]	Meta	386	0.5[e], 10[f]
C(10 %)[c]	Farrell [75]	CE, ERG, SAP, sometimes FP	3	66.7

(continued)

Table 5.5 (continued)

Drug	Study/design/year	Screening tests used	N	Prevalence (%)
HC	Wang [31]	NG	156	1.3
HC	Wallace [2]	NG	2,000	3
HC	Mavrikakis [14]/ prospective case series[g]	CE, CV, SAP, ERG	400	0.5
HC	Nebbioso [85]	NG	50	<1–40, depending on method
HC	Levy [20]	CE	1,207	0.08[e], 0.4[f]
HC	Yam[d] [51]	Meta	4,415	<1.0
HC	Elder [12]	CE, CV, SAP, VA	262	1.5
HC	Morand [80]	NG	403	0
HC	Finbloom [34]	CE, CV, CT	29	0
HC	Kobak [30]	CE, SAP	50	16
HC	Petri [81]	NG	104	1.0
HC	Mititelu [40]	CE	>2,000	<0.35
HC	Mackenzie [90]/1983	NG	900	0
HC	Mikkelsen cited in Morsman [91]	NG	338	0
HC	Rynes [79]	CE, SAP, VA	99	4
HC	Mantyjarvi [19]	CE, VA, CV, TS	63	1.6
HC	Johnson [92]	CE, VA, AG, CV, SAP, FP, FA	9	0
HC	Morsman [91]	CE, VA, CV, SAP, AG	73	0
HC	Frenkel [93]	NG	~100	0
HC	Morsman[d] [91]	Meta	1,547	0.32
HC	Shearer[b] [17]	CE, VA, VF, CV, FA	94	1
HC	Elder [12]	SAP	262	1.9 (95 % CI 1.6–2.2 %)
HC	Runge [95]	NG	101	0
HC	Grierson [33]	CE, AG	758	0
HC	Spalton [63]	CE, SAP, FP	82	0
HC(17 %)[c]	Neubauer [4]	CE, CV, EOG, AG	93	40.8 Mild, 4.3 advanced
HC(42 %)[c]	Bernstein[d] [5]	Meta	386	0[e], 2.7[f]
HC(90 %)[c]	Farrell [75]	CE, ERG, SAP, sometimes FP	26	34.6
Both (breakdown not given)	Easterbrook [94]	CE, AG, sometimes SAP	1,650	3.8

CV is color vision testing. CT means cone thresholds. ERG means electroretinogram. KVF stands for kinetic visual field testing. SAP stands for static automated perimetry. AG refers to the amsler grid. EOG is electrooculogram. NG means not given. FP is fundus photography. Mild retinopathy means pigmentary macular changes without Amsler or 10-2 VF defects [4]. Advanced means bull's-eye with visual field defects [4]. CE means clinical examination. DA represents dark adaptation test. LPT stands for light photo-stress test. VA means visual acuity. TS is tangent screen testing

[a] Means based on macular changes not peripheral retinopathy

[b] Specifies visual field (VF) as Harrington-flocks charts

[c] Means the series mixes chloroquine and hydroxychloroquine and the percentage in parentheses is the proportion taking the indicated drug

[d] Indicates review of other series "meta" means a meta-analysis of several studies using different methods of screening for retinopathy

[e] Is definite retinopathy

[f] Is probable retinopathy

[g] Represents all patients followed 6 years or more

Given its historical importance, it is important to consider its methodologic flaws that were as significant as those of other, less-heeded studies. The method of accruing cases was self-reporting of eye problems by patients, despite the fact that hydroxychloroquine retinopathy is frequently asymptomatic, and despite the fact that many symptomatic patients have no retinopathy. In studies in which self-reporting and examination by clinicians has been performed in parallel, the results of self-reporting have not accurately reflected the findings of examination [96, 97]. In the words of Linton and colleagues, "One must be aware of the limited validity of such surveys" [97]. As with many other studies, there was no standardized examination of the patients, nor a standardized definition for retinopathy. In addition, the study was biased by the nature of the sample, which was taken from the National Data Bank of Rheumatic Disease, a registry that only includes patients willing to complete a 28-page questionnaire. Many of the results reported from the study are not observations but are extrapolations based on modeling, a method useful for generating hypotheses, but of doubtful strength to form a basis for public health recommendations. The revised American Academy of Ophthalmology recommendations for screening 4AQ retinopathy are largely based on the epidemiologic conclusions of this flawed study [98].

Beyond the flawed point estimates for prevalence and incidence, there is even less information regarding changes in prevalence over time. Anecdotal observations have published that modern rates of hydroxychloroquine retinopathy are lower in the contemporary era than in the 1960s and 1970s, when dosing was frequently higher, durations of drug use longer, and the proportions using hydroxychloroquine rather than chloroquine were reversed [99, 100]. However, others have anecdotally observed the opposite [101].

Inconsistency of Authors on Assumed Prevalence of Hydroxychloroquine Retinopathy

The discussion of prevalence by the same authors can be inconsistent over time. For example, an author wrote that "visually-significant changes with retinopathy are actually very rare. They are virtually never seen in the first 5 years of usage at doses under 6.5 mg/kg, and are in fact very infrequent even among longer users" [102]. However, 6 years later the same author wrote that the prevalence of retinopathy among those taking the drug for over 5 years was 1 % and even higher with longer duration use. A 1 % prevalence was the implicit threshold at which a recommended universal screening program was considered to be justified [98]. There is nothing wrong with changing one's mind as the evidence dictates, but the reader is advised to reflect on how solid the evidential base can be that apparently comports with both views held by the same expert.

5.3   Summary of Key Points

- The prevalence of hydroxychloroquine among properly dosed patients is much less than 1 %.
- Although the prevalence of chloroquine retinopathy among properly dosed patients is much lower than among overdosed patients, good estimates for prevalence are lacking.
- The prevalence of hydroxychloroquine retinopathy is less than the prevalence of chloroquine retinopathy.
- Those who advocate universal screening for 4AQR do so because they believe the best estimate for prevalence of 4AQR is greater than 1 % among all users of these drugs for greater than 5 years. A prevalence of 1 % has been assumed to be a rate at which screening makes sense.

- If all persons were properly dosed according to IBW, such that prevalence of retinopathy drops to much less than 1 %, it would be difficult to support universal screening.
- It follows that a cost-effective screening program should emphasize proper dosing based on IBW.

References

1. Rothermich NO. Coming catastrophes with chloroquine? Ann Intern Med. 1964;61:1203–5.
2. Wallace DJ. Antimalarials-the 'real' advance in lupus. Lupus. 2001;10:385–7.
3. Bunch TW, O'Duffy JD. Disease modifying drugs for progressive rheumatoid arthritis. Mayo Clin Proc. 1980;55:161–79.
4. Neubauer AS, Samari-Kermani K, Schaller U, Welge-Luben U, Rudolph G, Berninger T. Detecting chloroquine retinopathy: electro-oculogram versus color vision. Br J Ophthalmol. 2003;87:902–8.
5. Bernstein HN. Ophthalmologic considerations and testing in patients receiving long-term antimalarial therapy. Am J Med. 1983;75:25–34.
6. Lawrence JS. Prevalence of rheumatoid arthritis. Ann Rheum Dis. 1961;20:11–7.
7. Marmor MF. Comparison of screening procedures in hydroxychloroquine toxicity. Arch Ophthalmol. 2012;130:461–9.
8. Lai TYY, Ngai JWS, Chan WM, Lam DSC. Visual field and multifocal electroretinography and their correlations in patients on hydroxychloroquine therapy. Doc Ophthalmol. 2006;112:177–87.
9. Browning DJ. Hydroxychloroquine and chloroquine retinopathy: screening for drug toxicity. Am J Ophthalmol. 2002;133:649–56.
10. Symmons D, Turner G, Webb R, Asten P, Barrett E, Lunt M, Scott D, Silman A. The prevalence of rheumatoid arthritis in the United Kingdom: new estimates for a new century. Rheumatology. 2002;41:793–800.
11. Helve T. Prevalence and mortality rates of systemic lupus erythematosus and causes of death of SLE patients in FInland. Scand J Rheumatol. 1985;14:43–6.
12. Elder M, Rahman AMA. Early paracentral visual field loss in patients taking hydroxychloroquine. Arch Ophthalmol. 2006;124:1729–33.
13. Almony A, Garg S, Peters RK, Mamet R, Tsong J, Shibuya B, Kitridou R, Sadun AA. Threshold amsler grid as a screening tool for asymptomatic patients on hydroxychloroquine therapy. Br J Ophthalmol. 2005;89:569–74.
14. Mavrikakis I, Sfikakis PP, Mavrikakis E, Rougas K, Nikolaou A, Kostopoulos C, Mavrikakis M. The incidence of irreversible retinal toxicity in patients treated with hydroxychloroquine—a reappraisal. Ophthalmology. 2003;110:1321–6.
15. Tobin DR, Krohel G, Rynes RI. Hydroxychloroquine-seven-year experience. Arch Ophthalmol. 1982;100:81–3.
16. Wolfe F, Marmor MF. Rates and predictors of hydroxychloroquine retinal toxicity in patients with rheumatoid arthritis and systemic lupus erythematosus. Arthritis Care Res. 2010;62:775–84.
17. Shearer RV, Dubois EL. Ocular changes induced by long-term hydroxychloroquine (Plaquenil) therapy. Am J Ophthalmol. 1967;64:245–52.
18. Rynes RI, Krohel G, Falbo A, Reinecke RD, Wolfe B, Bartholomew LE. Ophthalmologic safety of long-term hydroxychloroquine treatment. Arthritis Rheum. 1979;22:832–6.
19. Mantyjarvi M. Hydroxychloroquine treatment and the eye. Scand J Rheumatol. 1985;14:171–4.
20. Levy GD, Munz SJ, Paschal J, Cohen HB, Prince KJ, Peterson T. Incidence of hydroxychloroquine retinopathy in 1,207 patients in a large multicenter outpatient practice. Arthritis Rheum. 1997;40:1482–6.
21. Bergholz R, Schroeter J, Ruther K. Evaluation of risk factors for retinal damage due to chloroquine and hydroxychloroquine. Br J Ophthalmol. 2010;94:1637–42.
22. Heravian J, Saghafi M, Shoeibi N, Hassanzadeh S, Shakeri MT, Sharepoor M. A comparative study of the usefulness of color vision, photostress recovery time, and visual evoked potential tests in the early detection of ocular toxicity from hydroxychloroquine. Int Ophthalmol. 2011;31:283–9.
23. Bonanomi MT, Dantas NC, Medeiros FA. Retinal nerve fiber layer thickness measurements in patients using chloroquine. Clin Exp Ophthalmol. 2006;34:130–6.
24. Percival SPB, Behrman J. Ophthalmological safety of chloroquine. Br J Ophthalmol. 1969;53:101–9.
25. Fleck BW, Bell AL, Mitchell JD, Thomson BJ, Hurst NP, Nuki G. Screening for antimalarial maculopathy in rheumatology clinics. Br Med J. 1985;291:782–5.
26. Tanga L, Centofanti M, Oddone F, Parravano M, Parisi V, Ziccardi L, Kroegler B, Perricone R, Manni G. Retinal functional changes measured by frequency-doubling technology in patients treated with hydroxychloroquine. Graefes Arch Clin Exp Ophthalmol. 2011;249:715–21.
27. Bartel PR, Roux P, Robinson E, Anderson IF, Brighton SW, Van der Hoven HJ, Becker PJ. Visual function and long-term chloroquine treatment. S Afr Med J. 1994;84:32–4.
28. Bray VJ, Enzenauer RJ, Enzenauer RW, West SG. Antimalarial toxicity in rheumatic disease. J Clin Rheumatol. 1998;4:168–9.
29. Bailey LA, Hiltz JW. Ocular complications of chloroquine therapy. Can Med Assoc J. 1965;6:508–13.

30. Kobak S, Deveci H. Retinopathy due to antimalarial drugs in patients with connective tissue diseases: are they so innocent? A single center retrospective study. Int J Rheum Dis. 2010;13:e11–5.

31. Wang C, Fortin PR, Li Y, Panaritis T, Gans M, Esdaile JM. Discontinuation of antimalarial drugs in systemic lupus erythematosus. J Rheumatol. 1999; 26:808–15.

32. Wasko MCM, Hubert HB, Lingala VB, Elliott JR, Luggen ME, Fries JF, Ward MM. Hydroxychloroquine and risk of diabetes in patients with rheumatoid arthritis. JAMA. 2007;298:187–93.

33. Grierson DJ. Hydroxychloroquine and visual screening in a rheumatology outpatient clinic. Ann Rheum Dis. 1997;56:188–90.

34. Finbloom DS, Silver K, Newsome DA, Gunkel R. Comparison of hydroxychloroquine and chloroquine use and the development of retinal toxicity. J Rheumatol. 1985;12:692–4.

35. Voipio H. Incidence of chloroquine retinopathy. Acta Ophthalmol (Copenh). 1966;44:349–54.

36. Marks JS, Power BJ. Is chloroquine obsolete in treatment of rheumatic disease? Lancet. 1979;1: 371–3.

37. Scherbel AL, Mackenzie AH, Nousek JE, Atdjian M. Ocular lesions in rheumatoid arthritis and related disorders with particular reference to retinopathy-A study of 741 patients treated with and without chloroquine drugs. N Engl J Med. 1965; 273:360–6.

38. Henkind P, Rothfield NF. Ocular abnormalities in patients treated with synthetic antimalarial drugs. N Engl J Med. 1963;269:434–9.

39. Banks CN. Melanin: blackguard or red herring? Another look at chloroquine retinopathy. Aust N Z J Ophthalmol. 1987;15:365–70.

40. Mititelu M, Wong BJ, Brenner M, Bryar PJ, Jampol LM, Fawzi AA. Progression of hydroxychloroquine toxic effects after drug therapy cessation. New evidence from multimodal imaging. Arch Ophthalmol. 2013;131:1187–97.

41. Jekel JF, Elmore JG, Katz DL. Epidemiology, biostatistics, and preventive medicine. Philadelphia: WB Saunders; 1996. p. 216–7.

42. Vitale S, Maguire MG, Murphy RP, Hiner CJ, Rourke L, Sackett C, Patz A. Clinically significant macular edema in type I diabetes. Ophthalmology. 1995;102:1170–6.

43. Easterbrook M. Ocular effects and safety of antimalarial agents. Am J Med. 1988;85:23–9.

44. Sundelin SP, Terman A. Different effects of chloroquine and hydroxychloroquine on lysosomal function in cultured retinal pigment epithelial cells. APMIS. 2002;110:481–9.

45. Easterbrook M. Clinical characteristics of hydroxychloroquine retinopathy. Evid Based Ophthalmol. 2011;12:132–3.

46. Xiaoyun MA, Dongyi HE, Linping HE. Assessing chloroquine toxicity in RA patients using retinal nerve fiber layer thickness, multifocal electroreti-

47. Shinjo SK, Junior OOM, Tizziani VAP, Morita C, Kochen JAL, Takahashi WY, Laurindo IMM. Chloroquine-induced bull's eye maculopathy in rheumatoid arthritis: related to disease duration? Clin Rheumatol. 2007;26:1248–53.

48. Kishimoto M, Deshpande GA, Yokogawa N, Buyon JP, Okada M. Use of hydroxychloroquine in Japan. J Rheumatol. 2012;39:1296.

49. Houpt JB. A rheumatologist's verdict on the safety of chloroquine versus hydroxychloroquine. Liability in off-label prescribing. J Rheumatol. 1999;26:1864–6.

50. Marmor MF, Carr RE, Easterbrook M, et al. Recommendations on screening for chloroquine and hydroxychloroquine retinopathy. Ophthalmology. 2002;109:1377–82.

51. Yam JCS, Kwok AKH. Ocular toxicity of hydroxychloroquine. Hong Kong Med J. 2006;12:294–304.

52. Bourke B, Jones S, Rajammal AK, Silman A, Smith R. Hydroxychloroquine and ocular toxicity recommendations on screening. The Royal College of Ophthalmologists; 2009. p. 1–9. www.rcophth.ac.uk. Accessed 13 Apr 2014.

53. Blythe C, Lane C. Hydroxychloroquine retinopathy: is screening necessary? Intensive screening is not necessary at normal doses. Br Med J. 1998;316:716–7.

54. Coyle JT. Hydroxychloroquine retinopathy [letter to the Editors]. Ophthalmology. 2001;108:243–4.

55. Albert DA, Debois LKL, Lu KF. Antimalarial ocular toxicity, a critical appraisal. J Clin Rheumatol. 1998;4:57–62.

56. Fielder A, Graham E, Jones S, Silman A, Tullo A. Royal college of ophthalmologists guidelines: ocular toxicity and hydroxychloroquine. Eye. 1998;12: 907–9.

57. Jones SK. Ocular toxicity and hydroxychloroquine: guidelines for screening. Br J Dermatol. 1999;140: 3–7.

58. Cox NH, Paterson WD. Ocular toxicity of antimalarials in dermatology: a survey of current practice. Br J Dermatol. 1994;131:878–82.

59. Carr RE, Henkind P, Rothfield N, Siegel IM. Ocular toxicity of antimalarial drugs-long-term follow-up. Am J Ophthalmol. 1968;66:738–44.

60. Nylander U. Ocular damage in chloroquine therapy. Acta Ophthalmol (Copenh). 1966;44:335–8.

61. Fuld H. Retinopathy following chloroquine therapy. Lancet. 1959;2:617–8.

62. Maksymowych W, Russell AS. Antimalarials in rheumatology: efficacy and safety. Semin Arthritis Rheum. 1987;16:206–21.

63. Spalton DJ, Roe GMV, Hughes GRV. Hydroxychloroquine, dosage parameters and retinopathy. Lupus. 1993;2:355–8.

64. Adam MK, Covert DJ, Stepien KE, Han DP. Quantitative assessment of the 103 hexagon multifocal electroretinogram in detection of hydroxychloroquine retinal toxicity. Br J Ophthalmol. 2012;96: 723–9.

65. Michaelides M, Stover NB, Francis PJ, Weleber RG. Retinal toxicity associated with hydroxychloroquine and chloroquine: risk factors, screening, and progression despite cessation of therapy. Arch Ophthalmol. 2011;129:30–9.

66. Bernstein HN. Ocular safety of hydroxychloroquine. Ann Ophthalmol. 1991;23:292–6.

67. Semmer AE, Lee MS, Harrison AR, Olsen TW. Hydroxychloroquine retinopathy screening. Br J Ophthalmol. 2008;92:1653–5.

68. Blomquist PH, Chundru RK. Screening for hydroxychloroquine toxicity by Texas ophthalmologists. J Rheumatol. 2002;29:1665–70.

69. Falcone PM, Paolini L, Lou PL. Hydroxychloroquine toxicity despite normal dose therapy. Ann Ophthalmol. 1993;25:385–8.

70. Thorne JE, Maguire AM. Retinopathy after long term, standard doses of hydroxychloroquine. Br J Ophthalmol. 1999;83:1201–2.

71. Bienfang D, Coblyn JS, Liang MH, Corzillius M. Hydroxychloroquine retinopathy despite regular ophthalmologic evaluation: a consecutive series. J Rheumatol. 2000;27:2703–6.

72. Easterbrook M. An ophthalmological view on the efficacy and safety of chloroquine versus hydroxychloroquine. J Rheumatol. 1999;26:1866–7.

73. Mavrikakis M, Papazoglou S, Sfikakis PP, Vaiopoulos G, Rougas K. Retinal toxicity in long term hydroxychloroquine treatment. Ann Rheum Dis. 1996;55:187–9.

74. Payne JF, Hubbard III GB, Aaberg Sr TM, Yan J. Clinical characteristics of hydroxychloroquine retinopathy. Br J Ophthalmol. 2010;95:245–50.

75. Farrell DF. Retinal toxicity to antimalarial drugs: chloroquine and hydroxychloroquine: a neurophysiologic study. Clin Ophthalmol. 2012;6:377–83.

76. Maturi RK, Yu M, Weleber RG. Multifocal electroretinographic evaluation of long-term hydroxychloroquine users. Arch Ophthalmol. 2004;122:973–81.

77. Browning DJ. Impact of the revised American academy of ophthalmology guidelines regarding hydroxychloroquine screening on actual practice. Am J Ophthalmol. 2013;155:418–28.

78. Kellner U, Renner AB, Tillack H. Fundus autofluorescence and mfERG for early detection of retinal alterations in patients using chloroquine/hydroxychloroquine. Invest Ophthalmol Vis Sci. 2006; 47:3531–8.

79. Rynes RI. Ophthalmologic safety of long-term hydroxychloroquine sulfate treatment. Am J Med. 1983;75:35–9.

80. Morand EF, McCloud PI, Littlejohn GO. Continuation of long term treatment with hydroxychloroquine in systemic lupus erythematosus and rheumatoid arthritis. Ann Rheum Dis. 1992;51:1318–21.

81. Petri M. Hydroxychloroquine use in the Baltimore Lupus Cohort: effects on lipids, glucose and thrombosis. Lupus. 1996;5:S16–22.

82. Percival SPB, Meanock I. Chloroquine: ophthalmological safety and clinical assessment in rheumatoid arthritis. Br Med J. 1968;3:579–84.

83. Flach AJ. Improving the risk-benefit relationship and informed consent for patients treated with hydroxychloroquine. Trans Am Ophthalmol Soc. 2007; 105:191–7.

84. Sfikakis PP, Mavrikakis M. Ophthalmologic monitoring for antimalarial toxicity. J Rheumatol. 2004;31:1011–2.

85. Nebbioso M, Grenga R, Karavitas P. Early detection of macular changes with multifocal ERG in patients on antimalarial drug therapy. J Ocul Pharmacol Ther. 2009;25:249–58.

86. Elman A, Gullberg R, Nillson E, Rendahl I, Wachtmeister L. Choroquine retinopathy in patients with rheumatoid arthritis. Scand J Rheumatol. 1975;5:161–6.

87. Mackenzie AH. An appraisal of chloroquine. Arthritis Rheum. 1970;13:280–91.

88. Hobbs HE, Eadie SP, Somerville F. Ocular lesions after treatment with chloroquine. Br J Ophthalmol. 1961;45:284–97.

89. Butler I. Retinopathy following the use of chloroquine and allied substances. Ophthalmologica. 1965;149:204–8.

90. Mackenzie AH. Dose refinements in long-term therapy of rheumatoid arthritis with antimalarials. Am J Med. 1983;75:40–5.

91. Morsman CDG, Livesey SJ, Richards IM, Jessop JD, Mills PV. Screening for hydroxychloroquine retinal toxicity: is it necessary? Eye. 1990;4: 572–6.

92. Johnson MW, Vine AK. Hydroxychloroquine therapy in massive total doses without retinal toxicity. Am J Ophthalmol. 1987;104:139–44.

93. Frenkel M. Safety of hydroxychloroquine. Arch Ophthalmol. 1982;100:841.

94. Easterbrook M. Long-term course of antimalarial maculopathy after cessation of treatment. Can J Ophthalmol. 1992;2:237–9.

95. Runge LA. Risk/benefit analysis of hydroxychloroquine sulfate treatment in rheumatoid arthritis. Am J Med. 1983;75:52–6.

96. Patty L, Wu C, Torres M, Azen S, Varma R, Los Angeles Latino Eye Study Group. Validity of self-reported eye disease and treatment in a population-based study: the Los Angeles Latino Eye Study. Ophthalmology. 2012;119:1725–30.

97. Linton KL, Klein BE, Klein R. The validity of self-reported and surrogate-reported cataract and age-related macular degeneration in the Beaver Dam Eye Study. Am J Epidemiol. 1991;134: 1438–46.

98. Marmor MF, Kellner U, Lai TYY, Lyons JS, Mieler WF. Revised recommendations on screening for chloroquine and hydroxychloroquine retinopathy. Ophthalmology. 2011;118:415–22.

99. Spalton DJ. Retinopathy and antimalarial drugs-the British experience. Lupus. 1996;5:S70–2.

100. Blomquist PH. Screening for hydroxychloroquine toxicity. Comp Ophthalmol Update. 2000;1: 245–50.
101. Rodriguez-Padilla JA, Hedges III TR, Monson B, Srinivasan V, Wojtkowski M, Reichel E, Duker JS, Schuman JS, Fujimoto JG. High-speed ultra-high-resolution optical coherence tomography findings in hydroxychloroquine retinopathy. Arch Ophthalmol. 2007;125:775–80.
102. Marmor MF. The dilemma of hydroxychloroquine screening: new information from the multifocal ERG. Am J Ophthalmol. 2005;140:894–5.

Natural History of Hydroxychloroquine and Chloroquine Retinopathy

Abbreviations

4AQR	4-aminoquinoline retinopathy
4AQs	4-aminoquinolines (chloroquine and hydroxychloroquine)
BAL	British anti-Lewisite
C	Chloroquine
EOG	Electro-oculogram
ERG	Electroretinogram
FAF	Fundus autofluorescence
HC	Hydroxychloroquine
mfERG	Multifocal electroretinogram
RA	Rheumatoid arthritis
RPE	Retinal pigment epithelium
SAP	Standard automated perimetry
SD-OCT	Spectral domain optical coherence tomography
SLE	Systemic lupus erythematosus
VF-25	Visual function 25 questionnaire

This chapter covers the natural history of chloroquine and hydroxychloroquine retinopathy. There is no evidence to suggest that the natural histories of these maculopathies differ from each other. Therefore, all the statements in this chapter apply to both drugs. Hydroxychloroquine and chloroquine will be referred to as 4-aminoquinolines (4AQs) and the retinopathy that they can cause will be termed 4-aminoquinoline retinopathy (4AQR). Commonly used abbreviations in this chapter are collected in "Abbreviations" for reference. Each term will be first used in its full form, along with its abbreviation.

6.1 Clinical Setting and Picture for Development of Chloroquine and Hydroxychloroquine Retinopathy

Although scenarios vary in which chloroquine and hydroxychloroquine retinopathy occur, certain characteristics are common. Most patients with retinopathy have been overdosed, and height and weight have not been checked to determine the ideal body weight (IBW) (see Chap. 7) [1, 2]. Occasionally renal or hepatic insufficiency has not been noted and an adjustment to dosing made to account for these characteristics. These most common mistakes led Morsman to write, "Examining the patient's medical records is more useful than examining their eyes" [3]. In other cases, appropriate screening tests have been performed but misinterpreted as normal (see Chap. 8) [1]. Many patients have been screened at appropriate intervals, but the diagnosis of retinopathy has been missed (see Chap. 9) [1, 4, 5]. Although it is true that cases of 4AQR can occur in which everything has been done correctly, in most cases a failure analysis will indicate that the condition is iatrogenic.

D.J. Browning, *Hydroxychloroquine and Chloroquine Retinopathy*,
DOI 10.1007/978-1-4939-0597-3_6, © Springer Science+Business Media New York 2014

6.2   Symptoms

Symptoms have been reported in 3–71 % of patients taking 4AQs [6–8]. Comparisons across case series are fraught with pitfalls because different examiners expend different amounts of effort eliciting symptoms. Symptoms can be expressed spontaneously by the patient or elicited by questioning by the clinician. When subgrouped in this way, half are in each category [6]. The common symptoms associated with chloroquine and hydroxychloroquine use and their relative frequencies are noted in Table 6.1. Trouble with reading is the most common symptom [9].

The frequency of symptoms increases in patients who develop 4AQR, but many patients with retinopathy are asymptomatic [6, 9–14]. Easterbrook reported that 14 % of patients had symptoms at the stage where only relative paracentral scotomata were found, but 60 % of patients with absolute paracentral scotomata

had symptoms [10, 15]. Thus, 40–86 % of patients with retinopathy are asymptomatic, depending on the stage of retinopathy [9, 10]. Patients often have retained excellent single-letter visual acuity scores, but have reading difficulties because of loss of paracentral photoreceptors [16]. In a study in which the visual function-25 (VF-25) questionnaire was given to patients with chloroquine retinopathy, the median composite score of patients was 33.9, the range being 10–81.9 [4].

A failure analysis of cases of 4AQR showed a median delay of 12 months between the onset of symptoms referable to 4AQR and cessation of 4AQs [4]. Although some observers are enthusiastic about the usefulness of symptoms as a screening item [5], most have found symptoms to be unhelpful in detecting retinopathy. On the other hand, noting symptoms is inexpensive. Therefore, the clinician would do well to search for new symptoms at each visit by a patient taking 4AQs. New symptoms warrant increased

Table 6.1 Symptoms in patients taking 4-aminoquinolines and patients with 4-aminoquinoline retinopathy

Class of patient	Drug	N	Symptom	%	Study
Taking 4AQs	C	198	Trouble reading	16.2	Percival [17]
			Blurred images	8.6	
			Haloes	1.0	
			Grittiness	6.1	
		28	Blurred vision, colored rings, lack of accommodation	6.8	Reed [18]
		165	Haloes	7.3	Hobbs [19]
		165	Blurring	5.5	
		165	Halos and visual disturbances	1.3	
	C or HC	56	Haloes	12.5	Henkind [6]
			Difficulty adjusting to sunlight	7.1	
			Blurred vision	7.1	
			Vague awareness of eyes	7.1	
			Eyes tired	5.4	
			Diplopia	3.6	
			Dim vision	3.6	
		437	Decrease vision or blurred vision	2.9	Bray [7]
	HC	758	Blurred vision, photophobia, lachrymation, red circles, lack of accommodation, diplopia	1.1	Grierson [20]
		25	Nyctalopia, color vision problems, glare	2.0	Chen [21]

(continued)

Table 6.1 (continued)

Class of patient	Drug	N	Symptom	%	Study
4AQR	C	8	Trouble reading	6.3	Okun [22]
			Photophobia	6.3	
			Blurred distance vision	7.5	
			Peripheral field defects	3.8	
			Floaters/flashes of light	2.5	
		16	Blurred vision	3.1	Araiza-Casillas [23]
			Lack of accommodation	1.3	
			Decreased peripheral vision	1.0	
	C or HC	3	Trouble reading	100	Hickley [24]
			Lack of accommodation	100	
			Decreased color vision	6.7	
		16	Trouble reading	6.3	Michaelides [9]
			Decreased color vision	1.3	
			Nyctalopia	1.3	
			Blurred distance vision	1.0	
	HC	7	Decreased vision	4.3	Payne [25]
			Flashing lights	1.4	
			Decreased color contrast	2.9	
			Disappearing letters	1.4	
		13	Change in color perception	NG	Bienfang [26]
			Trouble finding a seat in a dim room		
			Scotomata on a TV screen		
		6[a]	Decreased or distorted vision	100	Bienfang [5]
		7	Blurred vision	42.9	Mititelu [8]
			Shimmering lights	28.6	
			Trouble with night vision	28.6	
			Trouble reading	14.3	

NG is not given. C is chloroquine. HC is hydroxychloroquine
[a]Means the patients in this series may also have been counted in the series Bienfang [26]

suspicion of retinopathy and the need for review of risk factors such as daily dosing based on IBW [15].

6.3   Signs of 4-Aminoquinoline Retinopathy

6.3.1   Visual Acuity

Visual acuity does not change in premaculopathy and may be excellent in advanced retinopathy with a bull's-eye lesion and dense paracentral scotomata [4–6, 9, 22, 27–29]. Decrease in visual acuity secondary to chloroquine or hydroxychloroquine indicates advanced maculopathy and progression from a paracentral to a central scotoma on standard automated perimetry (SAP) [30]. Approximately 8.6 % (17 of 198) of patients with 4AQR have less than 20/20 best corrected visual acuity in one or both eyes [17].

Easterbrook suggested that visual acuity is a useful factor for predicting progression of retinopathy. His idea is that if patients have visual acuity of 20/20, then there is a good chance that the relative scotoma will not progress [31]. On the other hand, he estimates the probability at greater than 50 % that further deterioration in the retinopathy will occur if the visual acuity is less than 20/20 at the time that retinopathy is diagnosed [14].

Table 6.2 Stages of 4-aminoquinoline retinopathy

Characteristic	Premaculopathy	Early maculopathy	Advanced maculopathy
Visual field	Scotoma to red target only	Scotoma to red or white target	Absolute scotoma to white object
Symptoms	Rare	Sometimes	Usually present
Visual acuity	Not affected	Rarely affected	More often affected, but can be normal
Macula	Pigment stippling or loss of foveal reflex at worst[a]; often normal	Pigment stippling or loss of foveal reflex[a]	Bull's-eye lesion
Reversibility	Usually	Sometimes	No
Onset or progression after cessation of drug	Rare	Uncommon	Possible

Parts of this table are taken from Yam [62] and Bray [7]
[a]Indicates that other observers consider that loss of foveal reflex does not occur in 4AQR [15]

6.3.2 Stages of 4-Aminoquinoline Retinopathy

Much of the early literature on chloroquine and hydroxychloroquine retinopathy contained observations and interpretations that are now recognized as erroneous. For example, macular edema and subretinal fluid were thought to be early signs of chloroquine retinopathy, but more sophisticated examination techniques, including spectral domain optical coherence tomography (SD-OCT), have shown that edema and subretinal fluid do not occur in 4AQR [6, 15, 18, 19, 32–36]. Nonspecific pigmentary changes of the macula were often attributed to 4AQR, but now it is thought that many of these observations reflected the common presence of pigmentary mottling in aging patients [6, 32, 37–39]. Peripheral retinopathy was claimed by some observers to predate central and paracentral changes, but it is now known that the order of changes is the reverse [40, 41]. A case of peripheral onset chloroquine retinopathy without maculopathy was reported, but not shown, and there remains doubt that this represented true chloroquine retinopathy [42]. Bull's-eye macular lesions were reported to go away with cessation of treatment, but subsequent experience suggests that these were mistaken observations, and that bull's-eye lesions do not go away [43, 44]. Although early observers claim to have had patients with bull's-eye lesions without scotoma or visual loss [32, 33], these reports probably represent mistakes as well. The presence of a bull's-

eye lesion is always accompanied by an annular scotoma and usually by symptoms [6, 45, 46].

Patients with 4AQR have been categorized in several ways. Some authors categorize by groupings of factors. In this classification, patients are classified first based on funduscopic changes, and then are further subdivided into subgroups based on which ancillary tests are abnormal. A second system classification is probabilistic. Retinopathy is graded as possible (also called questionable), probable, or definite [46]. The former method has the problem of uncertain reproducibility, as most studies do not report test-retest statistics using chosen definitions. The latter methodology depends on the panel of graders, which raises the issue of generalizability. Both problems limit the applicability of the information generated to a clinical setting and suffer from the lack of standardization across observers. For example, case 2 illustrated in a paper by Okun and colleagues is termed early chloroquine retinopathy [22], yet the photograph (Fig. 2 from that reference) shows a definite bull's-eye maculopathy, which would imply that it is an advanced case in most categorizations [47]. Table 6.2 lists commonly understood characteristics of the three major stages of retinopathy: premaculopathy, early maculopathy, and advanced maculopathy (see also Chap. 4).

There are varying definitions of premaculopathy (see Chap. 4) [7, 25, 38, 46, 48–54]. Some definitions specify that patients are asymptomatic but have macular pigmentary changes that are difficult to separate from normal aging changes [7, 25, 52, 54–57]. One common definition is the

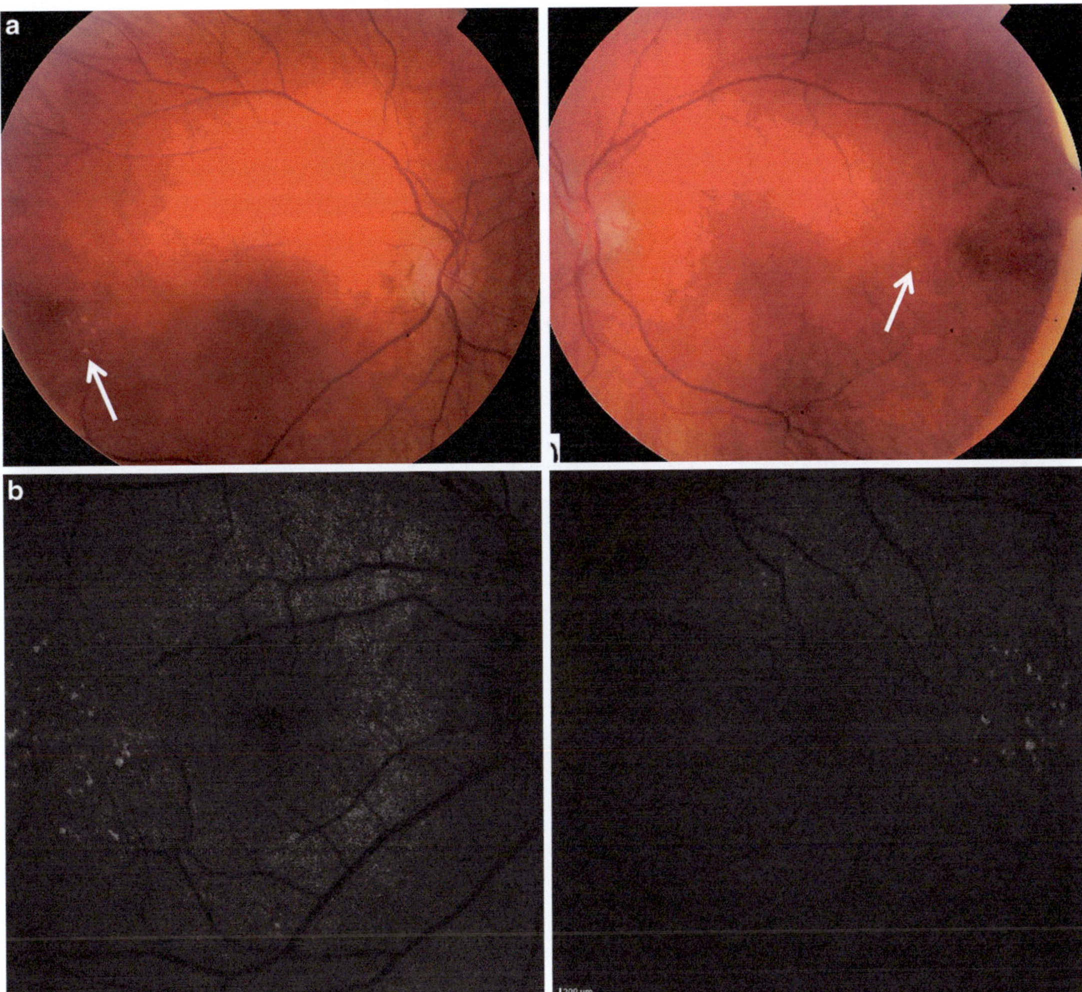

Fig. 6.1 This 38-year-old woman had been taking hydroxychloroquine at a dose of 400 mg/day for 21 years for systemic lupus erythematosus. She had no visual complaints and was seen for routine retinopathy screening evaluations. Her height was 66 inches and her weight 210 pounds. She had no liver or renal disease. (**a**) Her maculas had some drusen temporally, but no stigmata of hydroxychloroquine retinopathy were present. (**b**) Fundus autofluorescence imaging was normal bilaterally. (**c**) Relative paracentral scotomata were present on three consecutive 10-2 visual fields using a white target. (**d**) Multifocal electroretinography was normal bilaterally based on normal amplitudes in all rings and a normal R1/R2 ratio. (**e**) Spectral domain optical coherence tomography showed slight decreased reflectivity of the pericentral retinal pigment epithelial layer (*yellow arrows*) bilaterally. Although her daily dosage of hydroxychloroquine was 5.94 mg/kg based on an ideal body weight of 148 pounds, a typically nontoxic dosage, it was recommended that she decreased her hydroxychloroquine daily dosage to 300 mg. She had no relapse in lupus activity. She was asked to return for a recheck in 6 months rather than 1 year

presence of central or pericentral scotomata to a red test object without an accompanying scotoma to a white test object [32, 34, 41, 58]. Others define this stage in a similar way as having a relative but not an absolute paracentral scotoma [10]. Some add to this definition those patients who lose the foveal reflex during therapy, a questionable additional criterion given the lack of any evidence that foveal reflex assessment is reproducible [17, 38]. Another definition is a state of interference at the metabolic level that has not yet produced morphologic changes and that is reversible [17]. An example of premaculopathy is shown in Fig. 6.1.

From zero to 14 % of patients with premaculopathy were found to have ophthalmic symptoms in various studies [7, 10]. Reversibility (see next

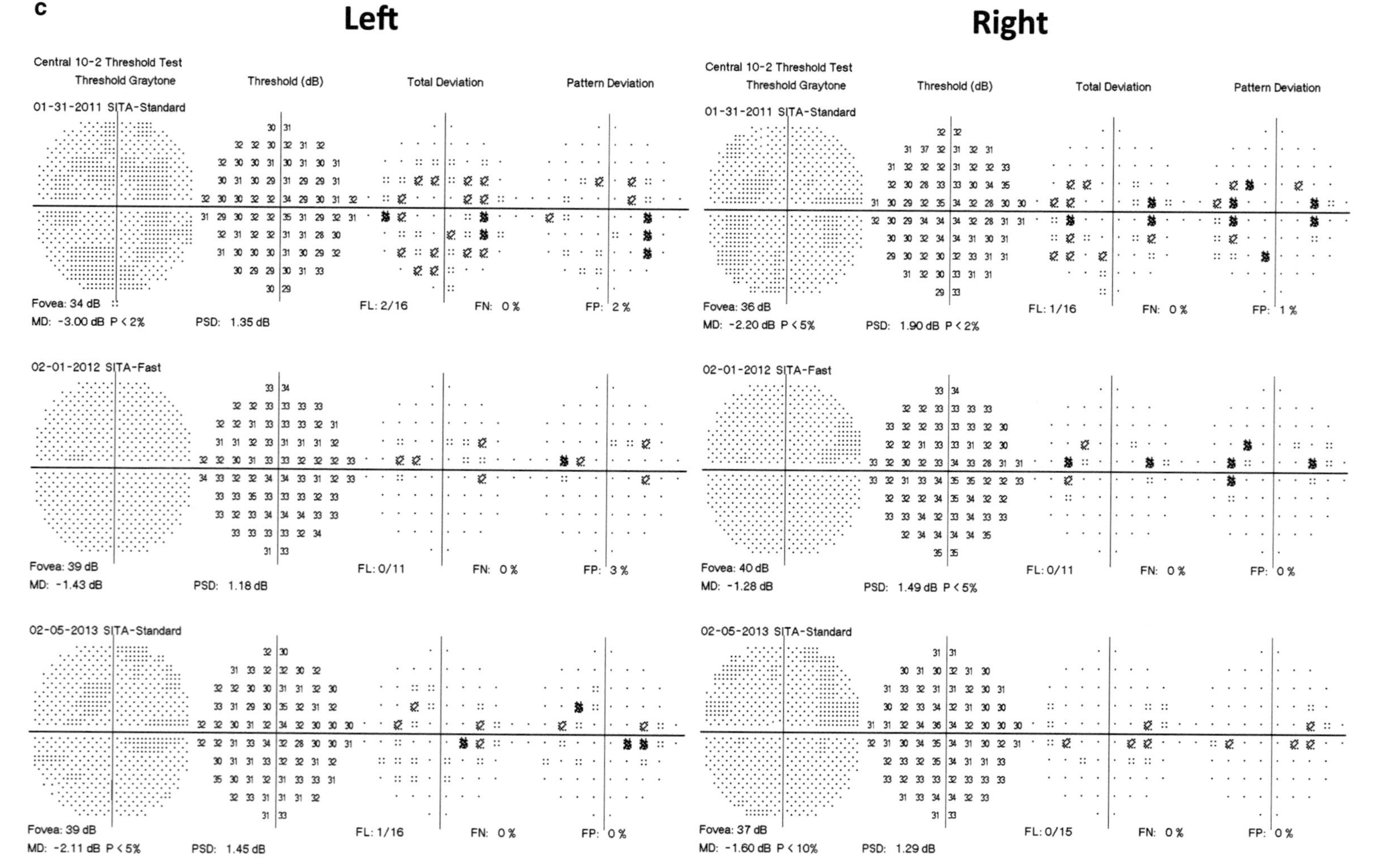

Fig. 6.1 (continued)

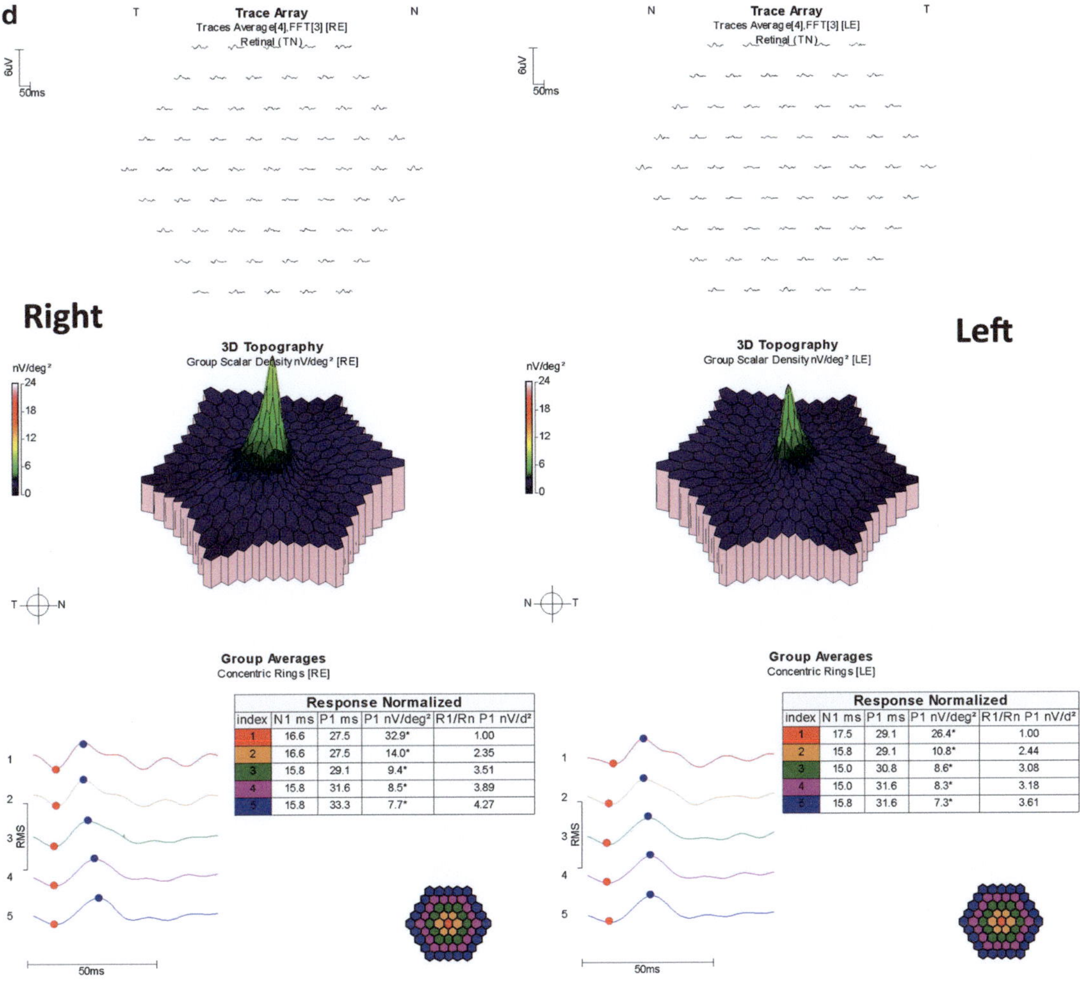

Group Averages — Concentric Rings [RE]

	Response Normalized			
index	N1 ms	P1 ms	P1 nV/deg²	R1/Rn P1 nV/d²
1	16.6	27.5	32.9*	1.00
2	16.6	27.5	14.0*	2.35
3	15.8	29.1	9.4*	3.51
4	15.8	31.6	8.5*	3.89
5	15.8	33.3	7.7*	4.27

Group Averages — Concentric Rings [LE]

	Response Normalized			
index	N1 ms	P1 ms	P1 nV/deg²	R1/Rn P1 nV/d²
1	17.5	29.1	26.4*	1.00
2	15.8	29.1	10.8*	2.44
3	15.0	30.8	8.6*	3.08
4	15.0	31.6	8.3*	3.18
5	15.8	31.6	7.3*	3.61

Fig. 6.1 (continued)

section) has been claimed for some patients at this stage of retinopathy, but documentation has been scant in support of this assertion [32, 41, 54, 58–60]. For example, Easterbrook reported on 44 eyes with relative paracentral scotomata after taking chloroquine or hydroxychloroquine [10]. Over a period of at least 4 years of follow-up, 5 (11 %) showed a decrease in size of the relative scotomas, but no eye returned to a normal visual field [10]. In a primate model of chloroquine retinopathy, histopathologic changes are evident before funduscopic changes occur [61].

The rate at which premaculopathy develops in hydroxychloroquine and chloroquine users has not been clearly defined in light of the variability of the definitions. Estimates of 3.3–17 % have been published for hydroxychloroquine users and 5.6 % for chloroquine users [7, 57].

There are few definitive case reports in which premaculopathy has progressed to advanced retinopathy (Fig. 6.2) [7, 57]. More frequently reported is progression to a more severe stage of retinopathy short of a bull's-eye maculopathy [10]. For example, of 44 eyes having relative paracentral scotomas that were followed at least 4 years, 4 (9 %) showed an increase in size of the relative scotomas, and 2 (4 %) showed progression from relative to absolute scotomas [10]. Fine macular stippling has no prognostic value with respect to subsequent unequivocal retinopathy. Many older normal patients have this finding [17, 57]. Cessation of 4AQs at the stage of

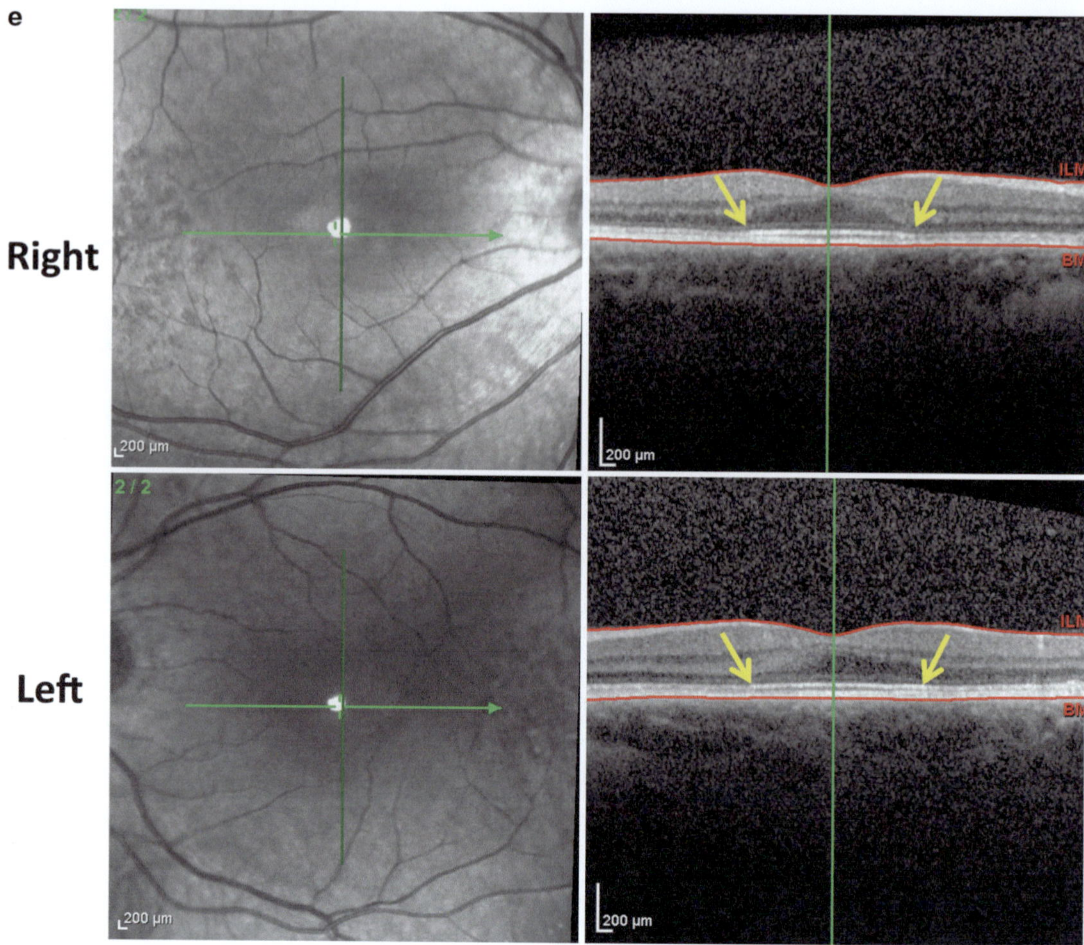

Fig. 6.1 (continued)

premaculopathy generally has a good prognosis, although exceptions occur (Fig. 6.2) [7, 10].

Patients with premaculopathy can pose a dilemma for clinicians who do not wish to discontinue a beneficial drug but also wish to avoid the harm of retinopathy (Fig. 6.1). In such cases close follow-up and assuring that toxic dosing, the only modifiable risk factor, does not occur may be the best that can be done.

Early retinopathy is more advanced than premaculopathy but is also inconsistently defined, leading to numerous cases that might be placed in either category [29, 63]. Patients often do not have symptoms at this stage [64]. Some authors term this moderate rather than early retinopathy [65]. The presence of a relative scotoma to a white test object is part of the usual definition [11].

Some have included a minimum duration criterion, e.g., treatment for at least 9 months [66]. Fundus changes can be present, but no bull's-eye lesion [22, 67]. In a primate retina model of chloroquine retinopathy, definite histopathological changes predated fundus changes [9, 61, 68]. Some authors describe patients in this group as having color vision problems and yet no visual field defects [29]. Various components of this stage include blunting or loss of the foveal reflex, parafoveal retinal pigment epithelial (RPE) irregularity, and parafoveal depigmentation (Fig. 6.2) [65, 69–71]. Loss of a foveal reflex is not a reliable sign since patients can have retinopathy and retain a foveal reflex [31]. Moreover, these changes can be seen in normal patients as they age [63]. Although some have said that early fundus

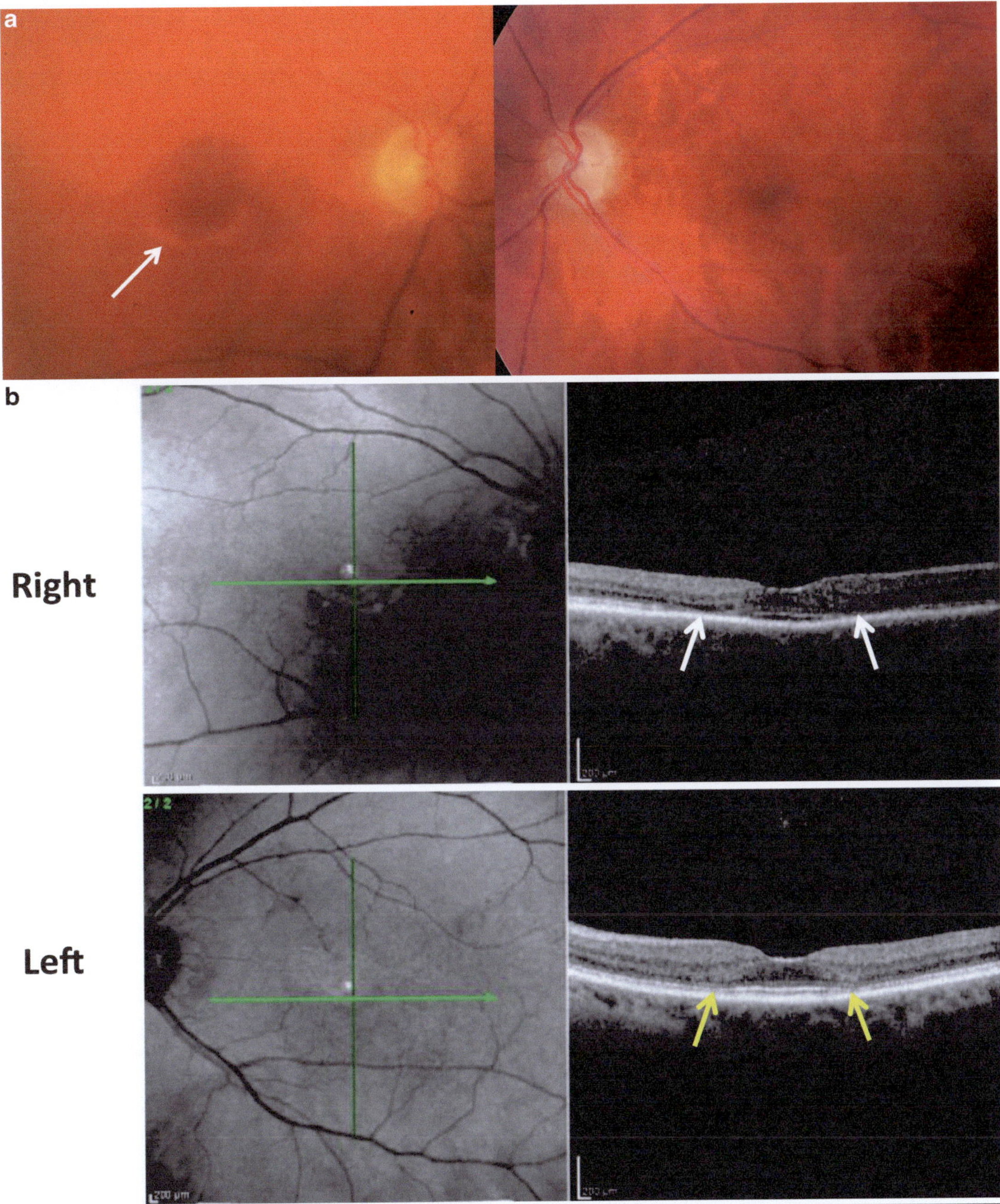

Fig. 6.2 Images of a 69-year-old woman with systemic lupus erythematosus who had taken hydroxychloroquine at a dosage of 400 mg/day from 1995 until 2006 when the drug was stopped secondary to retinopathy. She had no renal or liver disease. Her height was 5 feet 11 inches and her actual body weight 187 pounds; her ideal body weight 173 pounds. (**a**) She had a bull's-eye macular lesion of the right eye (*white arrow*) consistent with advanced retinopathy and mild, nonspecific retinal pigment epithelial (RPE) mottling of the left macula consistent with early maculopathy. (**b**) Spectral domain optical coherence tomography (SD-OCT) of the right eye shows loss of the outer segments and inner segment/outer segment junction in the perifovea (*white arrows*). In the left eye the inner segment/outer segment junction is attenuated but not lost (*yellow arrows*). (**c**) Fundus autofluorescence images show a hypo-autofluorescent ring around the fovea of the right eye corresponding to RPE atrophy. In the left eye there is a subtle locus of hyperautofluorescence (*orange arrow*). (**d**) Multifocal electroretinogram (mfERG) in the retina view (since the patient faces the observer, the patient's right eye is the *left panel*). The averaged N1P1 amplitudes for rings R1 and R2 are subnormal, but the R1/R2 ratio is normal for the right eye. All of the N1P1 amplitudes are low-normal for the left eye and the R1/R2 ratio is normal. (**e**) 10-2 visual fields over time for the right eye show development of a ring scotoma that improves once the drug is stopped (2006). (**f**) 10-2 visual fields over time for the left eye showing parallel changes to the right eye. The scotoma depth is not as great in this eye. Note that the mfERG, SD-OCT, and 10-2 VFs agree in their indication of severity of retinopathy

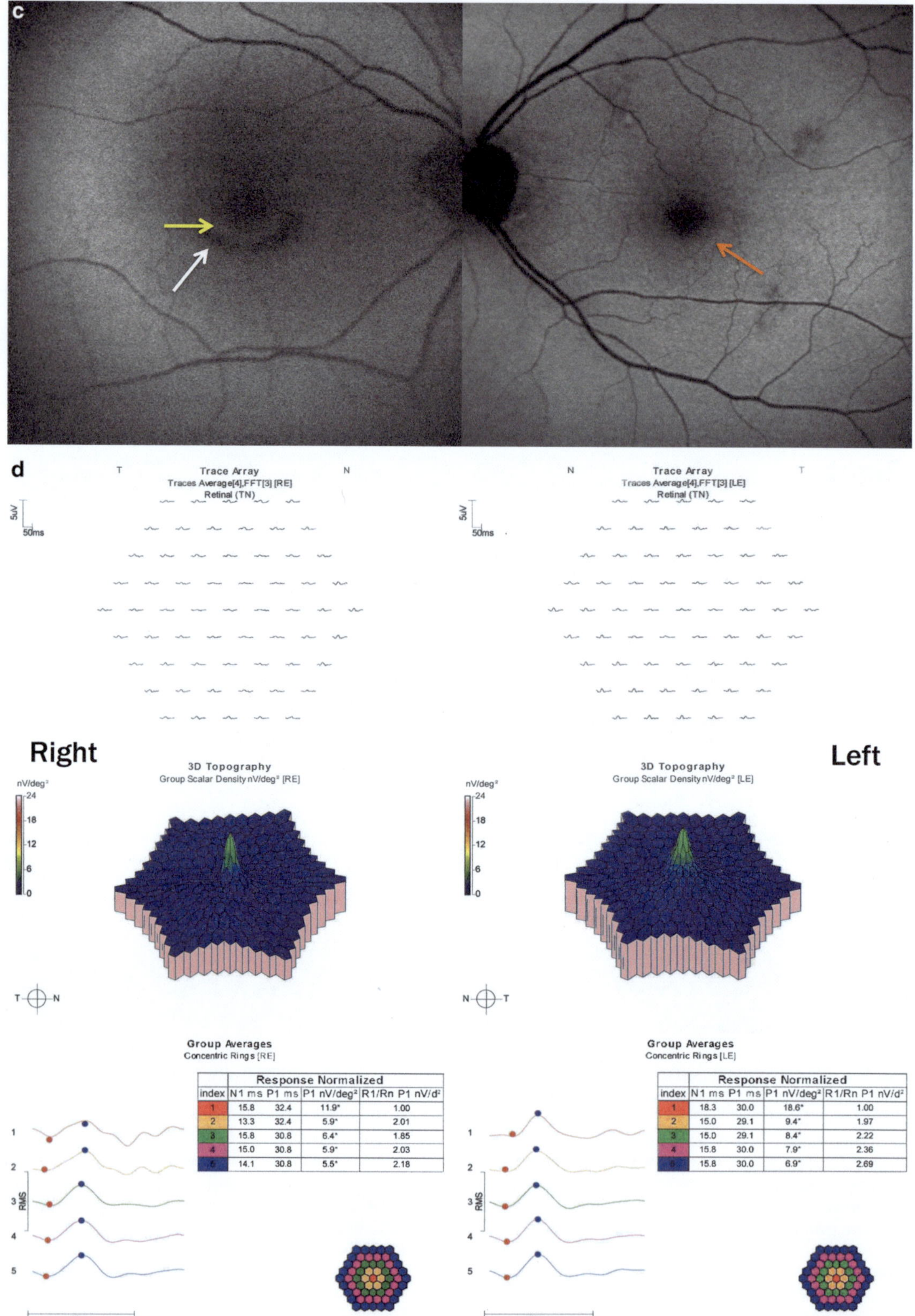

Fig. 6.2 (continued)

e

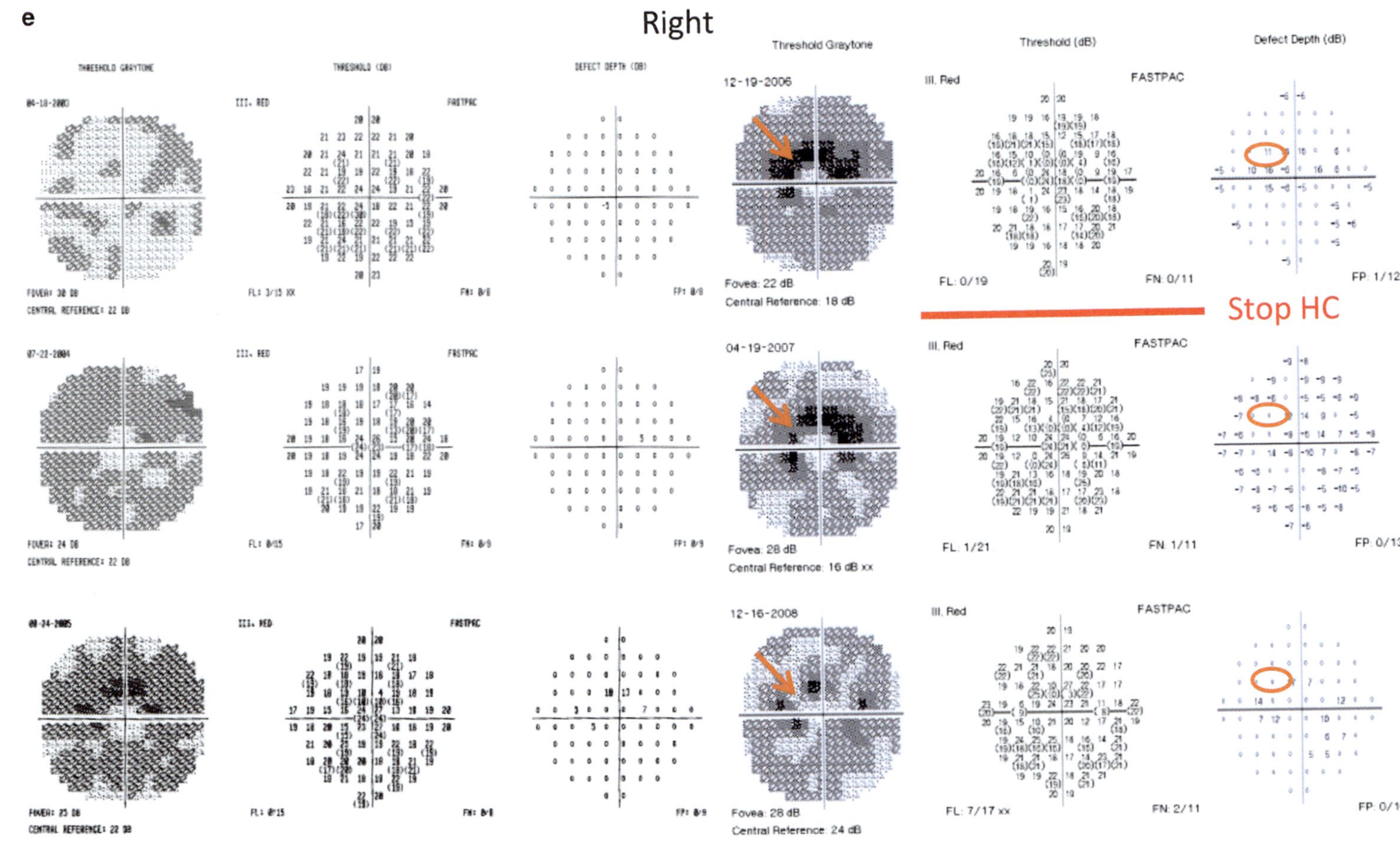

Fig. 6.2 (continued)

Left

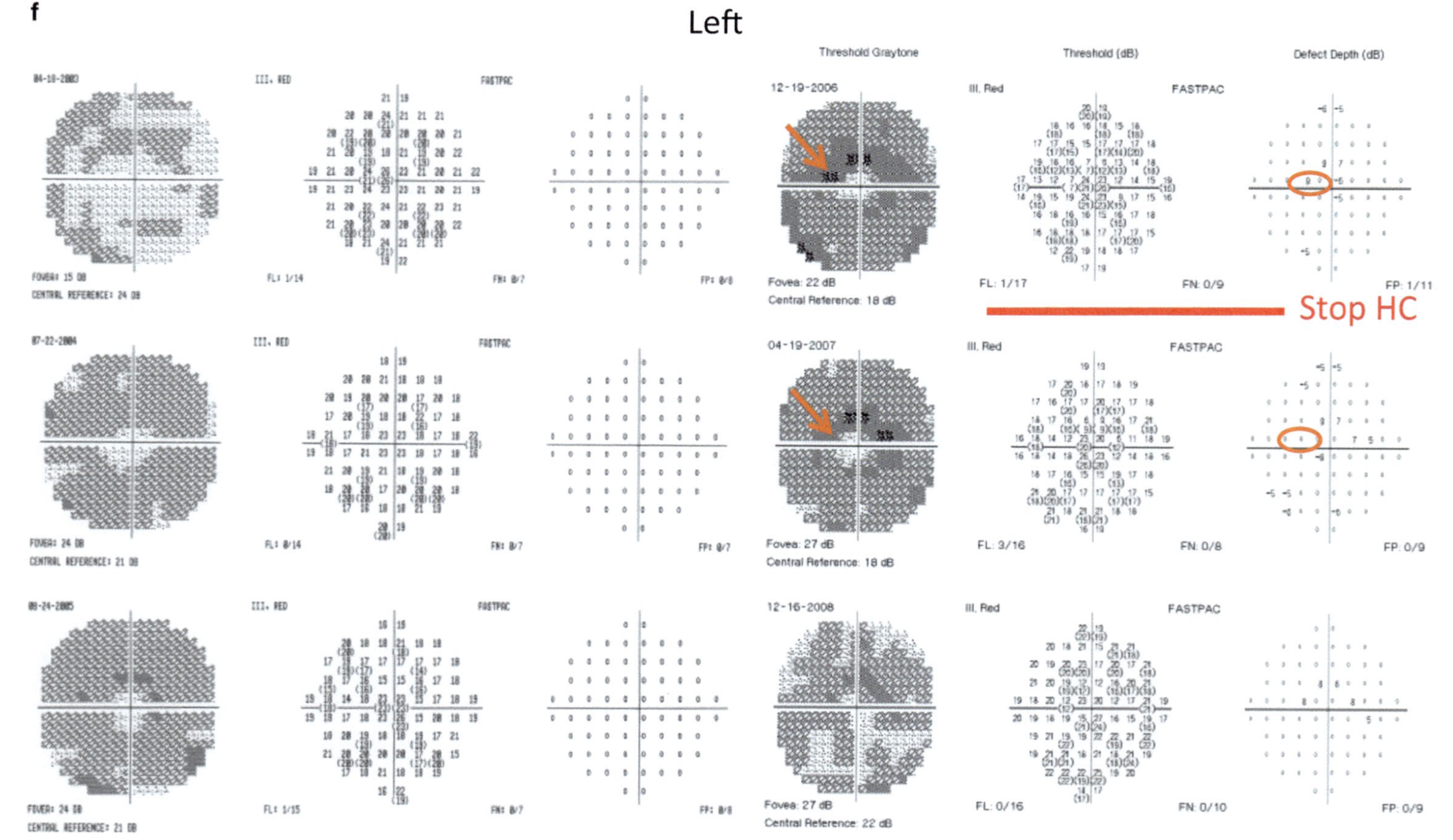

Fig. 6.2 (continued)

changes are reversible in up to 50 % of such cases [54], skepticism is appropriate as there has been no photographic documentation to analyze [53]. Patients with early retinopathy may have multifocal electroretinographic (mfERG) abnormalities with or without visual field abnormalities (Fig. 6.2) [29].

With cessation of 4AQs, regression of scotomas is said to be less frequent than if scotomas are only present to a red test object [32]. Fundus changes are often absent at this stage. The mean onset of this stage in a series of four patients from among 262 screened was 3.5 years [72]. Over 4 years of follow-up of 44 such patients, there were no patients who progressed to loss of visual acuity [10].

The presence of an absolute paracentral scotoma is more advanced than the presence of a relative white scotoma. Sixty per cent of such patients will have symptomatic color vision problems, dropped letters, or symptomatic field loss [10]. Over a period of at least 4 years of follow-up, 63 % of such eyes will lose central visual acuity, and 13 % will experience a visual acuity decline from 20/40 or better to 20/200 [10].

The classically recognized bull's-eye lesion of 4AQR signifies a very advanced stage of retinopathy that never reverts to normal [31, 46, 52, 62, 71, 73–75]. Patients at this stage will have more severe mfERG abnormalities [29]. The earliest that a bull's-eye lesion has developed after beginning 4AQ therapy has not been established. There is a report of a lesion developing after 10 months of taking HC at 400 mg/day after a normal baseline examination, but photodocumentation was not provided [76]. Early fundus changes can progress to a bull's-eye lesion within 3 years [77].

The bull's-eye lesion has been described as having a hyperpigmented center with a surrounding hypopigmented ring [38, 54, 78, 79]. Occasionally, the lesion forms a circle (e.g., Fig. 6.2 and case 1 of Weiner and colleagues [80]). However, the lesion is usually horizontally oval, with more RPE atrophy in the inferior half of the oval (Fig. 6.2) [5, 50, 51, 81]. The earliest and broadest zone of RPE atrophy is often found in the inferotemporal quadrant [50, 80, 82]. The central zone in which the RPE remains intact is not oval, however, but rather more circular (Fig. 6.5) [30, 83]. Correspondingly, the density of the associated scotoma is often greater for the superior paracentral visual field (Figs. 6.2 and 6.4). Most cases of 4AQR are symmetrical, but asymmetrical cases have been reported (Fig. 6.2) (Fig. 4, [9, 11, 20, 22, 25, 33, 77, 81, 84, 85]). Asymmetry may be detected in ancillary testing as well. For example, Maturi noted mfERG abnormalities in one eye but not the fellow eye in four patients taking hydroxychloroquine and suspected of having early retinopathy [86]. Similarly, Amsler grid testing can show asymmetric scotomata [87].

How Big are 4-Aminoquinoline Retinopathy Bull's-Eyes and How Variable are the Dimensions?

Table 6.3 shows the range of dimensions of bull's-eye lesions seen in 4-aminoquinoline retinopathy based on a review of 20 cases published with photographs [16, 22, 25, 29, 33, 51, 69, 80, 82, 83, 86, 88–93]. Each photograph included both the macular legion and the optic disc, which was used as an internal caliper in which the vertical diameter of the disc was assumed to be 1.8 mm.

Table 6.3 Dimensions of 4-aminoquinoline bull's-eye maculopathy

Dimension	Median (mm)	IQR (mm)	Range (mm)
Outer horizontal diameter	2.9	(2.2–3.7)	(1.6–4.3)
Outer vertical diameter	1.9	(1.8–2.4)	(1.4–3.3)
Inner horizontal diameter	1.1	(0.9–1.7)	(0.5–2.1)
Inner vertical diameter	0.9	(0.7–1.3)	(0.3–1.8)

The distributions of measurements were not normal; therefore, nonparametric statistics are given. mm means millimeters. IQR means interquartile range

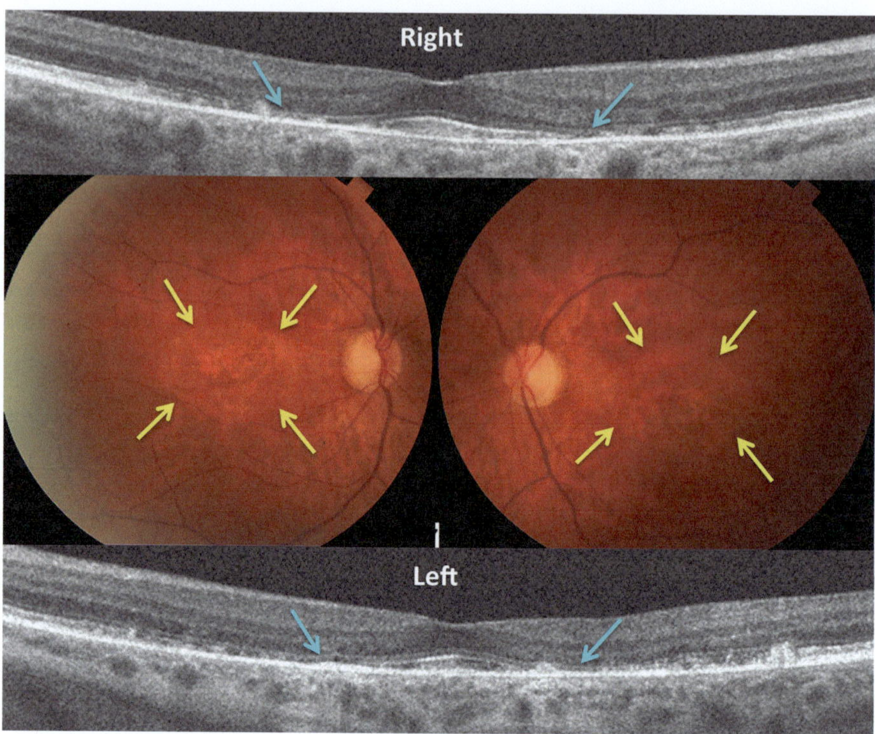

Fig. 6.3 Images of a 63-year-old woman with age-related maculopathy, no autoimmune diseases, and no history of 4-aminoquinoline usage, showing that a bull's-eye maculopathy is not specific to 4-aminoquinoline retinopathy. Both maculas have a bull's-eye lesion of retinal pigment epithelial atrophy (*yellow arrows* denote the peripheral borders). The spectral domain optical coherence tomogra-phy images show analogous changes to those seen in 4-aminoquinoline retinopathy, with perifoveal loss of the inner segment/outer segment junction (*blue arrows*). The presence of drusen in this case distinguishes the pattern from what would otherwise be compatible with the picture of 4-aminoquinoline retinopathy

Bull's-eye lesions are not specific for 4AQR [94]. They can occur in cone dystrophy, Stargardt disease, resolved central serous retinopathy, and age-related macular degeneration (Fig. 6.3) [94].

At an even more advanced stage, the central zone of spared RPE also becomes atrophic [28, 65, 83]. For unknown reasons, the fovea seems resistant to toxicity compared to the parafovea [8].

At the end-stage, mid-peripheral and eventually peripheral RPE atrophy and granulation develop, as well as arteriolar narrowing [22, 29, 40]. As with the paramacular fundus changes, the mid-peripheral fundus changes typically develop first and more extensively in the inferior fundus (Fig. 6.4). Visual field loss becomes more global with mid-peripheral breakout of the formerly paracentral scotomata [22, 29].

6.4   Reversibility

An impetus for screening to detect hydroxychloroquine and chloroquine retinopathy is that with cessation, the retinopathy might regress. Many suggestions of such a possibility have been published [6, 8, 33, 43, 95, 96]. Occasionally patients with asymptomatic minor macular lesions, relative scotomas, and sometimes electroretinogram (ERG) abnormalities (variations of premaculopathy or early maculopathy) have shown reversal of abnormalities upon discontinuation of 4AQs [6, 43, 60, 80, 96–100]. For example, in one study reversibility was claimed in 59 of 64 (92.2 %) patients on chloroquine with premaculopathy as defined by perception of paracentral scotomata to a red test object [17].

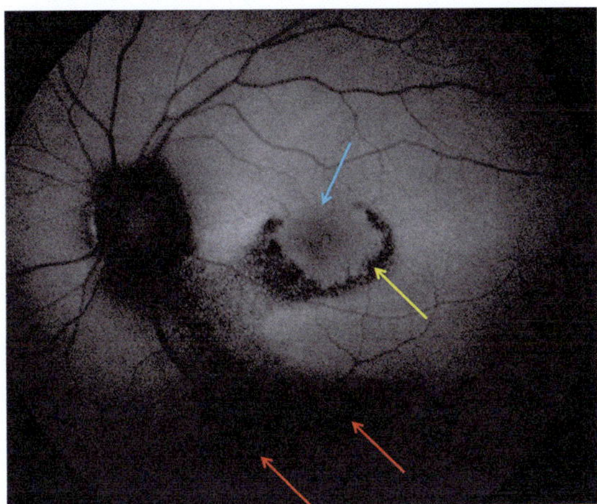

Fig. 6.4 Fundus autofluorescence image of a 46-year-old woman with systemic lupus erythematosus who had taken chloroquine for 17 years at a dosage of 500 mg/day. Based on her actual body weight, which was ideal, she had been overdosed at 8.8 mg/kg/day and had received a cumulative dose of 3,102 g of hydroxychloroquine. The preferential damage to the inferior paramacula is shown with the incomplete RPE atrophic annulus (*yellow arrow*). The superior paramacula from ten to one o'clock is spared (*blue arrow*).The inferior mid-peripheral atrophic zone is more pronounced than the superior (*red arrows*)

However, since premaculopathy is a fuzzy concept and difficult to prove, it is equally difficult to prove that an event represents true reversion to normal, rather than simply noise in testing with reversion to normal due to variability of discerning paracentral red scotomas.

Other studies claiming reversibility of perimetric scotomas likewise may be misinterpreting test-retest variability as reversibility of an abnormality [43, 53]. For example, several of the cases of reversibility were described at a time when tangent screen visual field testing was commonly used. It is a subjective, poorly standardized method for which reproducibility has not been shown [99]. Carr and colleagues followed 25 patients with 4AQR and found that after cessation of drugs three (12 %) had reversal of macular changes, 16 (64 %) had no change, and 6 (24 %) had worsening [101]. This report did not show photographs to document the asserted reversion of mild macular abnormalities back to normal. The authors suggested that an abnormal electrooculogram (EOG) at the time of drug cessation might predict progression of maculopathy, which seems doubtful given lack of confidence in the test to aid in diagnosis of 4AQR (see Chap. 8) [101]. In one report of reversible maculopathy, retinal sensitivity to proprietary red stimuli was measured, making it difficult for others to replicate the findings [48]. In cases in which mild macular pigmentary mottling has been claimed to reverse over 10 years of follow-up, a degree of skepticism is warranted in the absence of photographs because of the test-retest variability of funduscopy [96].

More convincing are reports of scotomas on 10-2 VF testing regressing upon cessation of 4AQs [25, 72, 102]. Easterbrook studied 67 patients with field defects due to 4AQs, 37 of whom were followed for at least 4 years after diagnosis and cessation of 4AQs [10]. He found that if stopped at the stage of relative paracentral scotomas, 75 % of 22 such patients were stable, 11 % showed improvement, and 9 % showed worsening of their visual field defects [10]. Of 15 patients with absolute scotomas, none regressed and 63 % got worse, with enlarging scotomas and loss of visual acuity [10, 14].

Besides the various types of perimetry, other ancillary tests used to detect 4AQR, such as mfERG and EOG, yield noisy measurements. Without discipline in interpretation, random variation in test results can be misrepresented either as toxicity in the first place, or as reversal of toxicity when the test is repeated after cessation of 4AQ consumption (see Chap. 8). An example of this phenomenon was published by Lyons and Severns [71]. A 47-year-old woman was presented who had taken hydroxychloroquine for 9 years with a cumulative dosage of 1,300 g. Her mfERG at baseline was normal, but 2 years later it was abnormal. On the basis of this test result, hydroxychloroquine was discontinued, and a follow-up mfERG 1 year later had returned to normal [71]. This sequence was interpreted as recovery of retinal function, yet in the absence of corroborating evidence from a more reliable test such as SD-OCT, it could have been a reflection of measurement variability with the mfERG [103]. The proper response in this case would be to do the test again in short order and see if it fluctuates again into the abnormal range or not [104]. More generally, one must determine the limits of repeatability for the test (see Chap. 8). The clinician needs to know what change in the given type of measurement is required to be sure that the test result represents a real change and not just measurement variability.

If 4-aminoquinoline toxicity can be reversed, it is probable that the earlier it is detected, the better the chance. Because mfERG is thought to be more sensitive than other methods of detection, mfERG studies have been used to examine the issue. Reversibility has been claimed when toxicity was detectable by mfERG but before it was detectable by other modalities [71, 86, 105]. The solidity of the claims is weakened by the poor reproducibility of mfERG studies (see Chap. 8).

Not all observers are convinced that reversibility is a characteristic of 4-aminoquinoline toxicity [5, 51]. In a series of 16 cases of retinopathy followed over time, Michaelides and colleagues did not find evidence of regression of retinopathy in any [9]. None of Bienfang's five cases followed for at least 4 years after diagnosis improved [5]. In a series of 6 cases followed for signs of regression, Payne and colleagues reported that 5 (83.3 %) did not improve [25]. Once a bull's-eye lesion is recognizable in the macula, the retinopathy has reached a point of irreversibility whether or not the drug is stopped, although there may be minor decrease in the breadth of the scotoma (Fig. 6.4) [14, 23, 80, 104].

6.5   Delayed Onset Retinopathy

Several cases of chloroquine and hydroxychloroquine retinopathy have been described in which the drug was stopped at a time when the eyes were normal, yet the retinopathy developed subsequently (Table 6.4) [22, 35, 54, 78, 96, 106, 107]. Delays ranging from 1 to 9 years have been reported. A similar case involving quinacrine has been reported [107]. The causal link in several of these cases is weak. Two of them involve therapy for malaria, for which dosing is lower. Three of them involve males, for which 4AQR is rare based on typical IBWs. Two of them had nonspecific macular pigmentary changes and normal visual fields. The case reported by Ehrenfeld seems unequivocal [78], but delayed-onset retinopathy is extremely rare.

6.6   Progression of Retinopathy

Progression of retinopathy despite cessation of a 4AQ is a fact based on many documented cases (Figs. 6.5 and 6.6) [5, 9, 10, 22, 35, 36, 69, 77, 78, 96, 100, 109–111]. The prevalence of progression of retinopathy despite cessation of drug use is not known, but it is not rare [69]. In one series of 16 patients in whom chloroquine was stopped when early retinopathy was diagnosed, 8 (50 %) progressed over 5 or more years of follow-up [69]. The study looked for characteristics predicting progression of retinopathy with early C retinopathy. Age at the time of diagnosis, cumulative dose of chloroquine, duration of chloroquine use, mean serum creatinine, mean serum ALT, and mean serum AST were no different between patients who did and did not progress [69]. Duration of underlying RA was associated with progression [69].

The risk of progression may depend on the stage at which the drug is stopped. The probability of progression seems to be less if cessation of the drug occurs earlier [10, 31]. Cases with severe fundus autofluorescence (FAF) changes at presentation have been observed to have a poorer prognosis for continued progression despite cessation of 4AQ [112]. In a survey of 68 patients with chloroquine retinopathy suing the manufacturer, serial visual acuity data were available in 19, of whom one improved after stopping drug, six remained unchanged, and 12 progressively worsened [109]. In five cases the worsening continued for more than 5 years after discontinuing the chloroquine. Easterbrook reported on his experience with 217 patients having 4AQR; two-thirds of patients who showed progression of retinopathy had less than 20/20 vision, abnormal color vision, and absolute scotomas [113].

Table 6.4 Characteristics of patients with delayed-onset 4-aminoquinoline retinopathy

Study	Age (years)	Gender	Drug	Total duration (years)/ interval after cessation (years)	Daily dose (mg)	Cumulative dose (g)	VA (R, L)	VF	Fundus exam (R,L)
Ehrenfeld [78]	50	F	C	8/7	250	730	0.33, 0.5	PS	Bull's-eye lesion
Scherbel [106]	41	M	HC	4.7/1.5	400	852	1/1	N	Macular pigmentary granularity
Scherbel [106]	57	M	HC	2/4	400	312	1/1	N	Macular pigmentary granularity
Burns [35]	14	F	C	3/5	250–750	458	0.33, 0.67	Unable	Bull's-eye lesion
Burns [35]	51	F	C	2/4	750	547	0.33, 1	PS	Bull's-eye lesion
Sassani [96, 108]	47	M	C	2/9	Not known	Not known	0.05, 0.05	CS	Bull's-eye lesion

PS is paracentral scotoma; CS is central scotoma; C is chloroquine; HC is hydroxychloroquine; F is female; M is male; unable means the patient was not able to cooperate with VF testing; VA is visual acuity; R is right; L is left; visual acuities are given in decimal format; total duration is number of years of drug treatment; interval after cessation is number of years after cessation of drug that retinopathy appeared

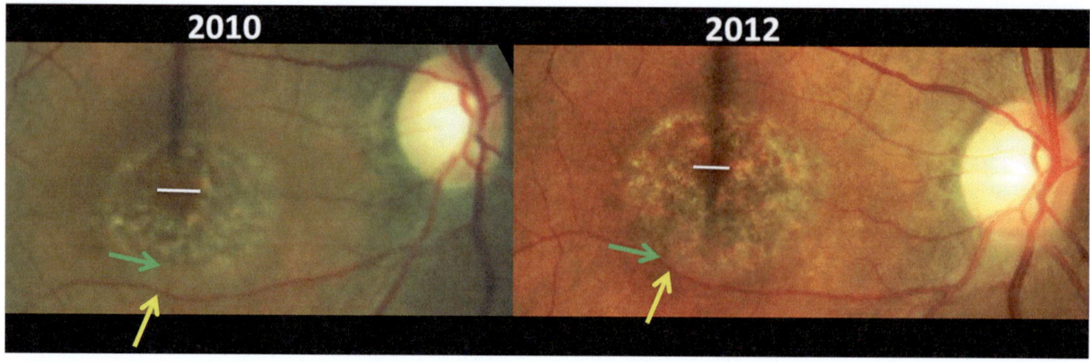

Fig. 6.5 This 60-year-old woman with rheumatoid arthritis had taken hydroxychloroquine at a dose of 6.9 mg/kg/day based on nonobese actual body weight for 3.5 years. She had liver disease from hepatitis C infection. Visual acuity dropped under observation from 20/30 in each eye in 2006 to 20/70 right, 20/100 left in 2010 when a bilateral bull's-eye maculopathy was recognized and hydroxychloroquine was stopped. Over the subsequent 2 years off the drug her visual acuity remained stable at 20/70 right, dropped to 20/200 left, but the extent of her maculopathy increased. The fundus photograph shows that the central spared zone has shrunk (white bars) and the edge of the bull's-eye has moved outward (*green arrow* relative to the retinal vessel at the *yellow arrow*). Similar growth was present in the left eye (not shown). Other cases have been published in which the dimensions of the annular ring of RPE atrophy around the fovea increased with time after the patient stopped taking the 4AQ ([88], Fig. 26.2)

6.7   Treatment of Retinopathy

Proposed treatments of chloroquine and hydroxychloroquine retinopathy have included corticosteroids, oxygen therapy, ascorbic acid, ammonium chloride, and dimercaprol (BAL) [28, 111]. Corticosteroids and oxygen therapy had no beneficial effects [28].

Ascorbic acid can increase release of chloroquine from melanin-containing tissues, but short-term experiments suggest that the effect is clinically unimportant. Ammonium chloride increases excretion of chloroquine, but only when it is given concurrently with chloroquine. Its effect on stored chloroquine seems clinically unimportant [114]. None of these treatments has been shown to be effective, and none are currently used [111].

6.8   Prognosis

The prognosis for 4AQR has been deduced mainly from experience with chloroquine retinopathy, for which more cases with longer follow-up have been reported [31]. It is assumed, but has not been shown, that prognostic factors for hydroxychloroquine retinopathy are similar. Several observers have noted that the prognosis in 4AQR depends on the duration of drug consumption and extent of the retinopathy at the time the drug is stopped [12, 31, 69]. Reversal of retinopathy is possible, but rare, in patients with premaculopathy. Once symptoms referable to retinopathy are present, reversal is probably not possible, but progression is unlikely if the patient has normal visual acuity, normal color vision, and relative rather than absolute paracentral scotomas [31]. If patients have less than 20/20 visual acuity, abnormal color vision testing, absolute rather than relative scotomas on 10-2 testing, and pigment epithelial dropout on fluorescein angiography then two-thirds will show progression of retinopathy over 8.5 years of follow-up [31]. Once a bull's-eye lesion is present, it is agreed that reversal is impossible, although some decrease in size of scotomas is possible (Fig. 6.6) [12].

The final visual acuity outcome in patients with chloroquine and hydroxychloroquine retinopathy depends on how early the retinopathy is detected and the drug is stopped, as well as how long the follow-up has been. In one case series of 68 patients with chloroquine retinopathy suing the manufacturer of the drug, 35 (51.4 %) had visual acuity at last follow-up of less than 20/200 and 14 (20.5 %) had visual acuity below counting fingers [109].

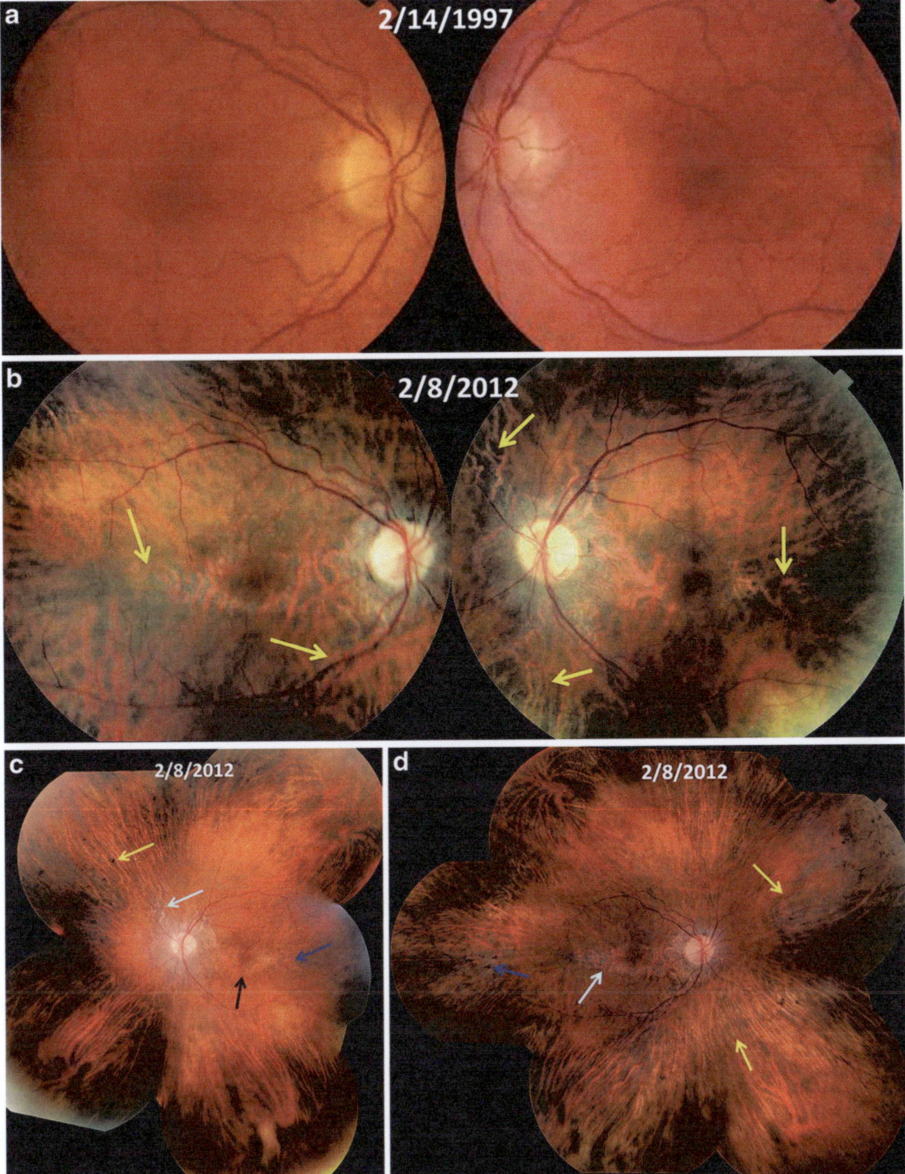

Fig. 6.6 Ancillary studies of a 46-year-old woman with systemic lupus erythematosus who had taken chloroquine for 17 years at a dosage of 500 mg/day. Based on her actual body weight, which was ideal, she had been overdosed at 8.8 mg/kg/day and had received a cumulative dose of 3,102 g. This is the same patient whose fundus autofluorescence image was shown in Fig. 6.4. (**a**) When she was first diagnosed with chloroquine retinopathy her maculas were normal. (**b**) Over the next 15 years she developed bilateral bull's-eye maculopathies. The retinal pigment epithelial (RPE) atrophy extended from the typical annular zones encircling the macula out into the mid-periphery (*yellow arrows*). Peripapillary RPE atrophy also developed. (**c**) Montage fundus photograph of the left eye shows mid-peripheral bone spicule pigmentation (*yellow arrow*). The arterioles are narrowed. The bull's-eye lesion is noted by the *black arrow* with extension of RPE atrophy temporally (*blue arrow*) and peripapillary radiating streaks of RPE atrophy. (**d**) Montage fundus photograph of the right eye shows mid-peripheral zones of RPE atrophy (*yellow arrows*), a bull's-eye lesion that extends temporally (*white arrow*), and mid-peripheral bone spicule pigmentation (*blue arrow*). (**e**) Spectral domain optical coherence tomography (SD-OCT) shows perifoveal loss of the outer nuclear layer, inner segment/ outer segment (IS/OS) junction, and RPE (*yellow arrows*), an intact zone of IS/OS junction and RPE in the fovea (*orange arrows*), and transition zones (*red circled areas*). (**f**) Abnormal multifocal electroretinograms of both eyes. The N1P1 amplitudes are abnormally low for rings R1 to R3 in both eyes. The R1/R2 ratio cannot be calculated in either eye because the machine-drawn cursors are unreliably drawn (*red circled areas*) at such small amplitudes. The individual hexagonal waveforms are attenuated in both eyes in a generalized fashion. (**g**) Serial 10-2 visual fields of the right eye from 1995 through 2012. The first definitively abnormal field was in 11/5/1996, in which a superior paracentral scotoma developed. The fundus was normal at this time. The drug was stopped, but progressive field loss continued through 8/8/2012 (*red arrows* and *blue arrows*)

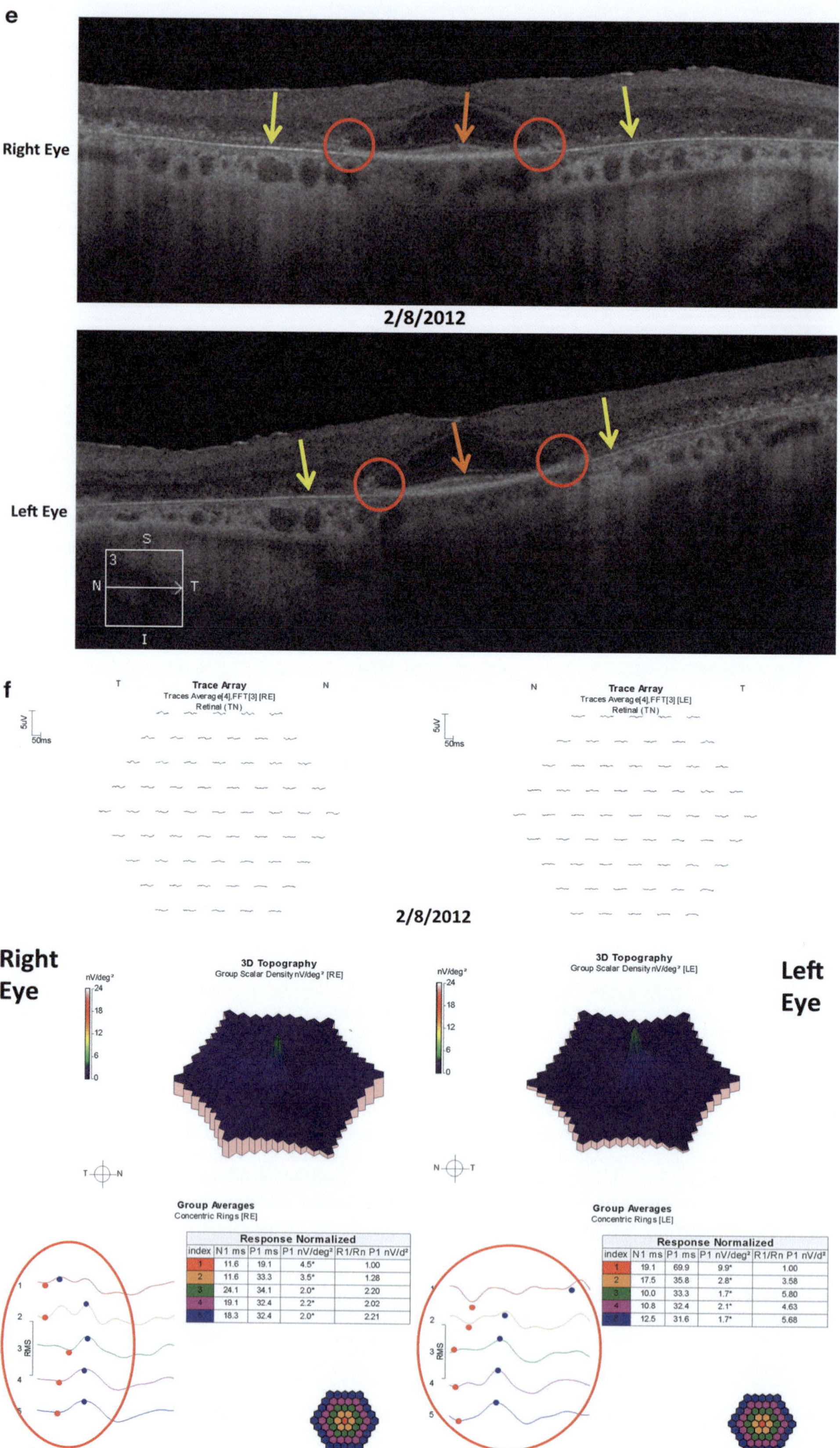

Group Averages — Concentric Rings [RE]

	Response Normalized			
index	N1 ms	P1 ms	P1 nV/deg²	R1/Rn P1 nV/d²
1	11.6	19.1	4.5*	1.00
2	11.6	33.3	3.5*	1.28
3	24.1	34.1	2.0*	2.20
4	19.1	32.4	2.2*	2.02
5	18.3	32.4	2.0*	2.21

Group Averages — Concentric Rings [LE]

	Response Normalized			
index	N1 ms	P1 ms	P1 nV/deg²	R1/Rn P1 nV/d²
1	19.1	69.9	9.9*	1.00
2	17.5	35.8	2.8*	3.58
3	10.0	33.3	1.7*	5.80
4	10.8	32.4	2.1*	4.63
5	12.5	31.6	1.7*	5.68

Fig. 6.6 (continued)

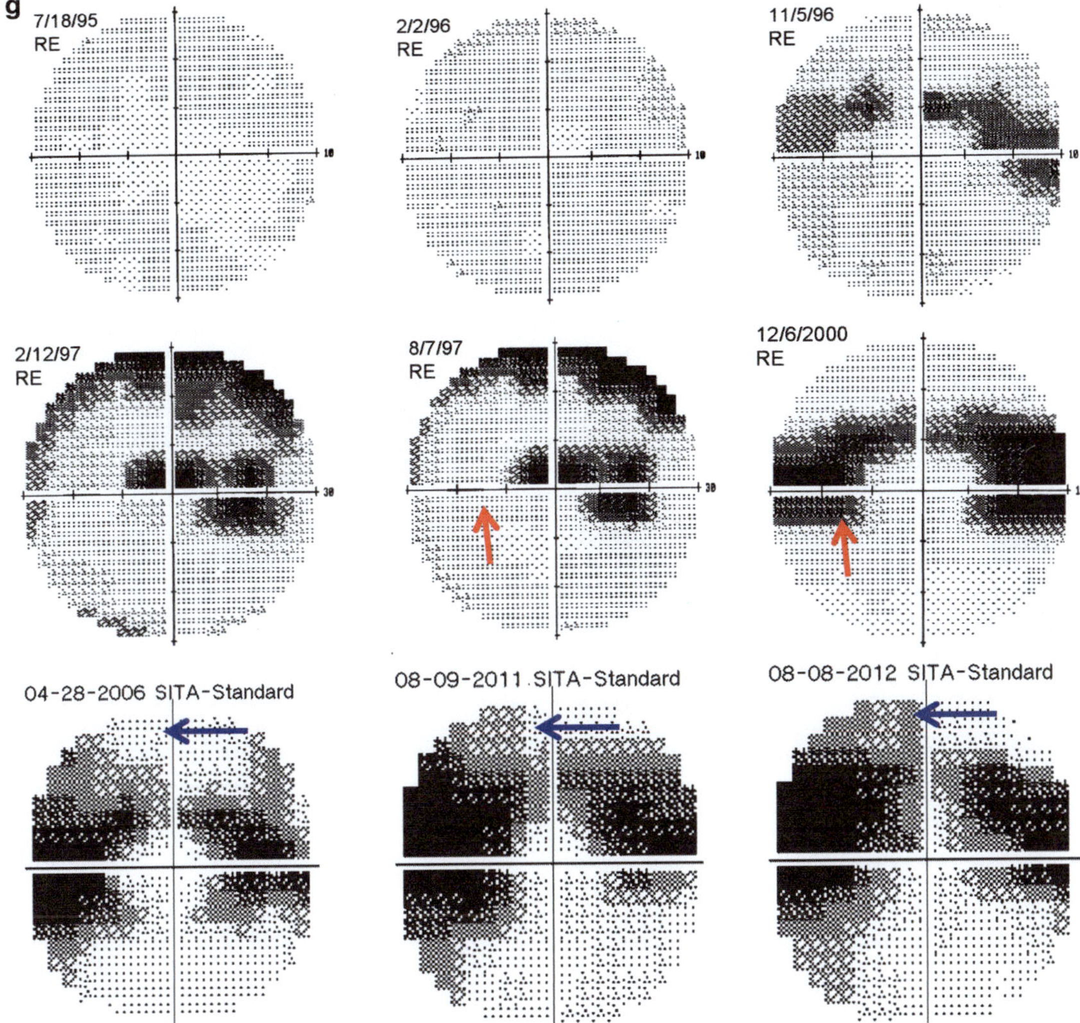

Fig. 6.6 (continued)

6.9 Summary of Key Points

- Most clinically serious cases of 4AQR are iatrogenic, arising from overdosing based on IBW, missed screening, or tardy recognition of evidence of toxicity from ancillary testing.
- Fewer than 15 % of patients taking 4AQs without retinopathy have visual symptoms.
- Between 15 and 60 % of patients with 4AQR have symptoms, which become more common as retinopathy advances.
- At least 40 % of patients with 4AQR are asymptomatic.

- Decreased visual acuity is an insensitive indicator of 4AQR; its presence implies advanced retinopathy.
- Older literature contains some erroneous observations. 4AQR does not cause macular edema. Bull's-eye maculopathy always causes a paracentral scotoma and is never reversible.
- Claims of reversibility of 4AQR are difficult to substantiate when they depend on tests with unknown or large test-retest variability, such as mfERG and tangent screen perimetry. In general, reversibility occurs more often in premaculopathy than in early retinopathy and does not occur in advanced retinopathy.

- Delayed-onset retinopathy can occur, but is rare.
- Progression of retinopathy is more likely and the prognosis poorer the more advanced the stage at which the drug is stopped.
- Two-thirds of patients with cessation of the drug at a point where visual acuity is less than 20/20, color vision is affected, and paracentral scotomata are absolute will show progression.
- There is no treatment for 4AQR.

References

1. Browning DJ. Hydroxychloroquine and chloroquine retinopathy: screening for drug toxicity. Am J Ophthalmol. 2002;133:649–56.
2. Browning DJ. Impact of the revised American academy of ophthalmology guidelines regarding hydroxychloroquine screening on actual practice. Am J Ophthalmol. 2013;155:418–28.
3. Morsman CDG, Livesey SJ, Richards IM, Jessop JD, Mills PV. Screening for hydroxychloroquine retinal toxicity: is it necessary? Eye. 1990;4:572–6.
4. Bergholz R, Ruther K, Tillack H, Joussen AM, Schroeter J. Ophthalmologic screening history and vision-targeted health status of patients suffering from chloroquine maculopathy. Ophthalmologe. 2013. doi:10.1007/s00347-012-2657-1.
5. Bienfang D, Coblyn JS, Liang MH, Corzillius M. Hydroxychloroquine retinopathy despite regular ophthalmologic evaluation: a consecutive series. J Rheumatol. 2000;27:2703–6.
6. Henkind P, Rothfield NF. Ocular abnormalities in patients treated with synthetic antimalarial drugs. N Engl J Med. 1963;269:434–9.
7. Bray VJ, Enzenauer RJ, Enzenauer RW, West SG. Antimalarial toxicity in rheumatic disease. J Clin Rheumatol. 1998;4:168–9.
8. Mititelu M, Wong BJ, Brenner M, Bryar PJ, Jampol LM, Fawzi AA. Progression of hydroxychloroquine toxic effects after drug therapy cessation. New evidence from multimodal imaging. Arch Ophthalmol. 2013;131:1187–97.
9. Michaelides M, Stover NB, Francis PJ, Weleber RG. Retinal toxicity associated with hydroxychloroquine and chloroquine: risk factors, screening, and progression despite cessation of therapy. Arch Ophthalmol. 2011;129:30–9.
10. Easterbrook M. Long-term course of antimalarial maculopathy after cessation of treatment. Can J Ophthalmol. 1992;27:237–9.
11. Mavrikakis I, Sfikakis PP, Mavrikakis E, Rougas K, Nikolaou A, Kostopoulos C, Mavrikakis M. The incidence of irreversible retinal toxicity in patients treated with hydroxychloroquine—a reappraisal. Ophthalmology. 2003;110:1321–6.
12. Tehrani R, Ostrowski RA, Hariman R, Jay WM. Ocular toxicity of hydroxychloroquine. Semin Ophthalmol. 2008;23:201–9.
13. Lozier JR, Friedlander MH. Complications of antimalarial therapy. Int Ophthalmol Clin. 1989;29:172–8.
14. Easterbrook M. Ocular effects and safety of antimalarial agents. Am J Med. 1988;85:23–9.
15. Easterbrook M. Screening for antimalarial toxicity. Can J Ophthalmol. 1993;28:51–2.
16. Kellner U, Kellner S, Weinitz S. Chloroquine retinopathy:lipofuscin- and melanin-related fundus autofluorescence, optical coherence tomography and multifocal electroretinography. Doc Ophthalmol. 2008;116:119–27.
17. Percival SPB, Behrman J. Ophthalmological safety of chloroquine. Br J Ophthalmol. 1969;53:101–9.
18. Reed H, Karlinsky W. Delayed onset of chloroquine retinopathy. Can Med Assoc J. 1967;97:1408–11.
19. Hobbs HE, Eadie SP, Somerville F. Ocular lesions after treatment with chloroquine. Br J Ophthalmol. 1961;45:284–97.
20. Grierson DJ. Hydroxychloroquine and visual screening in a rheumatology outpatient clinic. Ann Rheum Dis. 1997;56:188–90.
21. Chen E, Brown DM, Benz MS, Fish RH, Wong TP, Kim RY, Major JC. Spectral domain optical coherence tomography as an effective screening test for hydroxychloroquine retinopathy (the "flying saucer" sign). Clin Ophthalmol. 2010;4:1151–8.
22. Okun E, Gouras P, Bernstein H, von Sallmann L. Chloroquine retinopathy-A report of eight cases with ERG and Dark-Adaptation findings. Arch Ophthalmol. 1963;63:93–105.
23. Araiza-Casillas R, Cardenas F, Morales Y, Cardiel MH. Factors associated with chloroquine-induced retinopathy in rheumatic diseases. Lupus. 2004;13:119–24.
24. Hickley NM, Al-Maskari A, McKibbin M. Chloroquine and hydroxychloroquine toxicity. Arch Ophthalmol. 2011;129:1506–7.
25. Payne JF, Hubbard III GB, Aaberg Sr TM, Yan J. Clinical characteristics of hydroxychloroquine retinopathy. Br J Ophthalmol. 2010;95:245–50.
26. Bienfang DC. Screening for hydroxychloroquine retinopathy. Arch Ophthalmol. 2007;125:1585.
27. Anderson C, Blaha GR, Marx JL. Humphrey visual field findings in hydroxychloroquine toxicity. Eye. 2011;25:1535–45.
28. Ormrod JN. Two cases of chloroquine-inducted retinal damage. Br Med J. 1962;1:918–9.
29. Kellner U, Kraus H, Foerster MH. Multifocal ERG in chloroquine retinopathy: regional variance in retinal dysfunction. Graefes Arch Clin Exp Ophthalmol. 2000;238:94–7.
30. Maturi RK, Folk JC, Nichols B, Oetting TT, Kardon RH. Hydroxychloroquine retinopathy. Arch Ophthalmol. 1999;117:1262–3.

31. Easterbrook M. The ocular safety of hydroxychloroquine. Semin Arthritis Rheum. 1993;23:62–7.

32. Mackenzie AH. An appraisal of chloroquine. Arthritis Rheum. 1970;13:280–91.

33. Henkind P, Carr RE, Siegel IM. Early chloroquine retinopathy: clinical and functional findings. Arch Ophthalmol. 1964;71:157–65.

34. Maksymowych W, Russell AS. Antimalarials in rheumatology: efficacy and safety. Semin Arthritis Rheum. 1987;16:206–21.

35. Burns RP. Delayed onset of chloroquine retinopathy. N Engl J Med. 1968;275:693–6.

36. Hobbs HE, Sorsby A, Freedman A. Retinopathy following chloroquine therapy. Lancet. 1959;274:478–80.

37. Fleck BW, Bell AL, Mitchell JD, Thomson BJ, Hurst NP, Nuki G. Screening for antimalarial maculopathy in rheumatology clinics. Br Med J. 1985;291:782–5.

38. Giorgi D, Rosati C, Verrastro G, Grandinetti F. What's the right patient management for early diagnosis of hydroxychloroquine retinal toxicity? Recenti Prog Med. 1996;87:308.

39. Jones SK. Ocular toxicity and hydroxychloroquine: guidelines for screening. Br J Dermatol. 1999;140:3–7.

40. Butler I. Retinopathy following the use of chloroquine and allied substances. Ophthalmologica. 1965;149:204–8.

41. Percival SPB, Meanock I. Chloroquine: ophthalmological safety and clinical assessment in rheumatoid arthritis. Br Med J. 1968;3:579–84.

42. Pasadhika S, Fishman GA. Effects of chronic exposure to hydroxychloroquine or chloroquine on inner retinal structures. Eye. 2009;24:340–6.

43. Crews SJ. Chloroquine retinopathy with recovery in early stages. Lancet. 1964;284:436–8.

44. Marks JS, Power BJ. Is chloroquine obsolete in treatment of rheumatic disease? Lancet. 1979;1:371–3.

45. Kolb H. Electro-oculogram findings in patients treated with antimalarial drugs. Br J Ophthalmol. 1965;49:573–90.

46. Wolfe F, Marmor MF. Rates and predictors of hydroxychloroquine retinal toxicity in patients with rheumatoid arthritis and systemic lupus erythematosus. Arthritis Care Res. 2010;62:775–84.

47. Marmor MF, Chien FY, Johnson MW. Value of red targets and pattern deviation pots in visual field screening for hydroxychloroquine retinopathy. JAMA Ophthalmol. 2013;131:476–80.

48. Carr RE, Gouras P, Gunkel RD. Chloroquine retinopathy. Early detection by retinal threshold test. Arch Ophthalmol. 1966;75:171–8.

49. Marmor MF, Kellner U, Lai TYY, Lyons JS, Mieler WF. Author response. Ophthalmology. 2012;119:207–8.

50. Marmor MF. Comparison of screening procedures in hydroxychloroquine toxicity. Arch Ophthalmol. 2012;130:461–9.

51. Missner S, Kellner U. Comparison of different screening methods for chloroquine/hydroxychloroquine retinopathy: multifocal electroretinography, color vision, perimetry, ophthalmoscopy, and fluorescein angiography. Graefes Arch Clin Exp Ophthalmol. 2012;250:319–25.

52. Albert DA, Debois LKL, Lu KF. Antimalarial ocular toxicity, a critical appraisal. J Clin Rheumatol. 1998;4:57–62.

53. Rynes RI. Ophthalmologic safety of long-term hydroxychloroquine sulfate treatment. Am J Med. 1983;75:35–9.

54. Banks CN. Melanin: blackguard or red herring? Another look at chloroquine retinopathy. Aust N Z J Ophthalmol. 1987;15:365–70.

55. Bernstein HN. Ophthalmologic considerations and testing in patients receiving long-term antimalarial therapy. Am J Med. 1983;75:25–34.

56. Easterbrook M. The use of Amsler grids in early chloroquine retinopathy. Ophthalmology. 1984;91:1368–72.

57. Bernstein H. Ocular safety of hydroxychlotoquine sulfate (Plaquenil). South Med J. 1992;85:274–9.

58. Adams EM, Yocum DE, Bell CL. Hydroxychloroquine in the treatment of rheumatoid arthritis. Am J Med. 1983;75:321–6.

59. Rynes RI. Antimalarial drugs in the treatment of rheumatological diseases. Br J Rheumatol. 1997;36:799–805.

60. Rynes R. Ophthalmologic considerations in using antimalarials in the United States. Lupus. 1996;5:S73–4.

61. Rosenthal AR, Kolb H, Bergsma D, Huxsoll D, Hopkins JL. Chloroquine retinopathy in the rhesus monkey. Invest Ophthalmol Vis Sci. 1978;17:1158–75.

62. Yam JCS, Kwok AKH. Ocular toxicity of hydroxychloroquine. Hong Kong Med J. 2006;12:294–304.

63. Neubauer AS, Samari-Kermani K, Schaller U, Welge-Luben U, Rudolph G, Berninger T. Detecting chloroquine retinopathy: electro-oculogram versus color vision. Br J Ophthalmol. 2003;87:902–8.

64. Mills PV, Beck M, Power BJ. Assessment of the retinal toxicity of hydroxychloroquine. Trans Ophthalmol Soc UK. 1981;101:113.

65. Cruess AF, Schachat AP, Nicholl J, Augsburger JJ. Chloroquine retinopathy-Is fluorescein angiography necessary? Ophthalmology. 1985;92:1127–9.

66. Bernstein HN. Ocular safety of hydroxychloroquine. Ann Ophthalmol. 1991;23:292–6.

67. Hanna B, Holdeman NR, Tang RA, Schiffman JS. Retinal toxicity secondary to Plaquenil therapy. Optometry. 2008;79:90–4.

68. Kobak S, Deveci H. Retinopathy due to antimalarial drugs in patients with connective tissue diseases: are they so innocent? A single center retrospective study. Int J Rheum Dis. 2010;13:e11–5.

69. Shinjo SK, Junior OOM, Tizziani VAP, Morita C, Kochen JAL, Takahashi WY, Laurindo IMM. Chloroquine-induced bull's eye maculopathy in rheumatoid arthritis: related to disease duration? Clin Rheumatol. 2007;26:1248–53.

70. Arden GB, Kolb H. Antimalarial therapy and early retinal changes in patients with rheumatoid arthritis. Br Med J. 1966;1:270–3.

71. Lyons JS, Severns ML. Using multifocal ERG ring ratios to detect and follow Plaquenil retinal toxicity: a review. Doc Ophthalmol. 2009;118:29–36.

72. Elder M, Rahman AMA. Early paracentral visual field loss in patients taking hydroxychloroquine. Arch Ophthalmol. 2006;124:1729–33.

73. Shearer RV, Dubois EL. Ocular changes induced by long-term hydroxychloroquine (Plaquenil) therapy. Am J Ophthalmol. 1967;64:245–52.

74. Warner AE. Early hydroxychloroquine macular toxicity. Arthritis Rheum. 2001;44:1959–61.

75. Graniewski-Wijnands HS, Van Lith GHM, Vijfvinkel-Bruinenga S. Ophthalmological examination of patients taking chloroquine. Doc Ophthalmol. 1979;48:231–4.

76. Alarcon GS. How frequently and how soon should we screen our patients for the presence of antimalarial retinopathy? Arthritis Rheum. 2002;46:561.

77. Salu P, Uvijls A, van den Brande P, Leroy BP. Normalization of generalized retinal function and progression of maculopathy after cessation of therapy in a case of severe hydroxychloroquine retinopathy with 19 years follow-up. Doc Ophthalmol. 2010;120:251–64.

78. Ehrenfeld M, Nesher R, Merin S. Delayed-onset chloroquine retinopathy. Br J Ophthalmol. 1986;70:281–3.

79. Smith JL. Chloroquine macular degeneration. Arch Ophthalmol. 1962;68:186–90.

80. Weiner A, Sandberg MA, Gaudio AR, Kini MM, Berson EL. Hydroxychloroquine retinopathy. Am J Ophthalmol. 1991;112:528–34.

81. Hart WM, Burde RM, Johnston GP, Drews RC. Static perimetry in chloroquine retinopathy-Perifoveal patterns of visual field depression. Arch Ophthalmol. 1984;102:377–80.

82. Labriola LT, Jeng D, Fawzi AA. Retinal toxicity of systemic medications. Int Ophthalmol Clin. 2012;52:149–66.

83. Kearns TP, Hollenhorst RW. Chloroquine retinopathy. Arch Ophthalmol. 1966;76:378–84.

84. Mavrikakis M, Papazoglou S, Sfikakis PP, Vaiopoulos G, Rougas K. Retinal toxicity in long term hydroxychloroquine treatment. Ann Rheum Dis. 1996;55:187–9.

85. Marks JS. Chloroquine retinopathy: is there a safe daily dose? Ann Rheum Dis. 1982;41:52–8.

86. Maturi RK, Yu M, Weleber RG. Multifocal electroretinographic evaluation of long-term hydroxychloroquine users. Arch Ophthalmol. 2004;122:973–81.

87. Almony A, Garg S, Peters RK, Mamet R, Tsong J, Shibuya B, Kitridou R, Sadun AA. Threshold amsler grid as a screening tool for asymptomatic patients on hydroxychloroquine therapy. Br J Ophthalmol. 2005;89:569–74.

88. Schwartz SG, Mieler WF. Retinal and choroidal manifestations of systemic medications. In: Arevalo JF, editor. Retinal and choroidal manifestations of selected systemic diseases. New York: Springer; 2013. p. 479–92.

89. Lai TYY, Chan WM, Li H, Lai RYK, Lam DSC. Multifocal electroretinographic changes in patients receiving hydroxychloroquine therapy. Am J Ophthalmol. 2005;140:794–807.

90. Gorovoy I, Gorovoy JB. Advances in ophthalmic monitoring for hydroxychloroquine toxicity. J Clin Rheumatol. 2013;19:46–7.

91. Korah S, Kuriakose T. Optical coherence tomography in a patient with chloroquine-induced maculopathy. Indian J Ophthalmol. 2008;56:511–3.

92. Lin RC, Cantrill HL, Mieler WF. Retinal toxicities caused by systemic medications. Retin Physician. 2013;4:49–52.

93. Akman F, Cerman E, Yenice O, Kazokoglu H. Two cases with chloroquine and hydroxychloroquine maculopathy. Marmara Med J. 2011;24:68–72.

94. Weise EE, Yannuzzi LA. Ring maculopathies mimicking chloroquine retinopathy. Am J Ophthalmol. 1974;78:204–10.

95. Wolfensberger TJ. Toxicology of the retinal pigment epithelium. In: Marmor MF, Wolfensberger TJ, editors. The retinal pigment epithelium. New York: Oxford University Press; 1998. p. 621–47.

96. Brinkley JR, Dubois EL, Ryan SJ. Long-term course of chloroquine retinopathy after cessation of medication. Am J Ophthalmol. 1979;88:1–11.

97. Nosik RA, Weinstock FJ, Vignos PJ. Ocular complications of chloroquine: series and case presentation with simple method for early detection of retinopathy. Am J Ophthalmol. 1964;58:774–8.

98. Schmidt B, Muller-Limmroth W. Electroretinographic examinations following application of chloroquine. Acta Ophthalmol Suppl. 1962;70:245–51.

99. Tobin DR, Krohel G, Rynes RI. Hydroxychloroquine-Seven-year experience. Arch Ophthalmol. 1982;100:81–3.

100. Finbloom DS, Silver K, Newsome DA, Gunkel R. Comparison of hydroxychloroquine and chloroquine use and the development of retinal toxicity. J Rheumatol. 1985;12:692–4.

101. Carr RE, Henkind P, Rothfield N, Siegel IM. Ocular toxicity of antimalarial drugs-long-term follow-up. Am J Ophthalmol. 1968;66:738–44.

102. Thorne JE, Maguire AM. Retinopathy after long term, standard doses of hydroxychloroquine. Br J Ophthalmol. 1999;83:1201–2.

103. Browning DJ, Lee C. The coefficient of repeatability for multifocal electroretinography measurements in normal volunteers and patients taking hydroxychloroquine. Scientific poster 483. Presented at: American Academy of Ophthalmology 2013 Annual Meeting, Nov 14–19 2013, New Orleans; 2013.

104. Marmor MF, Carr RE, Easterbrook M, et al. Recommendations on screening for chloroquine and hydroxychloroquine retinopathy. Ophthalmology. 2002;109:1377–82.

105. Moschos MN, Moschos MM, Apostopoulos M, Mallias JA, Bouros C, Theodossiadis GP. Assessing hydroxychloroquine toxicity by the multifocal ERG. Doc Ophthalmol. 2004;108:47–53.

106. Scherbel AL, Mackenzie AH, Nousek JE, Atdjian M. Ocular lesions in rheumatoid arthritis and related disorders with particular reference to retinopathy-A study of 741 patients treated with and without chloroquine drugs. N Engl J Med. 1965;273:360–6.

107. Browning DJ. Bull's-eye maculopathy associated with quinacrine therapy for malaria. Am J Ophthalmol. 2004;137:577–9.

108. Sassani JW, Brucker AJ, Cobbs W, Campbell C. Progressive chloroquine retinopathy. Ann Ophthalmol. 1983;15:19–22.

109. Ogawa S, Kurukatani N, Shibaike N, Yamazoe S. Progression of retinopathy long after cessation of chloroquine therapy. Lancet. 1979;313:1408.

110. Farrell DF. Retinal toxicity to antimalarial drugs: chloroquine and hydroxychloroquine: a neurophysiologic study. Clin Ophthalmol. 2012;6:377–83.

111. Dubois EL. Antimalarials in the management of discoid and systemic lupus erythematosus. Semin Arthritis Rheum. 1978;8:33–51.

112. Kellner U, Renner AB, Tillack H. Fundus autofluorescence and mfERG for early detection of retinal alterations in patients using chloroquine/hydroxychloroquine. Invest Ophthalmol Vis Sci. 2006;47:3531–8.

113. Easterbrook M. Clinical characteristics of hydroxychloroquine retinopathy. Evid Based Ophthalmol. 2011;12:132–3.

114. McChesney EQ, Fitch CD. 4-Aminoquinolines. In: Peters W, Richards WHG, editors. Antimalarial drugs II. Current antimalarials and new drug developments. Berlin: Springer; 1984. p. 3–60.

Risk Factors for Hydroxychloroquine and Chloroquine Retinopathy

Abbreviations

ABW	Actual body weight
ADD	Adjusted daily dose
4AQR	4-Aminoquinoline retinopathy
4AQs	4-Aminoquinolines (chloroquine and hydroxychloroquine)
C	Chloroquine
HC	Hydroxychloroquine
IBW	Ideal body weight
RA	Rheumatoid arthritis
RPE	Retinal pigment epithelium
SD	Standard deviation
SLE	Systemic lupus erythematosus

The main risk factors for hydroxychloroquine and chloroquine retinopathy are the drug used (chloroquine being riskier), high daily dose, increasing cumulative doses and durations of drug ingestion, greater age, preexisting macular abnormalities, obesity, and renal or liver dysfunction [1–7]. Plausible additional risk factors that have not been sufficiently investigated include predisposing or protective genetic mutations. For example, ABCA4 variants have been proposed as increasing the risk for retinopathy [8].

The disease for which the patient takes the medicine has been inconsistently associated with risk. In some reports systemic lupus erythematosus (SLE) has been observed to be associated with increased risk [9–13], but in other series rheumatoid arthritis (RA) was considered to be more predisposing to retinopathy [14], and in others the risk seemed unrelated to the underlying disease [15–18]. Where SLE has been found to predispose to retinopathy, it was not ruled out that associated and confounding renal dysfunction was responsible [19]. There is no convincing evidence that the disease for which the 4AQ is taken has a clinically important influence on susceptibility to 4AQR. Many reports pool all patients taking 4AQs together under the assumption that the disease for which the drug is taken is immaterial to the risk of retinopathy [1, 16, 20].

Light exposure has been considered as a risk factor, but insufficient evidence has been adduced to rank it as important relative to the other factors [5, 21]. It can also be considered insufficiently investigated. Beyond the relative importance of particular risk factors, the additive risk of multiple concomitant risk factors has been noted [14].

Certain associations have been put forth, but may not be true risk factors. For example, the proportion of female patients with 4-aminoquinoline retinopathy (4AQR) is higher than the proportion of male patients. It may be that this increased risk follows from the smaller median height and weight of females who do not generally receive a lower prescribed dose. That is, the gender risk factor may reflect an underlying dosing risk factor. Similarly, obesity per se is not a risk factor, but is associated with overdosing, which is common in short, obese persons [22]. There are other risk factors that are not widely acknowledged, but demonstrable by particular examples. Among these would be preexisting visual field abnormalities that

D.J. Browning, *Hydroxychloroquine and Chloroquine Retinopathy*,
DOI 10.1007/978-1-4939-0597-3_7, © Springer Science+Business Media New York 2014

confound interpretation of visual fields obtained in screening for retinopathy.

Screening guidelines suggest frequency of follow-up depending on whether patients fall into low- or high-risk groups [4, 23]. The presence of a risk factor places a patient in a high-risk group. This categorization is of little practical use, because such a high percentage of patients possess at least one risk factor [7, 14]. A study of 109 patients in a Veterans Affairs Medical Center found that 87 % had one risk factor and 47 % had two or more [24]. In a survey of 3,995 rheumatologic patients who had taken hydroxychloroquine, 81.5 % had at least one risk factor [15]. In the series of Bergholz and colleagues, the low-risk group constituted only 3.9 % of the patients screened. Perhaps this fact explains why, in practice, clinicians ignore the recommendations of guidelines to omit screening after the baseline examination until the fifth year of follow-up in low-risk patients [25]. Instead they consistently choose follow-up at least as frequently as once a year for all patients [25].

Commonly used abbreviations in this chapter are collected in "Abbreviations" for reference. Each term will be first used in its full form, along with its abbreviation.

The relative frequency of various risk factors in patients screened for 4AQR and in patients with 4AQR is shown in Table 7.1.

Table 7.1 Frequency of risk factors in patients taking 4-aminoquinolines and patients with 4-aminoquinoline retinopathy

Risk factor	Class of patient	Study	Number of patients	Percent with risk factor
Duration >5 years	4AQs	Flach [24]	109	13.8
		Gupta [27]	62	85
		Lyons [91]	62	29
		Missner [70]	20	30
	4AQR	Michaelides [26]	16	93.8
		Mititelu [28]	7	71.4
		Shinjo [78]	16	50
		Anderson [125]	15	93.3
		Payne [39]	7	100
		Bienfang [58]	6	83.3
Daily dosage >6.5 mg/kg/d based, on IBW, HC	4AQs	Bray [29]	10	80.0
	4AQR	Michaelides [26]	16	56.2
		Mititelu [28]	7	85.7
		Payne [39]	7	42.9
Daily dosage >6.5 mg/kg/d, based on ABW, HC	4AQs	Flach [24]	109	8.3
		Michaelides [26]	16	25
		Gupta [27]	62	19
		Lyons [91]	62	8.1
		Neubauer [35]	93	2.2
		Elder [52]	262	0.38
	4AQR	Mititelu [28]	7	57.1
		Anderson [125]	15	46.7
		Payne [39]	7	100
		Bienfang [58]	6	66.7
Daily dosage >4.0 mg/kg/d, C	4AQs	Bonanomi [30]	34	53.0
		Xiaoyun [93]	60	100
		Neubauer [36]	93	2.2
Daily dosage >3.0 mg/kg/d, C	4AQR	Shinjo [78]	16	100

(continued)

Table 7.1 (continued)

Risk factor	Class of patient	Study	Number of patients	Percent with risk factor
Age >60 years	4AQs	Flach [24]	109	58
		Gupta [27]	62	85
		Elman [31]	270	29
		Elder [52]	262	1.2
		Missner [70]	20	25
	4AQR	Michaelides [26]	16	75.0
		Anderson [125]	15	46.7
		Payne [39]	7	42.8
		Bienfang [58]	6	66.7
		Mititelu [28]	7	28.6
Obesity	4AQR	Michaelides [26]	16	12.5
		Mititelu [28]	7	0
Preexisting retinal disease	4AQs	Flach [24]	109	34.9
		Gupta [27]	62	12
	4AQR	Michaelides [26]	16	12.5
		Mititelu [28]	7	0
		Payne [39]	7	14.2
Renal dysfunction	4AQR	Michaelides [26]	16	0
		Mititelu [28]	7	28.6
		Payne [39]	7	14.2
		Bienfang [58]	6	0
Liver dysfunction	4AQR	Michaelides [26]	16	0
		Mititelu [28]	7	0
Renal or liver disease	4AQs	Flach [24]	109	33
		Gupta [27]	62	33

Class of patient refers to whether the study looked at patients taking 4-aminoquinolines or patients with 4-aminoquinoline retinopathy. 4AQ is 4-aminoquinoline. 4AQR is 4-aminoquinoline retinopathy. IBW is ideal body weight. ABW is actual body weight. C is chloroquine. HC is hydroxychloroquine

7.1 Age

The inconsistent reports regarding the effects of age on risk of 4AQR suggest that it is a weak factor. Some have reported no effect [18, 28, 30]. Many have reported that increasing age increases the risk of hydroxychloroquine and chloroquine retinopathy [14, 31]. In reports showing an association, the most commonly asserted threshold for increased risk is 60 years [15, 23], although some have posited ages 40 [17, 32], 50 [6, 31], 65 [33], or 70 [34] years as more appropriate.

There is no rational basis for any of these thresholds [35]. The evidence to support associations of increased susceptibility to 4AQR with age is indirect. For example, a documented case of hydroxychloroquine retinopathy occurred in a patient taking less than 6.5 mg/kg/d. The patient happened to be older than 60 years. Because dosing was appropriate and there were no other risk factors, age was hypothesized to be a relevant predisposing factor [35]. In other studies the age of patients with and without retinopathy has not been compared [36].

It is probable that risk increases incrementally and continuously with age rather than reaching a threshold at which risk suddenly increases. Evidence for this comes from articles in which the median age for patients developing hydroxychloroquine and chloroquine retinopathy is greater than that of patients without retinopathy taking these drugs [14, 37]. In a multivariable analysis of risk factors associated with hydroxychloroquine retinopathy, age was not a significant predictor after other variables were taken into account [15]. Although Elman suggested that age less than 50 implies no need to screen [31], enough patients under age 50 have been reported with retinopathy that younger age does not excuse screening in published guidelines.

There may be multiple mechanisms by which increased age adds to the risk of 4AQR. For example, renal function decreases with age. As decreased renal function is a risk factor for 4AQR, increased age may just be an indirect risk factor working through the proximate factor of diminished renal function [22]. Likewise, effectiveness of hepatic metabolism of 4AQs may decrease with age, although this has not been investigated.

7.2   Gender

More than 90 % of cases of 4AQR occur in females [1, 28, 38, 39], but the relevant factor for this preponderance is the lower heights and ideal body weights (IBWs) of females with no adjustment of dosing. That is, the risk factor is the overdosing and not the gender.

A calculation illustrates this point. The average height of women in the US population is $65 \pm SD3.5$ inches and that of men is $69 \pm SD2.8$ inches. The IBW at which a typical hydroxychloroquine (HC) dose of 400 mg/d becomes toxic based on a threshold of 6.5 mg/kg/d is 135 pounds, which corresponds to a height of 5 ft 3 inches using the National Heart Lung and Blood Institute Table of IBW (Table 7.2). If one assumes that the distribution of IBWs is normal, then the concept of a Z-score is applicable (see Chap. 8). The Z-score tells where, along the normal distribution, a value of the independent variable (in this case height) lies. It is calculated by the formula $Z = (X - \mu)/\sigma$, where X is the value of the variable (in this case, 63 inches), μ is the mean value of the normal distribution (in this case, 65 inches), and σ is the standard deviation of the distribution (in this case, 3.5 inches). The Z-score for a height of 5 feet 3 inches (63 inches) would be $Z = (X - \mu)/\sigma = (63-65)/3.5 = -0.5714$. Looking this score up in a standard table of Z-scores shows that 28.4 % of women will be overdosed with typical 400 mg/d dosing of hydroxychloroquine. The analogous calculation of a Z-score for men yields a score of -2.14 which implies that only 1.6 % of men will be overdosed with typical hydroxychloroquine dosing. Similar calculations for the other algorithms of IBW in common use yield height cut-points ranging from 62 to 68 inches at which typical dosing represents overdosing (Table 7.2) [40].

Table 7.2 Algorithms for ideal body weight used in the literature regarding 4-aminoquinoline retinopathy

Study	Algorithm for ideal body weight (in kg) in women	Height below which 400 mg/d daily dosing of HC is an overdose
Easterbrook [40]	$45.5 + 2.3 \times$ every inch over 5 ft	5 ft 7 in.
Easterbrook [48], Vine [87][a]	$1.364 \times$ (height in inches) $- 32.273$	5 ft 9 in.
Easterbrook [48], Vine [87][b]	$1.506 \times$ (height in inches) $- 31.319$	5 ft 2 in.
Browning [42]	$1.9467 \times$ (height in inches) $- 61.05$	5 ft 3 in.
Bergholz [14]	$[2.54 \times$ (height in inches) $- 100] \times 0.85$	5 ft 8 in.
Walvick [43]	Referenced, but formula not given	5 ft 4 in.
Michaelides [26]	$(1.07 \times$ weight (in kg)) $- 148 \times$ (weight^2/ $(100 \times$ height (m))^2)	Depends on ABW

ABW is actual body weight. HC is hydroxychloroquine
[a]Means that the Metropolitan Life Insurance Table for Women, Small Frame was used for this row
[b]Means that the Metropolitan Life Insurance Table for Women, Large Frame was used for this row

---

Ideal, Lean, and Top Normal Body Weight

The fact that fat does not collect appreciable quantities of 4AQs has led to wide recognition that dosing should be based on an index that excludes the fatty component of body weight [2]. Most authors who discuss the issue use the terms IBW, lean body weight, and top normal body weight synonymously [2, 40–45], although some do not [46]. In cases where distinctions are made, the algorithms for lean body weight exclude more fat that algorithms for IBW [45]. Algorithms for IBW may yield weights that are higher or lower than top normal body weight for any given height [47]. Readers should be aware of these semantic differences as they read the literature on 4AQR. The various algorithms for lean, ideal, and top normal body weight can yield differences in weight as great as 20 pounds for a given height with implications on frequency of calls to prescribing doctors to adjust dosing [47]. Some authors have changed their preferred IBW algorithm over time, which can make comments written in one report inapplicable to those in the second one [48, 49].

7.3   Daily Dose Adjusted for the Lesser of Ideal and Actual Body Weight (Adjusted Daily Dose)

The importance of adjusted daily dose (ADD) is suggested by the rarity of retinopathy in patients who take 4AQs for malaria prophylaxis (a low-dose use, see Chap. 2) and the frequency of overdosing among patients with retinopathy who take the drugs for chronic autoimmune diseases (a higher-dose use) [6, 29, 50]. However, the evidence to support the role of ADD is not ironclad. Patients developing retinopathy do not always have higher mean daily doses than patients without retinopathy. For example, in one study involving both 4AQs, 18 patients with retinopathy had a mean daily dosage that was significantly higher than 84 patients without retinopathy. For patients on chloroquine, the mean daily doses were 5.35 ± 0.26 mg/kg (IBW)/d ($n = 10$) and 3.97 ± 1.2 mg/kg (IBW)/d ($n = 34$) for the cases with and without retinopathy, respectively. For those on hydroxychloroquine, the mean daily doses were 8.39 ± 0.42 mg/kg (IBW)/d ($n = 8$) and 6.90 ± 0.23 mg/kg (IBW)/d ($n = 50$) for the cases with and without retinopathy, respectively [2]. However, in a different study that involved both 4AQs, the mean ADDs were not different between patients with and without retinopathy [14].

There is considerable overlap in the daily dosing of patients with and without retinopathy. Many patients taking toxic doses never develop retinopathy, and rarely do patients taking subtoxic doses develop retinopathy. Levy and colleagues reported on 302 patients taking 6.5 mg/kg/d or more based on actual body weight (ABW). Only one of them developed retinopathy [51]. An example of such a patient is shown in Fig. 7.1. There have been between approximately 20 cases in which retinopathy developed despite adjusted daily dosing in the range less than 6.5 mg/kg (IBW)/d [1, 26, 52–59]. This implies considerable individual variability in sensitivity to retinopathy [60].

A range of maximal safe daily doses can be found in the literature ranging from 3 to 5.1 mg/kg/d for chloroquine and from 6 to 7.8 mg/kg/d for hydroxychloroquine (see Chaps. 2 and 3) [2, 61–63]. The most commonly cited toxic thresholds are 3.5 mg/kg(IBW)/d for chloroquine and 6.5 mg/kg (IBW)/d for hydroxychloroquine (see Table 3.2).

It is important to normalize dosing by the lesser of IBW and ABW [29, 64, 65]. The importance of calculating daily dose based on IBW has been known for a long time although it is often not done and is often done inaccurately [66–70]. In the obese person, much of the body weight is

a

Right Eye

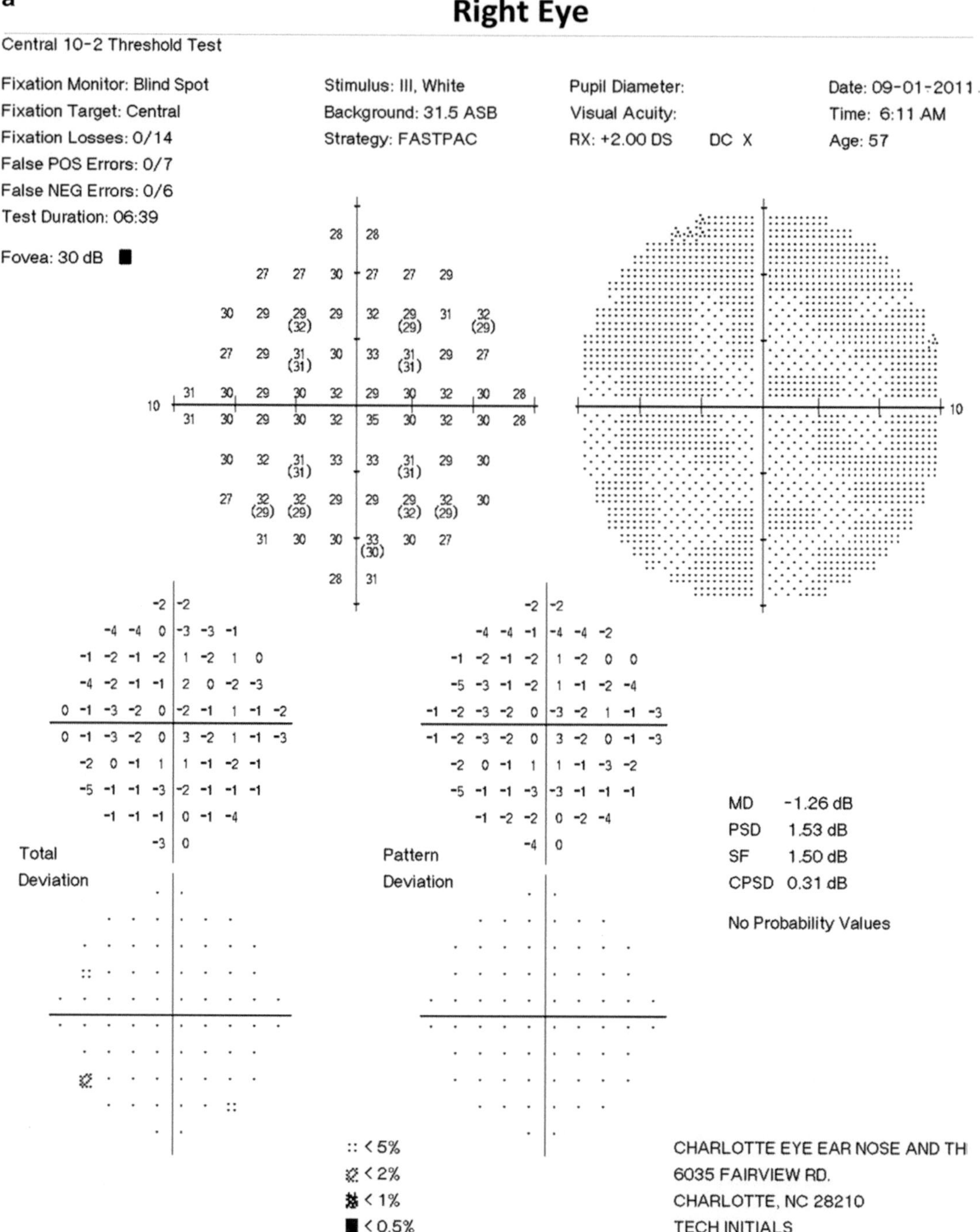

Fig. 7.1 This 57-year-old woman on hydroxychloroquine for Sjogren's syndrome was 5 feet 1 inch in height, and weighed 112 pounds. She had been taking 400 mg of hydroxychoroquine per day for 4 years yielding a cumulative dose of 681 mg and an adjusted daily dose of 7.9 mg/kg (actual body weight). In this case, the adjusted daily dosing was based on actual body weight because it is less than ideal body weight. Despite toxic dosing, both her 10-2 visual fields (VFs) and her multifocal electroretinogram (mf ERG) testing were normal in both eyes. (**a**) Normal 10-2 VF of the right eye. (**b**) Normal 10-2 VF of the left eye. (**c**) Normal mf ERG of both eyes. The display is shown in the retina view (as though the patient was looking at the reader, so that the display for the right eye is on the *left* side of the figure). Based on the toxic dosing, a request was made to her internist to consider reducing the dose of hydroxychloroquine

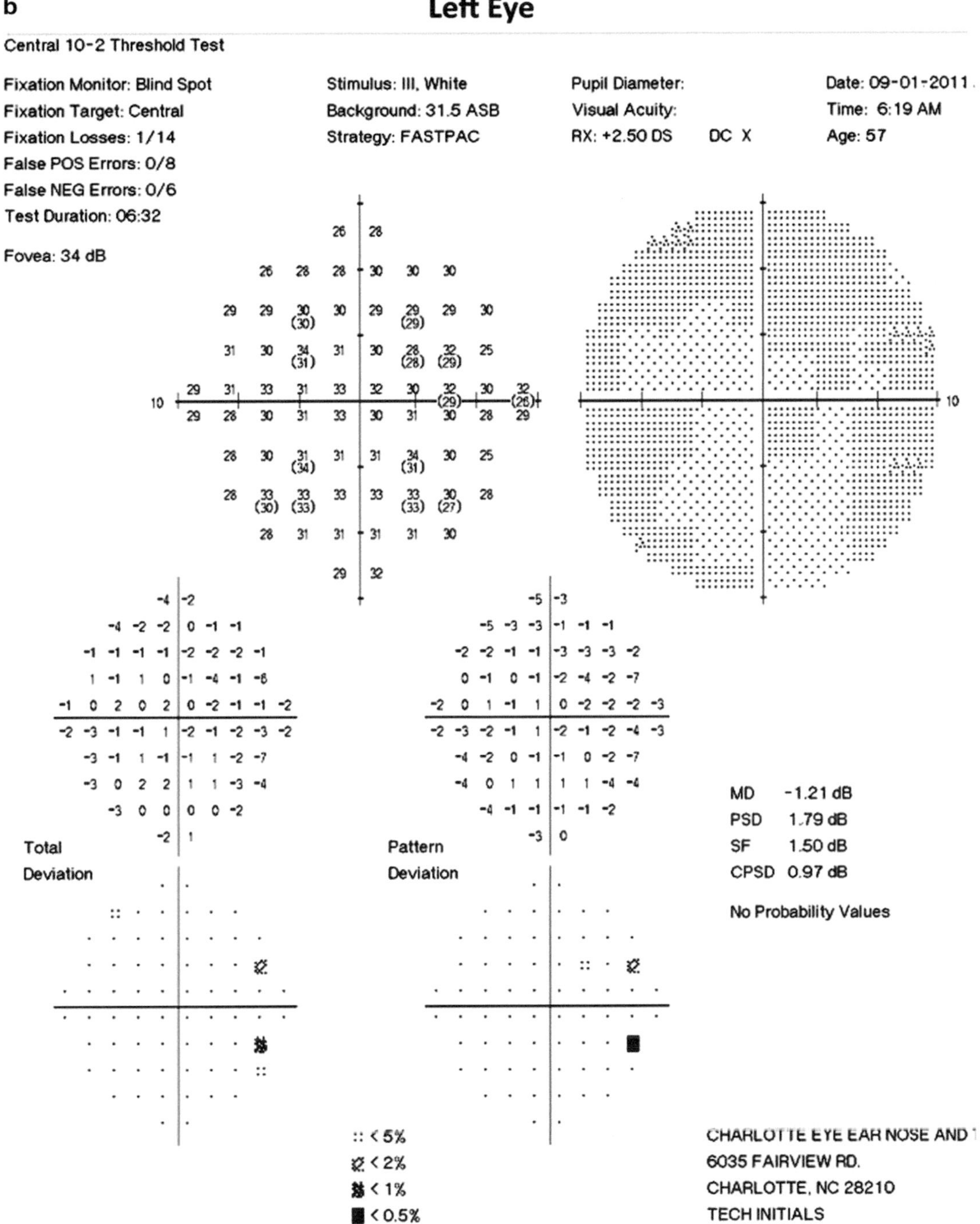

Fig. 7.1 (continued)

fat, into which 4AQs do not distribute much (see Chap. 2), and a false sense of safe dosing may be engendered [14]. Less well known is adjusting the dose for ABW when ABW is less than IBW [25].

A flow chart (Fig. 7.2) will help the clinician who screens for hydroxychloroquine retinopathy. To reduce dosing, an easy method is to exclude dosing for 1 or 2 days of the week—typically the

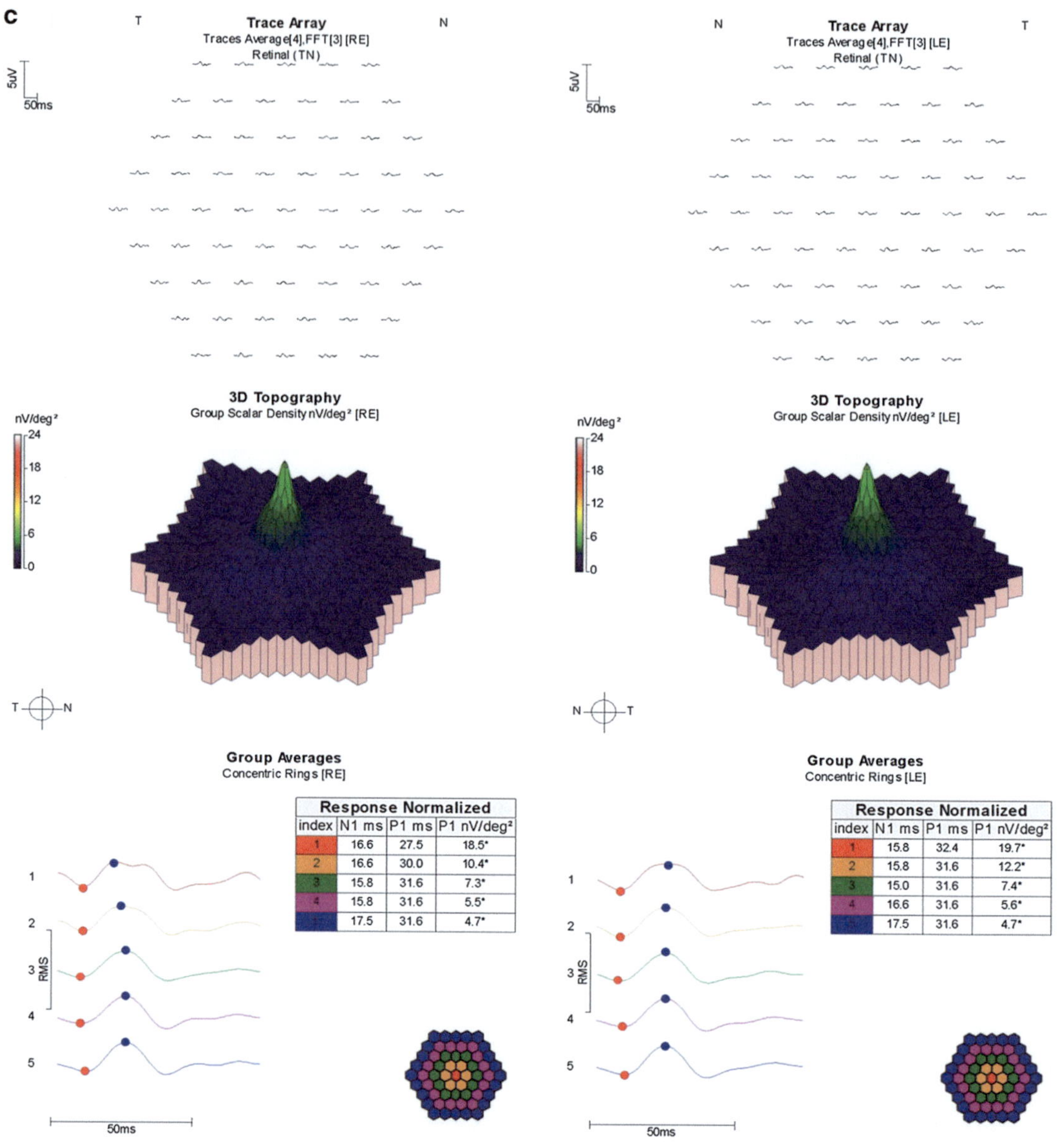

Fig. 7.1 (continued)

weekend. Because of the long half-life of hydroxychloroquine, no important fluctuations in plasma hydroxychloroquine concentrations are effected by this method. The average daily dose is calculated by adding the total weekly dose and dividing by seven.

In clinical practice, guidelines for regulating dosing based on IBW frequently get translated into guidelines based on height. These transla-tions are based on an underlying assumption by the issuer as to which algorithm for IBW should be used. For example, Schwartz states that 400 mg/d of HC is safe unless a patient is shorter than 5 feet 2 inches [71]. This is equiva-lent to choosing the Metropolitan Life Insurance Table for Women of Medium Build, Top of Range algorithm relating height and IBW. Marmor makes an analogous statement that

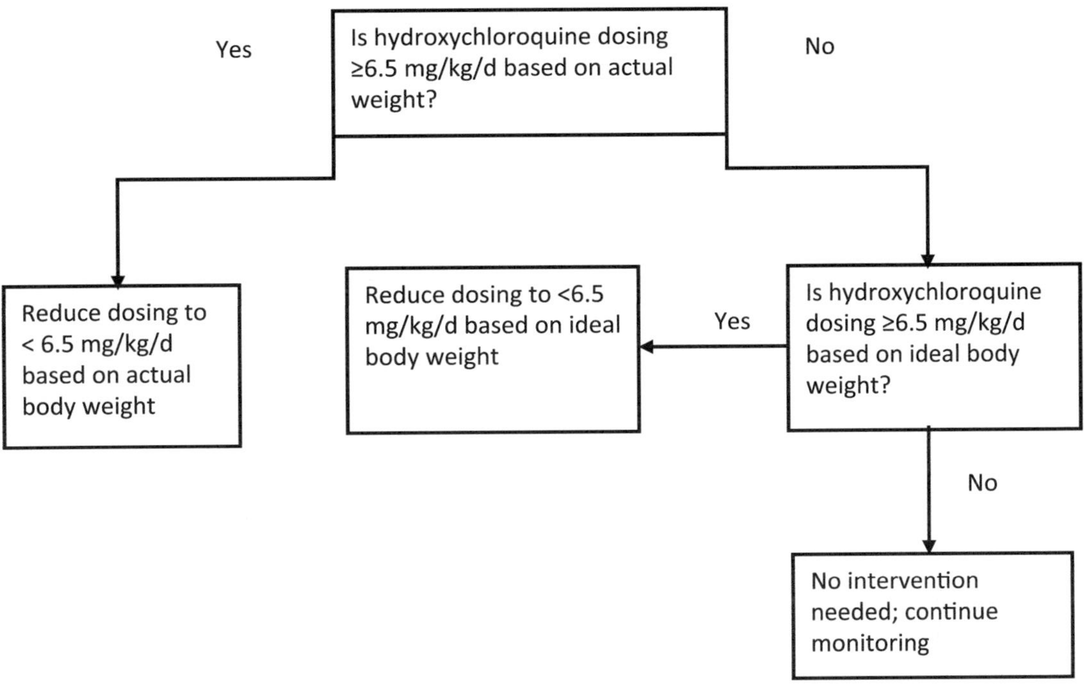

Fig. 7.2 Flow chart for avoiding pitfalls in daily dosing of hydroxychloroquine

women of height less than 5 feet 7 inches are overdosed when taking hydroxychloroquine 400 mg/d. Implicit in his comment is a preference for a different algorithm relating height and IBW than the one favored by Schwartz [46, 47]. There is no evidence to guide the clinician in choosing an algorithm, but the choice has consequences. Choosing an algorithm associated with a lighter IBW (e.g., the one favored by Marmor) for a given height will lead to lower dosing, but will imply that the screening eye doctor will need to call prescribing physicians more often to adjust dosing downward. Choosing a "heavier" algorithm will allow higher doses for patients, but calls to change dosing downward will be fewer [47].

When the ADD is 6.5 mg/kg/d or less, the risk of development of retinopathy is extremely low [33, 72]. Mackenzie reported that he had never seen a case of 4AQR in a patient taking less than 6.5 mg/kg/d of hydroxychloroquine or 3.5 mg/kg/d of chloroquine [2]. His sample size

for making this statement was 900 patients. Bernstein reported on 1,500 patients and noted that he had never seen a case of hydroxychloroquine retinopathy if the patient took less than 6.5 mg/kg/d and had been taking drug for less than 10 years [72, 73]. Levy reported that of 1,556 patients taking hydroxychloroquine, the only patient with definite toxicity was taking greater than 6.5 mg/kg/d [51]. In the only prospective study, 526 patients taking hydroxychloroquine at doses less than or equal to 6.5 mg/kg (ABW)/d were followed for 6 years with no cases of retinopathy. Subsequently two of these patients developed retinopathy after 6.5 and 8 years of retinopathy, respectively [74]. Had they been dosed based on IBW, presumably the incidence of retinopathy would have been even less. Since this report there have been at least 15 cases that violate his threshold [54–58, 75, 76], but this is as good a practical threshold for safety as has been found and has been widely adopted.

> **Is 6.5 a Magic Number for Hydroxychloroquine Dosing?**
>
> Much has been made of the cut-point of 6.5 mg/kg/d based on IBW as a threshold for increasing risk, but it is probably disadvantageous to see this as a clear dichotomy. There is no question that cases of 4AQR can occur in appropriately dosed patients (see Fig. 6.1) [1, 53, 54, 58]. Scientifically, the risk increases in a continuous manner, although it may be nonlinear. The dosage of 6.5 mg/kg/d may represent an inflection point of sorts, although even this has not been established. From a clinician's perspective, the take-home message is that risk can always be decreased by reducing daily dosage. The difficult task is determining how far one can reduce the risk of toxicity and not lose the therapeutic efficacy of the drug in treating the autoimmune disease [47]. Large rheumatologic case series in which attention was paid to keeping daily doses below 6 mg/kg (ABW)/d have reported no hydroxychloroquine retinopathy [77]. Therefore, one can expect that if dosing falls below 6.5 mg/kg/d, the risk of retinopathy continues to decrease.

Among reports of retinopathy for which daily dosing by IBW has been reported, rates of overdosing range from 12.8 to 100 % (Fig. 7.1) [1, 20, 25, 30, 33, 39, 51, 63, 65, 66, 78]. The percentage of patients overdosed depends on the algorithm for IBW that is used [47]. The most common daily dosages prescribed are 400 mg/d for hydroxychloroquine and 250 mg/d for chloroquine [16, 25, 47, 69]. In the author's series of 433 patients taking hydroxychloroquine screened for retinopathy for whom daily dosing was determined, 60 % were taking 400 mg/d. Grierson reported that 611 of 758 (81 %) of patients taking hydroxychloroquine were given 400 mg/d [69]. These commonly prescribed daily doses are in the toxic range for many women of small stature and low IBW and many taller women with an asthenic somatotype and lower ABW than IBW based on height. In the latter situation, it is the ABW that should be used for calculating daily dosing, and not the IBW [25].

In failure analyses of cases of 4AQR, overdosage is the most common problem and the most important problem, because it is remediable [1, 20, 33, 40, 79, 80]. Lowering daily dosage is a good response to data that suggest but do not prove retinopathy [23, 24, 62]. The general principle guiding clinical practice in prescribing 4AQs should be to find the smallest effective dose [31, 80, 81].

It is common among rheumatologists to temporarily prescribe 4AQs at higher than equilibrium dosages in order to raise blood concentrations to therapeutic levels rapidly (see Chap. 2) [16, 61]. However, the intention to reduce dosing once therapeutic blood concentrations can be forgotten. The ophthalmologist or optometrist screening the patient for retinopathy can usefully raise the issue with the prescribing physician.

Higher daily doses raise the risk of retinopathy and lead to retinopathy earlier than lower daily doses [2, 23, 79]. When 4AQs are prescribed in the treatment of graft-versus-host disease, higher doses than are typically used for rheumatological indications may be used, and the risk of retinopathy within a short period of time increases [23]. In these cases a calculated judgment has been made that the risk of retinopathy is overridden by the higher risk of other morbidity or mortality should the transplanted organ fail. The patient needs to be involved in this decision-making.

There is controversy over the relative importance of daily dosage compared to cumulative dosage as the most significant risk factor [15, 20, 61, 66, 82]. Some have interpreted the data to indicate that daily dose is more important than cumulative dose [2, 12, 29, 30, 41, 63, 73, 83–87]. Others have concluded the opposite [15, 58, 88–91]. The author's viewpoint is that there are only two modifiable risk factors—choice of

4AQ (chloroquine or hydroxychloroquine) and daily dosage. Therefore, in the absence of incontrovertible evidence to the contrary, the physi-

cian should err on the side of assuming that daily dosage is important, and adjust it to a typically safe range.

The Distinction Between Finding No Association and Showing That an Association Does Not Exist

Several investigators have failed to find evidence linking daily dose to retinopathy, but Wolfe and colleagues went further than the others in their reasoning. They stated, "Our study showed that most current patients receive 400 mg daily irrespective of weight, and suggests that this dosage is reasonable in clinical practice insofar as the published guidelines for dose/kg do not have a proven relationship to the risk of toxicity" [15]. When one considers that they lacked daily dosing information in 39.3 % of their patients with retinopathy, one might have expected more circumspection. Moreover, daily dosage is the only variable that can be altered with a potential influence on the risk of retinopathy in patients taking hydroxychloroquine. Their statement goes too far. They clearly have changed their minds over the years when writing on the topic, and were on more solid ground when they placed emphasis on the daily dose [15, 23, 92].

7.4 Cumulative Dose

The evidence regarding the role of cumulative dose of 4AQs and 4AQR is inconsistent. There are many studies reporting no association across various indices of retinopathy. Mackenzie found no correlation of 4AQR and cumulative dose once daily dose was taken into account [33]. Bonanomi and colleagues found no association of cumulative dose of chloroquine and retinal nerve fiber layer (RNFL) thinning [30]. Lai and colleagues found no correlation of cumulative dose of hydroxychloroquine with 10-2 VF mean defect or pattern standard deviation [89]. In investigating relationships of cumulative dose and 24 mfERG variables (N1 and P1 amplitudes and N1 and P1 latencies for rings R1–R6), Xiaoyun and colleagues found only one correlation of cumulative dose of chloroquine and a subcategory of mfERG responses, a rate expected based on the role of chance [93]. Almony found no relationship of cumulative dose with development of scotomas by threshold Amsler grid testing in patients taking hydroxychloroquine [88]. Other studies have also found no association of cumulative dose and hydroxychloroquine reti-

nopathy [14, 20, 94]. Many patients take enormous cumulative doses and do not develop retinopathy [87].

On the other hand, several studies have reported that cumulative dose is associated with 4AQR. Lyons and Severn, using an mfERG definition of retinopathy, found that hydroxychloroquine retinopathy depended on cumulative dose, but not daily dose [91]. Patients who had received 1,250 g or more of hydroxychloroquine had a 50 % probability of showing mfERG abnormalities and a risk of having mfERG abnormalities that was 2.8 times that of patients having lower cumulative doses [95]. Lai and colleagues found that cumulative dose correlated with mfERG N1-P1 amplitudes for rings 1 through 3 [89]. Wolfe and Marmor found an association between 4AQR based on funduscopy and perimetry with cumulative dose [15]. A significant negative correlation was found between cumulative dose and global RNFL thickness as measured by scanning laser polarimetry (Spearman's rank correlation coefficient $=-0.59$, $P<0.001$) [93].

There has been considerable variability in the reported cumulative doses of patients with and without retinopathy (Table 7.3) [96]. There are many patients with high cumulative doses 4AQs

Table 7.3 Thresholds for cumulative dose of 4-aminoquinolines associated with increased risk of retinopathy

Study	Drug	Cumulative dose at which risk of retinopathy increases to an important degree (g)	Cumulative dose at which risk of retinopathy increases to an important degree (g/kg ABW)
Banks [6]; Reed [99]; Voipio [11]; Carr [100]	C	100	NG
Marmor [4, 101, 102]; Labriola [22]	C	460	NG
Shinjo [78]	C	1,000	NG
Ben Zvi [103]	C	NG	1
Manufacturer's literature [6]	C	NG	1.6
Arden [104]	C	NG	8
Grierson [69]; Mills [105]; Tanenbaum [19]; Okun [106]; Marks [107]	C, HC	200	NG
Elman [31]; Johnson [87]; Nylander [98]; Ehrenfeld [108]; Mackenzie [33]	C, HC	300	NG
Elner [52]	HC	250	NG
Maturi [109]; Warner [75]; May [110]	HC	500	NG
Tobin [94]	HC	750	NG
American College of Rheumatology [34]	HC	800	NG
Wolfe [15]; Ben Zvi [103]; Marmor [4, 101, 102]; Mackenzie [2]; Albert [5]	HC	1,000	NG
Lyons [91]	HC	1,250	NG
Ben Zvi [103]	HC	NG	1
Arden [104]	HC	NG	14.4

Thresholds are often subjective impressions by authors based on the totality of their data. ABW is actual body weight. C is chloroquine. HC is hydroxychloroquine

who do not develop retinopathy and some patients who have taken low cumulative doses who do develop retinopathy [87]. This could imply individual variability in sensitivity to developing retinopathy [60]. However, it could also reflect the change over time in the definitions used for 4AQR [97]. For example, Nylander included patients with mild pigmentary retinal changes often associated with age alone in his cases of retinopathy [98]. Baseline studies were often not performed in the older reports making it impossible to exclude preexisting conditions simulating 4AQR [97]. The net effect may have been to falsely attribute toxicity to 4AQ use, which would lower the cumulative dose at which retinopathy risk increased.

As with ADD, it is probably incorrect to think of risk from cumulative dose as dichotomous. Rather, the risk probably monotonically increases with increasing cumulative doses. For example, Ehrenfeld states that for chloroquine the risk of retinopathy first appears at 100 g total dose, becomes significant at 300 g total dose, and

increases further at 900 g total dose [108]. Nylander reported a discernible increased risk of chloroquine retinopathy when cumulative dose exceeded 300 g, which increased to a 56 % risk of chloroquine retinopathy at cumulative doses exceeding 900 g [98].

Cumulative dose and daily dose may interact (Fig. 7.3). It is possible to develop retinopathy with a low cumulative dose if the daily dose is high enough [2]. If the cumulative dose increases, the daily dose that can produce retinopathy probably diminishes [2]. If a safe daily dose is used, truly massive cumulative doses are frequently not associated with any evidence of toxicity and there is probably no upper limit for cumulative dosage above which use of 4AQs should be discontinued [2, 87].

Some authors have proposed that patients take no more than certain maximal lifetime doses of 4AQs [2, 6]. For chloroquine the proposed lifetime doses have ranged from 300 to 600 g [6, 11, 98, 104]. Others have suggested that this is an unnecessary constraint as long as the daily dose is in a safe range [2].

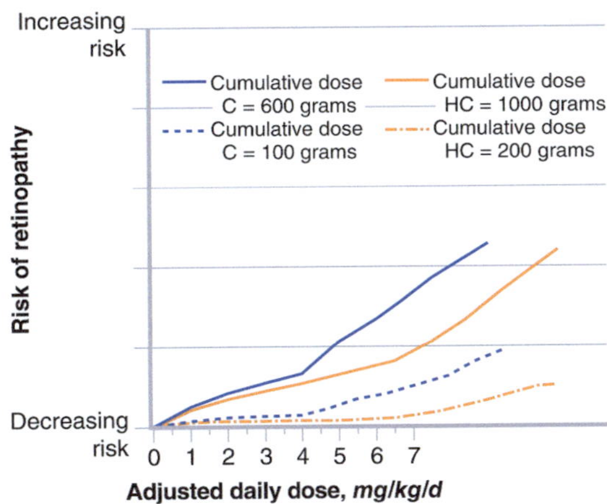

Fig. 7.3 Hypothesized interaction of cumulative dose and adjusted daily dose (ADD). At any given cumulative dose, there seems to be an inflection point for ADD at approximately 3.5–4.0 mg/kg/d for chloroquine and 6.5 mg/kg/d for hydroxychloroquine

Besides having a role with respect to risk of developing retinopathy, cumulative dose may affect the risk of progression of retinopathy. Shinjo studied 27 patients who developed early chloroquine retinopathy based on a funduscopic definition. The patients' medication was stopped and the patients were followed to determine whether or not a bull's-eye lesion developed. There was an insignificant difference in cumulative dose of C therapy in the two groups. The average cumulative doses were 923.4 ± 595.3 g and 591.0 ± 547.0 g in the bull's-eye and no bull's-eye groups, respectively ($P = 0.13$) [78].

7.5   Duration

Duration of treatment is correlated to cumulative dose through the conversion factor of daily dose. For this reason it is unsurprising that studies finding cumulative dosing associated with retinopathy also find duration of treatment associated and vice versa. For example, Wolfe and Marmor found that both cumulative dose and duration of treatment were associated with retinopathy [15]. Adjusted for age, gender, dose, IBW, and education, the odds ratio for retinopathy for each 5 year increase in duration of hydroxychloroquine therapy was 1.4 (95 % confidence interval 1.1–1.8) [15]. When duration of treatment was dichotomized into greater than or equal to 7 years and less than 7 years, the longer duration group had an odds ratio for developing retinopathy of 5.1 compared to the shorter duration group (no confidence interval given) [15]. Similarly, just as a number of studies have found no association between cumulative dose and 4AQR, the same studies discount duration as a relevant risk factor [78, 90].

The minimum duration of treatment with 4AQ treatment associated with retinopathy depends on daily dose. At higher doses the minimum duration is shorter. Yam has stated that the shortest duration of hydroxychloroquine associated with retinopathy was 1.9 months [38]. For chloroquine, the shortest duration of use associated with retinopathy was 7 months in an overdosed patient [12]. Others have asserted that the risk of retinopathy increases above durations ranging from 1 to 10 years [11, 20, 35, 74, 78, 98, 106]. The most commonly cited duration associated with increased risk of 4AQR is 5–6 years [20, 35, 74, 78].

In a prospective cohort study, none of 400 patients taking hydroxychloroquine at recommended doses for at least 6 years developed retinopathy before 6 years [74]. With more extended follow-up, one developed retinopathy at 6.5 years and another at 8 years. The authors concluded that there is no reason to screen for retinopathy in patients taking recommended doses of hydroxychloroquine before 6 years of drug use [74]. In a similar vein, Easterbrook recommended baseline screening and repeated screening after 9 years of therapy in patients taking hydroxychloroquine at less than 6.5 mg/kg(IBW)/d [63].

In an analogy to suggestions for a maximal lifetime cumulative dosing, some authors have suggested a lifetime maximal duration of 4AQ treatment. Butler has suggested that chloroquine treatment not extend beyond 3 years [111]. Others think that this is an unnecessary constraint as long as a safe daily dose is used [2].

7.6   Renal Dysfunction

In case series, the proportions of patients with 4AQR who have renal dysfunction is higher than in patients without retinopathy, but the differences do not reach statistical significance because renal dysfunction is relatively rare [14, 78]. Although few cases of 4AQR in patients with renal disease have been reported, it is likely that this area is understudied, especially as so many patients with SLE have renal disease and receive 4AQs.

Approximately 60 % of hydroxychloroquine is excreted by the kidneys (see Chap. 2). Therefore, renal dysfunction can lead to toxicity even if dosing is correct [72]. Renal disease is part of the spectrum of SLE with moderate to severe renal dysfunction seen in an estimated 20 % of patients [112, 113]. Patients with lupus have a probability of 14.3–18.2 % for a doubling of serum creatinine after 10 years of disease [114]. In patients taking 4AQs for SLE, presence of renal dysfunction should be specifically sought. Moreover, it is important to check for ongoing reduction in renal function in addition to baseline renal insufficiency as the underlying disease can induce renal dysfunction over time, even when it is not present initially [14].

7.7   Liver Dysfunction

Thirty to seventy nine percent of a 4AQ is metabolized by the liver (see Chap. 2). Therefore, patients with hepatic dysfunction can develop retinopathy at doses and after durations not normally associated with toxicity (Fig. 7.2). SLE is associated with subclinical hepatic dysfunction in approximately 20 % of cases, clinical liver dysfunction in from 1 to 16 %, and is a cause of death in an estimated 3 % of cases with SLE [113, 115–117]. Therefore, attention to this historical point is important in screening for risk factors for retinopathy.

7.8   Preexisting Maculopathy

Labeling preexisting maculopathy a risk factor is not quite accurate, because it is not known that having macular degeneration or another maculopathy makes a patient more susceptible to 4AQR although in isolated cases it has been suspected [39]. Nevertheless, it does make determination of onset of 4AQR more difficult, because from baseline the macula is already abnormal [22, 63]. Some have recommended excluding patients with preexisting maculopathy from taking 4AQs [36, 63]. Others recommend allowing therapy to see if it is effective, and if so, allow therapy at a low maintenance dose with regular monitoring [63]. It has been suggested that color fundus photography and fluorescein angiography may be useful to document a baseline appearance of the fundus in such cases [118]. In situations in which a clinician inherits a patient without information regarding a preexisting maculopathy, attribution of signs from a preexisting maculopathy to 4AQR may occur. For example Figs. 2 and 3 of Weisinger appear to represent macular degeneration with geographic atrophy rather than true 4AQR [119].

In one series, preexisting maculopathy severe enough to prevent screening and to disqualify patients from taking hydroxychloroquine was found in 3.1 % of patients [69]. Exactly where a preexisting maculopathy becomes so severe as to prevent recognition of drug toxicity is a judgment call, especially as an estimated 23–72.8 % of persons over the age of 65–80 have some degree of pigmentary abnormalities of the macula [31, 120–122].The statistics on preexisting maculopathy are suspect, and probably not appropriate for generalization, as they vary widely depending on who the observer is. For example, in another study, Smith reported pigmentary macular changes in only 0.4 % of 500 patients with RA not taking 4AQs [123].

7.9   Genetic Predisposition and Protection

It has been noted that some patients develop 4AQR at low cumulative and daily doses and others show no toxicity despite a high cumulative and daily dose [37, 87]. This raises the possibility of a genetic predisposition or protective effect [124]. Shroyer investigated six patients with chloroquine retinopathy and two with hydroxychloroquine retinopathy and found that two of the patients taking chloroquine were heterozygous for an ABCR missense mutation previously associated with Stargardt disease [8]. Genetic testing of patients being considered for 4AQ therapy is not routinely done.

7.10 Preexisting Visual Field Abnormalities

Preexisting visual field abnormalities may make it difficult to interpret the visual fields obtained in screening for 4AQR. In this sense, considering preexisting visual field abnormalities as a risk factor is analogous to considering preexisting maculopathy as a risk factor. Examples include visual field abnormalities associated with stroke (Fig. 7.4) and glaucoma. Having glaucoma as a comorbidity is a risk factor for 4AQR because it predisposes clinicians to following 30-2 or 24-2 visual fields rather than the preferred 10-2 visual fields. Detecting early scotomata from 4AQs with 20-2 or 24-2 visual field testing is less sensitive than 10-2 VF testing [1, 125]. In patients with

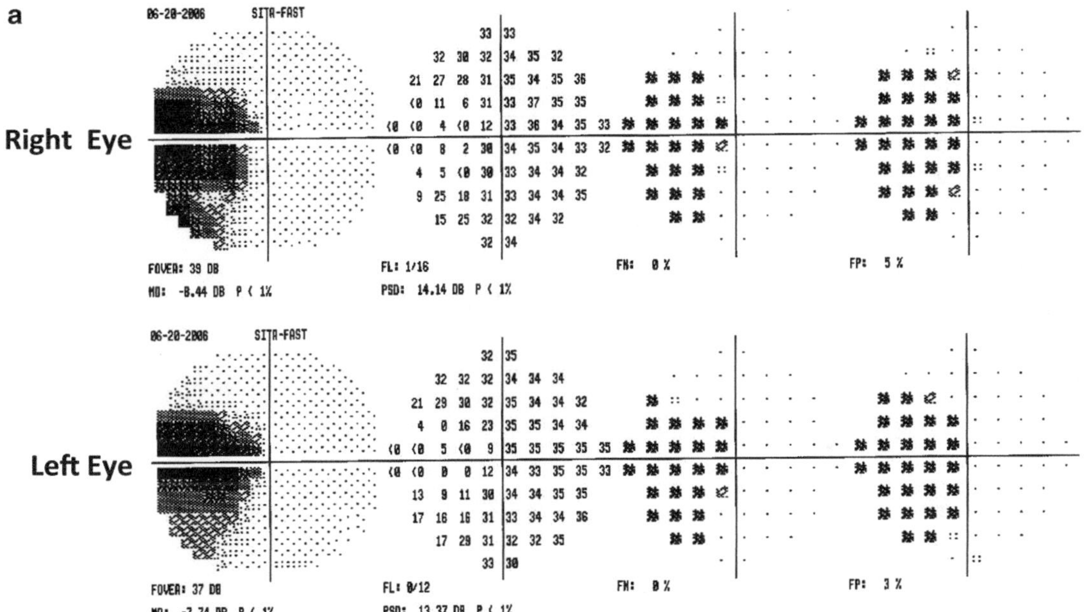

Fig. 7.4 These are visual fields and fundus images from a 60-year-old woman with rheumatoid arthritis. She had been on hydroxychloroquine at a dosage of 6.9 mg/kg/d based on non-obese actual body weight for 3.5 years. She had liver disease with hepatitis C infection. She had suffered a right occipital stroke in 2000 that left her with a homonymous left paracentral scotoma. (**a**) Baseline 10-2 visual fields (10-2 VFs) with a III, white test object from 2006 demonstrating a left homonymous paracentral scotoma attributed to her old stroke. Visual acuity at this time was 20/30 in each eye. (**b**) Three sequential 10-2 VFs of the left eye from 2006, 2007, and 2008. The fields from 2006 and 2007 are similar, but the field from 2008 shows a typical annular scotoma of hydroxychloroquine retinopathy superimposed on the preexisting field defect from the stroke. This was not recognized by the screening clinician who attributed the observed changes entirely to the old stroke. The fundus examination was normal. Hydroxychloroquine was continued. Similar superimposed changes of hydroxychloroquine were seen in the 10-2 VF of the right eye (not shown). (**c**) When the patient returned in 2010 the visual acuity had dropped to right 20/70, left 20/100, and a bilateral bull's-eye maculopathy was noted, as shown. (**d**) Fluorescein angiogram showed typical window defects with a bull's-eye shape. The annular defect was broader inferiorly (*orange arrows*) than superiorly (*yellow arrows*). (**e**) Time domain (Stratus) OCT of both maculas showing marked thinning and paracentral loss of retinal pigment epithelium bilaterally. Comment: this case illustrates the effects of three risk factors on development of hydroxychloroquine retinopathy. The first risk factor illustrated is a toxic daily dose (6.9 mg/kg/d based on a non-obese actual body weight). The second is the effect of concomitant liver disease. The patient had hepatitis C infection with liver dysfunction. Finally, she had preexisting visual field defects from her previous occipital stroke that confounded proper interpretation of her 10-2 VF testing and delayed the diagnosis of hydroxychloroquine retinopathy until a bull's-eye maculopathy developed 2 years later

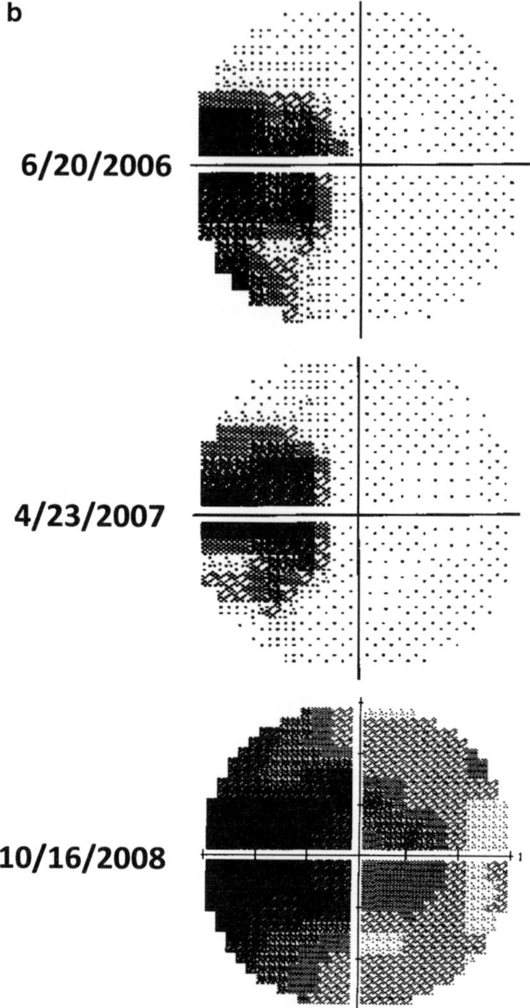

Fig. 7.4 (continued)

glaucoma who take chloroquine or hydroxychloroquine, it is advisable to follow the glaucoma with either the 30-2 or 24-2 VF and to screen for 4AQR separately with 10-2 VFs.

7.11 More Speculative Risk Factors

Smoking and exposure to sunlight have been linked to 4AQR, but few studies have critically examined these purported links, and they are currently considered to be tenuous [2, 12, 83].

One electroretinographic study in rats exposed to toxic doses of hydroxychloroquine found that continuous light exposure exacerbated changes whereas continuous darkness delayed them [126]. The location of the damage in the retina suggests that exposure to light may be important. Without much evidential basis, some have suggested that patients with 4AQR attempt to reduce their light exposure [33]. Diseases associated with breakdown of the blood/retina barrier have been suspected of increasing the risk of 4AQR, but the scant evidence available suggests that such is not the case [18].

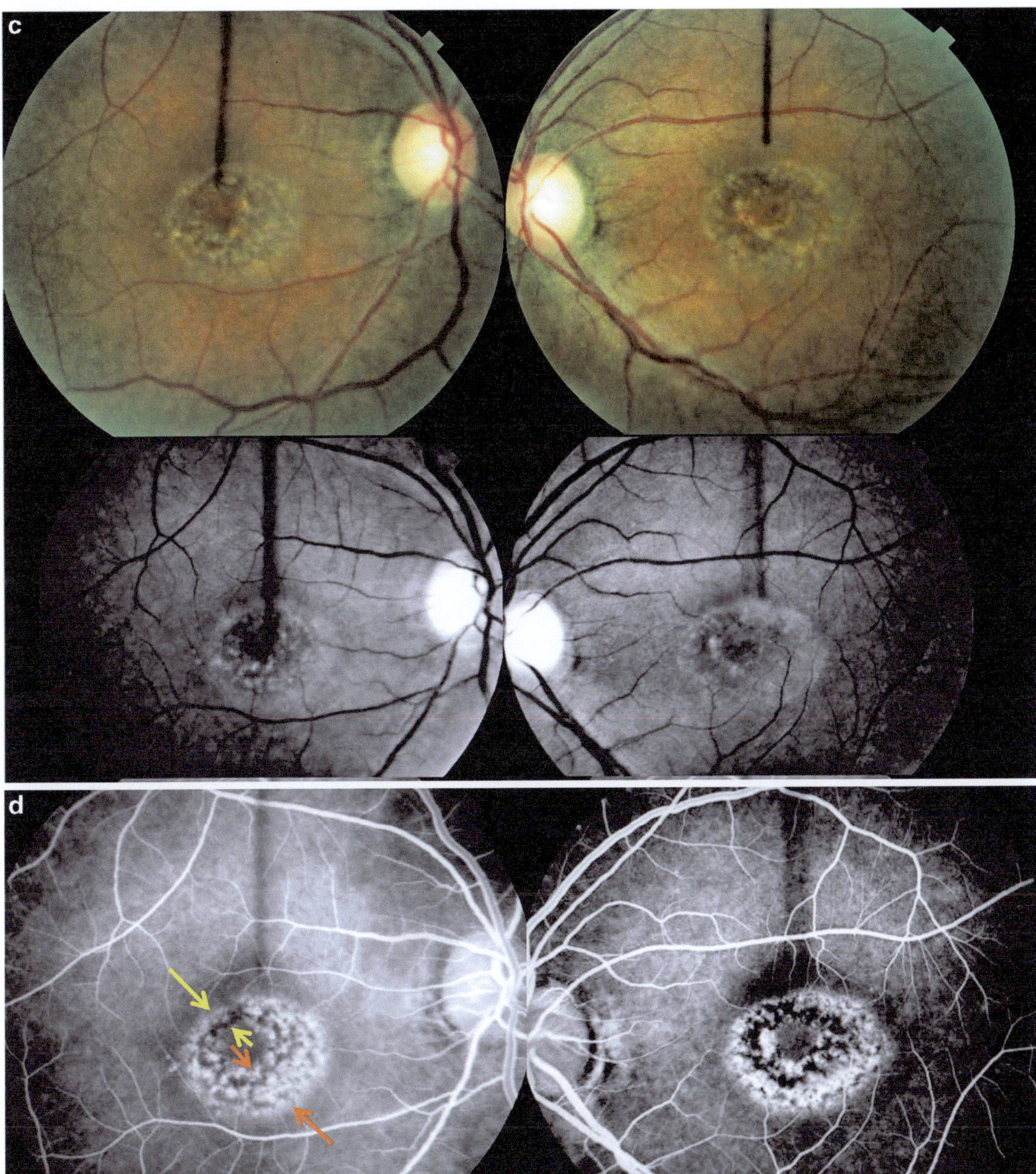

Fig. 7.1 (continued)

7.12   Combinations of Risk Factors

Bernstein analyzed the known experience with hydroxychloroquine retinopathy through 1992 and concluded that no case of retinopathy had occurred in a patient taking 6.5 mg/kg (IBW)/d or less for fewer than 10 years [72]. Although a few such cases have since been reported, they are rare, and the concept of a combined risk factor that includes daily dose plus duration (or its surrogate, cumulative dose) is useful to the screening clinician (Fig. 7.3) [54].

To assess the relative importance of the multiple risk factors for hydroxychloroquine retinopathy, a multivariable model is helpful, but only if

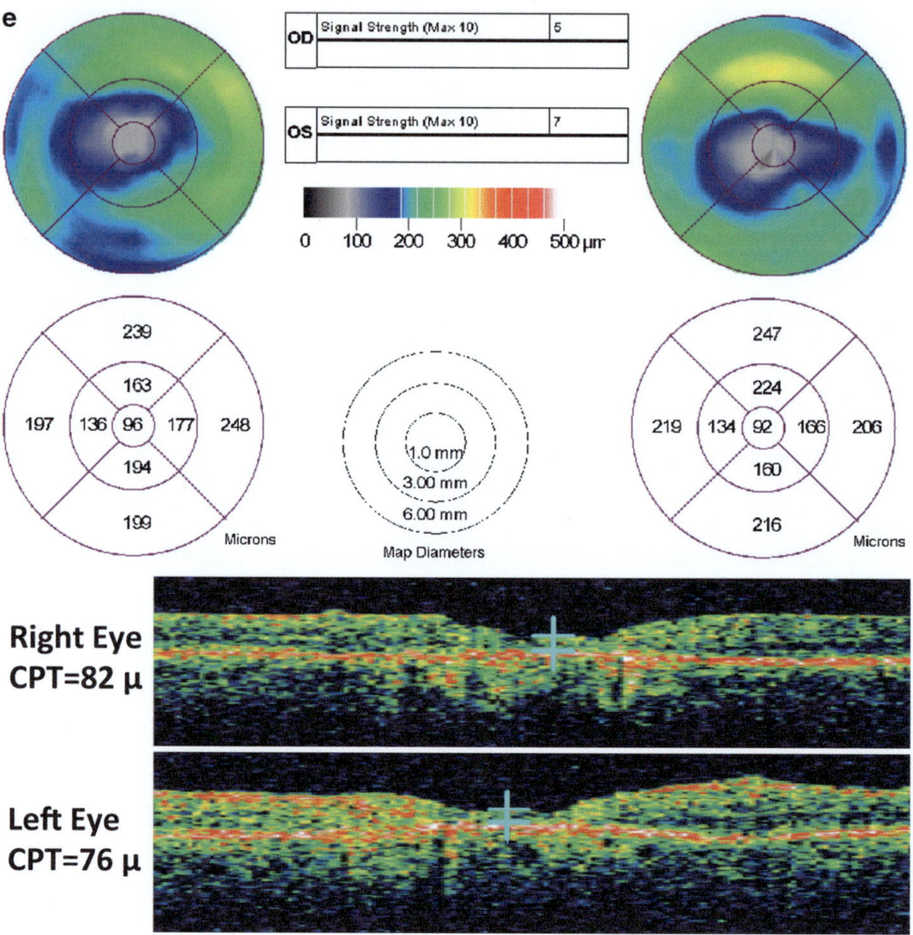

Fig. 7.4 (continued)

applied to a sample relatively free of bias. If applied to a biased sample, unreliable outcomes will be the result [15].

7.13 Summary of Key Points

- The risk factors for 4AQR are drug used; ADD; cumulative dose and its surrogate, duration of use; age; preexisting macular abnormalities; renal dysfunction; and hepatic dysfunction.
- Indirect risk factors include female gender and obesity. The more direct risk factor in these cases is ADD.
- Over 80 % of patients taking 4AQs have a risk factor for retinopathy.

- The risk associated with age probably increases continuously rather than increasing suddenly at some arbitrary threshold.
- Most physicians prescribe identical doses for all patients. For hydroxychloroquine this is 400 mg/d. For chloroquine this is 250 mg/d.
- IBW, lean body weight, and top normal body weight are often used as synonyms, but occasionally distinctions are made. When distinctions are made, lean body weight is the lowest index.
- IBW is related to height by multiple algorithms that can differ by as much as 20 pounds for a given height. Pay attention to the algorithm used in different papers. No evidence suggests that one algorithm is superior.

- The thresholds associated with unacceptably increased risk of 4AQR are 3.5 mg/kg (IBW)/d for chloroquine and 6.5 mg/kg (IBW)/d for hydroxychloroquine.
- Trade-offs exist in the choice of IBW algorithms. "Lighter" algorithms will lead to lower dosing, but require more phone calls to prescribing physicians to change dosing. "Heavier" algorithms will allow higher dosing, but will lead to fewer calls to prescribing physicians to change dosing.
- The general principle guiding clinical practice in prescribing 4AQs should be to find the smallest effective dose. Risk can always be decreased by reducing daily dosage.

References

1. Browning DJ. Hydroxychloroquine and chloroquine retinopathy: screening for drug toxicity. Am J Ophthalmol. 2002;133:649–56.
2. Mackenzie AH. Dose refinements in long-term therapy of rheumatoid arthritis with antimalarials. Am J Med. 1983;75:40–5.
3. Lee AG. Hydroxychloroquine screening. Who needs it, when, how, and why? Br J Ophthalmol. 2005;89:521–2.
4. Marmor MF, Kellner U, Lai TYY, Lyons JS, Mieler WF. Revised recommendations on screening for chloroquine and hydroxychloroquine retinopathy. Ophthalmology. 2011;118:415–22.
5. Albert DA, Debois LKL, Lu KF. Antimalarial ocular toxicity, a critical appraisal. J Clin Rheumatol. 1998;4:57–62.
6. Banks CN. Melanin: blackguard or red herring? Another look at chloroquine retinopathy. Aust N Z J Ophthalmol. 1987;15:365–70.
7. Semmer AE, Lee MS, Harrison AR, Olsen TW. Hydroxychloroquine retinopathy screening. Br J Ophthalmol. 2008;92:1653–5.
8. Shroyer NF, Lewis RA, Lupski JR. Analysis of the ABCR (ABCA4) gene in 4-aminoquinoline retinopathy: is retinal toxicity by chloroquine and hydroxychloroquine related to Stargardt disease? Am J Ophthalmol. 2001;131:761–6.
9. Shearer RV, Dubois EL. Ocular changes induced by long-term hydroxychloroquine (Plaquenil) therapy. Am J Ophthalmol. 1967;64:245–52.
10. Burns RP. Delayed onset of chloroquine retinopathy. N Engl J Med. 1968;275:693–6.
11. Voipio H. Incidence of chloroquine retinopathy. Acta Ophthalmol (Copenh). 1966;44:349–54.
12. Dubois EL. Antimalarials in the management of discoid and systemic lupus erythematosus. Semin Arthritis Rheum. 1978;8:33–51.
13. Rothfield N. Efficacy of antimalarials in systemic lupus erythematosus. Am J Med. 1988;85:53–6.
14. Bergholz R, Schroeter J, Ruther K. Evaluation of risk factors for retinal damage due to chloroquine and hydroxychloroquine. Br J Ophthalmol. 2010;94:1637–42.
15. Wolfe F, Marmor MF. Rates and predictors of hydroxychloroquine retinal toxicity in patients with rheumatoid arthritis and systemic lupus erythematosus. Arthritis Care Res. 2010;62:775–84.
16. Rynes RI. Ophthalmologic safety of long-term hydroxychloroquine sulfate treatment. Am J Med. 1983;75:35–9.
17. Finbloom DS, Silver K, Newsome DA, Gunkel R. Comparison of hydroxychloroquine and chloroquine use and the development of retinal toxicity. J Rheumatol. 1985;12:692–4.
18. Kobak S, Deveci H. Retinopathy due to antimalarial drugs in patients with connective tissue diseases: are they so innocent? A single center retrospective study. Int J Rheum Dis. 2010;13:e11–5.
19. Tanenbaum L, Tuffanelli DL. Antimalarial agents: chloroquine, hydroxychloroquine, and quinacrine. Arch Dermatol. 1980;116:587–91.
20. Marmor MF. Comparison of screening procedures in hydroxychloroquine toxicity. Arch Ophthalmol. 2012;130:461–9.
21. Mackenzie AH. An appraisal of chloroquine. Arthritis Rheum. 1970;13:280–91.
22. Labriola LT, Jeng D, Fawzi AA. Retinal toxicity of systemic medications. Int Ophthalmol Clin. 2012;52:149–66.
23. Marmor MF, Carr RE, Easterbrook M, et al. Recommendations on screening for chloroquine and hydroxychloroquine retinopathy. Ophthalmology. 2002;109:1377–82.
24. Flach AJ. Improving the risk-benefit relationship and informed consent for patients treated with hydroxychloroquine. Trans Am Ophthalmol Soc. 2007;105:191–7.
25. Browning DJ. Impact of the revised American academy of ophthalmology guidelines regarding hydroxychloroquine screening on actual practice. Am J Ophthalmol. 2013;155:418–28.
26. Michaelides M, Stover NB, Francis PJ, Weleber RG. Retinal toxicity associated with hydroxychloroquine and chloroquine: risk factors, screening, and progression despite cessation of therapy. Arch Ophthalmol. 2011;129:30–9.
27. Gupta G, Greenberg PB, Tsiaras WG. The prevalence of high-risk factors and adherence to screening guidelines for hydroxychloroquine retinopathy in a cohort of US veterans. Scientific poster 461. Presented at: American Academy of Ophthalmology 2005 Annual Meeting, Oct 17–18, Chicago; 2005.

28. Mititelu M, Wong BJ, Brenner M, Bryar PJ, Jampol LM, Fawzi AA. Progression of hydroxychloroquine toxic effects after drug therapy cessation. New evidence from multimodal imaging. Arch Ophthalmol. 2013;131:1187–97.

29. Bray VJ, Enzenauer RJ, Enzenauer RW, West SG. Antimalarial toxicity in rheumatic disease. J Clin Rheumatol. 1998;4:168–9.

30. Bonanomi MT, Dantas NC, Medeiros FA. Retinal nerve fiber layer thickness measurements in patients using chloroquine. Clin Exp Ophthalmol. 2006; 34:130–6.

31. Elman A, Gullberg R, Nillson E, Rendahl I, Wachtmeister L. Chloroquine retinopathy in patients with rheumatoid arthritis. Scand J Rheumatol. 1976; 5:161–6.

32. Farrell DF. Retinal toxicity to antimalarial drugs: chloroquine and hydroxychloroquine: a neurophysiologic study. Clin Ophthalmol. 2012;6:377–83.

33. Mackenzie AH. Antimalarial drugs for rheumatoid arthritis. Am J Med. 1983;75:48–58.

34. American College of Rheumatology Ad Hoc Committee on Clinical Guidelines. Guidelines for monitoring drug therapy in rheumatoid arthritis. Arthritis Rheum. 1996;39:723–31.

35. Tehrani R, Ostrowski RA, Hariman R, Jay WM. Ocular toxicity of hydroxychloroquine. Semin Ophthalmol. 2008;23:201–9.

36. Neubauer AS, Samari-Kermani K, Schaller U, Welge-Luben U, Rudolph G, Berninger T. Detecting chloroquine retinopathy: electro-oculogram versus color vision. Br J Ophthalmol. 2003;87:902–8.

37. Kellner U, Renner AB, Tillack H. Fundus autofluorescence and mfERG for early detection of retinal alterations in patients using chloroquine/hydroxychloroquine. Invest Ophthalmol Vis Sci. 2006;47:3531–8.

38. Yam JCS, Kwok AKH. Ocular toxicity of hydroxychloroquine. Hong Kong Med J. 2006;12:294–304.

39. Payne JF, Hubbard III GB, Aaberg Sr TM, Yan J. Clinical characteristics of hydroxychloroquine retinopathy. Br J Ophthalmol. 2010;95:245–50.

40. Easterbrook M. Clinical characteristics of hydroxychloroquine retinopathy. Evid Based Ophthalmol. 2011;12:132–3.

41. Terrell III WL, Haik KG, Haik Jr GM. Hydroxychloroquine sulfate and retinopathy. South Med J. 1988;81:1327–8.

42. Browning DJ. Reply to defining ideal body weight. Am J Ophthalmol. 2002;134:935–6.

43. Walvick MD, Walvick MP, Tongson E, Ngo CH. Hydroxychloroquine: lean body weight dosing. Ophthalmology. 2011;118:2100.

44. Pautler SE. Hydroxychloroquine dosages should be calculated using lean body mass. Arch Ophthalmol. 2007;125:1303.

45. Pai MP, Paloucek FP. The origin of the "Ideal" body weight equations. Ann Pharmacol. 2000;34:1066–9.

46. Marmor MF. Efficient and effective screening for hydroxychloroquine toxicity. Am J Ophthalmol. 2013;155:413–4.

47. Browning DJ. Reply to Impact of the revised American Academy of Ophthalmology guidelines regarding hydroxychloroquine screening on actual practice. Am J Ophthalmol. 2013;156:410–1.

48. Easterbrook M. Current concepts in monitoring patients on antimalarials. Aust N Z J Ophthalmol. 1998;26:101–3.

49. Easterbrook M. Defining ideal body weight. Am J Ophthalmol. 2002;134:935.

50. Bruce-Chwatt LJ. Chloroquine blindness? Lancet. 1968;2:1039.

51. Levy GD, Munz SJ, Paschal J, Cohen HB, Prince KJ, Peterson T. Incidence of hydroxychloroquine retinopathy in 1,207 patients in a large multicenter outpatient practice. Arthritis Rheum. 1997;40:1482–6.

52. Elder M, Rahman AMA. Early paracentral visual field loss in patients taking hydroxychloroquine. Arch Ophthalmol. 2006;124:1729–33.

53. Thorne JE, Maguire AM. Retinopathy after long term, standard doses of hydroxychloroquine. Br J Ophthalmol. 1999;83:1201–2.

54. Falcone PM, Paolini L, Lou PL. Hydroxychloroquine toxicity despite normal dose therapy. Ann Ophthalmol. 1993;25:385–8.

55. Weiner A, Sandberg MA, Gaudio AR, Kini MM, Berson EL. Hydroxychloroquine retinopathy. Am J Ophthalmol. 1991;112:528–34.

56. Raines MF, Bhargava SK, Rosen ES. The blood-retinal barrier in chloroquine retinopathy. Invest Ophthalmol Vis Sci. 1989;30:1726–31.

57. Wang C, Fortin PR, Li Y, Panaritis T, Gans M, Esdaile JM. Discontinuation of antimalarial drugs in systemic lupus erythematosus. J Rheumatol. 1999; 26:808–15.

58. Bienfang D, Coblyn JS, Liang MH, Corzillius M. Hydroxychloroquine retinopathy despite regular ophthalmologic evaluation: a consecutive series. J Rheumatol. 2000;27:2703–6.

59. Easterbrook M. Hydroxychloroquine retinopathy. Ophthalmology. 2001;108:2158–9.

60. Vu BLL, Easterbrook M, Hovis JK. Detection of color vision defects in chloroquine retinopathy. Ophthalmology. 1999;106:1799–804.

61. Tett S, Cutler D, Day R. Antimalarials in rheumatic diseases. Baillieres Clin Rheumatol. 1990;4:467–89.

62. Easterbrook M. Dose relationships in patients with early chloroquine retinopathy. J Rheumatol. 1987; 14:472–5.

63. Easterbrook M. The ocular safety of hydroxychloroquine. Semin Arthritis Rheum. 1993;23:62–7.

64. Alarcon GS. How frequently and how soon should we screen our patients for the presence of antimalarial retinopathy? Arthritis Rheum. 2002;46:561.

65. Hickley NM, Al-Maskari A, McKibbin M. Chloroquine and hydroxychloroquine toxicity. Arch Ophthalmol. 2011;129:1506–7.

66. Chen E, Brown DM, Benz MS, Fish RH, Wong TP, Kim RY, Major JC. Spectral domain optical coherence tomography as an effective screening test for hydroxychloroquine retinopathy (the "flying saucer" sign). Clin Ophthalmol. 2010;4:1151–8.

67. Teoh SC-B, Lim J, Koh A, Lim T, Fu E. Abnormalities on the multifocal electroretinogram may precede clinical signs of hydroxychloroquine retinotoxicity. Eye. 2006;20:129–32.

68. Browning DJ, Fraser CM. Reply to abnormalities on the multifocal electroretinogram may precede clinical signs of hydroxychloroquine retinopathy. Eye. 2007;21:147.

69. Grierson DJ. Hydroxychloroquine and visual screening in a rheumatology outpatient clinic. Ann Rheum Dis. 1997;56:188–90.

70. Missner S, Kellner U. Comparison of different screening methods for chloroquine/hydroxychloroquine retinopathy: multifocal electroretinography, color vision, perimetry, ophthalmoscopy, and fluorescein angiography. Graefes Arch Clin Exp Ophthalmol. 2012;250:319–25.

71. Schwartz SG, Mieler WF. Retinal and choroidal manifestations of systemic medications. In: Arevalo JF, editor. Retinal and choroidal manifestations of selected systemic diseases. New York: Springer; 2013. p. 479–92.

72. Bernstein H. Ocular safety of hydroxychlotoquine sulfate (Plaquenil). South Med J. 1992;85:274–9.

73. Bernstein HN. Ocular safety of hydroxychloroquine. Ann Ophthalmol. 1991;23:292–6.

74. Mavrikakis I, Sfikakis PP, Mavrikakis E, Rougas K, Nikolaou A, Kostopoulos C, Mavrikakis M. The incidence of irreversible retinal toxicity in patients treated with hydroxychloroquine—a reappraisal. Ophthalmology. 2003;110:1321–6.

75. Warner AE. Early hydroxychloroquine macular toxicity. Arthritis Rheum. 2001;44:1959–61.

76. Easterbrook M. An ophthalmological view on the efficacy and safety of chloroquine versus hydroxychloroquine. J Rheumatol. 1999;26:1866–7.

77. Morand EF, McCloud PI, Littlejohn GO. Continuation of long term treatment with hydroxychloroquine in systemic lupus erythematosus and rheumatoid arthritis. Ann Rheum Dis. 1992;51:1318–21.

78. Shinjo SK, Junior OOM, Tizziani VAP, Morita C, Kochen JAL, Takahashi WY, Laurindo IMM. Chloroquine-induced bull's eye maculopathy in rheumatoid arthritis: related to disease duration? Clin Rheumatol. 2007;26:1248–53.

79. Akman F, Cerman E, Yenice O, Kazokoglu H. Two cases with chloroquine and hydroxychloroquine maculopathy. Marmara Med J. 2011;24:68–72.

80. Cox NH, Paterson WD. Ocular toxicity of antimalarials in dermatology: a survey of current practice. Br J Dermatol. 1994;131:878–82.

81. Hollander JE. The calculated risk of arthritis treatment. Ann Intern Med. 1965;62:1062–4.

82. Spalton DJ, Roe GMV, Hughes GRV. Hydroxychloroquine, dosage parameters and retinopathy. Lupus. 1993;2:355–8.

83. Scherbel AL, Mackenzie AH, Nousek JE, Atdjian M. Ocular lesions in rheumatoid arthritis and related disorders with particular reference to retinopathy-A study of 741 patients treated with and without chloroquine drugs. N Engl J Med. 1965;273:360–6.

84. Laaksonen AL, Koskiahde V, Juva K. Dosage of antimalarial drugs for children with juvenile rheumatoid arthritis and systemic lupus erythematosus. A clinical study with determination of serum concentrations of chloroquine and hydroxychloroquine. Scand J Rheumatol. 1974;3:103–8.

85. Fischer VW. Evolution of a chloroquine-induced cardiomyopathy in the chicken. Exp Mol Pathol. 1976;25:242–52.

86. Marks JS. Chloroquine retinopathy: is there a safe daily dose? Ann Rheum Dis. 1982;41:52–8.

87. Johnson MW, Vine AK. Hydroxychloroquine therapy in massive total doses without retinal toxicity. Am J Ophthalmol. 1987;104:139–44.

88. Almony A, Garg S, Peters RK, Mamet R, Tsong J, Shibuya B, Kitridou R, Sadun AA. Threshold amsler grid as a screening tool for asymptomatic patients on hydroxychloroquine therapy. Br J Ophthalmol. 2005;89:569–74.

89. Lai TYY, Ngai JWS, Chan WM, Lam DSC. Visual field and multifocal electroretinography and their correlations in patients on hydroxychloroquine therapy. Doc Ophthalmol. 2006;112:177–87.

90. Tzekov R. Ocular toxicity due to chloroquine and hydroxychloroquine: electrophysiological and visual function correlates. Doc Ophthalmol. 2005;110:111–20.

91. Lyons JS, Severns ML. Using multifocal ERG ring ratios to detect and follow Plaquenil retinal toxicity: a review. Doc Ophthalmol. 2009;118:29–36.

92. Marmor MF. New American Academy of Ophthalmology recommendations on screening for hydroxychloroquine retinopathy. Arthritis Rheum. 2003;48:1764–70.

93. Xiaoyun MA, Dongyi HE, Linping HE. Assessing chloroquine toxicity in RA patients using retinal nerve fiber layer thickness, multifocal electroretinography and visual field test. Br J Ophthalmol. 2010;94:1632–6.

94. Tobin DR, Krohel G, Rynes RI. Hydroxychloroquine-Seven-year experience. Arch Ophthalmol. 1982;100:81–3.

95. Lyons JS, Severns ML. Detection of early hydroxychloroquine retinal toxicity enhanced by ring ratio analysis of multifocal electroretinography. Am J Ophthalmol. 2007;143:801–9.

96. Ruther K, Foerster J, Berndt S, Schroeter J. Chloroquine/hydroxychloroquine: variability of retinotoxic cumulative doses. Ophthalmologe. 2007;104:875–80.

97. Maksymowych W, Russell AS. Antimalarials in rheumatology: efficacy and safety. Semin Arthritis Rheum. 1987;16:206–21.

98. Nylander U. Ocular damage in chloroquine therapy. Acta Ophthalmol (Copenh). 1966;44:335–8.

99. Reed H, Campbell AA. Central scotomata following chloroquine therapy. Can Med Assoc J. 1962;86:176–8.

100. Carr RE, Gouras P, Gunkel RD. Chloroquine retinopathy. Early detection by retinal threshold test. Arch Ophthalmol. 1966;75:171–8.

101. Marmor MF. Author reply. Ophthalmology. 2011;118:2099–100.
102. Marmor MF, Kellner U, Lai TYY, Lyons JS, Mieler WF. Authro reply. Ophthalmology. 2011;118:2101.
103. Ben-Zvi I, Kivity S, Langevitz P. Hydroxychloroquine: from malaria to autoimmunity. Clin Rev Allergery Immunol. 2012;42:145–53.
104. Arden GB, Kolb H. Antimalarial therapy and early retinal changes in patients with rheumatoid arthritis. Br Med J. 1966;1:270–3.
105. Mills PV, Beck M, Power BJ. Assessment of the retinal toxicity of hydroxychloroquine. Trans Ophthalmol Soc U K. 1981;101:109.
106. Okun E, Gouras P, Bernstein H, von Sallmann L. Chloroquine retinopathy-A report of eight cases with ERG and Dark-Adaptation findings. Arch Ophthalmol. 1963;63:93–105.
107. Marks JS, Power BJ. Is chloroquine obsolete in treatment of rheumatic disease? Lancet. 1979;1:371–3.
108. Ehrenfeld M, Nesher R, Merin S. Delayed-onset chloroquine retinopathy. Br J Ophthalmol. 1986;70:281–3.
109. Maturi RK, Yu M, Weleber RG. Multifocal electroretinographic evaluation of long-term hydroxychloroquine users. Arch Ophthalmol. 2004;122:973–81.
110. May K, Metcalf T, Gough A. Screening for hydroxychloroquine retinopathy. Br Med J. 1998;317:1388–9.
111. Butler I. Retinopathy following the use of chloroquine and allied substances. Ophthalmologica. 1965;149:204–8.
112. Rees EG, Wilkinson M. Serum proteins in systemic lupus erythematosus. Br Med J. 1959;24:795–8.
113. Dubois EL, Tuffanelli DL. Clinical manifestations of systemic lupus erythematosus. Computer analysis of 520 cases. JAMA. 1964;190:104–11.
114. Mosca M, Tani C, Aringer M, Bombardieri S, Boumpas D, Brey R, Cervera R, Doria A, Jayne D, Khamashta MA, Kuhn A, et al. European league against rheumatism recommendations for monitoring patients with systemic lupus erythematosus in clinical practice and in observational studies. Ann Rheum Dis. 2010;69:1269–74.
115. Runyon BA, LaBrecque DR, Anuras S. The spectrum of liver disease in systemic lupus erythematosus. Report of 33 histologically-proved cases and review of the literature. Am J Med. 1980;69:187–94.
116. Miller MH, Urowitz MB, Gladman DD, Blendis LM. The liver in systemic lupus erythematosus. Q J Med N Ser. 1984;53:401–9.
117. Kofman S, Johnson GC, Zimmerman HJ. Apparent hepatic dysfunction in lupus erythematosus. AMA Arch Intern Med. 1955;95:669–76.
118. Cruess AF, Schachat AP, Nicholl J, Augsburger JJ. Chloroquine retinopathy-Is fluorescein angiography necessary? Ophthalmology. 1985;92:1127–9.
119. Weisinger HS, Pesudovs K, Collin HB. Management of patients undergoing hydroxychloroquine (Plaquenil) therapy. Clin Exp Optom. 2000;83:32–6.
120. Dickinson AJ, Sparrow JM, Duke AM, Thompson JR, Gibson JM, Rosenthal AR. Prevalence of age-related maculopathy at two points in time in an elderly British population. Eye. 1997;11:301–14.
121. Morsman CDG, Livesey SJ, Richards IM, Jessop JD, Mills PV. Screening for hydroxychloroquine retinal toxicity: is it necessary? Eye. 1990;4:572–6.
122. Percival SPB, Behrman J. Ophthalmological safety of chloroquine. Br J Ophthalmol. 1969;53:101–9.
123. Smith JL. Chloroquine macular degeneration. Arch Ophthalmol. 1962;68:186–90.
124. Gonasun LM, Potts AM. In vitro inhibition of protein synthesis in the retinal pigment epithelium by chloroquine. Invest Ophthalmol Vis Sci. 1974;13:107–15.
125. Anderson C, Blaha GR, Marx JL. Humphrey visual field findings in hydroxychloroquine toxicity. Eye. 2011;25:1535–45.
126. Legros J, Rosner I, Berger C. Influence of the ambient light level on the ocular modifications induced by hydroxychloroquine in the rat. Arch Ophthalmol. 1973;33:417–24.

8

Ancillary Testing in Screening for Hydroxychloroquine and Chloroquine Retinopathy

Abbreviations

4AQs	4-Aminoquinolines (chloroquine and hydroxychloroquine)
4AQR	4-Aminoquinoline retinopathy
asb	Apostilb
C	Chloroquine
COR	Coefficient of repeatability
COV	Coefficient of variation
dB	Decibel
DTL	Dawson–Trick–Litzkow electrodes
ERG	Electroretinogram
FA	Fluorescein angiography
FDP	Frequency doubling perimetry
HC	Hydroxychloroquine
ICC	Intraclass correlation coefficient
ISCEV	International Society for Clinical Electrophysiology and Vision
MD	Mean defect
mfERG	Multifocal electroretinography
nm	Nanometer
RNFL	Retinal nerve fiber layer
SAP	Standard automated perimetry
S	Standard deviation of a sample of a normally distributed variable
SD-OCT	Spectral domain optical coherence tomography
SITA	Swedish Interactive Treatment Algorithm
TD-OCT	Time domain optical coherence tomography
X	Mean of a sample of a normally distributed variable

The most important function of screening patients taking hydroxychloroquine or chloroquine is to detect overdosing, which can be corrected in almost all cases. Of secondary importance is detecting retinopathy that may occur despite appropriate dosing. This function is less important because there is no guarantee that retinopathy, if detected, can be reversed (see Chap. 6). Nevertheless, the probability of reversing toxicity is higher if the condition is detected earlier.

Unfortunately, the signs of 4-aminoquinoline retinopathy (4AQR) detectable on routine clinical examination occur late in its progression. Visual acuity is not a useful variable in screening for antimalarial retinopathy if it is normal. One review reported sensitivity and specificity of a visual acuity criterion for detection of 4AQR of 22 % and 77 %, respectively [1]. There are many patients with advanced 4AQR with dense paracentral scotomas, yet normal visual acuity (see Chap. 6) [2]. Neither is funduscopy sensitive for 4AQR. The bull's-eye lesion of 4AQR spares the fovea until late, and earlier signs are nebulous. Detecting the earliest funduscopic change of 4AQR is dependent on the examiner's skill and experience, which varies [3–5].

For these reasons, ancillary testing is important [6]. Threshold perimetry (e.g., 10-2 visual field testing (10-2 VF)), multifocal electroretinography (mfERG), spectral domain optical coherence tomography (SD-OCT), and fundus autofluorescence imaging (FAF) can reveal abnormalities of macular function and structure. These abnormalities influence the frequency of

D.J. Browning, *Hydroxychloroquine and Chloroquine Retinopathy*, DOI 10.1007/978-1-4939-0597-3_8, © Springer Science+Business Media New York 2014

follow-up when inconclusive, and lead to cessation of the drug when conclusive. Familiarity with ancillary tests and their limitations helps in the optimal management of patients taking 4AQs.

Many ancillary tests have been proposed as useful for detecting 4AQR but have been eventually discarded, generally for one main reason and several lesser ones [7]. The most important reason is that the results of testing are too variable [6, 8–11]. Among currently popular tests, the mfERG has this drawback (Fig. 8.1). In 4AQR it takes a large change in the value of the measured variable to discern a disease-induced change. This makes serial tests over time difficult to interpret [7].

Among lesser reasons for discarding ancillary tests, the first is that the test may be too sensitive [12]. For example, in a study of contrast sensitivity testing in patients taking hydroxychloroquine, 44.4 % of patients taking 200 mg/day for 1–9 years had abnormalities on contrast sensitivity testing [13]. A test that suggests an abnormality in such a high percentage of cases when the preponderance of other evidence suggests no clinically important retinopathy is not useful.

An ancillary test may demonstrate large overlaps between normals and patients with retinopathy implying difficulty discriminating cases. This is a problem with red Amsler grid testing, color vision testing, electrooculography (EOG), and mfERG [3, 5, 6, 14, 15].

On the other hand, a test may be too insensitive. Loss of foveal reflex, fluorescein angiography, home Amsler grid testing, and global electroretinography (ERG) are examples of such tests [6, 16–19]. Many patients with reproducible 10-2 ring scotomas have crisp foveal reflexes, normal Amsler grids, and normal global ERGs rendering these tests of little use for screening purposes [6].

Some tests, such as macular photostress testing, are not standardized [20]. Performance statistics obtained by one investigator mean little to others because the test is done differently by different clinicians.

Other tests are not specific for the condition of interest. For example, 10 of 758 consecutive patients taking hydroxychloroquine and screened for retinopathy had positive red Amsler grid testing, but none of the 10 had retinopathy [21]. The rate of false positives was 100 %, an obviously unacceptable performance.

Lastly, some tests are not reimbursed by health care payers. Examples include contrast sensitivity testing and macular photostress testing. Lack of reimbursement is as strong a disincentive for test adoption as reimbursement is for adoption. For one or more of these reasons, all of the following tests have been embraced and subsequently discarded: color fundus photography, fluorescein angiography, dark adaptometry, global electroretinography, electrooculography, macular photostress testing, Amsler grid testing, tangent screen testing, and color vision testing [6, 7, 22–24].

Interpretation of ancillary testing is typically not scientific, always involves assumptions, and is often controversial. It is important to identify the underlying assumptions and definitions of retinopathy used by the interpreter to be able to compare interpretations. Easterbrook co-wrote the American Academy of Ophthalmology (AAO) guidelines for 4AQ screening in 2002, when Amsler grid testing was advocated [25]. No counter-revelatory evidence regarding the performance characteristics of the Amsler grid was published between 2002 and 2011, when the guidelines were rewritten by a different set of authors without Easterbrook [26]. The new guidelines dropped the Amsler grid recommendation. The facts had not changed, but the interpretation had.

Only static automated perimetry (SAP) has withstood 30 years of use as an ancillary test. Although widely adopted by clinicians, its performance has not been quantitatively evaluated in patients taking 4-aminoquinolines (4AQs). This test is covered in detail in Sect. 8.4. In the past decade mfERG, SD-OCT, and FAF have been introduced and lauded [26]. They have received the compliment of being more objective than 10-2 VF, but the claim is dubious for mfERG and FAF [26]. Although in the United States one or more of them is currently recommended for universal application where available [26], their ultimate niche is more likely to be selective [27].

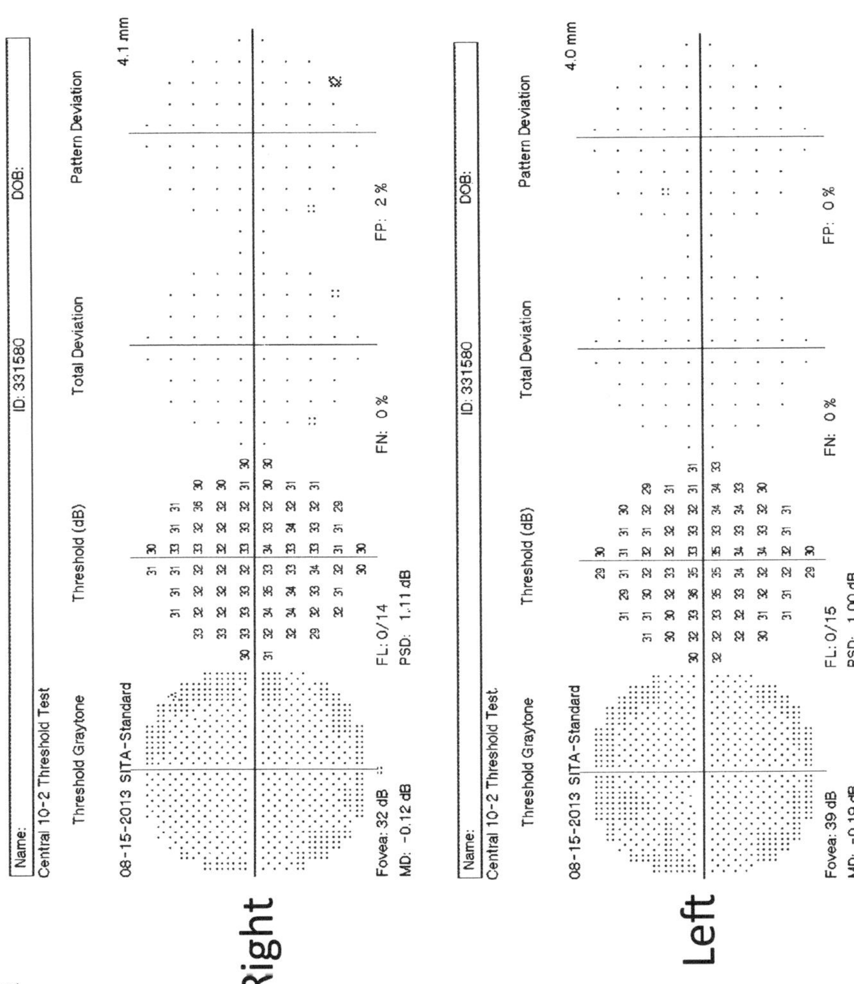

Fig. 8.1 Multifocal electroretinograms (mfERGs) on three consecutive visits in a 64-year-old woman with rheumatoid arthritis who was placed on hydroxychloroquine in 2007. She was 67 in. tall and weighed 185 lb. She had always taken 400 mg/day. Her best corrected visual acuity was 20/25 in both eyes secondary to early nuclear sclerotic cataracts. Her maculas at baseline were normal. She had no renal or liver disease. (**a**) Yearly 10-2 visual field testing with a III, red test object was normal for six consecutive years (this example was from 15 August 2013). When the American Academy of Ophthalmology revised guidelines were published, mfERG testing was begun. (**b**) mfERGs for three consecutive years shown in the retinal view (the left record in each study is from the right eye of the patient). Because of reductions in amplitudes noted in 2013, the question arose whether she had toxicity and needed to be taken off hydroxychloroquine. For example, note that the R_1 amplitude for the right eye was 27.6 nV/mm^2 on 15 August 2011 and 31.3 nV/mm^2 on 20 August 2012 (*red circled cells*). Compare this to the value of 16.2 nV/mm^2 (*red circled cell*) in study from

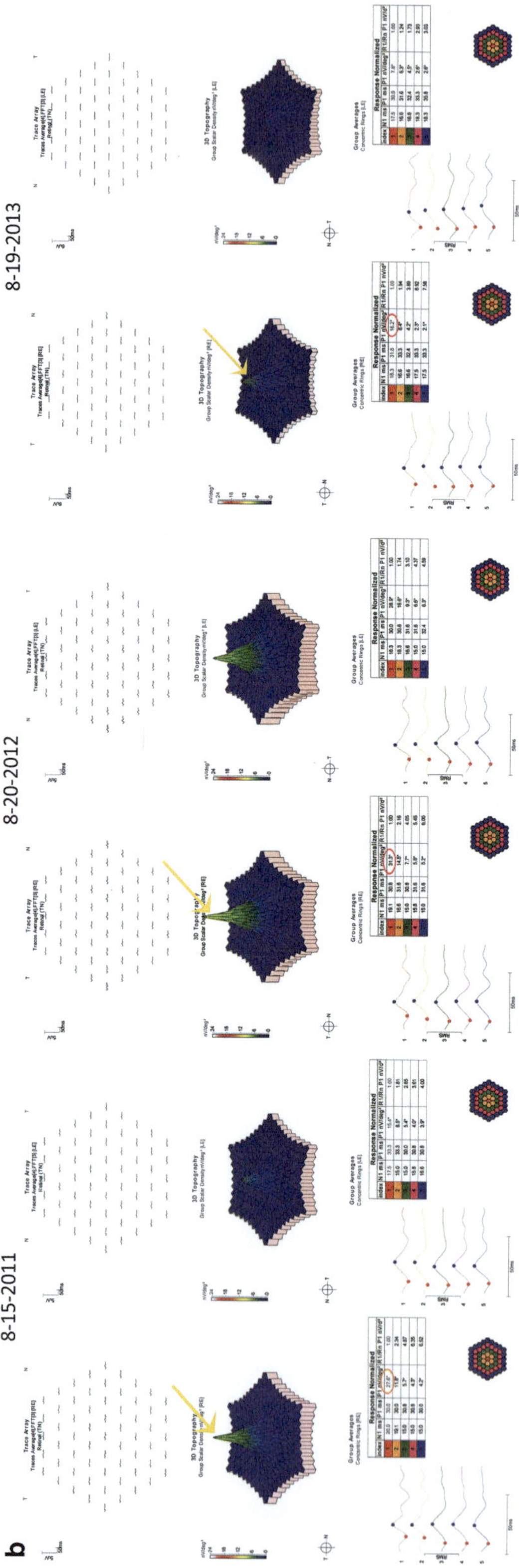

Fig. 8.1 (continued) 19 August 2013, a decrease of 41 %. Similar behavior is shown in the topographic surface map with a decreased amplitude shown in the last study (*yellow arrows*). The screening ophthalmologist worried that hydroxychloroquine retinopathy was responsible for the decreases. However, this change probably represents measurement variability. The coefficient of repeatability (COR) for R_1 is 60 %. The 41 % decrease in this case lies well within this COR

Ancillary testing is expensive. Because financial resources for health care are scarce, ophthalmologists need to judge whether a test adds sufficient value to the care of a patient to make obtaining it worthwhile. There can be a conflict of interest in fee-for-service systems of health care. An ophthalmologist or optometrist can profit by ordering more ancillary tests depending on the practice setting. Therefore, the topic is not only important to discuss, but also potentially inflammatory [28].

This chapter covers general principles of diagnostic testing and applies those concepts to their use in screening for 4AQR. Commonly used abbreviations in this chapter are collected in "Abbreviations" for reference. Each term will be first used in its full form, along with its abbreviation.

8.1 Defining Normal

For any ancillary test, it is necessary to decide what is considered abnormal. For a normally distributed variable, a common choice is that the value being measured lies more than two standard deviations from the mean value of a control group of clinically normal persons [7, 9, 29]. For a non-normally distributed variable, it may be that the value lies beyond the 5th or 95th or 99th percentile of a control group, or outside the range of the control group [23, 30]. The definition chosen will affect the frequency with which measurements are labeled abnormal.

These definitions are probabilistic and simply state where the given patient lies relative to a normative database. They do not make a diagnosis of retinopathy [31]. The clinician needs to understand that they imply that a certain percentage of normal patients will be classified as abnormal *by definition*. For example, suppose that an abnormal test result is defined as one in which the value lies beyond the 95th percentile of a group of controls not taking the drug. If the prevalence of 4AQR among those taking the drug is 1 %, and one applies the ancillary test to a random sample of 100 persons taking the drug, then on average six tests will be abnormal. Of these six, on average only one will have 4AQR. The other five persons labeled by the test as abnormal will in fact be normal, but happen to have measurements by the ancillary test that put them in a range *defined to be* abnormal.

The Normal Distribution

Many of the measurements made in ancillary testing for 4AQR either follow or are assumed to follow a normal distribution given by the formula

$$f(x) = \frac{1}{\sigma\sqrt{2\pi}} e^{\frac{(x-\mu)^2}{\sigma^2}},$$

where μ is the mean of the distribution, and σ is the standard deviation of the distribution.

Often a raw measurement is converted to a Z-score, defined by $Z = (X - \underline{X})/\underline{S}$. In this case $\underline{X}$ is the mean of the sample measurements and $\underline{S}$ is the standard deviation (SD) of the sample measurements. The Z-score shows how far a measurement is from the average value, expressed in units of standard deviations. A Z-score that is one, two, or three SDs from the mean value lies at a position encompassing 68, 95, and 99.7 % of the measurements for the sample, respectively. An example of the use of Z-scores arises in considering height, which determines the ideal body weight (IBW), an important concept in studies concerning 4AQR (see Chap. 7).

How *Not* to Define an Abnormal Ancillary Test

Legitimate methods for defining an abnormal ancillary test have been discussed. In all cases, the concept of a comparison of a test subject's value to the distribution of values from normal subjects is involved. Unfortunately, examples not to emulate have been published; studying one of these is instructive. For example, in a study of SD-OCT in 4AQR, the authors assert that the thickness of the outer nuclear layer is the most sensitive SD-OCT measurement to follow in detecting 4AQR [32]. As evidence they show a figure in which a scan from an eye with retinopathy is juxtaposed to two similar scans from eyes of normal subjects. They compare the thickness of the outer nuclear layer delineated by freehand of two scans from a single patient with 4AQR to the mean $\pm$ SD values from seven normal eyes. The thickness of the outer nuclear layer for one of the scans was 46.7 μm compared to 59.8 $\pm$ 7.1 μm for the normal subjects' scans [32]. The patient's value was 13.1 μm less than the mean value of the normals or 13.1 μm/7.1 μm = 1.84 standard deviations less than the sample mean of the normal subjects. Such an occurrence will happen on average 5.2 % of the time even in normal eyes.

There are several problems with the authors' approach:

- They don't define how their freehand method of delineating the outer nuclear layer was done. What were the landmarks? How reproducible was the method? No one can replicate the finding without these details.
- The sample of normals is small (seven).
- An unconventional cut-point for "abnormal" was used. A typical cut-point would be 2 standard deviations, not 1.84 standard deviations.
- The authors cherry-pick individual scans from the patient said to have 4AQR to compare to the normal controls. One wonders what the result of comparing all the scans in the raster would show. The authors reported that throughout the raster the thickness of the ONL of the affected patient was reduced compared to the normal subjects, but the size of the reductions was omitted. The size of the reductions may not have been inconsequential.

8.2 Principles Common to Ancillary Tests Used in Screening for 4-Aminoquinoline Retinopathy

To use an ancillary test for drug toxicity effectively, several pieces of information must be known:

- The values of the test in a normal population
- The values in the diseased population not taking the drug—for example, patients with rheumatoid arthritis (RA) and systemic lupus erythematosus (SLE)
- The intraindividual variability of the test
- A baseline value for the test in the patient before the drug is begun
- The performance characteristics of the test: sensitivity and specificity
- The prevalence of the toxicity (4AQR) in the population using the drug [9, 33]

In the case of chloroquine and hydroxychloroquine, the baseline test is frequently taken after the drug has already been started, which is less than satisfactory [34]. A tacit assumption has been made that the drug, in the absence of toxicity, has not changed the value of the test in the patient. This assumption may not be true. For example, for the mfERG, some investigators have claimed that taking hydroxychloroquine does change the values of the test measurements [35]. They distinguish this effect from true toxicity, by which they mean irreversible changes [36]. This also appears to be the case with the macular photostress test and the visual evoked potential (VEP) [20, 35–37].

Many studies on ancillary testing use normal subjects as a control group [38, 39]. This is flawed because the possibility exists that the diseases for which these drugs are used produce changes in the ancillary test independent of using the drug [9, 38]. For example, electrooculogram (EOG) values are affected by rheumatologic diseases [8, 9]. Intraindividual variability in normal subjects and patients with rheumatoid arthritis differs. The coefficient of variation (COV) is 10 % in the first, but 15 % of the second group [9]. Thus, a 30 % decrease in the Arden ratio would be necessary before one could conclude with 95 % confidence that the decrease represented a real change in the test as a result of taking a 4AQ and was not noise in the measurement (see Sect. 8.3) [9]. On the other hand, retinal nerve fiber layer (RNFL) thickness did not differ between patients with rheumatologic disease not taking aminoquinolines and normal subjects [40]. In the absence of a proper control group, evidence of a dose–response relationship between 4AQs and the test variable of interest can be helpful in increasing the probability that a purported effect is real [38].

The value of a diagnostic test is determined by its sensitivity, specificity, reproducibility, and cost. The first two characteristics, known as the performance characteristics of the test, are defined by referring to a 2×2 table that displays the true health status of the patient compared to the status as defined by the test (Fig. 8.1) [33, p. 891]. The usefulness of an ancillary test depends on the prevalence of the disease (see Chap. 5) as well as the sensitivity and specificity of the test. If a disease is rare, then there will be a number of patients who test positive for the disease but do not have it

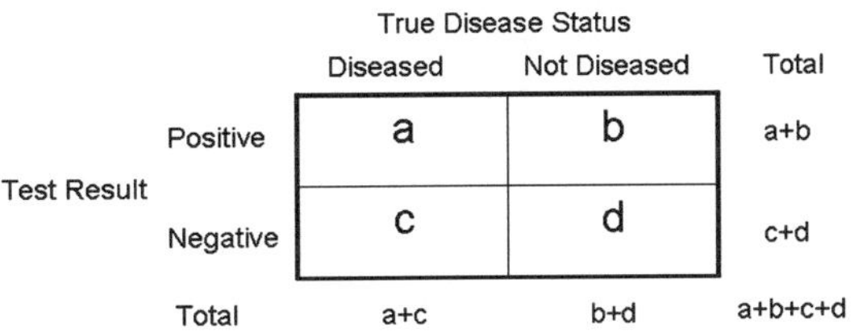

Fig. 8.2 2×2 table used in the definition of sensitivity and specificity

(false positives). The concepts of positive predictive value (PPV) and negative predictive value (NPV) capture the importance of disease prevalence in ancillary testing. The definitions of these terms and some corollaries follow.

- *Sensitivity*—The proportion of truly diseased patients deemed so by the test. In the symbols of Fig. 8.2, specificity equals $a/(a+c)$. Sensitivity is most important in screening for disease, because a clinician does not want to say mistakenly that a diseased patient is healthy. Therefore, high sensitivity in a test is desirable [41].
- *Specificity*—The proportion of truly nondiseased patients deemed so by the test. In the symbols of Fig. 8.2, specificity equals $d/(b+d)$. Specificity is most important in making a decision about beginning or stopping treatment, because a clinician does not want to risk side effects caused by treatment, or risk losing the benefit of effective treatment, based on an erroneously positive test. Therefore, high specificity in a test is desirable [41].
- *Positive predictive value (PPV)*—The probability that a patient has the disease in question if the ancillary test is positive; the equation for calculating this probability is

$$\text{Positive predictive value} = \left(\text{Sensitivity}\right)\left(\text{Prevalence}\right) \Big/ \left[\begin{array}{l}\left(\text{Sensitivity}\right)\left(\text{Prevalence}\right) \\ + \left(1-\text{Specificity}\right)\left(1-\text{Prevalence}\right)\end{array}\right]$$

- *Negative predictive value (NPV)*—The probability that a patient does not have the disease in question if the ancillary test is negative; the equation for calculating this probability is

$$\text{Negative predictive value} = \left(\text{Specificity}\right)\left(1-\text{Prevalence}\right) \Big/ \left[\begin{array}{l}\left(\text{Specificity}\right)\left(1-\text{Prevalence}\right) \\ + \left(1-\text{Sensitivity}\right)\left(\text{Prevalence}\right)\end{array}\right]$$

- *Likelihood ratio*—The ratio of the probability that a particular test result would occur in a patient with the disease compared to the probability that the result would occur in a patient without the disease [31]. Likelihood ratios come in two varieties—positive and negative. The positive likelihood ratio is defined as sensitivity/ $(1-\text{Specificity})$. For example, the sensitivity and specificity of 10-2 VF testing in patients with 4AQR has been reported to be 85.7 % and 92.5 %, respectively [42]. The positive likelihood ratio is therefore 0.857/0.075 or 11.4. In other words, this positive likelihood ratio means that an abnormal 10-2 VF is 11.4 times more likely in a patient with 4AQR than in a patient taking a 4AQ without retinopathy [31].

- *Odds*—The ratio of probability of having the disease to the probability of not having the disease. The probability of having the disease is usually estimated by the prevalence of the disease. In some cases, other information allows a more refined estimate of the probability of having the disease than the prevalence by Bayesian inference (see Sect. 8.4). The prevalence of hydroxychloroquine retinopathy in nonoverdosed patients after 6 years of therapy has been reported to be 0.5 % [43]. Therefore, the odds is 0.005/0.995 equals 0.005. As exemplified in this case, for small values of prevalence, the odds is approximately the prevalence. The odds is typically figured before and after an ancillary test. The pretest odds is based on the prevalence. The posttest odds is based on the pretest odds modified by the results of the ancillary test.

Specifically, posttest odds equals pretest odds times the positive likelihood ratio [31]. If the odds of having the disease is known, the probability of having the disease can be calculated as Odds/(Odds + 1) [31].

Defining the performance characteristics of an ancillary test implies that there is a gold standard against which the test can be compared, but in many cases there is no such standard. Instead, the gold standard may be the consensus of a panel of graders using some other method of assessment or a composite action such as discontinuation of therapy based on the totality of clinical evidence [21, 44]. Often, the gold standard is unreproducible. For example, the gold standard for mild retinopathy in some studies was presence of mild macular pigmentary changes alone, which will be dependent on the judgment of the examining clinician [34, 45]. In other cases the gold standard is another ancillary test, most often SAP [46–48]. The problem with this approach is that the new test has no chance of exceeding the test used as the gold standard in relative sensitivity or specificity. The best that the new test can do is match the performance of the ancillary test chosen as the gold standard. For example Adam and colleagues used the 10-2 VF as the gold standard for testing mfERG [47]. They found mfERG to have a sensitivity of 89 %. By the way the study was set up, 10-2 VF testing had 100 % sensitivity. Therefore the study design biased a comparison of relative sensitivity in favor of SAP [47]. Despite the inelegance of real life, the assumption of a gold standard for diagnosis is useful in understanding the underlying concept.

Is There a Gold Standard for 4AQR?

The literature is inconsistent on the issue of a gold standard for defining 4AQR (Table 8.1). Various gold standards are used, and in some cases none is defined. If there is no gold standard, then one cannot specify performance characteristics of an ancillary test of interest. This is a variation on the problem of defining 4AQR (see Chap. 4). Gold standards based on 10-2 VF interpretation alone are difficult to sustain because of the variation in interpretation of SAP by different clinicians.

Table 8.1 Published gold standards for 4-aminoquinoline retinopathy (4AQR)

Study	Gold standard
Farrell [16]	10-2 VF is abnormal and compatible fundus abnormalities (unspecified) are present
Adam [47]	Two of the three following are present: (1) 10-2 visual field defects, (2) compatible fundus abnormalities (unspecified), (3) compatible SD-OCT abnormalities (unspecified)
Elder [49], Easterbrook [48]	10-2 VF is abnormal
Fleck [45]	Compatible fundus pigmentary abnormalities to ophthalmoscopy
Michaelides [44], Grierson [21]	Based on the totality of the clinical evidence (e.g., for Michaelides, this is the history, examination, 10-2 VF, global ERG, mfERG, SD-OCT, and FA; for Grierson this is history, examination, and red Amsler grid testing)
Lee [12], Almony [17], Chen [50], Anderson [51]	None defined for early 4AQR

Published gold standards for 4AQR and documentation of absence of gold standards in some cases

Of the performance characteristics of an ancillary test, the sensitivity is more important when the damage incurred by missing the presence of the disease is high. Specificity receives more emphasis when the costs of intervention are high. In the case of 4AQR, the cost of missing the diagnosis is some degree of visual loss. The cost of intervention—either reduction of dosing or cessation of drug—is reactivation of quiescent autoimmune disease.

Sensitivity and specificity are characteristics of a test, but to apply these statistics in clinical practice, one must know the prevalence of the disease in the population being studied. As covered in Chap. 5, there are no reliable data on prevalence of 4AQR, thus an assumption of prevalence must be made based on the available crude estimates. One way to handle this situation, which this chapter employs, is to assume a range of plausible prevalences based on the imperfect data and conduct a sensitivity analysis over that range of values.

An Example of Calculating PPVs and NPVs and How They Are Used by the Clinician

The ability of treating rheumatologists to detect early maculopathy, before bull's-eye changes develop, has been proposed as a screening test for 4AQR [45]. The gold standard in this case was the findings of a single ophthalmologist [45]. The sensitivity and specificity of the rheumatologists for detecting maculopathy were 80.0 % and 89.3 %, respectively [45]. For a plausible range of prevalences of 4AQR, the calculated PPVs and NPVs are shown (Table 8.2). A recurring theme in the use of ancillary testing for 4AQR is illustrated—the dominating effect of prevalence on the PPVs and NPVs and the relative unimportance of small differences in performance characteristics of the ancillary test.

Table 8.2 Example of a spreadsheet calculation of positive and negative predictive values from sensitivity, specificity, and assumed prevalences

Assumed prevalence (%)	Sensitivity (%)	Specificity (%)	PPV (%)	NPV (%)
0.1	80.0	89.3	0.7	100
1	80.0	89.3	7	99.8
3	80.0	89.3	18.8	99.3
5	80.0	89.3	28.2	98.8

PPV is positive predictive value. *NPV* is negative predictive value

Regardless of the result of this single ancillary test, it would be unlikely for a clinician to stop the prescribed 4AQ. At the most, a positive test would increase the clinician's estimate of the probability of having 4AQR from 5 to 28.2 %—not enough to stop the medication. Instead, 28.2 % would become the new prior probability in a subsequent step of Bayesian inference. It is likely that another ancillary test would be applied to the patient. This test would have its own sensitivity and specificity, and a new PPV and NPV would be generated, which might be sufficient to change management.

When the definition of an abnormal test depends on a cut-point of a continuous variable, changes in the cut-point will change the sensitivity and specificity of the test. Receiver operating curve analysis may then offer the best choice of a cut-point that gives the best balance of sensitivity and specificity. However, not all authors go to the trouble to do this. For example, Lyons chose to maximize specificity of the mfERG in discriminating hydroxychloroquine retinopathy by defining an abnormal R_1/R_2 as lying above the 99th percentile for the normal population [52]. Had a lower percentile been chosen as the cut-point, the specificity would have been lowered but the sensitivity increased.

The Problems of Judging Usefulness of an Ancillary Test

To judge whether a test is useful in detecting retinopathy, it is necessary to apply it to patients who clearly do and others who clearly do not have retinopathy. If this rule is not followed, one can decide erroneously that a test is not useful. For example, Fleck and colleagues assessed the value of SAP with red targets using the Friedmann Mark 1 visual field analyzer against patients who were taking 4AQs but had no retinopathy [45]. There were some differences in the proportions of minor macular pigmentary abnormalities between the group of patients taking and not taking 4AQs, but the macular pigmentary changes could not be classified as severe enough to diagnose 4AQ retinopathy. When they found no difference in the proportion of scotomas within 10 deg of fixation between groups, they concluded that SAP and surveillance by ophthalmologists might not be required. The conclusion does not follow, however, because they did not test their screening program against any patient with definite retinopathy.

It is also necessary to apply a test to a sufficient number of patients who have 4AQ retinopathy to be able to reach a valid conclusion. An illustration of the pitfall here was the series of six patients with hydroxychloroquine retinopathy reported by Bienfang [4]. All six had color vision abnormalities. This led him to conclude that the test had high sensitivity [4]. Yet the result was probably an artifact of a small sample as other studies have not been able to replicate his observation [26].

An Erroneous Calculation of PPV and NPV in the Literature of 4AQR

Vu and colleagues have published PPV and NPV for various color vision tests in detecting chloroquine retinopathy that appear to be erroneous [53]. Consider the evidence: They report the results for a number of color vision tests including Ishihara, Spp-2, D-15, Dsat-15, CU, and AO-HRR tests. Only the results reported for the SPP-2 are reviewed here, but the same analysis applies to all the other results in the paper. They calculate PPV and NPV for the SPP-2 as 90 % and 91.7 %, respectively, which would make this test valuable to a clinician if true.

The authors do not disclose the prevalence of chloroquine retinopathy that they used in their calculation, but by working backward it can be determined. By taking the formula for PPV and rearranging, one can show that

$$\text{Prevalence} = (\text{PPV} - \text{PPV} \times S_p)/(S_n - \text{PPV} \times S_n - \text{PPV} \times S_p + \text{PPV}), \quad \text{where} \quad S_n = \text{sensitivity} \quad \text{and}$$

$S_p = $ specificity. They report S_n and S_p for SPP-2 as 93.3 % and 88 %, respectively [53]. Therefore,

$$\text{Prevalence} = \left(0.9 - 0.9 \cdot 0.88\right)/\left(0.933 - 0.9 \cdot 0.933 - 0.933 \cdot 0.88 + 0.9\right) = .626959.$$

The prevalence of chloroquine retinopathy is not 62.7 % (see Chap. 5). Using more realistic values, one can calculate low values for PPV for SPP-2 and all the other color vision tests. These values correspond with the clinical observation that color vision testing, when abnormal, is poorly predictive that chloroquine retinopathy is present.

A high NPV means that a test rarely misclassifies a person with 4AQR as unaffected, but provides no information about the risk of a healthy person having 4AQR. A high PPV increases the probability that the person has the disease. A low PPV means that many of the positive tests will be false positives, and that a more reliable follow-up test is needed. A test with a high PPV rarely misclassifies a person without 4AQR as having 4AQR but does not bear on the tendency to misclassify a person with 4AQR as healthy.

The PPV of a diagnostic test should not be used to evaluate the efficacy of the test when the pretest likelihood of the presence of disease is low (e.g.,10 % or less). Instead, in such a case the NPV is the appropriate concept to invoke. A high NPV confirms the entering clinical impression that disease presence is unlikely. The appropriate use of PPV is in a situation in which the pretest probability of presence of the disease is high (e.g., 90 % or greater). In this case, a high PPV supports the clinical impression that the disease is present. For cases with intermediate pretest probabilities, a combination of NPV and PPV can substantially improve clinical decision-making. For example, if the pretest probability of disease presence is 80 %, then a PPV of 90 % can improve one's confidence that disease is truly present.

Because the estimated prevalence of 4AQR is less than 10 % (see Chap. 5), the main use of a positive ancillary test is to raise the prior probability from a low value (the estimated prevalence) to a higher posterior probability which will become the prior probability for another ancillary test. If this next test is also positive, the resulting PPV may be sufficient to change management (i.e., stop the 4AQ). It would be rare for management to change based on the results of a single ancillary test.

Because chloroquine and especially hydroxychloroquine retinopathy are not common, often the statistics for sensitivity and specificity are based on small numbers of patients. For example, in one report assessing color vision testing, statistics were based on four cases of advanced retinopathy [34]. One way to determine the reliability of a published statistic for sensitivity or specificity is to calculate the marginal error assuming that an additional case were added to the data and that the test misclassified the case. How would the sensitivity or specificity statistic be affected? An example of such a calculation has been published [54]. The desired outcome is that the marginal sensitivity and specificity would not be much affected by misclassification of the next patient. In reports with small sample sizes, marginal sensitivity and specificity would be influenced, making the reported estimates of sensitivity and specificity suspect.

What Does It Mean When There Is No Gold Standard?

In some studies of ancillary tests, no attempt is made to define a gold standard and no action is taken as a result of applying the ancillary testing. The only aim appears to be to establish what proportions of patients have abnormalities in one or another of several tests. For example, Xiayun and colleagues compared 10-2 VFs, mfERGs, and RNFL thickness measurements with a scanning laser polarimeter in patients with rheumatoid arthritis (RA) taking chloroquine, patients not taking chloroquine, and normal subjects [40]. No patient was taken off chloroquine, leading the reader to infer that retinopathy was not diagnosed in any patient. The authors reported that mfERGs were abnormal in 42 of 60 (70 %), RNFL measurements were abnormal in 40 of 60 (66.7 %), and 10-2 VFs were abnormal in 2 of 60 (3.3 %).

The percentages are dependent on the definitions chosen for abnormality. In this case, the authors defined an abnormal mfERG as having a reduced N1 or P1 amplitude in either of ring R_1 or R_2 [40]. They defined an abnormal 10-2 VF as one with a paracentral point having less than a 1 % chance of being normal without regard to whether the abnormality persisted on repeat field testing [40]. The definition of an abnormal RNFL measurement was not given, but may have been compared to a proprietary table of normal values provided by the instrument manufacturer. Had the authors required R_1/R_2 to be greater than 2.6 (another common definition for mfERG abnormality [52]) for an mfERG to be labeled as abnormal, the percentage of abnormal results may have been lower than the 70 % reported. In the absence of a gold standard that implies a clinical action, it is hard to know what to do with the information reported. Similarly, Almony and colleagues never define a gold standard, reducing the clinical impact of their report [17].

The clinician would often like to know how much value is gained by performing an additional test, because the use of multiple ancillary tests is common in screening for 4AQR. This depends on the number of additional cases turned up by adding the additional test. A statistical rule termed the Rule of Three is used in analyses of these situations. It holds that if no additional patients out of n tested are detected with 4AQR by adding a test, then one can have 95 % confidence that the true rate of additional detection of 4AQR were the test to be applied universally to the population is no more than 3/n [55, 56].

8.3   Reproducibility of Ancillary Tests

All of the instruments used in ancillary testing for detecting 4AQR are subject to measurement error. There are many sources of variation in measurements including intra-observer test–retest variability, inter-observer variability, variability across different machines, short-term variation, and long-term variation. The clinician needs to know the size of the measurement error in order to properly interpret a change in a measurement. Reproducibility gives the clinician an idea of how trustworthy the test result is [57]. If a test has poor reproducibility, then one is not confident in making the diagnosis of 4AQR based on that test alone [23]. For example, mfERG is poorly reproducible, which is a source of controversy over how useful this test could be in screening for 4AQR (see Sect. 8.6). Other examples include fundus photography, tangent screen testing of central visual field using a red test object, and Amsler grid testing [10, 11, 58].

To motivate a way of approaching the problem of reproducibility, consider the mfERG as used to assess macular function in patients taking 4AQs. To take one index of interest, R_1/R_2, the clinician wishes to know how big a change in the R_1/R_2 ratio is required to consider that a change in the patient has truly occurred and not simply natural variation. The true value of a variable is not known. The measurements are attempts to estimate the true value. The best estimate of the true value is the mean of multiple measurements. Therefore, the study of the variability involves a study of the errors of the measurements from the mean values. For example, if two measurements S1 and S2 are made, the best estimate of the true value is (S1 + S2)/2. The estimated errors of the individual measurements would be

$$S1 - (S1 + S2)/2 = (S1 - S2)/2.$$
$$S2 - (S1 + S2)/2 = (S2 - S1)/2.$$

This points to the usefulness of plotting the difference in values of a pair of measurements against the average of the values, which is the basis of the Bland–Altman analysis [57]. From the Bland–Altman analysis comes the coefficient of repeatability (COR), which allows one to state how large a change in a measurement must occur to be 95 % confident that the change is real and not measurement variability (1.96×COR) [59, 60, p. 236]. This is the difference between any two measurements above which one can be 95 % confident that the change is real, and not due to measurement variability [57].

For example, in the measurement of ring-averaged mfERG amplitudes in normal volunteers from one study, the COR ranged from 17.4 to 30.3 % in rings R_1 to R_5 [61]. If we suppose that a baseline R_1 amplitude is 50 nV/deg^2, then we can be 95 % confident that a measurement of less than 32.9 nV/deg^2 at a follow-up visit represents a true diminution of the patient's R_1 amplitude because the greater than 17.1 nV/deg^2 decrement in voltage exceeds 1.96×17.4 % of the baseline measurement.

Test equipment improves continuously. Therefore, reproducibility depends on technology. For example, reproducibility with SD-OCT is better than with time domain OCT (TD-OCT) [62, 63]. Repeatability cannot be assessed by simply performing measurements on a sample of patients or eyes at times one and two and comparing the means and standard deviations of the groups at the two times, as has been done [64]. These statistics may be comparable, but this says nothing about the reproducibility, which is assessed by comparing measurements in each patient at times one and two [57].

Which Measure of Reproducibility Is Best?

There are other methods of assessing reproducibility besides the COR. Some studies use the COV defined as the standard deviation divided by the mean value of a set of repeated measurements usually expressed as a percentage [65]. When the COV is used, another statistic is often used—the smallest measurable change, defined as the measurement times the COV. Table 8.3 lists reproducibility data for various OCT machines for macular thickness using this conceptual framework.

Yet another method of assessing reproducibility is to calculate the intraclass correlation coefficient (ICC). This is a statistic that scales the test–retest variability (the undesirable variability) by the true variability of the quantity being measured across the subjects in the sample. The ICC has values ranging from 0 to 1. The closer the value is to 1, the more reproducible the measurement is. A typical ordinal scale for ICCs follows:

- Slight reproducibility—ICC between 0 and 0.2
- Fair reproducibility—ICC between 0.21 and 0.4
- Moderate reproducibility—ICC between 0.41 and 0.6
- Substantial reproducibility—ICC between 0.61 and 0.8
- Almost perfect reproducibility—ICC between 0.81 and 1.0 [65]

Reassuringly, different measures of reproducibility tend to vary together. Altemir and colleagues presented reproducibility data on SD-OCT measurements of RNFL and macular thickness as assessed by both COV and ICC. As Fig. 8.3 shows, the two measures were correlated ($r^2 = 0.7216$) [65].

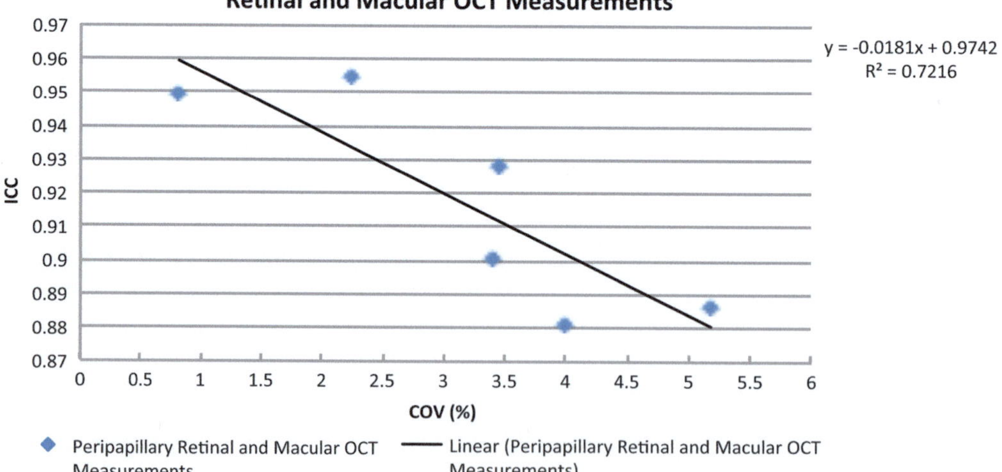

Fig. 8.3 Graph of intraclass correlation coefficient versus coefficient of variance in spectral domain optical coherence tomography measurements of macular thickness and retinal nerve fiber layer (RNFL) thickness. Data from Altemir [65]

All three methods of analyzing reproducibility are described in the literature covering ancillary testing in ophthalmology. There seems to be no consensus about which form of reproducibility analysis is superior, and attaining familiarity with each method is worth the effort required [66].

For some ancillary tests, the greatest challenge is distinguishing long-term fluctuation (LTF) from progressive change due to toxicity. This is the case with 10-2 VF testing and mfERG, but notably does not apply to SD-OCT [67, p. 86]. SD-OCT has a privileged position as the most reproducible ancillary test and the one with the smallest LTF.

8.4 Establishing a Prior Probability and Bayesian Inference

To properly use an ancillary test one should have in mind a prior probability of the patients having 4AQR. This will depend on multiple characteristics of the patient and a knowledge of the epidemiologic facts contained in Chap. 5. In the absence of other information, the best estimate of the prior probability is the prevalence of 4AQR among patients similar to the one under review.

Bayesian inference refers to modification of the clinician's estimate of the probability of having a disease based on the addition of further information. Thus, for example, if a patient is a 6 ft 4 in. male taking hydroxychloroquine 400 mg/day for 1 year, our initial estimate of the probability that he has hydroxychloroquine retinopathy is vanishingly low—perhaps 0.001 % or less. In such a circumstance, an initial 10-2 visual field with paracentral loci of increased threshold would be discounted given the entire clinical picture. The significance of such a field would be different if a female patient happened to be 5 ft tall and was in her 20th year of therapy on the same daily dose.

It is useful to formally state Bayes' theorem. If H is the hypothesis to which the evidence E refers, then the formula expressing Bayes' theorem is:

$$P(H \,/\, E) = \left[P(E \,/\, H) \times P(H) \right] / P(E),$$

where

$P(H)$ is the prior probability that H is true before we have the evidence E.

$P(H/E)$ is the probability that H is true after we know E.

$P(E/H)$ is the probability that the evidence E occurs when H is true.

$P(E)$ is the marginal likelihood of E, which is the probability of having that piece of evidence in a random person drawn from the population [68].

In the example we posited, the marginal probability is the probability that a random person taking a 10-2 VF would have paracentral loci of increased threshold.

The importance of Bayes' theorem for the clinician is that it refocuses attention away from the characteristics of the ancillary test and puts more emphasis on the probability of disease presence before the test is applied. In this way awareness of Bayes' theorem leads the clinician to screen those at higher risk and provides a rational basis for relative neglect of those at low risk, because in those patients extensive testing would represent an unwise expenditure of money [69, 70].

8.5 Static Automated Perimetry

Perimetry encompasses many methods, including tangent screen perimetry, kinetic perimetry with a Goldmann perimeter, and SAP, which is the standard method of testing the central visual field in screening for 4AQR. Advantages over the older methods include its standardization and greater sensitivity to visual field loss [71]. Testing protocols have been developed that allow gathering of data in an acceptable amount of time in ways less dependent on operator expertise, a significant variable in Goldmann perimetry [67, p. 89]. In the United States, and perhaps the world, the Humphrey visual field analyzer is the most commonly used instrument [67, p. 86]. The examples included in this book largely come from this instrument.

Static perimetry measures differential light sensitivity to a stimulus of varying intensity against a background of constant luminance. Luminance is the amount of light reflected or emitted from a surface. The unit of luminance is the apostilb (asb). One apostilb is the luminance of a perfectly diffusing surface that is emitting or reflecting 1 lumen/m²; other conversions are one apostilb (asb) = 0.3183 cd/m² = 0.1 millilambert

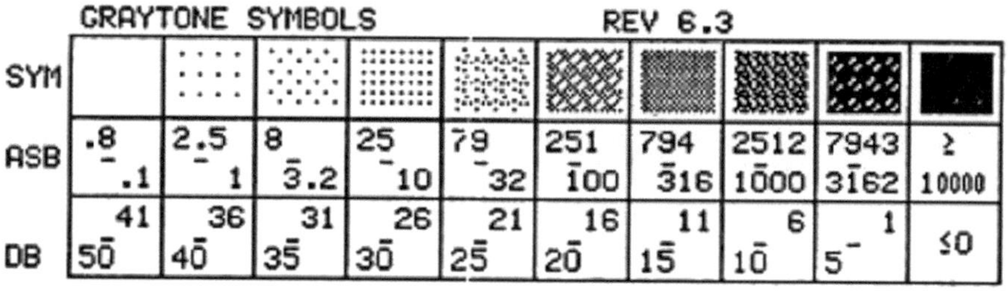

GRAYTONE SYMBOLS   REV 6.3

SYM										
ASB	.8 – .1	2.5 – 1	8 – 3.2	25 – 10	79 – 32	251 – 100	794 – 316	2512 – 1000	7943 – 3162	≥ 10000
DB	41 – 50	36 – 40	31 – 35	26 – 30	21 – 25	16 – 20	11 – 15	6 – 10	1 – 5	≤ 0

Fig. 8.4 Gray scale symbols used in the Humphrey 10-2 visual field plot. The symbol used in the gray scale visual field appears on the *top row*. The *second row* shows the stimulus brightness that corresponds to the gray scale symbol above it. The *third row* shows the strength of the neutral density filter interposed between the stimulus and the patient that corresponds to the stimulus strength and gray scale symbol listed above it

Table 8.4 Comparison of specifications of three static automated perimeters

Variable	Instrument		
	Humphrey visual field analyzer	Octopus 900 perimeter	Rodenstock peristat
Background luminance	31.5 asb	4 asb	3.1 asb
Stimulus size	III (4 mm²) or V	I, II, III, IV, V	III, V
Stimulus	White or red	White	Blue, green
Radius of tested VF	10, 24, or 30 depending on program	30	25
Number of tested points	68, 54, and 76 for the 10-2, 24-2, and 30-2	59	78
Minimal stimulus intensity	0.1 asb	0.1 asb	0.3 asb
Maximal stimulus intensity	10,000 asb	6,000 asb	10,000 asb
Step size of increasing stimulus intensity	3–4 dB steps	2–10 dB steps	2 dB steps

asb stands for apostilbs

[67, p. 90]. The maximal stimulus luminance of the Humphrey perimeter is 10,000 apostilbs. Lower luminances are achieved by interposing neutral density filters of increasing strength between the light bulb and the perimeter. The resulting stimulus intensity is measured in decibels (dB), where 10 dB is equivalent to 1 log unit of stimulus luminance, and 1 log unit is equivalent to a tenfold change in stimulus intensity.

Stimulus intensity and retinal sensitivity are related concepts that have inverted scales relative to each other. The highest stimulus intensity, 10,000 asb, corresponds to a retinal sensitivity of 0 dB. Failure to respond to this stimulus at a location is termed an absolute scotoma. The minimal stimulus intensity is 0.1 asb, which corresponds to a retinal sensitivity of 50 dB. An increase in retinal sensitivity of 10 dB corresponds to a reduction by a factor of 10 in stimulus intensity that is seen. Thus, a retinal sensitivity of 20 dB corresponds to recognition of a stimulus of intensity of 100 asb, calculated by 10,000 divided by 10 (corresponding to 10 dB of the 20 dB total) =1,000, which is divided by 10 again (corresponding to the other 10 dB of the 20 dB total) equaling 100. Therefore, in the parlance of visual field interpretation, a threshold with a higher number of decibels implies that the retina is more sensitive at that locus. Likewise, a threshold with a lower number of decibels implies less sensitivity at that location. Figure 8.4 shows the conversion scale of thresholds and gray scale shadings for the Humphrey visual field analyzer.

The three major commercial static perimetry instruments are the Humphrey Visual Field Analyzer, the Octopus perimeter, and the Rodenstock perimeter. Table 8.4 lists some differences in these instruments. The luminance values attached to the decibel scale are not standardized across different machines because the maximal

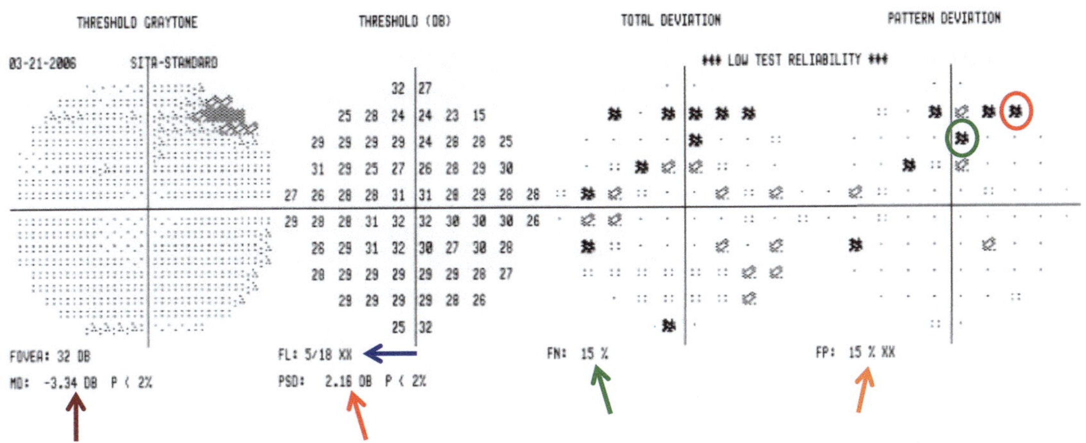

Fig. 8.5 Example of an unreliable 10-2 visual field (VF). This is the 10-2 VF from the right eye of a 79-year-old woman taking 200 mg/day of hydroxychloroquine for unspecified arthritis. There are many flags that this test is unreliable. The fixation losses were 5 of 18 trials (28 %) (*blue arrow*). The false negative responses were 15 % (*green arrow*). The false positive responses were 15 % (*orange arrow*). Therefore the accuracy of the various indicators of abnormality, such as the depressed mean defect (*brown arrow*), pattern standard deviation (PSD) (*red arrow*), and paracentral scotomas (*green-circled and red-circled locations*), must all be interpreted with skepticism

luminance for the different machines is not the same. The maximal luminance is brighter on the Humphrey Visual Field Analyzer than on the Octopus perimeter. A 20 dB stimulus on the Humphrey machine is the same brightness as a 10 dB stimulus on the Octopus machine.

The measured threshold at a given location using the Humphrey visual field analyzer is determined using an initial stimulus methodology followed by a pointwise bracketing methodology. The initial stimulus values are chosen by determining thresholds at four points in the visual field, one per quadrant, with each one 9 deg from the horizontal and vertical meridians. The initial stimulus is set at 25 dB and then stimulus intensities are changed in 4 dB steps until the threshold from seeing-to-nonseeing or nonseeing-to-seeing is crossed. Then the direction of change is reversed and the steps are reduced in size to 2 dB until the threshold is recrossed. The last-seen stimulus luminance is then recorded as the threshold for the location. From the thresholds at these four locations, initial stimulus strengths are determined by an algorithm based on the correlation of stimulus strengths at different locations in normals. The same bracketing strategy, termed the 4-2 strategy, is then applied to each location tested in a random order to reduce the probability of anticipation by the patient.

Threshold sensitivity at a retinal location cannot be precisely measured because it is a probabilistic concept. Instead, it is estimated by the strategy of bracketing. The threshold is the dimmest target identified 50 % of the time at a given location. When the frequency of seeing curve is steep, the estimate for the threshold is more reliable. When it is shallow, the estimate is less reliable [67, p. 91]. Threshold deviation refers to the difference between the patient's threshold sensitivity at a particular location and the age-matched normal retinal sensitivity for that location. A list of several terms and their definitions that are used in displays of SAP follow.

False positive—The instrument provides a sound cue with a subthreshold or no stimulus; if the patient responds, a false positive is recorded. In the SITA strategy, false positive implies the response occurred within the response time for the patient. A false positive rate greater than 33 % implies low reliability of testing [40, 49, 69, 71, 72, p. 102]. Others have used a stricter criterion, such as requiring a false positive rate less than 25 or 15 % to be considered reliable (Fig. 8.5) [39].

False negative—The instrument registers the threshold at a locus and then returns to test the same locus with a stimulus 9 dB brighter than the threshold stimulus determined previously. Failure of the patient to respond to this stimulus is a false negative. Fatigue is a common source of false negative responses. A false negative rate greater than 20–33 % implies low reliability of testing [40, 49, 67, 71, 72, p. 102]. Others have used a stricter criterion, such as requiring a false negative rate less than 15 % to be considered reliable (Fig. 8.5) [39].

Fixation losses—Maintenance of fixation can be tested by periodically retesting the location of the physiologic blind spot which has dimensions 5×7 deg (Heijl-Krakau method) or by using a video monitor to detect pupil movement. A fixation losses rate greater than 20 % is considered significant [40, 67, 71, 72, p. 102]. Others have used a stricter criterion, such as requiring a fixation loss rate less than 15 % to be considered reliable [39]. Some have used a looser criterion, such as requiring that fixation losses must be less than 33 % (Fig. 8.5) [49].

Sensitivity—A threshold expressed in decibels. A higher number indicates that the retina has a lower threshold for seeing, or that the retina is more sensitive, or that the retina sees a dimmer light.

Deviation plot—A map of sensitivity versus location. The numbers shown are the sensitivities in dB in some displays or a symbol in others that expresses the probability of measuring the observed sensitivity compared to age-matched normal subjects. A positive deviation implies that the retina was more sensitive at the given location than normal. A negative deviation means that the retina was less sensitive at the given location than normal.

Defect depth plot—A map of the amplitude of the deviations relative to the average age-adjusted sensitivities by location. A positive defect depth implies that a scotoma exists at the location. A negative defect depth implies that the retina at that location is more sensitive than normal. Deviations within 4 dB of expected are displayed on a defect depth plot as normal.

Total deviation plot—A plot in which the number appearing at each point is the difference in the light sensitivity for the patient compared to an age-matched normal subject. The numbers represent the stimulus expressed in decibels. The larger a negative number, the more abnormal and less sensitive the retinal sensitivity is at the given point.

Pattern deviation plot—A plot related to the total deviation plot in which the seventh largest deviation in the total deviation plot is subtracted from the deviation at each point [71]. The effect is to remove generalized depression of the visual field and reveal localized depressions (scotomas).

Pattern standard deviation (PSD)—A location weighted standard deviation of the threshold values that quantitates the variation of the hill of vision. In the vernacular of Octopus visual fields, the same concept is captured by the term "loss variance."

In SAP, the stimulus spot size is indicated by a roman numeral. The 10-2 VF stimulus typically has a spot size III which subtends 0.43 deg of visual field, small enough to detect small scotomas, and yet to be unaffected by refractive error [73, p. 8]. The stimulus duration is 0.2 s, which is shorter than the latency time of 0.25 s for voluntary eye movements, a necessary condition to prevent a saccade to follow a stimulus [73, p. 10]. The stimulus may be a red or a white light in the 10-2 VF. Results of visual field testing using the red light tend to be more sensitive and less specific than when using the white light [74, 75].

SAP is a subjective psychophysical test that depends on the cooperation, effort, and mental status of the patient [67, p. 91]. The effort involved in a visual field test is substantial. For a 30-2 visual field, the patient is presented with approximately 550 stimuli, which takes on average 15 min per eye. Although fatigue is less of a problem with the 10-2 VF, which takes on from 3 to 7 min per eye (Fig. 8.6), the problem of inattention is not trivial, especially among the older patients. However, the subjectivity is not confined to the patient. The perimetrist must monitor and coach the patient on attention and fixation. Some perimetrists do this more successfully than others, and the performance of a given perimetrist will vary over time.

The terms for visual field programs using the Humphrey Field Analyzer have the format

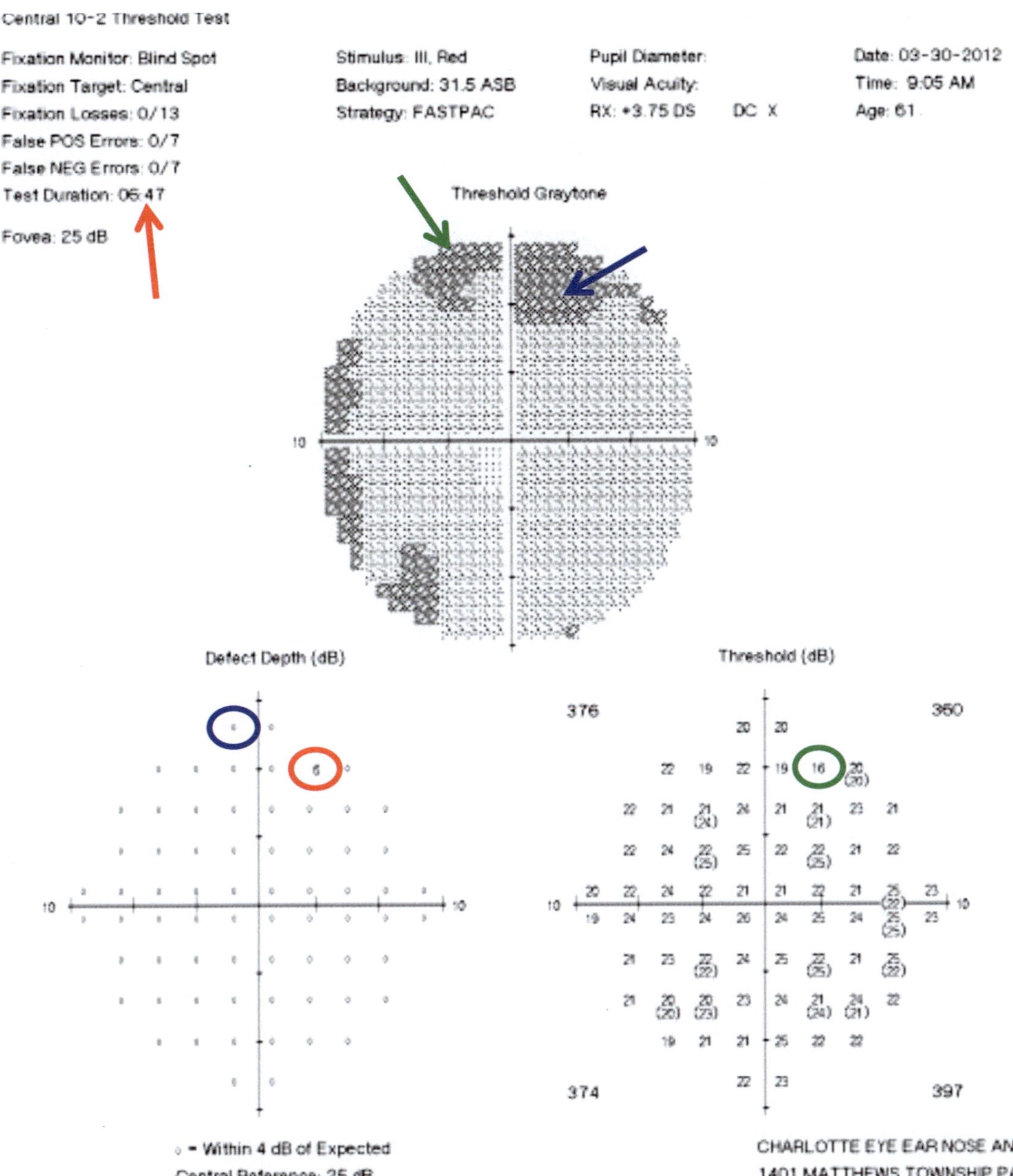

Fig. 8.6 This 10-2 visual field (VF) was done with the III, red light using the FASTPAC protocol. The field is normal, and illustrates several points to consider in interpreting such VFs. The test took 6 min, 47 s (*red arrow*). The gray scale commonly shows *dark areas* particularly near the edge of the visual field that are not worrisome, because the thresholds at the involved locations, as shown from the defect depth display, all lie within 4 dB of the expected thresholds for age-matched normal subjects. In the defect depth display, there is only one location with an abnormal threshold (*red-circled locus*). At this location the threshold was 16 dB (*green-circled locus*), which can be seen to be a higher threshold (reduced sensitivity) compared to its neighboring loci, which range from 19 to 23 dB. Note the inexact congruence of the gray scale and defect depth display. For example, on the gray scale display there appears to be a relative scotoma at the *green arrow*, but the defect depth display shows that the threshold at this location lies within 4 dB of normal as represented by the 0 at the location (*blue-circled location*)

"program $X-Y$". The X refers to the radius of visual field tested relative to fixation. Thus, a 10-2 visual field tests the field from fixation out to 10 deg from fixation. The Y implies that the test points lie on either side of the horizontal and vertical axes, not on the axes. The other possible value for Y is 1, in which case the test points lie on the axes. This latter protocol is not used [76].

The 10-2 VF test is the preferred program to use in screening for 4AQR [40, 72]. It tests 68 points at 2 deg intervals from fixation outward to 10 deg, which is the same area tested by the Amsler grid and is the region where the earliest scotomas of 4AQR appear [74]. The normal control value for retinal sensitivity at each point of the 10-2 VF is age-matched [6]. There are no published results of 10-2 VF testing with either white or red programs in patients taking 4AQs, although they were promised as an outcome of the prospective, multicenter North American Plaquenil Study, which apparently collapsed [6].

Although 10-2 VF testing is the most commonly used form of SAP, others have been used, including the Friedmann visual field analyzer with red targets, the Humphrey 24-2, 30-2, and macular visual field programs [23, 45, 77–80]. The Friedmann visual field analyzed tests 14 points within 10 deg of fixation compared to 68 test points for the 10-2 VF. The 24-2 and 30-2 programs extend testing further radially and suffer from the disadvantage that they minimize attention to the affected paracentral visual field [78, 79]. The macular visual field program tests 16 points in the central 5 deg of visual field at 2 deg intervals.

Commonly used variations of 10-2 VF protocols are the Swedish Interactive Threshold Algorithm (SITA) protocol with a white III target, the FASTPAC protocol with the red III target, or the FASTPAC protocol with the white I target [72, 75]. The literature often depicts threshold graytone visual field displays for the red and white target protocols, but only shows pattern deviation plots for the SITA protocol for white III targets [75]. In the SITA protocol symbols are shown with the probability of having a defect of the recorded size relative to an age-matched normal population (Fig. 8.4).

SITA is a program that determines whether to recheck thresholds at more points based on the results of selected rechecks at a small sample of points. SITA-standard is a program that is stricter in its requirements for reproducibility. SITA-FAST has looser criteria. SITA-standard takes approximately 50 % as long, and SITA-FAST approximately 20 % as long as older pre-SITA programs. In the FASTPAC protocol, the bracketing strategy for determining the retinal threshold is modified. The stimulus intensity is adjusted in 3 dB increments until the threshold is crossed once. This saves time compared to the 4-2 strategy. In normal or near normal fields, the test time is reduced approximately 40 %. The FASTPAC protocol with the red III target has a defect depth display. In this display, the more positive the defect depth the denser the scotoma (Fig. 8.6).

In following patients taking 4AQs, the clinician looks for changes in the 10-2 VFs over time. As with all ancillary tests, discriminating fluctuation in measurements from true changes reflecting retinopathy is important [67, p. 86]. Many have complained that 10-2 VFs are often variable, inconsistent, and difficult to confirm [30]. Fluctuation not associated with retinopathy has been subcategorized into short-term fluctuation (STF) and LTF. STF refers to variation in threshold during the course of a single visual field examination. The Humphrey visual field analyzer measures the threshold twice at 10 loci and displays the standard deviation of the repeated threshold determinations. Normally STF is less than 5 dB for the 10-2 VF [81]. STF greater than 5 dB suggests poor reliability [67, p. 93]. STF increases at the borders of scotomas and in patients who are inconsistent [82]. The variability of 10-2 VFs in some patients implies that SD-OCT or other ancillary tests may be more reliable and needed for making screening decisions (Fig. 8.7) [83]. It is rare to stop a patient from taking a 4AQ based on a single abnormal 10-2 VF, especially if adjusted dosing is appropriate.

LTF refers to variation between tests occurring over time (not within a single test) and does not include learning curve effects.

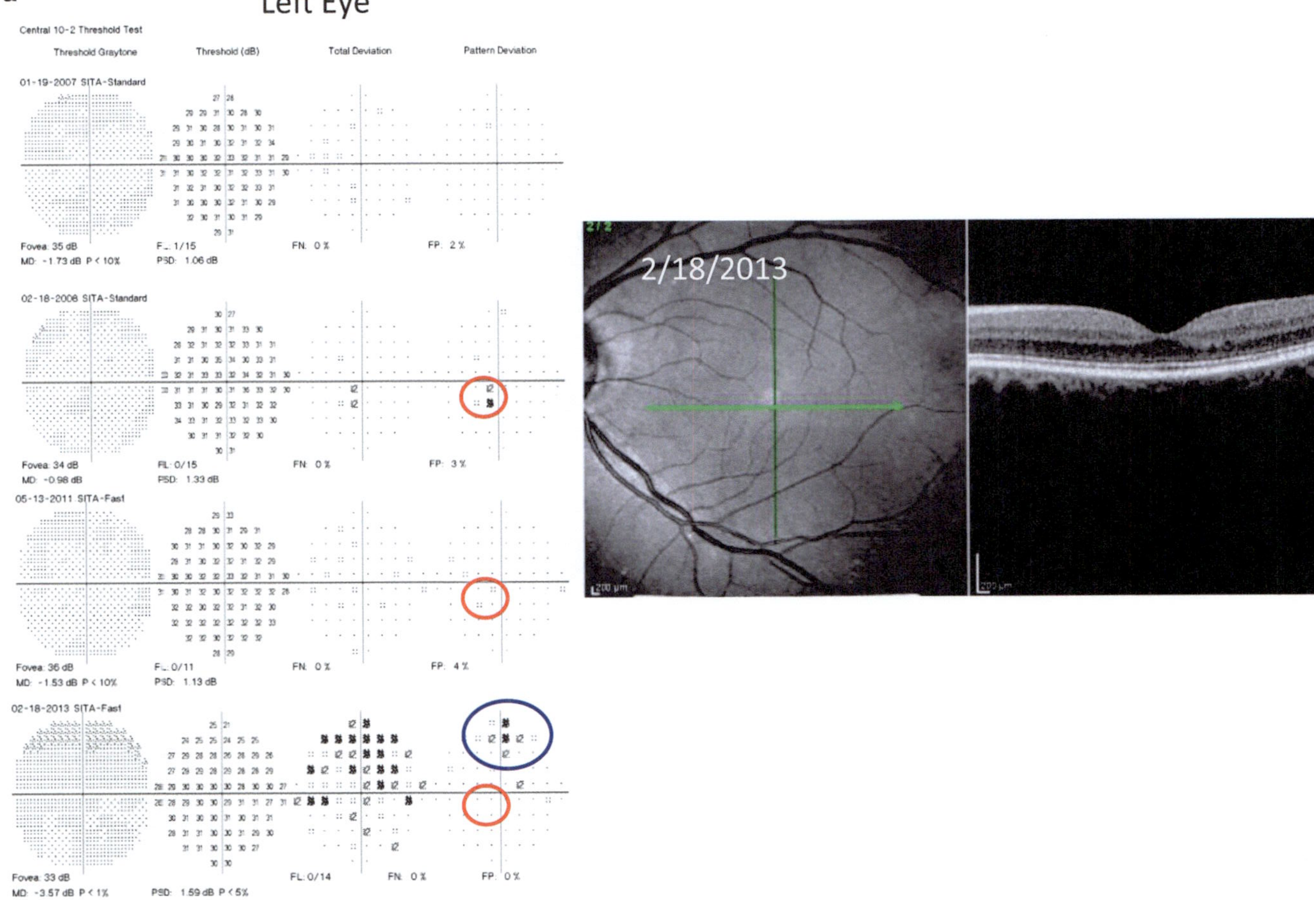

Fig. 8.7 10-2 visual fields and spectral domain optical coherence tomography (SD-OCT) of a 65-year-old female taking 400 mg/day of hydroxychloroquine since 2000 for arthritis. She was 67 in. tall, weighed 250 lb, and had no renal or liver disease. Her cumulative dose of hydroxychloroquine was 1,752 g. Her 10-2 VFs showed a number of scotomas that were not reproducible over time. Because she was on a nontoxic dose of hydroxychloroquine, and had a normal SD-OCT bilaterally, the medication was continued and the dosage not reduced. The cumulative dose of hydroxychloroquine placed her in a risk group indicating a need for yearly screening according to American Academy of Ophthalmology guide- lines, but in the presence of nontoxic daily dosing, the risk was still extremely low. (**a**) Serial 10-2 visual fields and an SD-OCT of the left eye. The locations circled in *red* show scotomatous points that vanish from one test to the next. The new scotomatous points that appear in the field of 18 February 2013 (*blue-circled area*) are not credible given the past history and the presence of a normal SD-OCT. (**b**) Serial visual fields and an SD-OCT of the right eye. The locations circled in *red* show scotomatous points that vanish over time. The new scotomatous points that appear in the field of 18 February 2013 (*blue-circled area*) are not credible given the past history and the presence of a normal SD-OCT

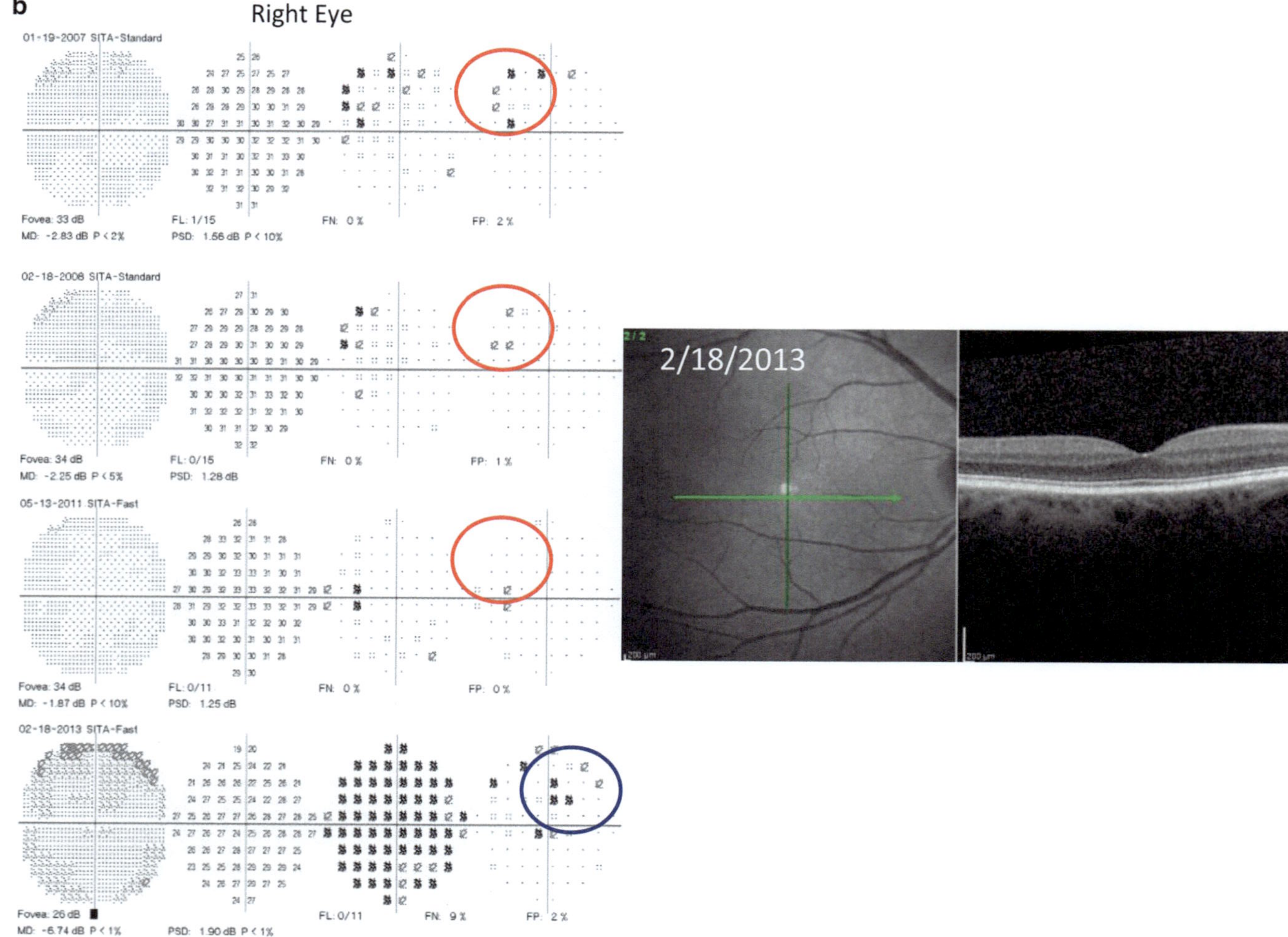

Fig. 8.7 (continued)

Two types of LTF are recognized—homogeneous and heterogeneous. Homogeneous LTF refers to variation over time throughout the visual field. Heterogeneous LTF refers to incongruous variation at different locations. LTF increases as the initial sensitivity of a location decreases and as distance of a location from the fovea increases [67, p. 94]. LTF limits the clinician's ability to detect subtle changes caused by 4AQR. In glaucoma, greater than 3–4 dB can indicate early glaucomatous damage. For example, Hoskins and colleagues studied how much change in sensitivity was necessary between a first and second visual field to predict that a third visual field would be decreased compared to the first field [84]. This analysis was based on 30-2 visual fields obtained in patients with glaucoma and minimal (mean sensitivity for the studied region was greater than 25 dB) or moderate (mean sensitivity for the studied region was 25 dB or less) visual field damage. In patients with minimal field damage a 4.7–5.6 dB change in mean sensitivity was required to have 95 % confidence that the negative trend would be confirmed in the third visual field. In patients with moderate visual field damage a 5.5–7.2 dB change in mean sensitivity was necessary for 95 % confidence [84]. Caution is necessary in extrapolating these results to patients taking 4AQs and tested with 10-2 VFs. In 10-2 VFs, estimates of LTF have not been published.

There are many variables relating to the patient that account for the common experience that some of them are unable to cooperate and provide reliable test results. Uncorrected refractive error can reduce sensitivity to a stimulus. A value attributed to this effect is 1.26 dB per diopter of uncorrected refractive error. Media opacification, most commonly from cataract, can reduce sensitivity. Miosis reduces sensitivity, becoming more of a problem when the pupillary diameter is less than 2.5 mm. Sensitivity to the visual stimulus is age-dependent, generally declining with increasing age. For the central visual field tested in chloroquine and hydroxychloroquine screening, a reduction of 0.5 dB per decade of age can be expected. There is a learning curve in visual field testing that affects results (Fig. 8.8).

Fatigue, psychological factors, and clarity and uptake of pretest instructions can influence the results of testing.

Visual field interpretation involves analysis of global indices and of local abnormalities. The definitions of the important global indices follow.

Mean deviation (MD)—A location-weighted mean of the values of the total deviation plot. It provides an overall index of the height of the hill of vision and is insensitive to localized scotomas. It is a good index for judging the size of diffuse loss of sensitivity as can be caused by cataract. Negative values mean subnormal overall sensitivity. The equation for mean deviation is

$$\mathrm{MD} = \left[\left(1/m\right) \sum_{i=1}^{m} \frac{x_i - z_i}{S_{1i}^2} \right] / \left[\left(1/m\right) \sum_{i=1}^{m} \frac{1}{S_{1i}^2} \right]$$

where x_i is the measured threshold of test location i, z_i is the normal reference threshold at location i, S_{1i}^2 is the variance of the normal field measurement at location i, and m is the number of tested locations excluding the blind spot. For the 30-2 visual field, $m = 76$ (19 points per quadrant). For the 24-2 visual field, $m = 56$. For the 10-2 visual field, $m = 68$. Mean deviation of SAP correlates with mfERG R_1 ring amplitude in patients taking hydroxychloroquine [72].

Pattern standard deviation (PSD)—A statistic that represents the unevenness of the hill of vision. This is an index of localized loss of sensitivity. It is calculated as the location-weighted standard deviation of all threshold values. It is insensitive to overall height of the hill of vision and is sensitive to localized scotomas.

Corrected pattern deviation (CPSD)—A statistic based on PSD but with a correction based on the STF.

SAP can be done with a white or a red test object. When of equal size, a white object is seen more easily than a red test object [67, p. 31]. Therefore 10-2 VF testing using the III, red test object is more sensitive but less specific than testing with a III, white test object [46, 74]. The sensitivity and specificity of the 10-2 VF using the III, red test object were 91.3 %

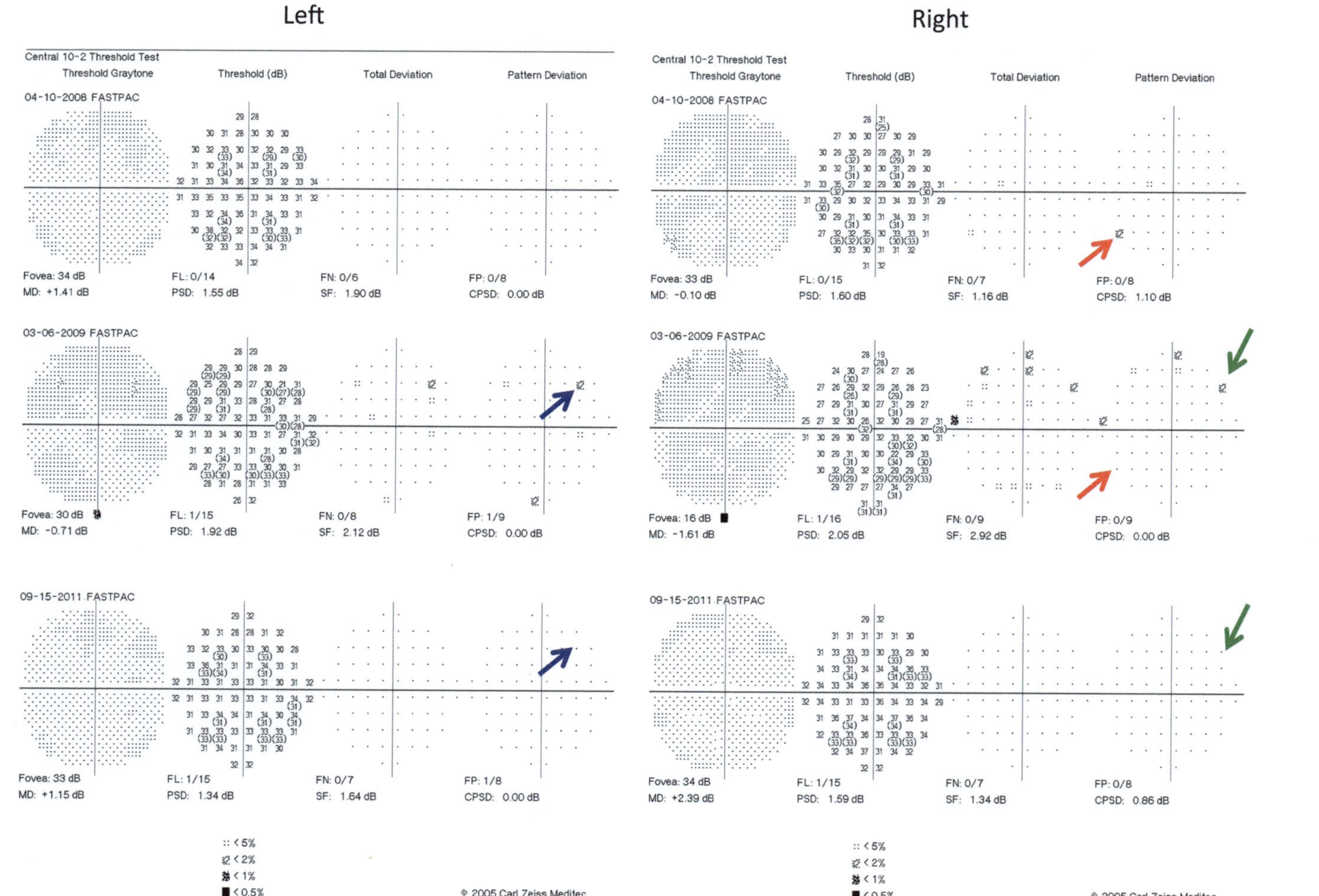

Fig. 8.8 This 70-year-old woman with systemic lupus erythematosus (SLE) had been taking 200 mg/day of hydroxychloroquine for 7 years. She was 66 in. tall and weighed 135 lb. Her visual fields showed improvement over the years, presumably as she became more accustomed to testing. Note that on serial fields the locations of high thresholds vanish (*blue arrows* for left eye, *red and green arrows* for right eye)

and 57.8 %, respectively. For testing with the 10-2VF using the III, white test object the sensitivity and specificity were 78 % and 84 %, respectively [74]. Clinicians disagree as to which test is preferable for screening with approximately equal numbers favoring the test with red and the test with white targets [75, 85]. To manage the problem of false positives, some have labeled scotomas in 10-2 VF testing as significant if they are reproducible 2 months later upon repeat testing [78].

In the 10-2 VF, the difference displays (total deviation plot and PSD plot) identify threshold values that deviate more than 4 dB from those of a sample of normal subjects [40]. The defect depth display of the same information shows the size of the scotoma at a point relative to the mean value for normal subjects at that point. A comparison of the two kinds of displays is shown in Fig. 8.9. Many observers have noted that 4AQR is easier to detect on the pattern-deviation plot than on the gray scale display (Fig. 8.10) [75, 78]. Less well recognized is that the gray scale display is more sensitive than the defect display if one uses the 10-2 VF with red III test objects (Fig. 8.11).

Interpretation of computerized visual fields in the context of screening for 4AQR is particularly difficult because one wishes to detect early field loss, which is the loss hardest to differentiate from normal physiologic variation [86]. The size of physiologic variability in visual field threshold increases with increasing eccentricity from fixation [81, 86]. Therefore, locus-invariant rules, e.g., that a threshold greater than 4 dB anywhere in the 10-2 is abnormal, do not reflect the complexity of normal threshold variability [86].

There are no consistent criteria for judging an SAP abnormality in 4AQR [30]. Unlike the situation in glaucoma care, there are no longitudinal programs for following 10-2 visual fields, and the sophistication of visual field interpretation is rudimentary. Lyons understates, "It has been difficult to develop clear criteria for abnormality" [30]. Marmor states

that "any points of parafoveal loss should be taken seriously; initiate retesting (or testing with the alternative color target) and, if consistent, initiate corroborative testing with objective modalities such as SD-OCT or mfERG" [75]. However, we do not know how often this leads to unnecessary retesting.

Different clinicians have different rules for declaring an abnormality in a 10-2 VF and a change in a visual field (Table 8.5). It is worth recalling that in any 10-2 VF with 68 test points, one can expect $0.05 \times 68 = 3.4$ points (that is, three or four points, on average) to be labeled with the $P < 0.05$ probability symbol [71]. Taking Marmor's dictum literally is therefore likely to lead to many unnecessary follow-up tests. Therefore, a more judicious evaluation of parafoveal loss is advisable. For example, two or three adjacent scotomatous points and scotomas that are unchanging over consecutive tests deserve more weight than a single scotomatous point in a decision to retest.

The MD and PSD indices provided with the 10-2 VF printout have not been useful in distinguishing patients taking 4AQs from healthy control subjects (Table 8.6) [89]. Comparison of these variables between patients taking 4AQs with and without retinopathy has not been reported, but comparisons across studies suggest that these indices may discriminate the categories, at least for cases of advanced retinopathy.

The pattern of scotomas in 4AQR has the shape of a complete or incomplete annulus in 87 % of cases and scattered islands of relative scotomas in 13 % of cases [78]. The eccentricity of the annular scotoma in 4AQR has varied across reports. Depending on the paper, it has been said to occur typically from 2 to 3 deg, 2 to 6 deg, 2 to 8 deg, or 4 to 9 deg from fixation [5, 18, 75, 78, 90, 91]. The different statements likely arise from the different techniques used to check visual field. The 4–9-deg band arose from tangent screen testing with a red object [5], whereas the 2–6-deg band arose from the 10-2 VF. Many cases of more advanced

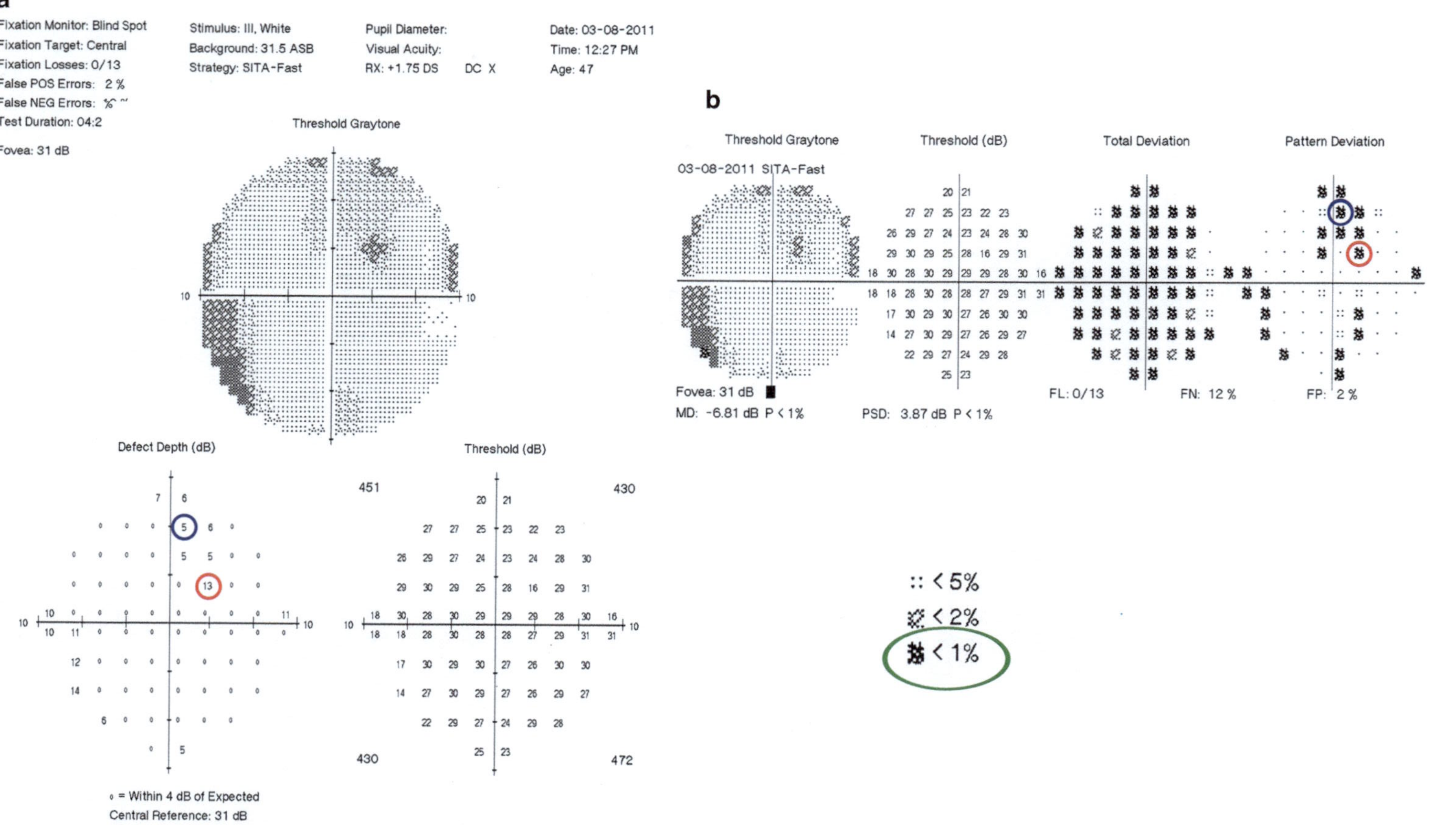

Fig. 8.9 Two data displays of the same information after 10-2 visual field testing. (a) The defect depth display shows the size of the difference between the patient's visual threshold for a given locus and the mean value for normal subjects at that locus. Only values that exceed 4 dB are shown, as departures less than or equal to 4 dB are considered to be within normal limits. In the defect display a positive number means that the patient has a subnormal retinal sensitivity or an abnormally high threshold compared to normals. A negative number means that the patient was more sensitive than normal subjects at the location. In the context of 4AQR screening, negative numbers are ignored. Sometimes they imply a trigger—happy patient who may show a high number of false positives. (b) The same information is shown using the threshold display, total deviation display, and pattern deviation display with probability symbols. The defect depths located at the *red-circled* and *blue-circled* locations both are seen in less than 1 % of normal subjects and thus both get the darkest shading in the PSD display (*green-circled symbol*) even though the values are different at the two locations (13 dB for the *red-circled location* and 5 dB for the *blue-circled location*)

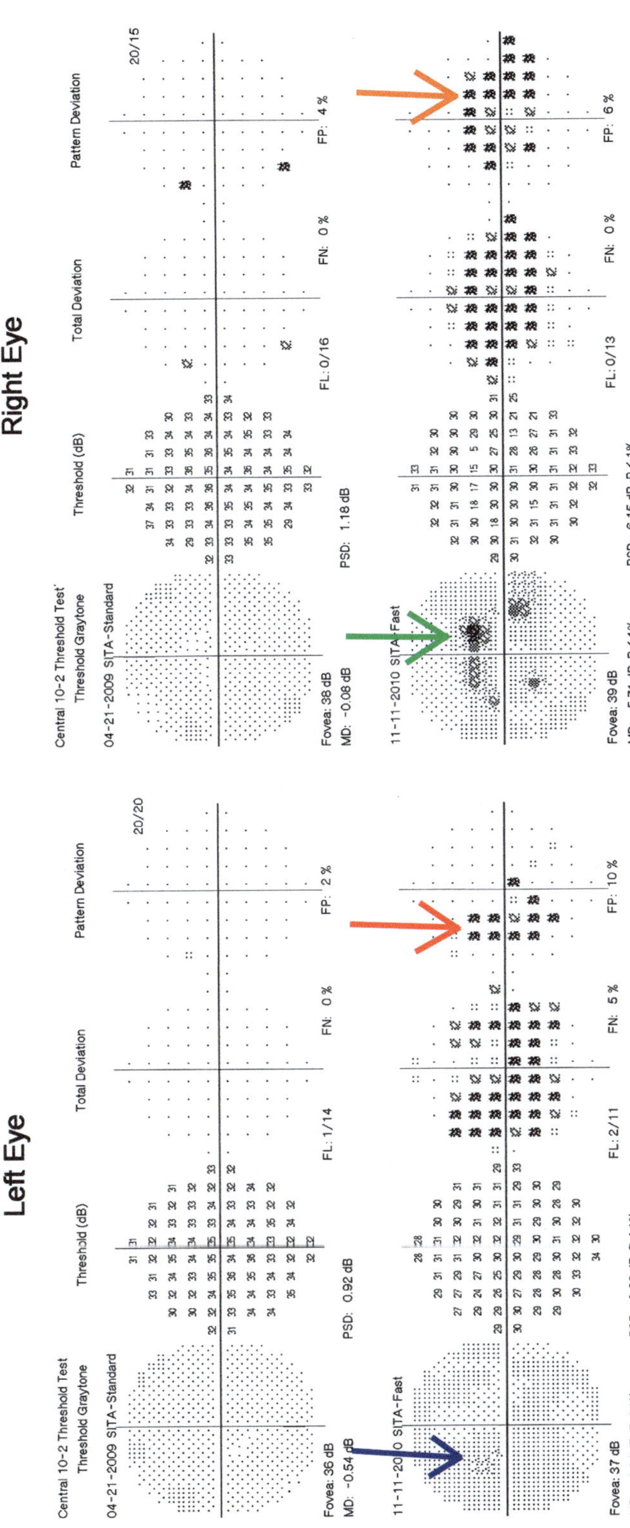

Fig. 8.10 10-2 visual fields (10-2 VFs) of a 37-year-old woman with SLE who had taken hydroxychloroquine 400 mg/day for 8 years. She had no renal or liver disease, but did have sickle cell anemia. Her height was 5 ft 6 in., and her actual body weight had been as low as 132 lb, which was less than her ideal body weight (IBW). Her daily dose adjusted for the lesser of ABW and IBW was 6.7 mg/kg. Her cumulative dose was 1,168 g. The 10-2 VFs show that a paracentral scotoma may be better visualized on the pattern deviation plot (*red arrow*) than the gray scale plot (*blue arrow*). This is not always the case. In the left eye, the paracentral scotoma is equally apparent on either display (*green and orange arrows*)

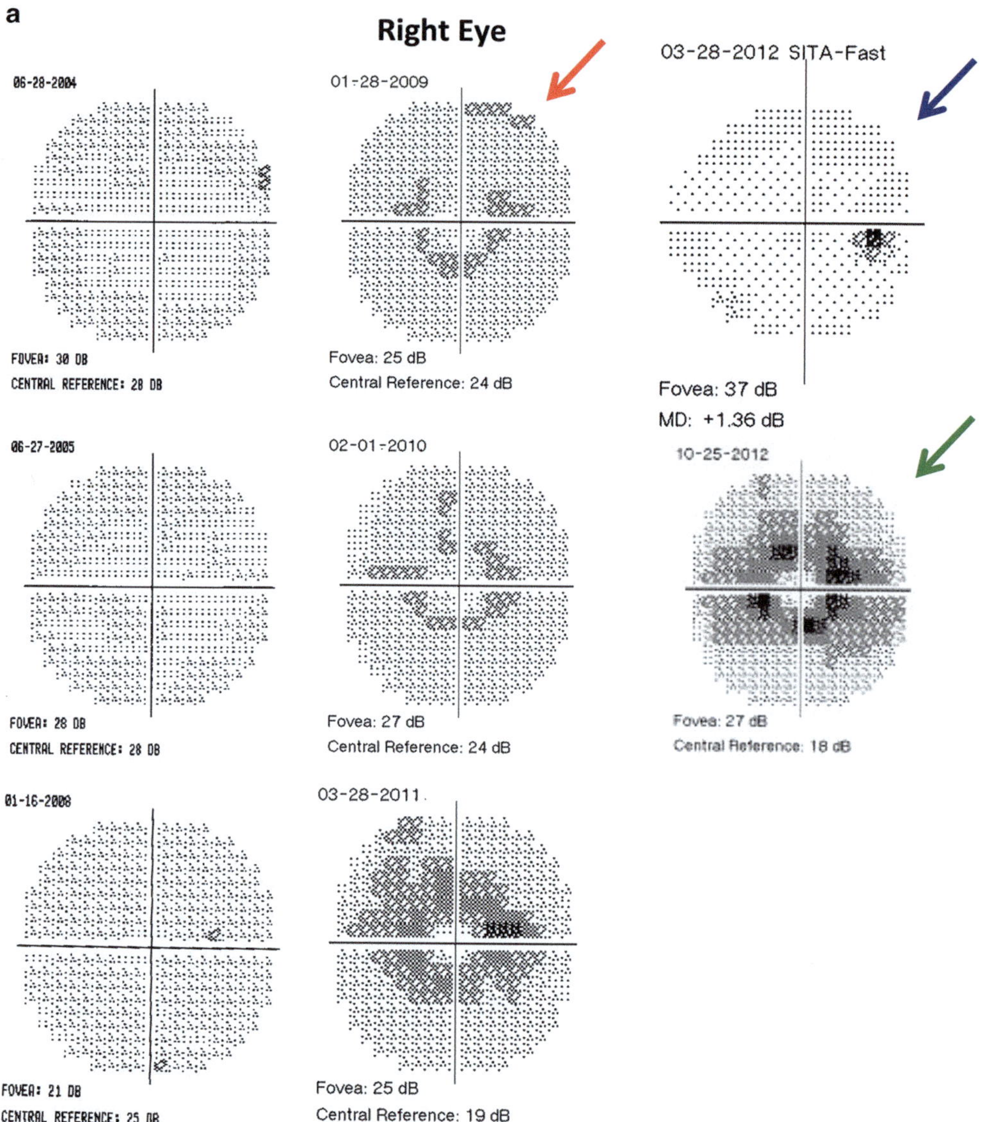

Fig. 8.11 Serial visual fields (VFs) and multifocal electro-retinograms (mfERGs) of the right eye of a 69-year-old woman with Wegener's granulomatosus treated with 400 mg/day of hydroxychloroquine for 17 years. She received a cumulative dose of 2,450 g. She was 63 in. tall, weighed 147 lb, and had an IBW of 135 lb. Her adjusted daily dose based on IBW was 6.52 mg/kg/day. (**a**) Gray scale display of the 10-2 VF using a red test object of size III. The first indication of retinopathy was on the field of 16 January 2008 when a right paracentral scotoma had developed. By 28 January 2009 there was a clear indication of a paracentral scotoma, which atypically began inferior to fixation (*red arrow*). Retinopathy should have been recognized and the drug stopped. Instead, the visual field was interpreted as normal and hydroxychloroquine continued for an additional 38 months before retinopathy was recognized on 28 March 2012 and the drug was stopped. Note another practice fraught with pitfalls—the mixing of different types of visual fields. The visual field of 28 March 2012 (*blue arrow*) was a 24-2 visual field which is not easily compared to the preceding 10-2 visual fields. Although the drug was stopped on 28 March 2012, the retinopathy progressed with worsening of the ring scotoma on 10-2 VF testing (*green arrow*). (**b**) Defect depth displays serial 10-2 VFs using a III, red test object showing the insensitivity of this display relative to that of the gray scale display. In (**a**), the retinopathy is easily discernible on the visual field of 28 January 2009, but the defect depth display does not depict the abnormality (*red arrow*). Instead the retinopathy is not discernible on this display until 28 March 2011. The PSD display of the 24-2 VF on 28 March 2012 shows that hydroxychloroquine retinopathy appears as a central scotoma rather than a ring scotoma as seen in the 10-2 VFs (*blue arrow*). The defect depths increase in amplitude from 28 March 2011 until 25 October 2012. Negative defect depths are ignored when interpreting 10-2 VFs obtained for 4AQR screening. Only positive defect depths correspond to depressed retinal sensitivity. (**c**) Serial mfERGs of the right eye of the patient. At the time the drug was stopped the R_1/R_2 ratio was 4.00 (*red-ringed value*), but at the follow-up mfERG of 25 October 2012 the R_1/R_2 ratio had decreased to normal. It reflected the progression of retinopathy centrally with progressive loss of response density in the central circular zone, R_1 (*orange-arrowed peak* in the topographic response density plot)

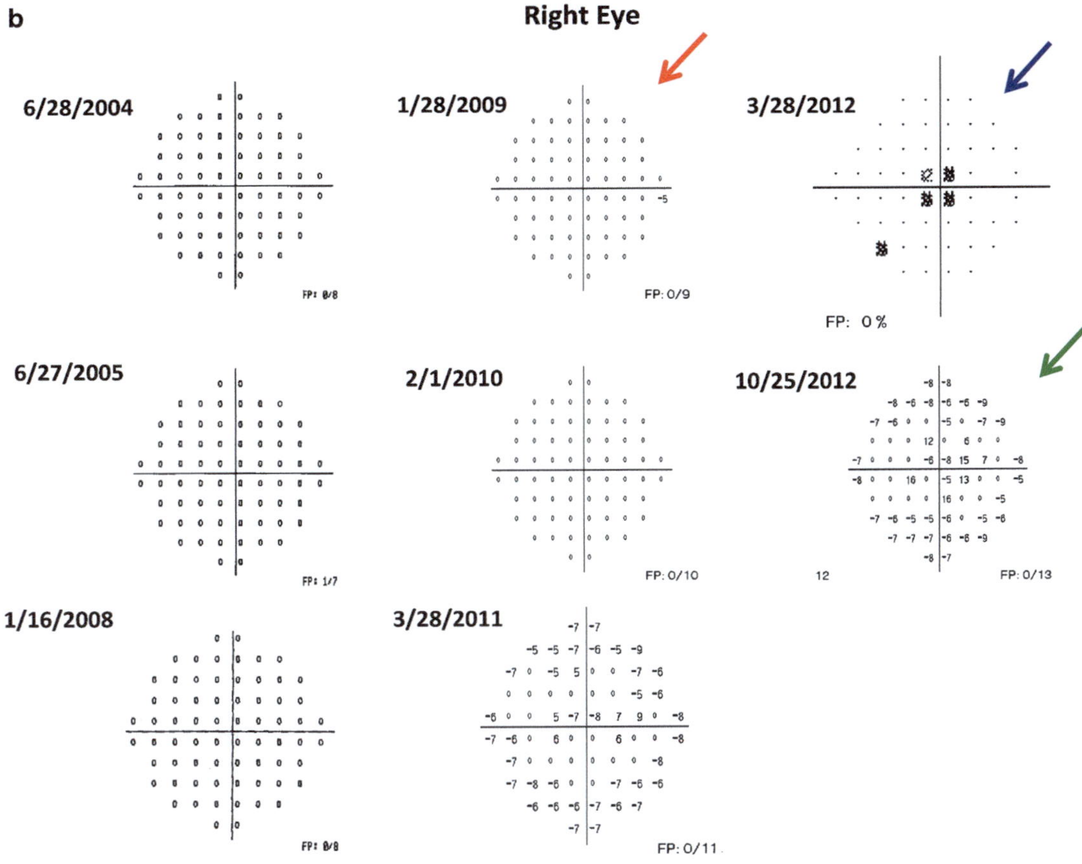

Fig. 8.11 (continued)

retinopathy produce scotomas that extend into the mid and far periphery; therefore the location of the scotoma depends on the stage of the retinopathy (see Chap. 6) [92].

Visual field defects often occur without symptoms or fundus changes [8]. The earliest 10-2 visual field changes tend to be superior paracentral scotomas (Fig. 8.12). Occasional exceptions are seen in which a paracentral scotoma develops first inferior to fixation (Fig. 8.11) [78, 93]. As retinopathy progresses, the density of the scotoma increases superiorly until a complete ring scotoma and eventually a central scotoma develops [38, 78].

The normal variability of static perimetric threshold values has been determined using the 30-2 program of the Humphrey Visual Field Analyzer, but not for the 10-2 program. Nevertheless, there is some information from the 30-2 VF data that can be applied to the interpretation of 10-2 VFs. The mean foveal threshold for a 50-year-old subject is 38 dB. In 95 normal subjects, the mean parafoveal threshold for points less than 6 deg from the fovea was $32.48 \pm SD$ 0.26 [81]. The interindividual variation of the foveal threshold was 1.7 dB. The best point estimate for the interindividual variation of the parafoveal threshold for points less than 6 deg from

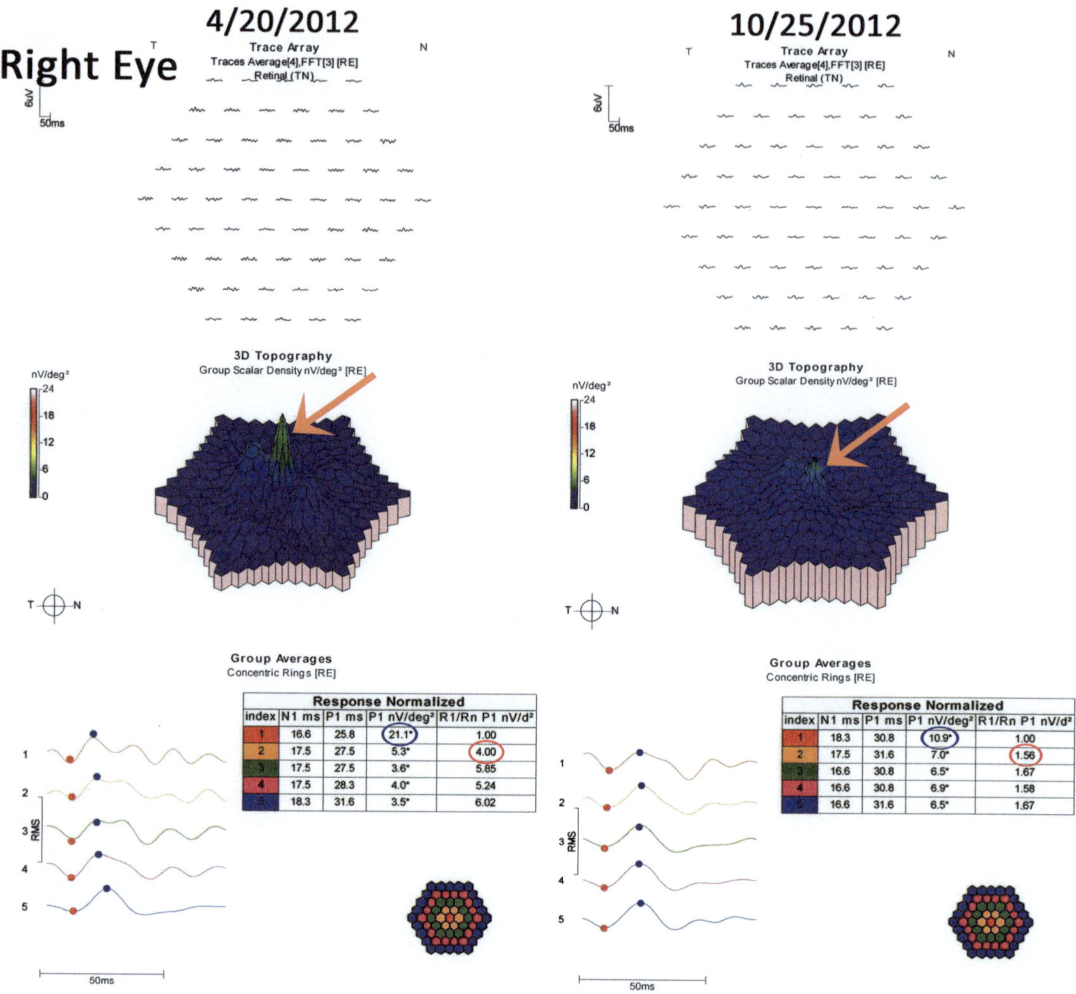

Left table (4/20/2012):

index	N1 ms	P1 ms	P1 nV/deg²	R1/Rn P1 nV/d²
1	16.6	25.8	21.1*	1.00
2	17.5	27.5	5.3*	4.00
3	17.5	27.5	3.6*	5.85
4	17.5	28.3	4.0*	5.24
5	18.3	31.6	3.5*	6.02

Right table (10/25/2012):

index	N1 ms	P1 ms	P1 nV/deg²	R1/Rn P1 nV/d²
1	18.3	30.8	10.9*	1.00
2	17.5	31.6	7.0*	1.56
3	16.6	30.8	6.5*	1.67
4	16.6	30.8	6.9*	1.58
5	16.6	31.6	6.5*	1.67

Fig. 8.11 (continued)

Table 8.5 Criteria for declaring a new scotoma and a change in a scotoma on 10-2 visual field testing

Study	Instrument	Program	Criterion for a new scotoma	Criteria for a scotoma change
Fleck [45]	Friedmann Visual Field Analyzer, Mark 1	Red target	Failure to see any of the 14 points within 10 deg of fixation in a repeatable manner	NG
Johnson [87]	Humphrey Visual Field Analyzer	10-2 VF, red target	Two or more adjacent points of 5 dB loss each or one point of 10 dB loss	NG
Xiaoyun [40]	Humphrey Visual Field Analyzer	10-2 VF, white target	Threshold for a point has <1 % chance of being normal	NG
Mititelu [88]	Humphrey Visual Field Analyzer	10-2 VF, white target	NG	NG

(continued)

Table 8.5 (continued)

Study	Instrument	Program	Criterion for a new scotoma	Criteria for a scotoma change
Mavrikakis [43]	Rodenstock	Central 25 deg, white target	Presence of two or more adjacent points of 0.8–1.2 log units increased threshold	1. For a single point scotoma, an increase in threshold of ≥1.4 log units 2. For a scotoma of area ≥2 adjacent points, an increase in threshold of ≥0.8 log units
Missner [23]	Octopus 2000 30 deg field Or Oculus Twinfield version 1.78	Central 30 deg, white target	No objective standard. Subjective grading by perimetrist: 0 = normal 1 = mild sensitivity reduction of central field 2 = relative pericentral scotoma 3 = absolute pericentral scotoma	NG

NG means not given

Table 8.6 Mean deviation and pattern standard deviation in normal subjects and patients taking 4-aminoquinolines

Study	Group	*N* (patients)	MD (dB)	PSD (dB)
Tanga [39]	Healthy controls	36	−1.27±0.89	1.04±0.16
	Patients taking HC for <36 months	26	−1.58±1.23	1.09±0.22
	Patients taking HC for >36 months	22	−2.00±1.39	1.26±0.42
Xiaoyun [40]	Patients with RA taking C	60	−1.38±1.29	2.02±1.85
	Patients with RA not taking C	30	−1.37±1.33	2.13±1.91
	Normal subjects	100	−1.40±1.35	2.09±1.88
Lai [72]	Patients taking HC	13	−1.31±1.35	1.98±2.00
Mititelu [88]	Patients with HC retinopathy	7[a]	−7.76±4.43	7.46±3.44

RA is rheumatoid arthritis. *C* is chloroquine. *HC* is hydroxychloroquine. *dB* is decibels
[a]indicates that one of the patients had 10-2 visual field testing with a red rather than white test object so that MD and PSD were not reported; therefore the means and standard deviations were calculated from six rather than seven patients

fixation was 1.83 dB [81]. Mavrikakis and colleagues have suggested, without showing data from patients taking 4AQs, that short-term variation does not exceed 0.5 log units (5 dB) for the 10-2 VF. Therefore, they argue that a change of 0.5 log units (5 dB) in a scotomatous point exceeds measurement variability and raises suspicion of further damage [43].

Some patients have greater than average variability on 10-2 VF testing. In such patients, SD-OCT and mfERG become more important. In a study of 39 patients taking 4AQs to a matched

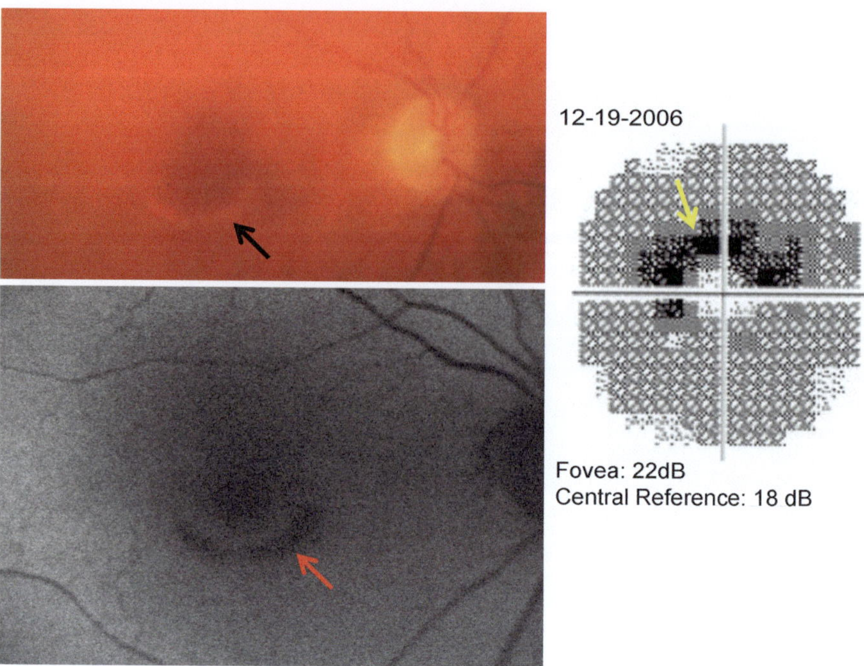

Fig. 8.12 Images showing that paracentral scotomas on 10-2 visual field testing usually begin superiorly. The patient was a 68-year-old female with SLE who had taken hydroxychloroquine 400 mg/day from 1995 to 2011. She was 5 ft 11 in. tall and weighed 183 lb. Her daily dose adjusted for IBW was 5.1 mg/kg. Her cumulative dose was 2,336 g. An inferior paracentral depigmented arc of RPE atrophy is seen on the fundus photograph (*black arrow*). A hypoautofluorescent arc corresponds to this lesion on fundus autofluorescence (FAF) imaging (*red arrow*)

control group of 16 patients not taking these drugs, there were no differences in the number of repeatably non-seen points within the central 10 deg using a red target [45].

The inter-test variation within a single individual for tests separated by 2 months (what was called LTF above) was 2.1 dB for the fovea in one study [81]. For the parafoveal points less than 6 deg from fixation, the intraindividual variation was $1.9 \pm SD$ 0.26 dB [81]. There was an age-dependent decline in the perimetric thresholds at each point of the visual field [81]. For the fovea, threshold value decreases on average 0.6 dB per decade of age. For parafoveal points less than 6 deg from fixation, the threshold value decreased on average by $0.52 \pm SD0.03$ dB per decade of age [81].

Many patients who take 4AQs are in an age group in which concomitant morbidity with glaucoma and epiretinal membranes can occur. These comorbidities can affect the 10-2 VF, making interpretation for 4AQR more difficult (Fig. 8.13). Occasionally the visual field changes accompanying 4AQR have been misinterpreted as glaucoma [80]. In such cases, the macular examination and the mfERG can be useful, as glaucoma does not typically affect them.

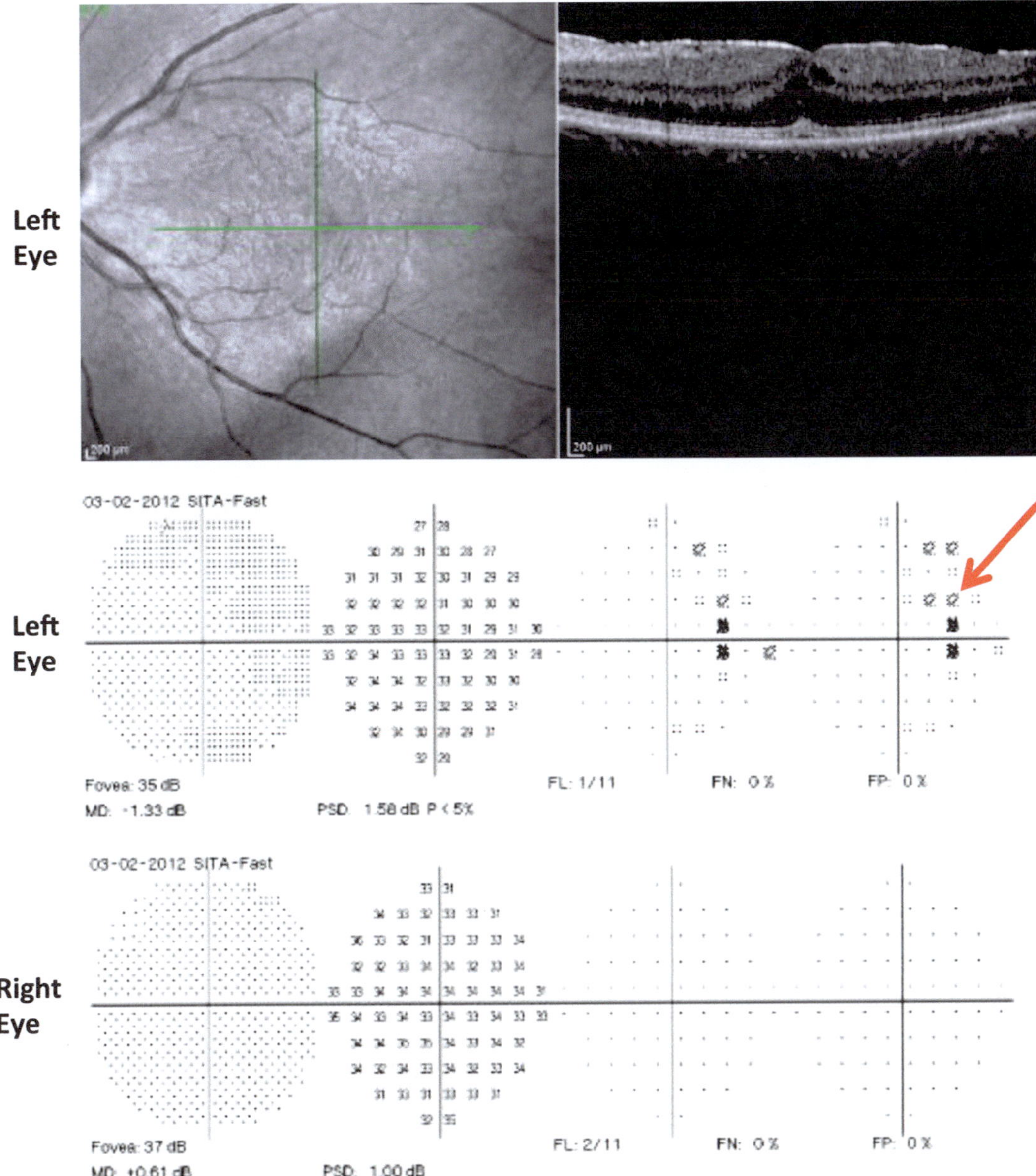

Fig. 8.13 The effect of an epiretinal membrane on the 10 2 visual field (10 2 VF). The patient was a 64 year old woman with mixed connective tissue disease. She had taken hydroxychloroquine from 1993 until 2013 on a regimen of alternating day 400 mg and 200 mg dosing. She was 5 ft 3 in. tall and weighed 162 lb. Her adjusted daily dose based on IBW was 4.9 mg/kg. Her cumulative dose was 2,190 g. (**a**) The spectral domain optical coherence tomogram shows an epiretinal membrane distorting the inner retinal contour. The 10 2 VF of the right eye is normal, but the left eye has a paracentral scotoma (*red arrow*). (**b**) The multifocal electroretinogram is normal and symmetric bilaterally. In cases of macular comorbidity, the use of several ancillary testing modalities can dissect the possible effect of the 4-aminoquinoline from the effects of the second condition

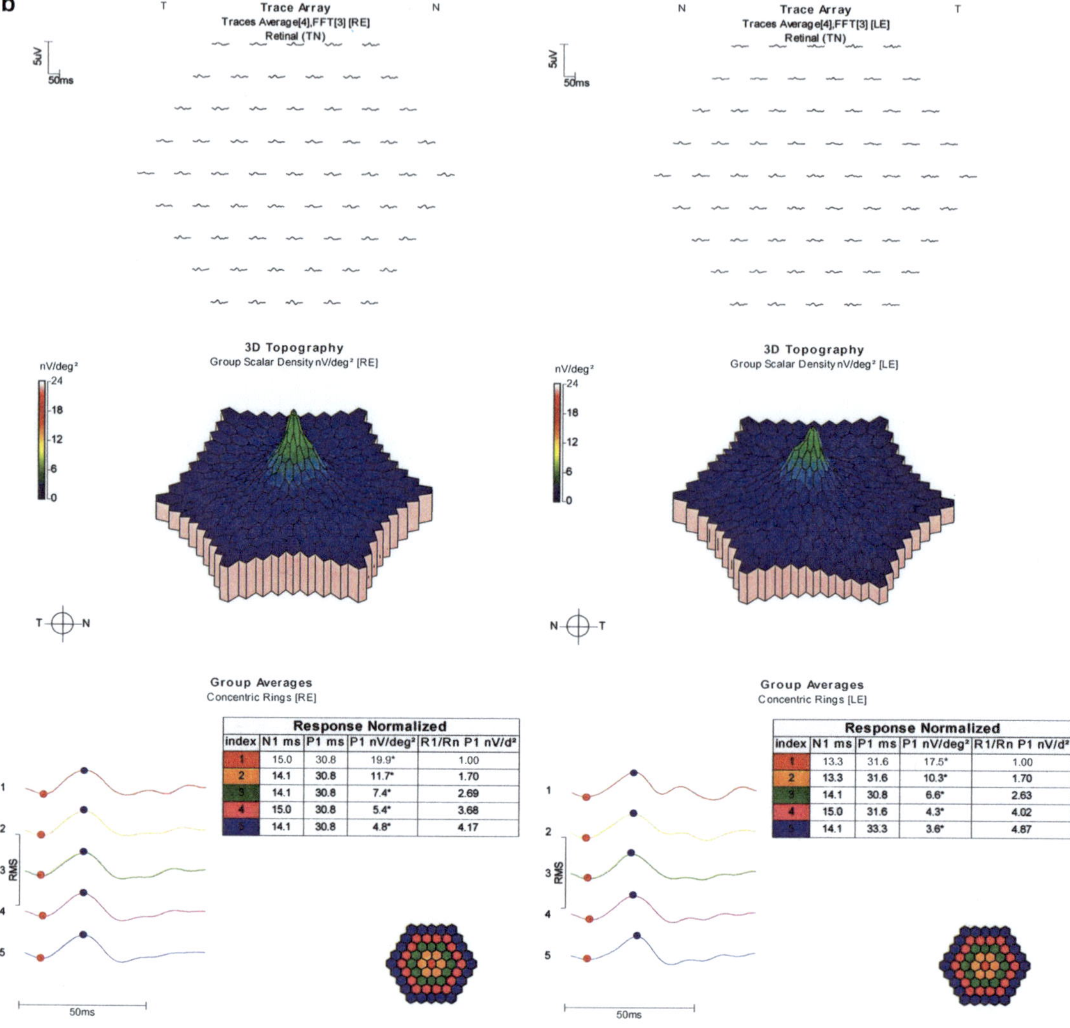

Fig. 8.13 (continued)

Misinterpreting the 10-2 Visual Field

Misinterpretation of 10-2 VFs is common in clinical practice (Fig. 8.14) [78, 79]. In failure analyses clinicians have been found to overlook characteristic visual field defects of 4AQR in 20–67 % of instances leading to delay in diagnosis and potentially worsening the prognosis of the patient [78, 79]. The misinterpretation occurs more commonly with 24-2, 30-2, and 40-2 visual fields than with 10-2 visual fields [78, 79, 94]. The 10-2 visual field obtained with the III, red test object yields deeper and broader scotomas with smaller zones of central sparing than the 10-2 VF with the III, white test object [75, 78].

The most common errors made in interpreting SAP for 4AQR screening are:

- Failure to recognize patterns of 4AQR on 10-2, 24-2, or 30-2 displays
- Not looking at pattern deviation plots but focusing instead on the gray scale plot in 10-2 VFs performed with a III, white test object
- Changing back and forth from 10-2 to 30-2 or 24-2 visual fields (Fig. 8.10)

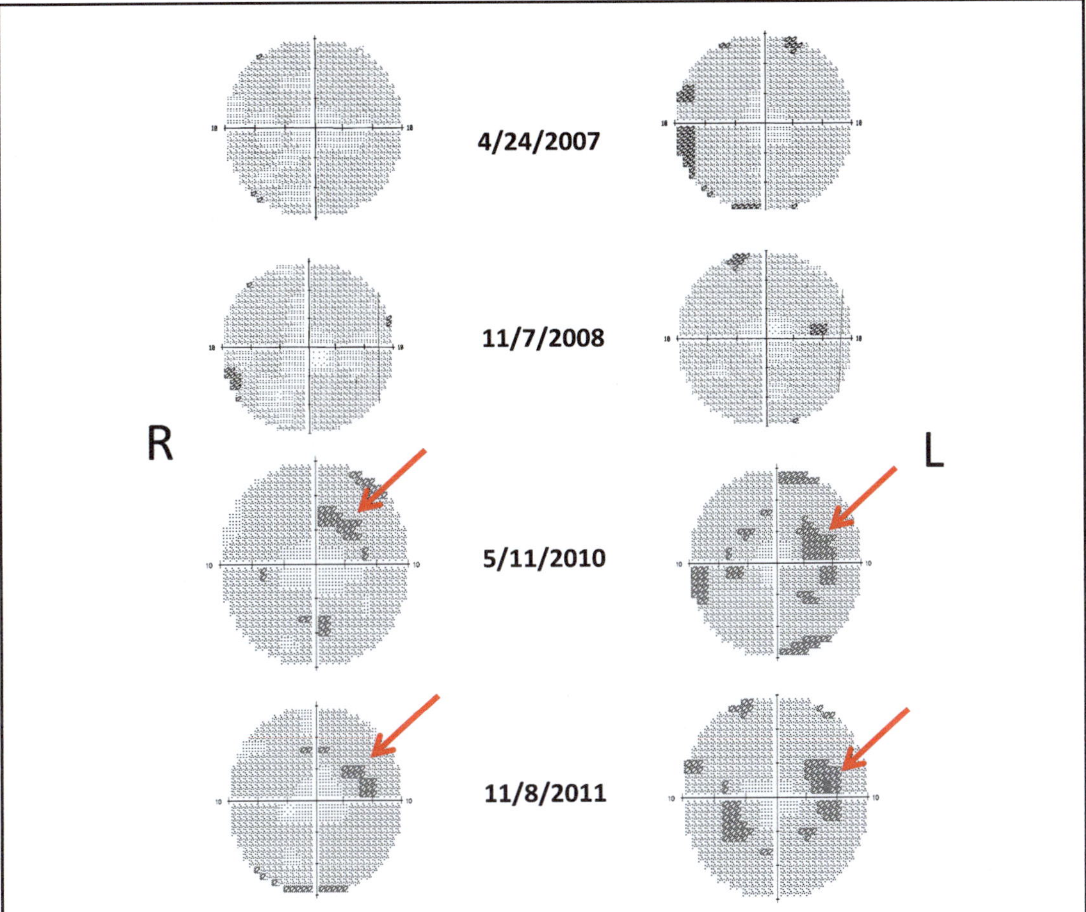

Fig. 8.14 Misinterpreted 10-2 visual fields in a 61-year-old woman taking 400 mg/day of hydroxychloroquine for rheumatoid arthritis. The ophthalmologist screening this patient read all of these fields as normal, but there are suspicious, reproducible paracentral scotomas (*red arrows*). These are in the zone typical of 4-aminoquinoline retinopathy (4AQR) (2–8 deg), have started superiorly (typical), and are symmetric (typical). The patient needs risk-factor assessment and a secondary ancillary test done to pursue the suspicion of toxicity. Unfortunately, none of the following data had been obtained: height, weight, date of starting therapy, or renal or liver status; nor had spectral domain optical coherence tomography, multifocal electroretinography (mfERG), or FAF, although all of these tests were available in the practice setting

Although the 10-2 VF is the preferred program to use in screening for 4AQR, many clinicians continue to use the 24-2 or 30-2 programs especially in cases where the patient has a concomitant disease such as glaucoma for which the 24-2 or 30-2 programs are more suitable [78, 83, 95]. In one clinic, the proportion of patients studied with the 10-2 VF was 79 %. Twenty-one percent of patients were tested with the 24-2 or 30-2 programs [78]. When the latter are used, 4AQR manifests as central rather than paracentral scotomas because of the compressed display of the visual field [78]. It is important not to switch back and forth from one program to another, because the ability to longitudinally compare visual fields over time is lost (Fig. 8.11) [78]. Authors differ in their preferences regarding the target color. Both red and white are acceptable choices. The main point is to be consistent unless one is specifically seeking a more sensitive (red test object) or specific (white test object) follow-up test because of a suspicion in need of confirmation or refutation [75, 78, 96].

In addition to SAP, blue-yellow perimetry has been proposed as a more sensitive ancillary test, but has not been adopted [97]. Frequency doubling perimetry (FDP) has been used in screening for 4AQR in an attempt to selectively isolate the function of low-redundancy magnocellular ganglion cells, which have been hypothesized to be a population of cells damaged earlier than others in the course of 4AQR [39]. Although the MD of FDP was reduced to a statistically significant extent in patients taking hydroxychloroquine compared to healthy controls, there was no clinical advantage to this modality compared to 10-2 VF testing with a white test object, which had a similar performance relative to controls. FDP has not been adopted as a standard screening test for 4AQR.

The most recent variation of threshold perimetry is microperimetry, in which there is an auto-tracking feature that approaches the objective of reproducibly placing the stimulus at a particular place in the fundus [98]. Preferential hyperacuity perimetry (PHP) measures visual acuity in the central 14 deg of the retina. The correlation of scotomas by PHP and 10-2 VF testing is variable. The sensitivity and specificity are unknown [51]. A customized form of SAP using red and blue test objects found that chloroquine caused elevated thresholds to red stimuli in a cumulative dose-dependent manner both at fixation and 5 deg eccentric to fixation. Perimetric thresholds were elevated in all patients with cumulative doses greater than 100 g. After cessation of drug the thresholds returned to normal over the course of 1 year [99]. None of these variations in SAP has been adopted clinically.

The sensitivity and specificity of 10-2 VF testing for 4AQR have not been well defined, primarily because the test itself is often the gold standard for making the diagnosis. Some evidence of sensitivity and specificity can be inferred from reports not specifically calculating these statistics. In one study of patients taking hydroxychloroquine without retinopathy, 10 % had abnormal 10-2 VFs compared to 11.4 % of rheumatology patient controls not taking 4AQs. This suggests an upper bound on speci-

ficity of 10-2 VF testing of 90 %. Patients with hydroxychloroquine retinopathy defined by fundus changes had a 37.5 % prevalence of abnormal 10-2 VFs, suggesting a low sensitivity. However, the definition of abnormal 10-2 VF was not given, making these inferences tenuous [20]. Another study reported on 39 patients taking 5.5–6.5 mg/kg/day of hydroxychloroquine for a mean of 1.5 years. No paracentral scotomas were observed to 10-2 VF testing using a red stimulus, suggesting a specificity higher than 90 % [100].

Easterbrook and Trope measured the sensitivity and specificity of 10-2 VF testing with red and white test objects against a gold standard defined as an abnormal Amsler grid verified by abnormal Tubinger perimetry in patients taking chloroquine [74]. They reported that 10-2 VF testing with a red test object was 91.3 % sensitive and 57.8 % specific. With 10-2 VF testing using a white test object the sensitivity and specificity were 78 % and 84 %, respectively. Only 19 of the 69 eyes in the study had no retinopathy, weakening the strength of the specificity statistics.

Browning and Lee measured the sensitivity and specificity of 10-2 VF testing in 121 patients taking 4AQs (predominantly hydroxychloroquine). In this study, fields done with red and white test objects were pooled. The gold standard was that the 4AQ was discontinued by the prescribing physician based on the totality of the evidence. Sensitivity and specificity were 85.7 % and 92.5 %, respectively [42]. Only 14 of the 121 eyes in this study had 4AQR, weakening the strength of the sensitivity statistic.

Table 8.7 shows the PPVs and NPVs for a plausible range of prevalences of 4AQR that a clinician might encounter. The NPVs are extremely high and the PPVs are rather low, regardless of the prevalence assumed. In these circumstances, a normal 10-2 VF is useful for confirming the absence of 4AQR. The most that a single abnormal 10-2 VF with a suggestive paracentral scotoma can do is raise the suspicion of 4AQR (increase the posttest probability of 4AQR compared to the pretest probability). By itself, this single test is not dispositive, and should not, by itself, lead to cessation of the 4AQ. With a revised posterior probability of 4AQR, another test should be applied, and if it is also positive,

Table 8.7 Positive and negative predictive values for 10-2 visual field testing over a plausible range of assumed prevalences

Assumed prevalence (%)	Sensitivity (%)	Specificity (%)	PPV (%)	NPV (%)
0.1	85.7	92.5	1.1	100
1	85.7	92.5	10.3	99.8
3	85.7	92.5	26.1	99.5
5	85.7	92.5	37.6	99.2

Sensitivity and specificity are from Browning and Lee [42]. *PPV* is positive predictive value. *NPV* is negative predictive value

then the second stage posterior probability may indeed be high enough to warrant cessation of the drug.

To summarize, SAP with the 10-2 VF is the most common ancillary test used in screening for 4AQR, but its performance characteristics and reproducibility remain insufficiently studied. Variability of interpretation of 10-2 VFs by screening physicians limits the test's usefulness in detecting toxicity. In most clinical scenarios, a single 10-2 VF has a low PPV and, if positive, can only indicate whether another test is indicated. A series of consistently positive 10-2 VFs or a single positive 10-2 VF buttressed by a positive mfERG, FAF image, or SD-OCT can make the case for cessation of a 4AQ. Better education of eye-care providers regarding limitations and nuances of interpretation may help, but probably should not preempt the message that attention to correct dosing is the most important part of examining patients taking 4AQs.

8.6 Multifocal Electroretinography

8.6.1 Fundamentals of Multifocal Electroretinography

mfERG is a method of recording local electrophysiologic responses from the central retina. It was invented by Sutter and Tran in 1992 [101]. The retina is stimulated by a pattern of hexagons turned on and off according to a pseudorandom sequence at a frequency of 75 hz [102]. At any given time a hexagon has a 50 % chance of being illuminated [103]. The signal attributable to the individual hexagons is mathematically extracted from a continuous recording of the electroretinogram by cross correlating the recording and the sequence of the on and off phases of the hexagons (Fig. 8.15) [104]. There are no direct recordings from retinal cells.

Typically the mfERG response that is analyzed is called the first-order kernel, a biphasic recording as exemplified in Fig. 8.16 [103]. The N1 wave is the initial downward deflection. The P1 wave is the upward deflection that follows the N1 wave. N1 is composed of contributions from cones [23, 103]. P1 is composed of contributions from cones as well as from amacrine and bipolar cells in the inner nuclear layer [23, 104, 105]. In general, the mfERG can detect a retinal lesion covering at least half the area of a hexagon from the projected image of the stimulation screen onto the retina [102]. Therefore, it is evident that an instrument using 103 hexagons will be more sensitive to small lesions than one using 61 hexagons [102, 106]. However, there is a price paid by increasing the number of hexagons. The more hexagons there are the lower the signal-to-noise ratio and the longer the necessary testing time to obtain a usable recording [102]. The hexagons are not all the same size, but rather increase in size with greater eccentricity to attempt to obtain uniform response densities [102]. Cone density diminishes as eccentricity increases which accounts for this necessity [107]. Recordings can be done monocularly or binocularly. The author's laboratory typically employs binocular testing unless there is a clinically evident tropia.

Peak-to-peak amplitude is measured as shown in Fig. 8.16. First-order kernel N1P1 amplitudes are measured from the trace recorded from each hexagon [109]. Another method of expressing amplitude is the scalar product response density, defined as the dot product between the normalized response template and each local response [109–111]. Corresponding points between a template waveform from a normal control population and from the subject's waveform are multiplied and each component multiplication is summed

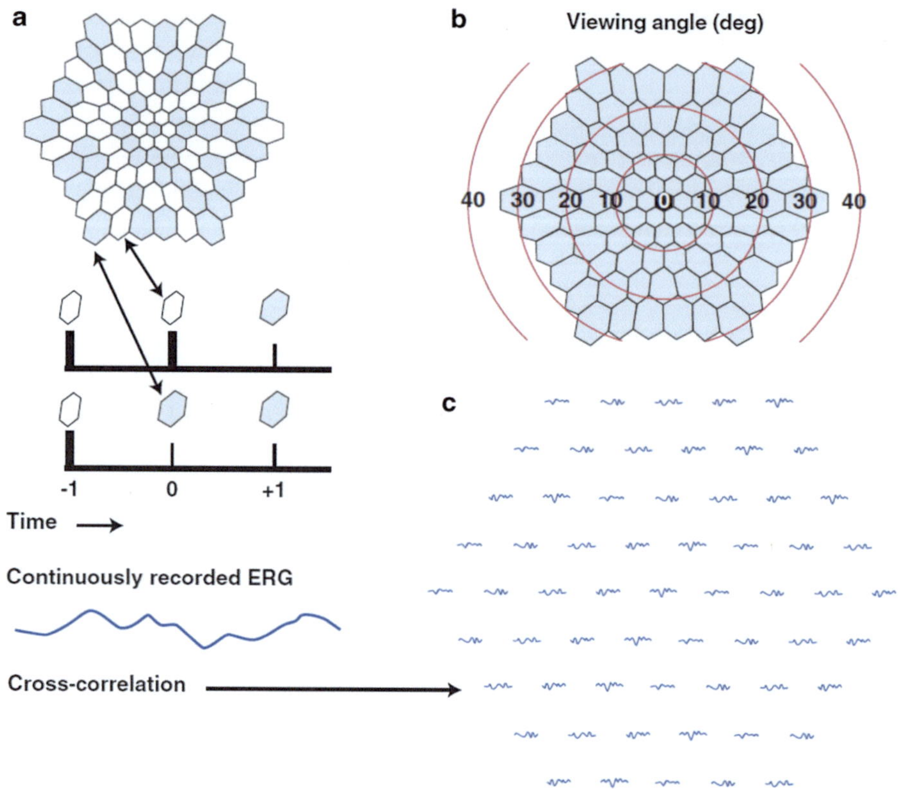

Fig. 8.15 Methodology of mfERG recording. (**a**) A screen of hexagons is illuminated with a pattern of stimulation. The frames typically change at a frequency of 75 Hz. The hexagons increase in area as distance from the center increases so as to make the voltage recorded over the area of the hexagon approximately equal across the hexagons. At any given time a hexagon has a 50 % probability of being illuminated. (**b**) The hexagons are grouped in rings concentric with the center. There are five or six rings depending on the number of hexagons, which is typically 61 or 103. (**c**) The electroretinogram is continuously recorded and by cross correlating the recorded signal with the pattern of stimulation the focal responses that arise from each hexagon can be extracted and displayed. Data from Hood [108]

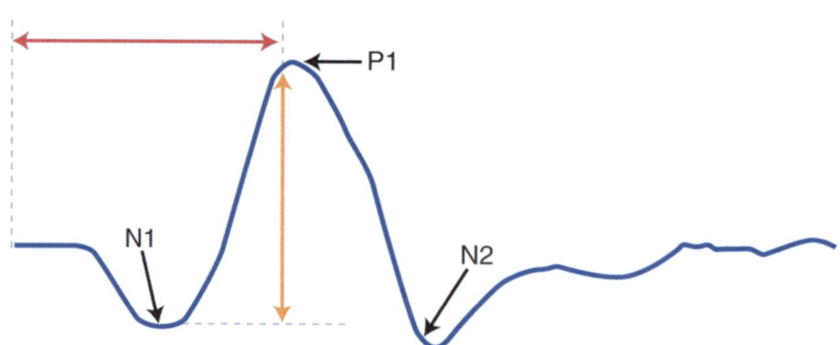

Fig. 8.16 Multifocal electroretinogram waveform. N1 arises from the cones. P1 arises from cones, bipolar, and amacrine cells. The *red arrow* denotes the P1 implicit time. The *orange arrow* indicates the N1P1 amplitude. Data from Hood [108]

to yield an overall number that is divided by the area of the hexagonal area [112]. The scalar product is affected by both amplitude and implicit time changes [112]. Scalar product amplitude is measured by the system's software. A less commonly used method of displaying the mfERG output involves root mean square analysis. Its disadvantage relative to the retinal response density is that it is the sum of both signal and noise [104]. Units of mfERG amplitude are commonly nV/deg^2 whether amplitude is expressed as peak-to-peak amplitude or scalar product amplitude [113]. What is termed the amplitude of the mfERG response by some [23] is termed the retinal response density by others [110].

There are variations in data displays of mfERG outputs. Data can be displayed in the retina format or the field format. The retina format means that one looks at the hexagons as one would look at a fundus photograph (imagine the patient facing you and you are looking at his fundus) (Fig. 8.12b). The field format means that one looks at the hexagons as one would look at a visual field printout (imagine that you are in the patient's position in a visual field instrument looking out at the bowl).

The eccentricity of the rings can vary. For the author's system using 61 hexagons covering a radius of approximately 30 deg of retina from the fovea, the angular subtense of the rings is:

- R_1—0–2.3 deg
- R_2—2.3–7.8 deg
- R_3—7.8–14.9 deg
- R_4—14.9–23.2 deg
- R_5—23.2–32.0 deg [107, 114]

For a system using 103 hexagons covering a radius of 40 deg, the subtense of the rings was:

- R_1—0–2.3 deg
- R_2—2.3–7.8 deg
- R_3—7.8–14.0 deg
- R_4—14.0–22.4 deg
- R_5—22.4–31.0 deg
- R_6—31.0–40.0 deg [115]

For a system using an unspecified number of hexagons covering a radius of 20 deg, the subtense of the rings was:

- R_1—0–2.5 deg
- R_2—2.5–5.0 deg
- R_3—5.0–10.0 deg
- R_4—10.0–15.0 deg
- R_5—15.0–20.0 deg [39]

Where this can matter is in the mean response densities averaged over a ring and in calculating ratios of average ring response densities [39, 52]. The use of ring ratios reduces noise in the measurements and increases sensitivity [52, 116]. It has been claimed, but not proven, that other advantages of ring ratios include invariance with respect to stimulus luminance, reference electrode placement, and anterior segment differences [52]. In calculating ring ratios, some authors consistently make the average ring 1 (R_1) response density the numerator and the paracentral ring response densities the denominator [52]. Others do the reverse with the average ring 1 response as the consistent denominator [39]. This makes comparisons across studies difficult.

Pitfalls in Data Displays

It is easy to confuse the data displays of the mfERG. As an example, Teoh shows the field format to display the hexagon waveforms and suggests a direct correspondence of the hexagons with reduced signal amplitudes with the areas of scotoma on the threshold visual field [117]. Instead, if the retina format for displaying the mfERG is chosen, the correspondence of the regions of the mfERG and the threshold visual field will be inverted.

8.6.2 Sources of Variability and Factors That Influence the Multifocal Electroretinogram

There are many variables in mfERG testing. There are different machines (e.g., VERIS, Roland, Metrovision, and Diagnosys), different numbers of hexagons (e.g., 61, 103, or 241), different luminances of the light and dark hexagons (e.g., 100–1,000 cd/m^2 for the bright hexagons and 0–3.5 cd/m^2 for the dark hexagons), number of rings (5 or 6), subtended angles of retina covered by the hexagons (from 20 to 50 deg), durations of light adaptation before testing (10–20 min), ambient illumination, distance of the screen from the test subject (24–40 cm), status relative to wearing refractive correction, dilation status, specifications of the band-pass filters (e.g., 3 Hz- and 300 Hz-), gain (e.g., 10,000–200,000), type of electrodes used (e.g., Burian-Allen contact lens electrodes, contact lens jet electrodes, gold foil, Dawson–Trick–Litzkow (DTL) electrodes, H-K loop sclera electrodes), use of CRT or LED displays, and frame stimulation rate [23, 35, 102, 108, 110, 117–127].

How to Compare mfERG Data Across Laboratories

There is so much variability in mfERG from laboratory to laboratory that investigators have studied methods for interlaboratory comparison. One method is to convert the raw data into Z-scores (see Sect. 8.1). In using the Z-score method, amplitudes more than minus two times the standard deviation below the mean are defined as abnormal and implicit times more than two times the standard deviation above the mean are defined as abnormal. Recall that for a normally distributed variable, 2.5 % of the values will lie more than 2 SDs above the mean and 2.5 % of the values will lie more than 2 SDs below the mean [128].

Increasing luminance increases response densities and decreases implicit times, but the relationship is modest with only a 20 % change in amplitude for a 3.3-fold change in luminance [107, 121]. Implicit time decreases less than 1.5 ms over the same change in luminance [107]. Amplitudes decrease with decreased stimulus contrast (e.g., from cataract), but implicit times do not change [115]. Pupillary dilation increases response amplitude by up to 50 % and decreases implicit time by as much as 17 % for 7 mm of dilation [125]. Therefore, International Society for Clinical Electrophysiology and Vision (ISCEV) guidelines recommend that mfERG recordings should be done with the patient's pupil dilated to improve the signal-to-noise ratio [125]. Other characteristics of patients also introduce variability. For example, a cataract acts as a neutral density filter and can decrease amplitude and increase implicit time [121].

The ambient illumination that is most conducive to a stable mfERG is that of a fully lighted room (1.6 log cd/m^2 = 36 cd/m^2) [129]. Changing from a fully lit to a dark room can change increase response amplitude 30 %; therefore room illumination should be constant throughout a study and from study to study [129]. Preadaptation of patients to light or dark conditions does not matter to a clinically significant degree and is not necessary in a clinical setting [129]. Nevertheless, patients should wait in a room with ordinary lighting, and not in a dark room, before recording the mfERG to avoid the potential problem of growing mfERG response amplitudes in the first minutes of a recording in a patient preadapted to dark conditions [129]. Contrast adaptation is not necessary before clinical mfERG recording for purposes of chloroquine and hydroxychloroquine retinopathy screening, because prerecording contrast adaptation did not significantly affect mfERG response amplitudes [130].

In one study, the mfERG P1 amplitude for the central macula was reduced up to 12 % with three diopters of optical defocus [131]. The N1 amplitude, and N1 and P1 implicit times were not similarly affected. In other studies, amplitudes were decreased and implicit times delayed as refractive error increased [102]. Therefore, to optimize recordings, wearing the full refractive correction is ideal during mfERG recording, although not required by ISCEV guidelines as the variance introduced by omission is not great [103, 112, 131].

Measurements at the hexagon level are less repeatable than ring averages, regional, or whole eye averages because of the lower signal-to-noise ratio and variations in the location of individual hexagons relative to the fovea [118, 132]. Among all the single hexagons, the reproducibility is best from the central hexagon [132]. In general, intrasession reproducibility is higher than intersession reproducibility and implicit times are more reproducible than amplitudes [105, 118, 127]. Intrasession reproducibility is better because electrode variability is eliminated [127].

In the clinical literature, it is frequently stated that 10-2 VF testing is subjective and mfERG is objective, as though the mfERG does not depend on patient input, but such is not the case. Patient fixation is necessary for a successful mfERG recording [104, 133]. To facilitate fixation stability, recordings are made in short segments and recordings with excessive blinking are rejected [112]. In view of the large number of uncontrolled variables that influence the mfERG, and the variability in methods of interpretation of the resulting waveforms, it is a reflection of hope rather than reality to term mfERG "a method of obtaining objective visual fields" [134].

Practical Issues in mfERG

There are many types of electrodes used for mfERG including JET contact lens, gold foil, carbon fiber, and DTL electrodes. There are pros and cons to each type of electrode in use for mfERG testing. The signal-to-noise ratio of DTL electrodes is worse than with Burian-Allen contact lens electrodes [102, 135]. However, Burian-Allen contact lens electrodes are associated with more stray light and introduce a prismatic effect on the stimulus illumination. DTL electrodes are more comfortable than Burian-Allen electrodes [135, 136]. With Burian-Allen electrodes, an air bubble can lodge between the electrode and the cornea.[121]H-K sclera loop electrodes are more comfortable to the patient than Burian-Allen contact lens electrodes [123]. In a study of the performance of various electrodes the contact lens electrode gave the largest response density, followed by gold foil, DTL, and carbon fiber electrodes. Coefficients of variation were similar for the contact lens, gold foil, and DTL electrodes but were significantly higher with the carbon fiber electrodes [137].

Another difficulty in applying published information on mfERGs is that much of it is specific to one machine or another. To make data between different machines and laboratories comparable, it has been suggested that data be normalized and then compared as percentage amplitude loss or percentage implicit time delay [138].

8.6.3 Normal Values and Reproducibility of the Multifocal Electroretinogram

Normal values for the mfERG vary across laboratories as shown in Table 8.8. Several themes emerge from a study of this table. First, the COV of amplitudes is 24–27 % compared to 3–6 % for the COV of implicit times across the rings. In a study that compared COVs of rings to those of ring ratios, the COV of ring ratios was smaller. The average COV for ring amplitudes over six

Table 8.8 Normal values of multifocal electroretinographic variables

Ring	Laboratory	Number in control group	Age range/mean	Mean amplitudes (nV/deg^2)	SD amplitudes (nV/deg^2)	Lower limit of normal (nV/deg^2)	Mean P implicit times (ms)	SD of implicit times (ms)
R_1	Moschos [110]	30	30–50/39	20.0				
	Author's laboratory	32	22–79/46	31.4	7.6	14.2	30.0	1.9
	Lai [35]	20	NG/41	103.1	17.7		27.1	1.3
	Kondo [122]	15	21–63/NG	12.2	2.7		NG	NG
	Kellner [139]	15	NG/NG	140[a]	31		NG	NG
	Tanga [39]	36	27–69/48	79.3	23.8		NG	NG
	Missner [23]	50	30–70/NG	137.7[a]	NG	74.5		
	Kretschmann [140]	30	22–58/31[a]	59[b]	NG	40[b]	32[b]	NG
R_2	Moschos [110]	30	30–50/39	15.0				
	Author's laboratory	32	22–79/46	17.0	4.1	8.8	29.7	1.2
	Lai [35]	20	NG/41	65.5	14.6		26.8	1.1
	Kellner [139]	15	NG/NG	72	13.5		NG	NG
	Tanga [39]	36	27–69/48	42.1	13.0		NG	NG
	Missner [23]	50	30–70/NG	70.3		46.2		
	Kretschmann [140]	30	22–58/31[a]	28[b]	NG	20[b]	30[b]	NG
R_3	Moschos [110]	30	30–50/39	12.8				
	Author's laboratory	32	22–79/46	10.5	2.6	4.8	29.8	1.1
	Lai [35]	20	NG/41	47.5	10.0		26.4	1.0
	Kellner [139]	15	NG/NG	50	11.5		NG	NG
	Tanga [39]	36	27–69/48	26.7	8.1		NG	NG
	Missner [23]	50	30–70/NG	44.7		26.6		
	Kretschmann [140]	30	22–58/31[a]	18[b]	NG	12[b]	30[b]	NG
R_4	Moschos [110]	30	30–50/39	10.0				
	Author's laboratory	32	22–79/46	7.7	2.0	3.4	30.2	1.1
	Lai [35]	20	NG/41	37.3	7.2		25.9	1.0
	Kellner [139]	15	NG/NG	40	8.5		NG	NG
	Tanga [39]	36	27–69/48	18.7	5.8		NG	NG
	Missner [23]	50	30–70/NG	37.2		20.9		
	Kretschmann [140]	30	22–58/31[a]	12[b]	NG	9[b]	30[b]	NG
R_5	Moschos [110]	30	30–50/39	10.0				
	Author's laboratory	32	22–79/46	6.3	1.7	3.4	30.3	0.9
	Lai [35]	20	NG/41	31.0	6.3		26.2	1.1
	Kellner [139]	15	NG/NG	35	7.5		NG	NG
	Tanga [39]	36	27–69/48	13.9	4.2		NG	NG
	Missner [23]	50	30–70/NG	32.8		17.9		
	Kretschmann [140]	30	22–58/31[a]	12[b]	NG	9[b]	32[b]	NG
R_6	Lai [35]	20	NG/41	26.7	5.4		26.3	1.2

NG means not given. "*a*" means median rather than mean. "*b*" means data extracted from Fig. 2 of Kretschmann [140]

Table 8.9 Reproducibility of multifocal electroretinography (mfERG)

MfERG variable	Level of measurement	Study	COV (%)	COR (%)	Subjects
Amplitude	Hexagon	Harrison [118]	10.5–47.3	NG	Normal subjects
	Central hexagon	Yoshii [121]	9.8	NG	Normal subjects
		Parks [123]	NG	12.2*	Normal subjects
		Kondo [122]	14.9		15 normal subjects 4 without AQR
		Bultmann [132]	10.4		Normal subjects
	Ring average for R_1	Browning [141]		51	Normal subjects
				60	Patients taking HC
				60	Patients taking HC
	Ring average for R_2	Bultmann [132]	9.3		Normal subjects
		Browning [141]		43	Normal subjects
				53	Patients taking HC
	Ring average for R_5	Parks [123]		28.4*	Normal subjects
	Ring average for R_1/R_2 ratio	Browning [141]		43	Normal subjects
				47	Patients taking HC
	Nasal or temporal hexagon from ring 3	Yoshii [121]	9.7		Normal subjects
	Ring averages	Harrison [118]	10.4–36.0		Normal subjects
Implicit time	Hexagon	Harrison [118]	2.2–4.3	NG	Normal subjects
	Central hexagon	Bultmann [132]	1.3		Normal subjects
	Ring average for R_2		1.4		Normal subjects
	Ring averages	Harrison [118]	3.1–30.3		Normal subjects

The *asterisk* indicates Parks and colleagues definition of coefficient of repeatability [123], which differs from the conventional definition [57] by a factor of 1.96; thus the Parks' figure has been multiplied by 1.96 to make the cells of the table comparable. *HC* is hydroxychloroquine

rings was 24.6 %, but for R_1 and R_5 based ring ratios, the COVs were 15.8 % and 11.2 %, respectively [47]. This theme is echoed in a study of COV across individual hexagons rather than ring averages in which the mean COV for all subjects and hexagonal areas was 29.2 ± SD 3.9 % [109]. Variability was higher for hexagons adjacent to the optic disc [109]. The author's data and that of others suggest that the COV of implicit times in normal subjects is approximately 1/10 to 1/4 that of amplitudes [105, 109, 120, 128].

The use of age-adjusted normal values is recommended, because amplitudes decrease with age due to optical and neural factors, but many studies do not adhere to this practice [47, 108, 115]. In one study, the amplitude of P1 decreased roughly 10.5 % per decade of increased age, whereas the implicit time increases by approximately 1 % per decade of increased age [102]. In another, amplitudes in normal subjects decreased 50 % between age 20 and 40, whereas implicit time increased from 25 to 29 ms from age 20 to 60 [16]. Use of ring ratios circumvents this problem because these are not dependent on age [47, 52].

Because the reproducibility of amplitude measurements is less than implicit time measurements, a greater change in serial amplitude measurements is required to be able to conclude that an actual change has occurred that is not noise in the measurement. A summary of reproducibility observations from selected studies is shown in Table 8.9.

A measurement analogous to repeatability was reported in a study of normal patients with two mfERGs recorded within 1 year of each other. This might be termed short-term variation. The mean difference in implicit time Z-scores was 0.36 ± 0.28. The mean difference in amplitude Z-scores was 0.85 ± 0.81 [118].

Browning and Lee studied the COR for R_1, R_2, and R_1/R_2 in 21 normal subjects and 44 patients taking hydroxychloroquine without retinopathy. For the normal subjects, the CORs were 51 %, 43 %, and 43 % for R_1, R_2, and R_1/R_2, respectively. For the patients taking hydroxychloroquine, the values were 60 %, 53 %, and 47 % [141]. Penrose looked at the COV for mfERG amplitudes in 20 normal controls and 11 patients on hydroxychloroquine. The values were 22 % and 29 %, respectively, suggesting that variability of mfERG amplitudes in patients taking hydroxychloroquine is similar to that of normals [142]. Other studies' estimates of COV for the central hexagon vary from 10 to 22 % [114, 121, 143]. For more peripheral rings, the COV is greater (up to 35 %) [144]. The variability of the mfERG reduces its usefulness [109].

Because of the variability of the mfERG across and within patients, several mfERGs should usually be done before deciding that drug should be stopped.

Otherwise, one might stop useful drugs based on a drop in mfERG amplitude that in reality reflected only intersession variability of the measurements [35, 36, 145, 146]. In fact, some investigators think that the sole purpose of the mfERG is to raise suspicion with other tests necessary to confirm or disconfirm presence of retinopathy [119, 145]. At the other end of the spectrum of 4AQR, the value of mfERG in more advanced retinopathy has been questioned; if a more reliable test such as SD-OCT shows 4AQR, mfERG adds little [35, 146].

It is important to look at the trace array of individual hexagonal signals and not simply inspect the three-dimensional response map and the ring averages [103]. Early 4AQR does not necessarily involve an entire parafoveal ring, and ring averages can swamp the effects at the hexagonal level [109].

Certain mfERG variables are age-dependent [113]. The response densities of individual hexagons can decrease from 5 to 12 % per decade of age [109]. Ring amplitudes decrease with age at approximately 11 % per decade [30, 113]. Both N1 and P1 implicit times decrease at approximately 1 % per decade [113]. This adds an additional level of complexity to mfERG analysis of patients taking 4AQs, because patients taking 4AQs as a group are often older than the normal population from which tables of normal mfERG values are derived. One method to circumvent this difficulty is to emphasize ring ratios, some of which are invariant with respect to age. For example, R_1/R_2, R_1/R_3, and R_1/R_4 have been reported to be invariant over age [30]. In particular, R_1/R_2 has been reported as particularly useful in assessing hydroxychloroquine toxicity with 2.6 used as a cut-point for classification of responses as abnormal or not [52]. Another advantage cited for ring ratio analysis has been better reproducibility than amplitude measurements [30]. Not all investigators have found this to be true.

8.6.4 Interpretation of Multifocal Electroretinograms

Interpretation of mfERGs may involve comparison of recordings from single hexagons or groups of hexagons with averaged recordings. A particularly common grouping is by concentric rings of hexagons around the fovea [135]. This is a useful methodology in detecting 4AQR because its morphology generally shows concentricity around the fovea.

As with any ancillary test used in a clinical situation, the results of the test depend on the definition of abnormality. These definitions are inconsistent across the literature. For example, Lyons defines an abnormal mfERG as one in which the R_1/R_2 ratio exceeded the upper limit of normal [52]. On the other hand, Maturi defined an abnormal mfERG as one with any abnormality of amplitude or implicit time in any of the rings [83].

Reductions in mfERG amplitudes are an earlier indicator of toxicity than clinical indicators. Visual acuity reductions were seen eyes with severely reduced mfERG amplitudes [30], but many eyes with less severely reduced mfERG amplitudes have normal visual acuity [139].

Some authors make a distinction between an effect of hydroxychloroquine on the mfERG and hydroxychloroquine toxicity [23, 77, 83]. Abnormalities of some aspect of the mfERG have been reported in 20–70 % of patients taking 4AQs, a broad range that renders it more difficult to define what represents toxicity [23, 40, 72, 77].

In a study of 20 patients taking 4AQs in nontoxic doses (but not specified with respect to actual or IBW), decreased amplitudes compared to age-matched normals were noted in 32.4 %, 54.3 %, and 32.4 % for rings R_1, R_2, and R_3, respectively [23]. A study of 13 patients taking hydroxychloroquine but without retinopathy reported a correlation between cumulative dosage and reduction in N1 and P1 amplitudes in rings R_1 to R_3 [35, 72]. When patients were taken off hydroxychloroquine and retested later, amplitudes improved [35]. Independently, others have shown that mfERG amplitudes improved when patients were taken off 4AQs [110]. Others disagree that these drugs affect the mfERG in patients without retinopathy. For example, three groups have found no difference in absolute ring responses of eyes from patients taking hydroxychloroquine without retinopathy and control subjects [39, 47, 141].

The general theme of all reports is that amplitudes are decreased and implicit times delayed in patients with 4AQR [23, 77, 83, 117]. Most investigators think that amplitudes are a more sensitive indicator of 4AQR than implicit times, and some do not measure implicit times [42, 44, 77]. For example, Michaelides found amplitude reductions alone approximately six times as often as implicit time increases alone in a case series of patients with hydroxychloroquine retinopathy [44].

Heterogeneity of mfERG abnormalities in 4AQR has been observed, prompting a classification of the types of changes seen [44]. The responses depend on the stage of retinopathy. In a study of 25 patients taking 4AQs for more than 1 year, some of whom had retinopathy and others who did not, amplitude reductions in R_2 were seen most commonly, followed by reductions in R_3, R_4, and R_1 [138]. Delayed implicit times were less common. The following patterns of mfERG response were observed:

- Pericentral pattern—reduced amplitudes in R_2 and R_3
- Central pattern—reduced amplitudes in R_1, R_2, and R_3
- Generalized pattern—reduced amplitudes in R_1 to R_5
- No mfERG response [138]

These patterns of response were consistent between two eyes of a single patient, but varied at the level of the patient [138]. Similar results were reported in a study of 12 patients taking hydroxychloroquine tested 1 and 2 years after an initial test. N1-P1 amplitudes were decreased in rings R_2 to R_4 with no changes in implicit times. Another study of three patients also reported that reduced amplitudes in rings R_2 and R_3 were the most striking mfERG responses to chloroquine retinopathy [139].

A similar classification system, but with the additional category of peripheral abnormalities, has been introduced by Lyons and coworkers. Reductions in mfERG amplitudes in a pericentral, full (i.e., throughout the tested retina), central, and peripheral patterns were reported in 62 %, 22 %, 5 %, and 11 % of patients using hydroxychloroquine, respectively [30, 52]. Only the first three patterns were arbitrarily deemed toxic by the authors. The reductions in mfERG amplitude were congruent with the retinal ring hexagons that correspond to the annular scotoma observed in chloroquine retinopathy [124].

Maturi proposed another system, similar to that of Lyons and colleagues, but allowing that peripheral abnormalities could be attributed to 4AQ retinopathy:

- Paracentral abnormality in amplitude or latency
- Abnormality in the central area alone
- Abnormality in the peripheral area alone
- Decrease in the entire tested area [83]

Missner and colleagues used a grading system that incorporated criteria based on both amplitudes and implicit times as follows:

- (Normal)—normal amplitudes and implicit times
- (Mild abnormality)—decrease in amplitude in ring 2 or increase in implicit time in two of rings 1–3
- (More marked abnormality)—decrease in amplitude in two of rings 1–3
- (Severe abnormality)—decrease in amplitudes in two or more rings and an increase in implicit time in three or more rings including rings 2 and 3 [23]

Marmor suggested another grading system that allowed as abnormal some responses within the normal ranges:

- Pattern #1—mfERG measurements are within laboratory reference ranges but there are diminished responses in areas of early damage;

ring responses are normal; and ring ratios show relative weakness of parafoveal rings.

- Pattern #2—Measurements show diminished central responses with greater diminution in the parafovea both on the trace arrays and in the ring ratios.
- Pattern #3—The central responses of the mfERG are decreased to the point that parafoveal predilection of damage cannot be recognized.
- Pattern #4—Severe depression of mfERG signals across the posterior pole [146].

The system does not specify how diminished the responses must be in Pattern #1 to qualify as abnormal.

A difficulty with all of these proposed grading systems is their subjectivity. How does one define a response as diminished if it lies within reference ranges? Does that mean in the bottom 30 % of normal? The bottom 40 %? Does it mean in comparison to an earlier measurement that was also in the normal range? How does one compare gradings across different instruments and laboratories? Without more details, the grading systems are not useful in the clinical setting.

The complexity of mfERG interpretation and its challenges for busy clinicians has led some to devise simpler methods of interpreting the mfERG. In a study of 23 patients taking hydroxychloroquine, Chang and colleagues tested a method based on the color difference plot provided in the mfERG display [119]. They developed a scoring system applied to this plot that agreed reasonably well with interpretations based on response amplitudes. Their opinion was that this method was simpler for the clinician to use. Other clinicians simply look at the display of waveforms and the topographic display of voltage densities and subjectively look for absence of a foveal peak and subjective flattening of individual hexagon waveforms [147, 148].

Of the many possible published ways to interpret mfERGs, we do not know which is the best. For example, Lyons recommends using R_1/R_2 ring ratios [30]. Yet Adam and colleagues found no difference between controls, hydroxychloroquine users without toxicity, and hydroxychloroquine users with toxicity using the R_1/R_2 ratio [47]. Instead they suggest that R_5/R_6 discrimi-

Table 8.10 Positive and negative predictive values for mfERG testing over a plausible range of assumed prevalences of 4AQR

Assumed prevalence (%)	Sensitivity (%)	Specificity (%)	PPV (%)	NPV (%)
0.1	92.9	86.9	0.7	100
1	92.9	86.9	6.7	99.9
3	92.9	86.9	18.0	99.7
5	92.9	86.9	27.2	99.6

Sensitivity and specificity are from Browning and Lee [42]. *PPV* is positive predictive value. *NPV* is negative predictive value

nates best between control eyes and eyes with hydroxychloroquine retinopathy [47]. To further complicate matters, the sensitivity of mfERG variables to the use of 4AQs is not uniform. For example, in one study of 20 patients taking hydroxychloroquine without retinopathy as determined by normal visual acuity, funduscopy, and static perimetry, the amplitudes were reduced in R_1 and R_2 in eight cases, but the R_1/R_2 ratios were increased in three cases [110].

Because the results of investigations involving mfERGs will depend on the definitions chosen to define abnormal, it is difficult to compare results across studies. Table 8.10 shows the sensitivity and specificity of mfERG based on a definition of low amplitudes of N1P1 in rings R_1, R_2, or R_3 or an R_1/R_2 ring ratio greater than 2.6 [42]. Also shown are PPVs and NPVs over the plausible range of prevalences the clinician might expect to encounter. As with 10-2 VF, the NPVs are extremely high and the PPVs are rather low, regardless of the prevalence assumed. As with 10-2 VF testing, in these circumstances, a normal mfERG is useful for confirming the absence of 4AQR. The most that a single abnormal mfERG consistent with 4AQR can do is raise the suspicion of 4AQR (increase the posttest probability of 4AQR compared to the pretest probability). With a revised posterior probability of 4AQR, another test should be applied, and if it is also positive, then the second stage posterior probability may indeed be high enough to warrant cessation of the drug. The variability of mfERG testing is too great and the usually applicable pretest probabilities of 4AQR are too low to base decisions to stop therapy on a single abnormal mfERG. The role of this test is to identify risk that should be further assessed with other testing [119].

There are certain clinical situations in which mfERG may be more useful as a means of screening for 4AQR. For example, a patient with a macular epiretinal membrane that affects both the 10-2 VF and SD-OCT can have an mfERG that is relatively unaffected and therefore can be used to follow outer retinal function (Fig. 8.13).

Interpreting the Multifocal Electroretinogram in the Clinic

A broad base of knowledge of the literature is helpful in analyzing an mfERG, but how about a distilled primer on how to do it? The method of interpreting the mfERG depends on whether it is the first or a subsequent study. For the first study, one inspects the waveforms for evidence of 60-cycle noise and for evidence of loss of fixation. Some instruments give an index of reliability of the study (Fig. 8.17). If the study is technically good and the amplitudes and implicit times are in the normal range, the test is read as normal. However, for subsequent studies, the results of the first study must be taken into account. One uses knowledge of the COV and the results of the first study to determine if a change greater than measurement variability has occurred. Therefore, it is possible that on the second and subsequent studies that the absolute measurements fall in the normal range, but evidence of toxicity exists by virtue of a decrease in amplitude or an increase in the R_1/R_2 ratio that exceeds measurement variability [114].

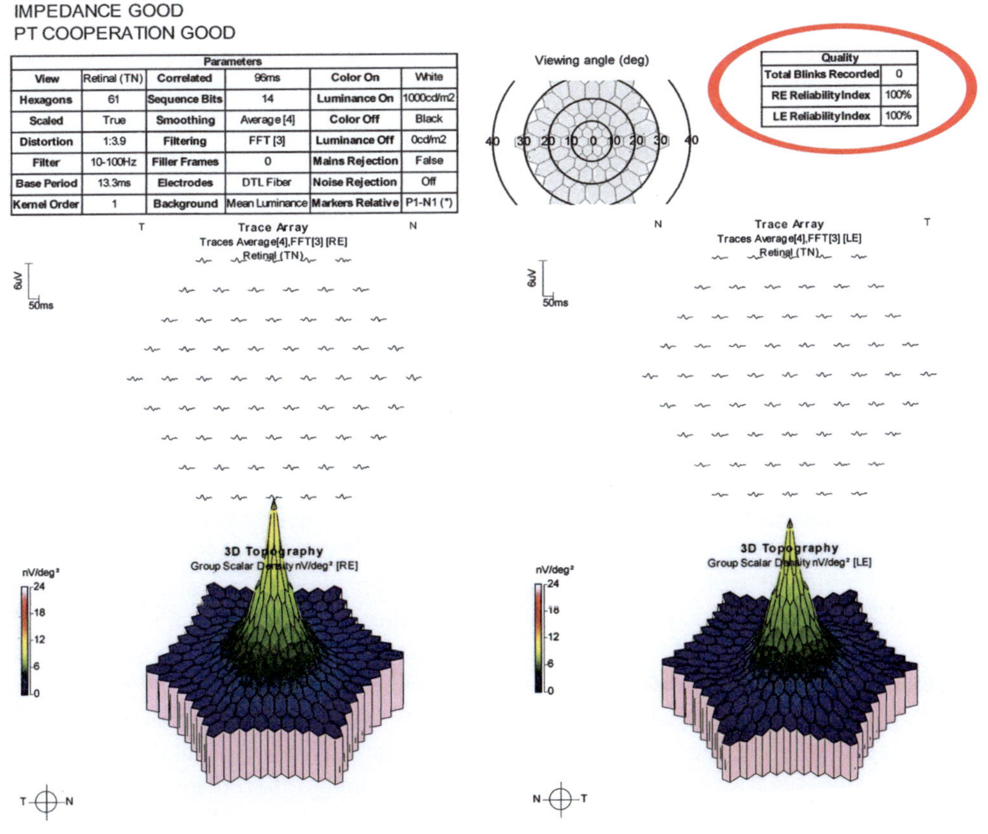

Fig. 8.17 Quality indicators for mfERG. The waveforms do not have 60-cycle noise. The topographic displays show no evidence of fixation loss. The machine determined quality indicators (*red-circled box*) are both 100 %. The technician noted good electrode impedance and patient cooperation

As an example, suppose that the baseline R_1 amplitude was 30 nV/deg^2 and that the COV is 15 %. We do not know where the patient's R_1 amplitude lies in the normal distribution of R_1 amplitudes. In the absence of any other information, the most probable assumption is that it is "average"—that is, to assume that it is the mean value for the population. Because the COV equals the standard deviation divided by the mean value, and because we know that 68.3 % of values lie within one standard deviation of the mean, we deduce that a decrease in amplitude of greater than $0.15 \times 30 = 4.5$ nV/deg^2 would be compatible with measurement error in 31.7 % ($=100 - 68.3$ %) of cases. On the other hand, a decrease in amplitude of greater than two standard deviations, i.e., $2 \times 0.15 \times 30 = 9.0$ nV/deg^2, would be compatible with measurement error in only 5 % of cases. This is a level of improbability at which most clinicians are willing to say a real decrease in R_1 amplitude has occurred—that is, not simply measurement error. We would conclude that there is evidence of 4AQR.

8.6.5 Summarizing the Role of Multifocal Electroretinography in Screening for 4-Aminoquinoline Retinopathy

mfERG as a screening modality for 4AQR is hampered by its high variability and the lack of uniformity in how it is performed and interpreted. The comparison groups used by different investigators are not the same, and the percentages of abnormalities depend on whether one compares to clinic-specific normals, literature normals, instrument-maker databases, age-matched or non age-matched normals, among other choices. Published statements that the "multifocal electroretinogram (mfERG) can be performed in standardized fashion with high sensitivity that has been verified in the literature" do not hold up to critical evaluation [149].

The mfERG has excellent sensitivity, but its specificity is lower than SD-OCT. In a situation of serial screening, reliance on mfERG is therefore saddled with a large number of false positive tests which must be followed with repeated testing leading to rapidly rising expense. For this reason, its blanket use in screening for 4AQ retinopathy is questionable, and selective application based on the clinical context is more prudent [27, 42].

8.7 Spectral Domain Optical Coherence Tomography

SD-OCT allows precise measurements of the macula and its layers (see Chap. 1, Table 1.2). When different observers measure macular thickness or RNFL thickness on the same patients or when the same observers measure the same patients at different times, the mean differences reported have been less than 3μ [150, 151]. Coefficients of variance for measurements of macular thickness and RNFL thickness by SD-OCT are consistently <4 % (Table 8.11). There is less information available regarding the COR for SD-OCT measurements total macular volume, but data from time domain optical coherence tomography measurements imply a value of 3 % of the measurement [152]; the COR for SD-OCT is probably even less.

In one study of SD-OCT in patients taking hydroxychloroquine, those without retinopathy showed thinning of the RNFL nasally compared to normal controls [154]. Thinning of the combined macular RNFL, ganglion cell layer (GCL), and inner plexiform layer (IPL) was present in both patients with advanced 4AQR and in patients taking hydroxychloroquine without retinopathy [154]. Advanced hydroxychloroquine retinopathy showed peripapillary RNFL thinning inferiorly, superiorly, and nasally [154]. A further study by the same investigators to define the affected layers of the inner retina more specifically showed no difference in perifoveal RNFL between patients taking hydroxychloroquine without other evidence of retinopathy compared to normals. However, there was a significant difference noted in the combined GCL + IPL thickness between the hydroxychloroquine group and normal controls [155]. The authors did not comment on the inner segment/outer segment (IS/OS) junction and retinal

Table 8.11 Reproducibility of macular thickness and retinal nerve fiber layer thickness measurements with SD-OCT

Study	Instrument	Macular thickness—intraobserver		Macular thickness—interobserver		Average RNFL—intraobserver		Average RNFL—interobserver	
		COV (%)	COR (µm)	COV (%)	COR (µm)	COV (%)	COR (µm)	COV (%)	COR (µm)
Altemir [65]	Cirrus	0.97	12.01	0.82	10.27	2.24	9.93	2.23	8.22
Menke [153]	Topcon					4.1[a]			9.4
Garcia-Martin [150]	Cirrus	1.2[a]			12.0[b]	4.4			7.5[b]
Menke [151]	Spectralis	0.54							
Wolf-Schnurrbus [63]	RTVue	2.77							
	Copernicus	3.50							
Ibrahim [212]	Stratus		17						
	Spectralis		5						
Hirasawa [213]	Topcon							1.7	2
Leung [214]	Topcon	0.9	6.3						
	Stratus	1.7	12.2						

[a]Average of intraobserver COV for two observers [150]
[b]Estimated from Fig. 2 of Garcia-Martin

pigment epithelial (RPE) changes in their patients with thinning of the GCL + IPL and funduscopic changes of 4AQR [154]. As with hydroxychloroquine retinopathy, chloroquine retinopathy is associated with a reduction in RNFL [38, 156]. Although measurements of RNFL thickness measured by SD-OCT can show differences across groups (e.g., normal subjects and patients with 4AQR), the author's experience has been that RNFL thickness measured by SD-OCT in an individual patient is an insensitive indicator of hydroxychloroquine retinopathy (Fig. 8.18). The overlap between normal subjects and patients with 4AQR is too large to allow clinically important discrimination. On the other hand, a series of studies that shows progressive thinning of the perifoveal can indicate 4AQR even before loss of the IS/OS junction (Fig. 8.19).

In other studies, SD-OCT findings in 4AQR include reduced thickness of the perifoveal outer nuclear layer and loss of the perifoveal cone outer segment tips (COST) and inner segment/outer segment (IS/OS) junction [32, 50, 146, 157–159]. Which change is the earliest has not been established with certainty, but thinning of the perifoveal outer nuclear layer thickness is a leading candidate [32, 160]. Although histopathology indicates that GCL effects occur early in toxicity (see Chap. 3), these changes are difficult to

appreciate in clinical SD-OCTs although their effects can be seen in averages taken over groups rather than in individual cases [154]. Because there are few data published on normal outer nuclear layer thickness by SD-OCT, it is unknown whether these observations are reproducible. In more advanced disease the central retinal structures are also damaged [159]. Examples of SD-OCT changes in 4AQR at different stages are shown in Fig. 8.20.

Although advanced cases of 4AQR are recognizable on TD-OCT, which shows loss of RPE, macular thinning, and increased perifoveal choroidal reflectivity, more subtle findings such as loss of the IS/OS junction can be missed [50, 117, 159, 161, 162].

Table 8.12 shows the sensitivity and specificity of SD-OCT based on a definition of loss of perifoveal IS/OS junction and RPE continuity [42]. Also shown are PPVs and NPVs over the plausible range of prevalences the clinician might expect to encounter. As with 10-2 VF, the NPVs are extremely high, regardless of the prevalence assumed. However, the PPVs are higher than for 10-2 VF and mfERG testing. In these circumstances, as was the case with the 10-2 VF and mfERG, a normal SD-OCT is useful for confirming the absence of 4AQR. However, in some contrast to 10-2 VF and mfERG testing, a single

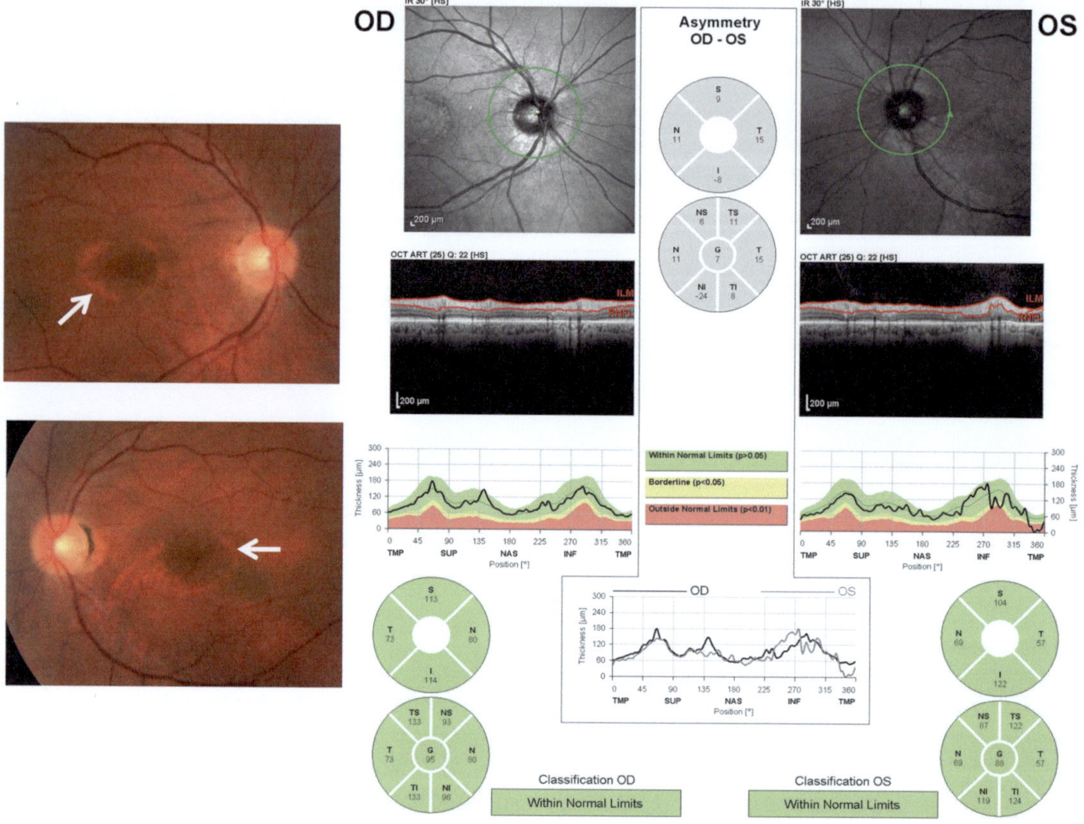

Fig. 8.18 This 60-year-old woman with rheumatoid arthritis had taken 400 mg/day of hydroxychloroquine from 1971 until 2000 when retinopathy was diagnosed and her medication stopped. When examined in 2012, both eyes showed a bull's-eye maculopathy (*left panel*, *white arrows*), yet her RNFL as measured with the Spectralis SD-OCT instrument was of normal thickness in all sectors bilaterally. The globally averaged nerve fiber layer thickness was 95 μm on the *right* and 88 μm on the *left* (*right panel*). Her 10-2 visual fields, macular SD-OCT line scans, FAF images, and multifocal electroretinograms were abnormal and typical for hydroxychloroquine retinopathy bilaterally (not shown)

abnormal SD-OCT consistent with 4AQR can do quite a lot to raise the suspicion of 4AQR, increasing the posttest probability above 60 % for plausibly low pretest probabilities. The variability of SD-OCT testing is so low, that it is probably the test of choice to follow a suspicious 10-2 VF or mfERG, and is an excellent first choice as an ancillary test [42].

Of the four ancillary tests currently considered to have high value in assessing presence or absence of 4AQ retinopathy, SD-OCT is the most reproducible and surpasses that of mfERG, 10-2 VF, and FAF testing [23, 42, 59, 63]. Together with sensitivity that approximates that of mfERG and 10-2 VF testing and superior specificity, the SD-OCT is probably more valuable than mfERG or FAF as an ancillary test to supplement the time-tested 10-2 VF.

8.8   Fundus Autofluorescence

Autofluorescence of the retinal pigment epithelium (RPE) arises from lipofuscin deposition in these cells secondary to their phagocytosis of photoreceptor outer segments (see Chap. 1) [156, 163]. Hyperautofluorescence is noted when an increased amount of lipofuscin is present in the

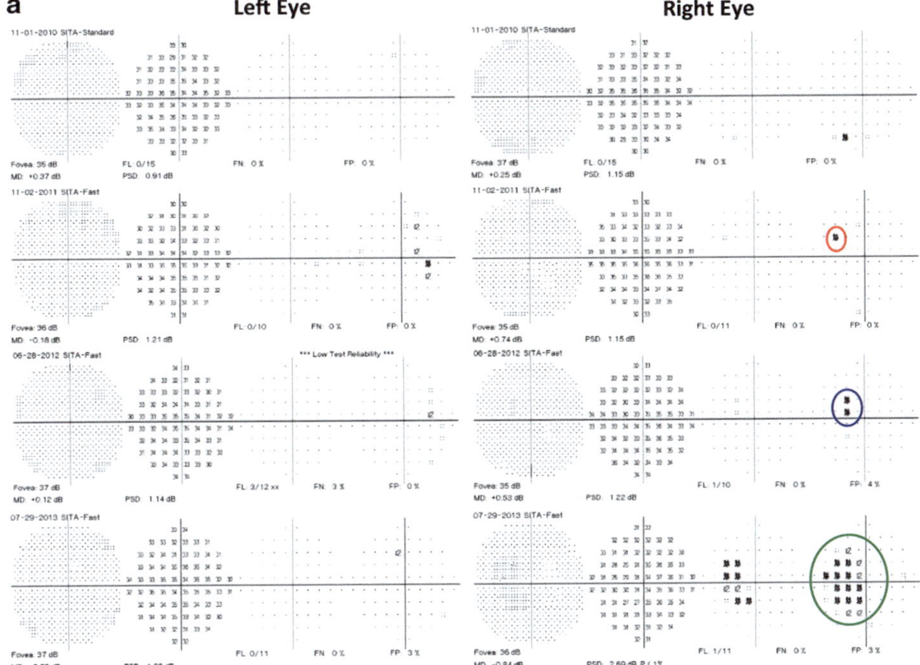

Fig. 8.19 A 61-year-old woman with SLE had been on hydroxychloroquine for 20 years. For 19 of those years she had been on 400 mg/day, but for the last year had been on 371 mg/day (400 mg/d for Monday through Saturday and 200 mg/day on Sunday). She was 62 in. tall and weighed 155 lb, but her weight fluctuated and had been as low as 120 lb for a year's duration. She reported renal disease from her lupus but did not know her serum creatinine. She denied liver disease. She had no preexisting maculopathy. Her optometrist had followed her with yearly 10-2 visual fields (10-2 VFs) and since the revised American Academy of Ophthalmology screening guidelines of 2011 with SD-OCT and since 2012 with mfERG. (**a**) All four 10-2 VFs of the left eye are normal. The 10-2 VF of the right eye from 1 November 2010 shows an isolated paracentral scotoma but at the follow-up 10-2 VF of 2 November 2011 that scotoma has resolved, but a new one (*circled in red*) has appeared. The follow-up 10-2 VF of 28 June 2012 is contiguous with the *red circled* one, and is larger, raising suspicion of retinopathy. The repeat 10-2 VF of 29 July 2013 is in the same location and larger indicating unequivocal retinopathy. (**b**) An mfERG from 28 June 2011 shows low amplitudes of the right eye for rings R_1 and R_2 (*circled red*) and of the left eye for rings R_1, R_2, and R_3 (*circled green*). The averaged waveforms for rings R_1 and R_2 in the right eye (*blue arrows*) and left eye (*green arrows*) are abnormal and there are flat waveforms in individual hexagons in each eye (*circled orange*). (**c**) An mfERG from 10 January 2013 has normal amplitudes of the ring averaged waveforms for R_1 and R_2 in right (*circled red*) and left (circled *green*) eyes. Such variability (compared to the previous mfERG) is common in mfERGs. The morphology of the ring averaged waveforms of the right eye is normal (*red arrows*). The morphology of the ring averaged waveform for R_1 of the left eye is still abnormal. Waveforms in individual hexagons are flat, but they are in different hexagons compared to the earlier study. (**d**) An mfERG from 28 July 2013 has low amplitudes for the ring averaged waveforms of R_1, R_2, and R_3 (*circled red*) of the right eye, but not the left eye. Waveforms from isolated hexagons in each eye are flat (*circled orange*). The variability of mfERG testing is highlighted. (**e**) False color maps of the macular SD-OCT show progressive perifoveal thinning of both maculas. Red sectors are in the bottom 1 % of expected sector thicknesses based on normals. Note that the inner superior sector thinned from 287 µm on 2 November 2011 to 278 µm on 28 June 2012 (*black arrow*) and that the outer temporal sector thinned from 235 µm on 28 June 2012 to 219 µm on 29 July 2013 (*dashed black arrow*). Similar changes occurred in the left eye (*solid* and *dashed blue arrows*). The "spread of red" captures the gestalt of progressive thinning over time in both eyes. (**f**) SD-OCT line scans show morphologic changes consistent with hydroxychloroquine retinopathy later than the false color map changes. The first unequivocal change is in the right eye at the 29 July 2013 study. The inner segment/outer segment junction is lost at the *yellow arrow*, and the outer nuclear layer thins (*orange arrow*). At this time the morphology of the SD-OCT line scans of the left eye is normal. (**g**) Simultaneously the fundus pictures are normal in both eyes. Fundus changes are late in hydroxychloroquine retinopathy. The *white arrows* indicate out-of-focus asteroid hyalosis particles in the vitreous. The fluorescein angiogram of the left eye is normal, but the right eye shows a window hyperfluorescent abnormality (*yellow arrows*) in the location that corresponds with the SD-OCT and 10-2 VF changes. (**h**) Simultaneous FAF photography of the right macula shows hyperautofluorescence (*white arrows*) in the location found to be abnormal on SD-OCT and corresponding to the 10-2 VF defect. FAF photography of the left eye is normal. To summarize the relative sensitivity and variability of the tests in this case, false color mapping on SD-OCT was the earliest so-called objective test abnormality with the morphologic line scan changes occurring later. The mfERG was too variable to bear much clinical decision-making weight. The 10-2 VF was equally sensitive to SD-OCT in showing a problem. The fluorescein abnormality was less extensive than the other abnormalities and the fundus photographs were normal. The patient was advised to discontinue her hydroxychloroquine

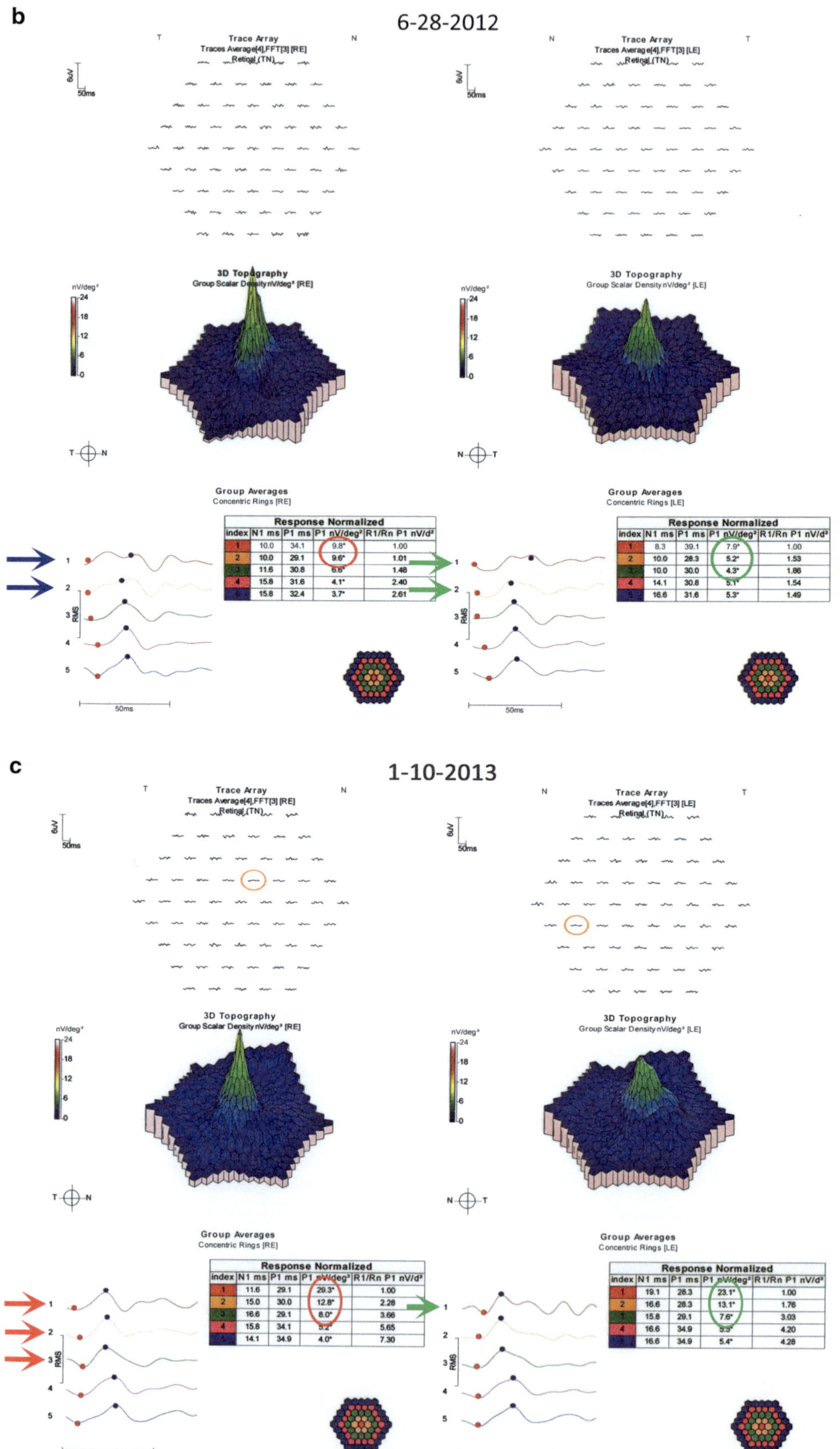

Fig. 8.19 (continued)

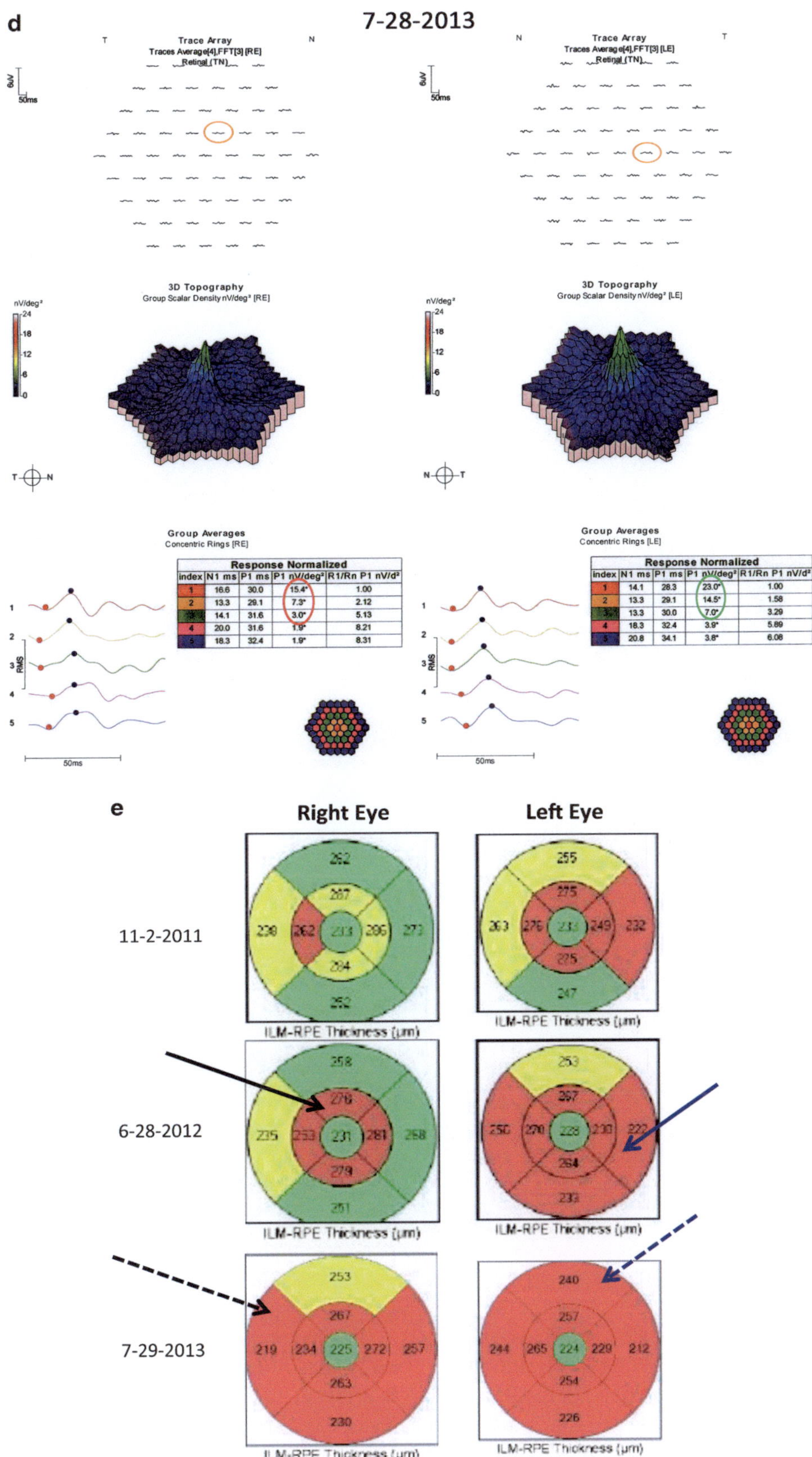

Right Eye — Response Normalized [RE]

index	N1 ms	P1 ms	P1 nV/deg²	R1/Rn P1 nV/d²
1	16.6	30.0	15.4*	1.00
2	13.3	29.1	7.3*	2.12
3	14.1	31.6	3.0*	5.13
4	20.0	31.6	1.9*	8.21
5	18.3	32.4	1.9*	8.31

Left Eye — Response Normalized [LE]

index	N1 ms	P1 ms	P1 nV/deg²	R1/Rn P1 nV/d²
1	14.1	28.3	23.0*	1.00
2	13.3	29.1	14.5*	1.58
3	13.3	30.0	7.0*	3.29
4	18.3	32.4	3.9*	5.89
5	20.8	34.1	3.8*	6.08

Fig. 8.19 (continued)

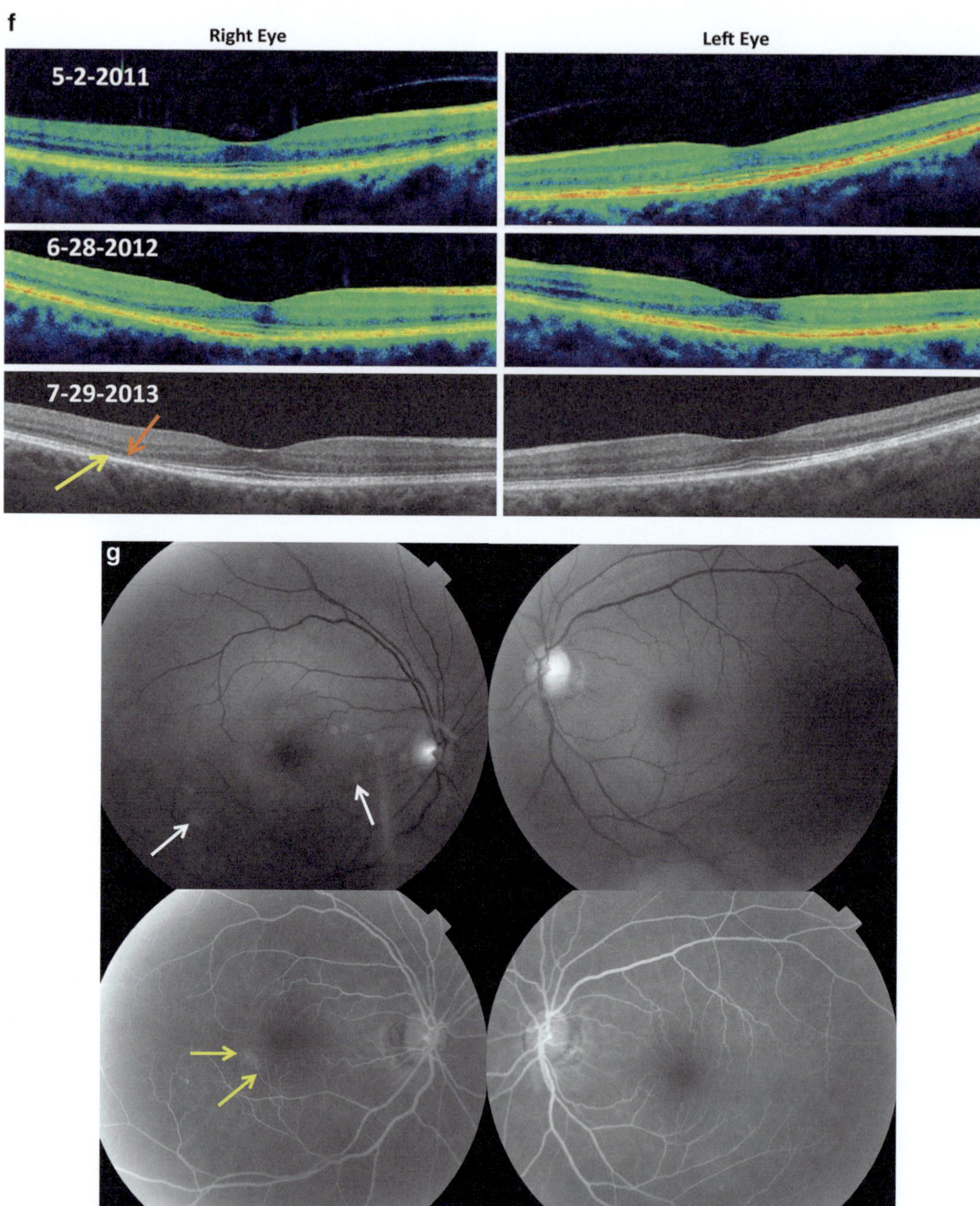

Fig. 8.19 (continued)

RPE. Hypoautofluorescence implies loss of RPE and overlying photoreceptors [138, 156, 164]. Retinal regions with increased lipofuscin appear hyperautofluorescent (a whiter color) and areas of RPE atrophy appear hypoautofluorescent (a darker color).

The membranous bodies found in pathological studies of animal models of 4AQR are autofluorescent, and may provide a link between microscopic and clinical observations (see Chap. 3) [165]. The changes in autofluorescence described in 4AQR are not specific for these diseases, but

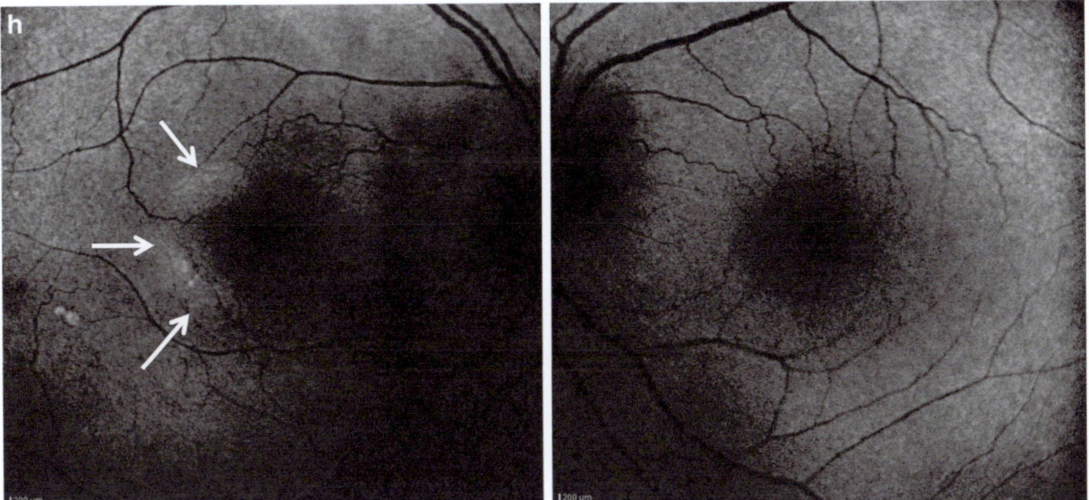

Fig. 8.19 (continued)

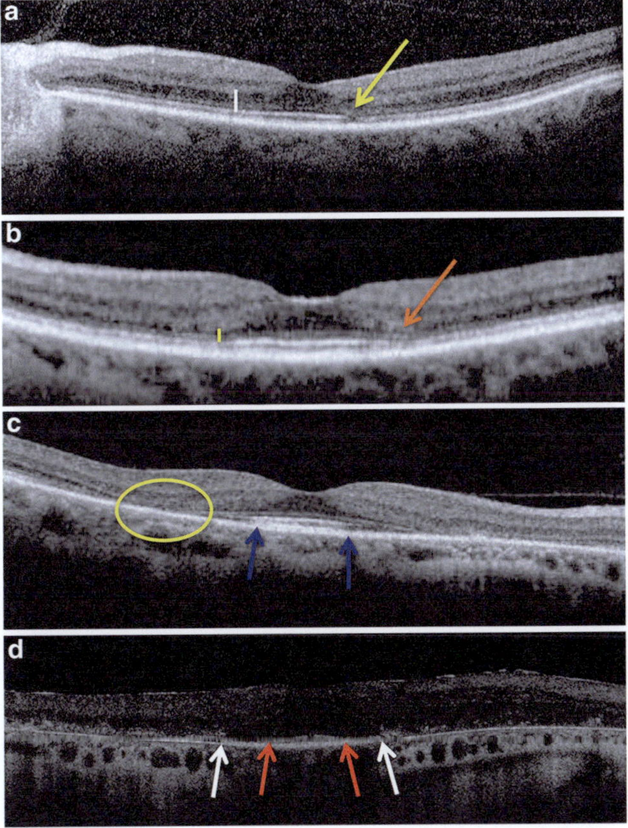

Fig. 8.20 Stages of 4AQR as reflected in spectral domain optical coherence tomography. (**a**) Early retinopathy manifests an attenuation of the temporal parafoveal inner segment/outer segment (IS/OS) junction (*yellow arrow*) and a thinned but present outer nuclear layer (*white bar*). The external limiting membrane is continuously present across the macula. (**b**) Slightly more advanced retinopathy shows attenuation of the IS/OS junction both nasally and temporally (*orange arrow*) and more thinning of the outer nuclear layer (*yellow bar*). The external limiting membrane is still continuous across the macula. (**c**) In even more advanced retinopathy the IS/OS junction, the external limiting membrane, and the outer nuclear layer have all been lost parafoveally (*yellow-circled zone*). Foveal IS/OS junction and retinal pigment epithelium (RPE) are coterminous where they stop (*blue arrows*). (**d**) In advanced retinopathy, the outer nuclear layer, external limiting membrane, IS/OS junction, and RPE have been lost more peripherally than the *white arrows*. The IS/OS junction has been lost more peripherally than the *red arrows*

are characteristic [156]. The regional abnormalities in autofluorescence usually mirror the locations of abnormalities in the mfERG and 10-2 VF [156].

FAF may be recorded with confocal scanning laser ophthalmoscopy (SLO) or by fundus photography using a camera fitted with special filters that excites with a green wavelength and records in the yellow-orange band of the spectrum. Instruments that use the first technique include the Heidelberg Retinal Angiograph and the Optos OCT SLO which use blue and green light, respectively. The confocal SLO technique has the advantage of isolating FAF from a single plane (e.g., the retina) and excluding signals from the lens. The fundus camera-based system sums fluorescence from many different planes simultaneously.

Two types of FAF are used in clinical studies. Melanin-related near-infrared autofluorescence imaging becomes apparent when an exciting light of wavelength 787 nm is shone on the fundus [156]. This leads to emission of radiation of wavelength 820 nm. Near-infrared autofluorescence images normally exhibit the greatest autofluorescence under the fovea with drop-off in the perifoveal region. On the other hand, lipofuscin-related FAF involves an exciting light of wavelength 488 nm with emitted radiation of wavelength greater than 500 nm [156]. Images of normal eyes show reduced autofluorescence in the fovea, greater amounts in the perifoveal region, and lesser amounts under the vascular arcades [156]. Both types of FAF imaging can be obtained with the Heidelberg Retinal Angiograph [32, 156].

The area of autofluorescence is larger than the area of funduscopic pigmentary change when both are present (Fig. 8.21) [138]. In patients with more advanced stages of FAF abnormalities,

Table 8.12 Positive and negative predictive values for spectral domain optical coherence tomography testing over a plausible range of assumed prevalences of 4AQR

Assumed prevalence (%)	Sensitivity (%)	Specificity (%)	PPV (%)	NPV (%)
0.1	78.6	98.1	4	100
1	78.6	98.1	29.5	99.8
3	78.6	98.1	56.1	99.3
5	78.6	98.1	68.5	98.9

Sensitivity and specificity are from Browning and Lee [42]. *PPV* is positive predictive value. *NPV* is negative predictive value

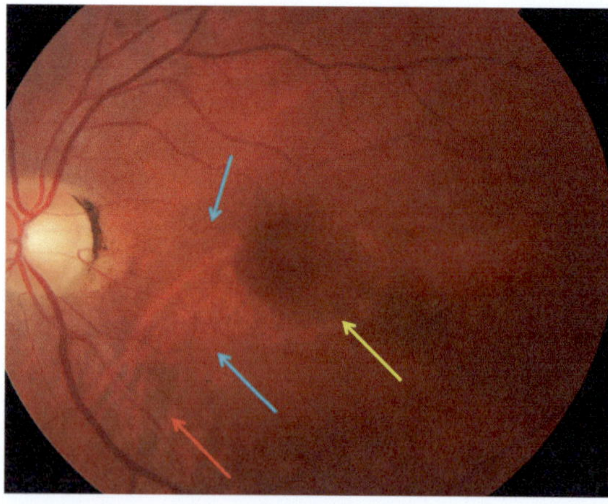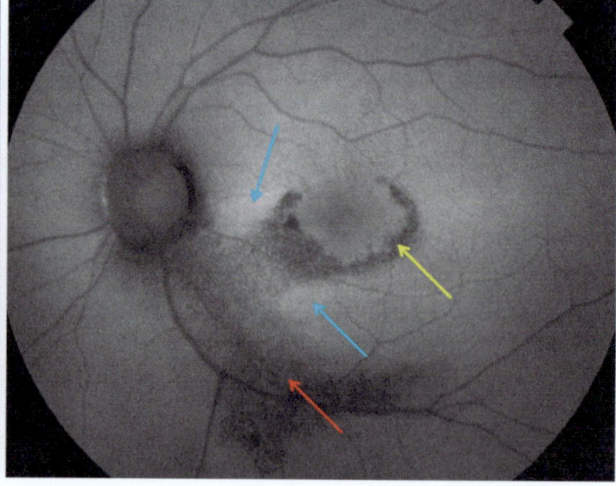

Fig. 8.21 These are fundus images of a 45-year-old woman with rheumatoid arthritis who had taken hydroxychloroquine for 20 years at a dosage of 400 mg/day. Based on her actual body weight, which was ideal, she had been overdosed at 6.9 mg/kg/day and had received a cumulative dose of 2,920 g of hydroxychloroquine. Comparison of her color fundus photograph (*left panel*) and FAF image (*right panel*) shows that FAF imaging is more sensitive. The RPE atrophic annulus can be seen in both images (*yellow arrows*). However, the hyperautofluorescent zones adjacent to the RPE atrophic areas (*blue arrows*) have no fundus photographic correlate. In addition, the area of more peripheral retinal atrophy that is clearly seen in the fundus autofluorescent image (*red arrow*) is more difficult to appreciate in the fundus photograph (*red arrow*)

progression of FAF changes has been noted after the 4AQ has been stopped, but the methods of judging borders of hyperfluorescence versus normal fluorescence involve freehand drawing, and are subjective [88, 138].

FAF has been reported to be less sensitive than mfERG and SD-OCT, and opinion pieces have echoed this view, but there are few data to support the suggestion [138, 146]. Although FAF is labeled as an objective test, its interpretation is subjective. As an example, certain examples of perifoveal hyperautofluorescence attributed to early hydroxychloroquine retinopathy could be interpreted otherwise (cf. Fig. 2 of Labriola et al. [166]). FAF has been reported to be more sensitive than funduscopy, but no color fundus photographs were published to allow more meticulous investigation of the claim [167].

Clinicians have been slow to adopt FAF for 4AQR screening despite advocacy by professional governing bodies [26, 27]. Although the reasons are unclear, it may reflect the subjectivity of interpreting the test and lack of information regarding sensitivity and specificity [27].

8.9   Fluorescein Angiography

Hydroxychloroquine and chloroquine retinopathy cause a bull's-eye hyperfluorescence in the early phases of the of the fluorescein angiogram (FA) with no late leakage (Fig. 8.22) [168, 169]. Although originally attributed to depigmentation of the RPE, later studies, including correlations with SD-OCT, show that the bull's-eye arises from a ring of RPE atrophy [168]. No large series have compared the relative sensitivity of FA to other ancillary screening tests. One study of the Kodachrome slide photography of 83 patients taking chloroquine found that FA was less sensitive than color fundus photography [22]. However, case reports of the reverse exist in which no color fundus photographic changes were present, but window hyperfluorescent defects were [80]. An unverified anecdotal remark is that FA is more useful in blonde fundi than darkly pigmented ones [43]. Another study reported that it was possible to have funduscopic

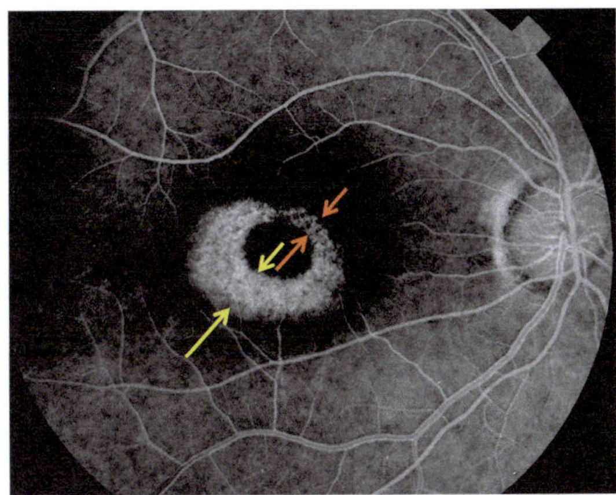

Fig. 8.22 Frame from the mid-phase fluorescein angiogram of the right eye of a patient with hydroxychloroquine retinopathy. The lesion is characterized by window-type hyperfluorescence. There is no late leakage. The depicted lesion shows the typical broader inferotemporal part of the annulus (compare *yellow arrows* to *orange arrows*)

changes without FA changes especially in patients with darkly pigmented fundi, which would be consistent with the statement that funduscopy is a more sensitive test than FA for detecting 4AQR [43].

An assertion has been published that FA is "almost always positive in the presence of a symptomatic scotoma," but no evidence exists to support the claim, and the author's personal experience is that the statement is false. The lack of sensitivity of FA relative to PHP has been reported in a series of nine cases [51]. FA changes are considered to be a less sensitive but more specific test for 4AQR than static perimetry [14, 170]. Fluorescein angiography is not a routine component of screening for 4AQR [25].

8.10   Amsler Grid

Screening strategies throughout medicine often feature a highly sensitive screening test that is inexpensive followed by a more specific test that is more expensive. Of the screening tests currently recommended for hydroxychloroquine retinopathy screening, none is inexpensive and none has a clearly superior sensitivity; therefore this strategy cannot be employed.

Table 8.13 Performance characteristics of versions of the Amsler grid

Study	Amsler grid test version	Gold standard for study	Number of eyes with scotomas present	Number of eyes with no scotomas present	Sensitivity (%)	Specificity (%)
Morin [177]	Standard	Static perimetry	27	NG	70	NG
Almony [17]	Standard	NG	2	54	3.6	NG
	Red	NG	5	51	8.9	NG
	Threshold	NG	25	31	45	NG
Grierson [21]	Red	Synthesis of all evidence	10	748	Unable to determine	98.7
Schuchard [179]	Standard using TA-300	SLO fundus perimetry	89	21	59.6	95.2
	Standard using SLO Amsler grid	SLO fundus perimetry	89	21	62.9	85.7
	Threshold using TA-300	SLO fundus perimetry	102	8	55.9	87.5
	Threshold using SLO Amsler grid	SLO fundus perimetry	102	8	60.8	100

SLO is scanning laser ophthalmoscope. TA-300 is Stereo Optical Corporation threshold Amsler grid system. Unable to determine means that no cases of retinopathy were detected, so sensitivity could not be calculated

However, there are many who have recommended use of the Amsler grid test, because it is inexpensive and adapted for regular use at home [4, 18, 29, 46, 100, 171–176]. Amsler grid testing was a recommended screening test in the 2002 version of the American Academy of Ophthalmology guidelines for hydroxychloroquine [25]. Unfortunately, as its poor sensitivity and specificity became known, it fell out of favor (Table 8.10) [83]. Its sensitivity is at best 69 % with cases reported in which it fails to show an abnormality despite a bull's-eye maculopathy [4, 177]. Its specificity has been reported to be 85–100 % [17, 21, 178, 179]. In the 2011 version of the American Academy of Ophthalmology guidelines for screening its use was not recommended because of these poor performance characteristics. Interestingly, the newly recommended screening tests (10-2 VF, mfERG, SD-OCT, and FAF) supplanting the Amsler grid had no published data on performance characteristics at the time [78, 87].

There are many versions of the Amsler grid test with different sensitivities and specificities (Table 8.13). There are advocates for each version [17, 100, 175]. The most common form of the grid involves a grid spanning 10 deg from

Table 8.14 Positive and negative predictive values for Amsler grid testing over a plausible range of assumed prevalences of 4AQR

Assumed prevalence (%)	Sensitivity (%)	Specificity (%)	PPV (%)	NPV (%)
0.1	70	98.7	5	100
1	70	98.7	35.2	99.7
3	70	98.7	62.5	99.1
5	70	98.7	73.9	98.4

Sensitivity and specificity are from Browning and Lee [42]. *PPV* is positive predictive value. *NPV* is negative predictive value

fixation when held at 14 in. Each square represents 1 deg of field. A total of 20 deg of central visual field is spanned [67, p. 34]. Usage of threshold Amsler grid testing with cross-polarizing filters may show larger size relative scotomas in approximately 13 % of patients tested [175]. There continue to be clinicians who use Amsler grid testing not so much because of its efficacy, but as part of an informed consent process [19, 180].

Table 8.14 shows the PPVs and NPVs for the Amsler grid using published sensitivity and specificity and a range of plausible prevalences.

As with the other ancillary tests, the NPVs are extremely high, regardless of the prevalence assumed. Therefore, a normal Amsler grid in a patient who can do the test and who has a low pretest probability of having 4AQR is reassuring that no retinopathy is present, and in such a situation no further testing is necessary. The PPVs are higher than for 10-2 VF and mfERG testing, but are suspect because the published performance characteristics upon which they are based are so variable. In these circumstances, the cost of the test becomes a factor. Amsler grid testing is inexpensive, and if positive, usefully increases a pretest probability that in turn may be used in applying an expensive and more reliable ancillary test such as SD-OCT. For patients who can use an Amsler grid, it is a useful test. However, many patients cannot use it and its variability is too high to make it the workhorse of a screening program.

8.11 Electrooculogram

In the electrooculogram (EOG), electrodes are connected at the inner and outer canthi and a ground electrode is attached to the ear or forehead. Voltages generated by the RPE are measured under conditions of dark adaptation and light adaptation [13, 15]. The cornea has a positive voltage relative to the RPE [181]. Basal RPE membrane permeability changes are responsible for the corneo-fundal potential difference [181]. A period of dark adaptation of 12–15 min leads to a recording of the trough value of the voltage between the electrodes [13]. Illumination is then increased and the light rise in the voltage measured is recorded. The light peak/dark trough ratio (Arden ratio) is calculated [182]. The test is done with dilated pupils [181]. The electrooculogram is hindered by both high intrasubject and intersubject variability [14, 183, 184].

The choice of the control group is important in EOG testing because some investigators have reported that autoimmune diseases cause the EOG to be reduced apart from taking 4AQs [9, 14, 183, 185]. However, not all have agreed [182, 184]. If the effect is real, the proper control group should be patients with rheumatologic disease not taking 4AQs rather than normal subjects. Some studies fail to observe this nuance [13, 186]. In one study, no difference was observed between patients taking hydroxychloroquine and normal subjects used as controls [13]. Conceivably, the underlying disease and the ingestion of hydroxychloroquine could have had canceling effects on the EOG. The disease could have caused the Arden ratio to increase by improving the RA but the hydroxychloroquine could have decreased the Arden ratio as a toxic effect [183].

All 4AQs have similar effects on the EOG, but they have been inconsistent [184]. In some reports the Arden ratio is decreased as soon as chloroquine is begun and generally begins to increase when chloroquine is stopped, returning to normal values in most cases within 9 months [8, 110, 186]. In other reports, chloroquine use in patients without retinopathy has not caused abnormalities in the EOG [15]. In rare cases in which both EOG and mfERG have been obtained, the EOG Arden ratio has decreased before the mfERG changes [110]. When changes in the EOG have been observed, duration of therapy with 4AQs has not influenced the decrease in the Arden ratio [184].

Many patients with mild chloroquine retinopathy have a normal EOG [15]. The lower limit of normal for the Arden ratio is 1.85, but a sufficiently large number of normal subjects not taking these drugs fall below this threshold to make it a poor discriminator of toxicity [5, 182, 186]. Not all authors agree with the choice of lower limit of normal. Some prefer 1.60, 1.70, or 1.80 as cut-points for abnormal [7, 8, 13, 34]. The variability of the EOG makes detection of 4AQR uncertain. Reported standard deviations of 0.2 in EOG testing suggest that a change in Arden ratio of 0.4 would be required to conclude that a true change in EOG had occurred [13]. Various investigators have arbitrarily chosen 15–30 % as the minimum decrease in the Arden ratio required to be considered a real change and not noise [5, 34]. A dual EOG criterion for retinopathy has been suggested—both a 15 % decline in the Arden ratio and a value less than 1.85 [5]. Even with

Table 8.15 Performance characteristics of the electrooculogram in screening for 4AQR

Study	Arden ratio cut-point for abnormal	Stage of retinopathy	Sensitivity (%)	Specificity (%)
Neubauer [34]	1.80	Mild	61	54
	1.60	Mild	32	82
	1.80	Advanced	50	54
	1.60	Advanced	50	82
Gouras [15]	1.80	Advanced	100	NG
	1.80	Mild	10	NG
Albert [1]	Review of pooled studies (NG)	Review of pooled studies (NG)	50	100

these more stringent criteria an 11 % false positive rate was reported in a study in which the gold standard for retinopathy was presence of a paracentral scotoma to tangent screen testing with a red test object [5]. Given the intrapatient variability, the preferred method of using the EOG is to take serial measurements [184].

In general, eye signs of 4AQR have not correlated well with the effects on the EOG [14, 46, 184]. Because the instrument is not widely available, and is variable and insensitive and nonspecific for 4AQR (Table 8.15), its use for screening has been abandoned in practice [7, 11, 25, 34].

Besides the use of EOG as a screening test, others have suggested that it is useful for predicting progression of retinopathy once 4AQs are discontinued [187]. Sparse evidence was adduced that a reduced Arden ratio at the time of discontinuation was predictive of progression of retinopathy [187]. To summarize, in 2014 the EOG is not used to screen for 4AQR or predict its probability of progression [178].

8.12 Global and Focal Electroretinography

In the global electroretinogram (ERG) the initial negative a-wave arises from hyperpolarization of photoreceptors. The b-wave arises from depolarization of proximal Muller cells processes and from on-bipolar cells. Oscillatory potentials derive from amacrine and bipolar cells of the inner retina [188]. The global ERG is hampered by high variability. Coefficients of repeatability

for various components of the global ERG in normal controls were measured by Birch and colleagues, who showed that the rod a-wave amplitude would have to change from baseline by 23 % to have 95 % confidence that a change had occurred (i.e., COR = 11.7 %). For the cone a-wave the necessary change was 37 %. For the rod b-wave amplitudes, the necessary change ranged from 46 to 51 % and for the cone b-wave the necessary change ranged from 35 to 55 %. The flicker fusion b-wave amplitude must change by 37 % for the clinician to be 95 % confident that the change is other than noise [189].

Although in animal experiments with rats and cats, ERG amplitudes decrease with increasing chloroquine doses, in a rhesus monkey model of chloroquine retinopathy, there was no global ERG effect despite clear histopathological changes [190]. In clinical practice global electroretinography is insensitive to 4AQR [2, 7, 43, 191, 192]. Many clinical cases have been reported with normal ERGs [2, 5, 8, 148]. In Marmor's series, 33 % of cases of definite retinopathy had normal global ERGs [146]. The global ERG can show abnormalities at a time when the visual acuity is normal, but usually shows changes only after the onset of paracentral scotomas to SAP [43, 92, 99, 193].

In cases of 4AQR with abnormal ERGs, the earliest effects are a decreased amplitude and increased implicit time of oscillatory potentials and an increase in the a-wave amplitude, followed by a decreased amplitude of both a- and b-waves at a slightly more advanced stage of retinopathy, and ultimately by extinction of both a- and b-waves and a retinitis pigmentosa-like result in extremely advanced retinopathy [7, 8, 43, 80, 194, 195]. The implicit time changes generally follow the amplitude effects [16]. Decreased amplitude of oscillatory potentials in patients taking 4AQs suggests inner retinal effects of these drugs [195]. Preferential loss of rod function compared to cone function has been described [92].

Focal electroretinograms have been reported to be abnormal in some cases of 4AQR, but are rarely done [80]. To summarize, the global and focal ERG are not useful tests in screening for 4AQR [11, 14, 16, 25, 44, 46, 195].

8.13 Color Vision Testing

Color vision testing can be performed with Ishihara plates, Hardy–Rand–Rittler (HRR) plates, the Farnsworth D-15 test, the Standard Pseudoisochromatic Plates-Part 2 (SPP-2), the City University (CU) color vision test, or with a computerized color vision test as described by Arden [34]. Eyes with earlier retinopathy, having relative scotomas and better visual acuity, have a higher proportion of tritan (blue-yellow) defects [34, 53, 97, 196]. Later, a protan (red-green) defect predominates in eyes with deeper scotomas and worse visual acuity [53, 173]. Tests designed to detect congenital red-green color abnormalities will be relatively insensitive for the detection of retinopathy [53]. Despite evidence that red-green errors occur later in the disease, approximately 63 % of ophthalmologists who screen for color vision deficits use the Ishihara plates [29, 85, 178].

A problem with color vision testing is that it is not standardized and is therefore poorly reproducible. For example, some clinicians score the Ishihara plate test dichotomously using different numbers of plates for cut-points [53]. Others use an informal method described as an assessment of whether the patient can recognize the plates as quickly as the examiner [197]. This may explain why some clinicians find it sensitive and valuable [2, 4, 173, 197–199], but many do not [7, 20, 26, 46, 170, 171, 200]. Moreover, common comorbidities such as cataract can confound color vision testing especially in the tritan axis, the axis affected by early 4AQR [53].

Many patients have normal color vision to conventional testing when they show clear toxicity by SAP and mfERG [23, 78, 83, 117]. From 14.3 to 22.3 % of patients with some degree of retinopathy have normal color vision [201, 202]. Even patients with advanced retinopathy and absolute scotomas can have normal color vision [46]. The scant data that has been published on the performance characteristics of color vision testing is reproduced in Table 8.16. When these sensitivities and specificities are applied to a plausible range of prior probabilities (0.1–5 %) for a patient to have 4AQR, the resulting PPVs do not exceed 36 % for any of the tests and the NPVs do not fall below 95 %. As a result, color vision tests alone rarely change clinical decision-making. A positive test will almost never be sufficient evidence alone to stop a patient's 4AQ and a normal test does nothing to alter a typically high pretest probability that 4AQR is not present. Color vision testing has been suggested as having prognostic value even if it does not have screening value. Supposedly, when color vision is affected, the prognosis is graver [6]. Few data exist to test this hypothesis.

To summarize, testing color vision is an insensitive method to screen for 4AQR and is not recommended although many clinicians continue to do so out of training and habit [2, 5, 11, 25, 46, 178, 202, 203].

8.14 Scanning Laser Polarimetry

The nerve fiber layer of the retina contains structures such as microtubules that are smaller than the wavelength of illuminating light. These structures retard the polarization of laser light that passes through the retina. The retardation is related to the thickness of the nerve fiber layer. Therefore by measuring the retardation of the polarization, it is possible to measure the RNFL thickness. The GDx-Nerve Fiber Layer Analyzer is one such commercially available instrument composed of a confocal scanning laser ophthalmoscope with an integrated polarization modulator.

Table 8.16 Performance characteristics of color vision tests

Color vision test	Cut-point for abnormality	Drug/stage of retinopathy	Sensitivity (%)	Specificity (%)
Ishihara[a]	≥5 Errors	C/Pooled early and advanced	43.3	96
SPP-2[a]	If age 20–60, any BY or RG error; if ≥60 years, ≥2 BY errors or ≥2 RG errors	C/Pooled early and advanced	93.3	88
D-15 [53]	≥2 Major crossings	C/Pooled early and advanced	16.7	96
Dsat-15 [53]	≥2 Major crossings	C/Pooled early and advanced	33.3	84
CU [53]	≥2 Errors on the chroma 4 plates or ≥1 error on the chroma 2 plates	C/Pooled early and advanced	20	92
AO HRR [53]	Any error on the screening plates supported by similar errors on the diagnostic plates	C/Pooled early and advanced	76.7	88
Computerized color vision test of Arden [34]	Protan axis abnormal	Both/mild	22	88
	Protan axis abnormal	Advanced	75	88
	Tritan axis abnormal	Mild	60	67
	Tritan axis abnormal	Advanced	100	67

BY means blue-yellow. RG means red-green. In data from Vu, the gold standard was bilateral irreversible and reproducible scotomas on both Amsler's grid and 10-2VF with fundus changes of RPE mottling or a bull's-eye maculopathy [53]. In data from Neubauer, mild retinopathy was defined as pigmentary macular changes without visual field defects; advanced retinopathy was defined as bull's-eye maculopathy with reproducible visual field defects [34]

There are two versions of the instrument—one with a fixed corneal compensator and one with a variable corneal compensator. The operator manually outlines the outer margin of the optic disc. From this outline a concentric band is drawn by the machine at 1.75 disc diameters from the center of the optic disc. Measurements are grouped into superior and inferior segments subtending 120 deg, a temporal segment subtending 70 deg, and a nasal sector subtending 50 deg. Average RNFL thickness for each sector and global thickness are automatically calculated [38].

The COV among normals for RNFL thickness using the version with a fixed corneal compensator has been estimated to be 17.6 %. Patients on chloroquine therapy have been reported to have a thinner RNFL on average, than normal controls matched for age and gender. The global RNFL thickness in normals was $72.1 \pm SD12.7$ μm compared to $60.6 \pm SD11.2$ μm for patients on chloroquine [38]. Increasing RNFL thinning was associated with increasing actual body weight adjusted daily dosages (Spearman rank correlation coefficient $=-0.45$; $P=0.007$) [38]. Results using a version of the instrument with a variable corneal compensator supported these findings [40]. In addition, the average RNFL thickness in patients taking chloroquine for RA was thinner than that of a control group of patients with RA who were not taking chloroquine. The average RNFL thickness of patients with RA not taking chloroquine did not differ from normal subjects without RA [40].

8.15 Multiple Other Failed or Unadopted Ancillary Tests

Serial fundus photography is an insensitive way to screen for 4AQR and is not routinely used [5]. It is highly variable as well, based on nonstandardized processing either of film and development or more recently by digital techniques [11]. Its theoretical use—to provide a baseline record for later comparison [25]—is outweighed by the large numbers of tests obtained for no benefit.

Dark adaptation is normal in cases with only macular changes, but may be diminished when disease is so advanced that peripheral retinopathy is apparent [2, 7, 8, 92, 204, 205]. At this time the global ERG can show decreased rod and cone amplitudes [92]. This test is not used clinically in the evaluation of patients with C or HC retinopathy [25].

Spatial contrast sensitivity has been proposed as a test for 4AQR [45]. A study comparing 39 patients taking chloroquine or hydroxychloroquine to 16 matched controls not taking these drugs found no differences between groups [45]. Another study compared 27 patients taking hydroxychloroquine to a control group of 28 patients not taking the drug. No definite cases of hydroxychloroquine retinopathy were included, but abnormal contrast sensitivity scores were found in 44.4 % of patients and 10.7 % of controls ($P<0.005$) [13]. The authors stated that discontinuing the drug led to improvements in contrast sensitivity testing. In third study, contrast sensitivity testing was associated with many false positive results and was plagued by high variability [29]. This test has not been adopted for clinical use [203].

The VEP P100 latency but not amplitude differed significantly between patients taking hydroxychloroquine without evidence of retinopathy and normal subjects [20]. Pattern VEP did not distinguish between patients taking hydroxychloroquine and controls not taking the drug. Abnormal responses were found in 2 of 27 (7.4 %) and 2 of 28 (7.1 %) of patients in the two groups, respectively [13]. In another series, VEP did not provide useful screening information [29]. This test is not used in screening for HC retinopathy.

Computerized visual acuity mapping defines visual field deficits in the central 10 deg of the visual field by flashing individual letters for 20 ms in a random sequence and location while the patient fixates on a central cross [92]. Published upper limits of normal for patients less than 50 years of age are less than two errors out of 100 trials. For patients of age 50 or greater, the upper limit of normal is five errors. This test is not useful in screening for 4AQ retinopathy.

A custom-built device using red light emitting diodes having adjustable luminosity has been tested. The test is performed at 2 m, at which distance the array of diodes subtends 2 deg. Patients are dark-adapted for 5 min. Then the luminosity at which the red lights are detected in a reproducible fashion is measured [45]. A study comparing 39 patients taking chloroquine or hydroxychloroquine to 16 matched controls not taking these drugs found no differences between groups. This test is not used clinically to screen patients.

The macular photostress test is based on the recycling of visual pigments between the photoreceptors and the RPE. Light causes release of retinaldehyde from the opsin moiety of photoreceptor outer segments with conversion of the 11-cis-retinal to all-trans-retinol. The RPE takes up the all-trans-retinol and converts it to 11-cis-retinal, which is cycled back to the photoreceptor outer segments [206]. Thus a bright light depletes the level of visual pigment in the photoreceptors, decreasing the sensitivity of the retina to further light until the RPE can replenish the depleted photopigment. In the macular photostress test the eye is illuminated with a bright light and the time required to attain the pre-dazzle level of visual acuity is measured. In normal subjects this time increases gradually with age [20, 64, 187]. The results of macular photostress testing in patients taking 4 AQs have been inconsistent. In one study patients taking 4AQs were found to have prolonged photostress recovery times compared to normal subjects [187]. No discriminative ability of the test to separate patients with and without retinopathy was reported [187]. In another study, the photostress recovery time was significantly prolonged in patients with fundus changes of retinopathy but not in those taking hydroxychloroquine without fundus changes in comparison to normal subjects [20]. A third study did not find it useful for screening [29]. A review of published evidence arrived at pooled estimates of sensitivity and specificity of 0 % and 71 %, respectively [1]. This lack of reproducible discriminatory ability and the lack of standardization of the test may account for the failure to be adopted in clinical practice [14].

Another test has been described in which a red light emitting diode or a white target in a perimeter is made to flicker at a variable frequency and the threshold frequency at which flickering is perceived to cease is determined. It has not proven useful in discriminating 4AQR and has been abandoned as a potentially useful test [29, 207].

8.16 Relative Sensitivity and Specificity of Ancillary Screening Tests for 4-Aminoquinoline Retinopathy

There has been little testing of the relative sensitivity and specificity of ancillary testing for the detection of 4AQR. However, there have been many oblique observations made from case series where serendipitously multiple tests were available for the same patient at the same time [23]. As of 2012 the consensus view was that the relative sensitivity of ancillary tests in detecting 4AQR had not been determined [146, 208]. The order of relative sensitivity of the tests depends on the definitions chosen for abnormal, about which there has been no agreement. For example, in interpreting mfERG testing one can examine ring ratios in which R_1 or R_5 is the internal reference standard (the denominator) and the interpretations depend on the choice made [47]. Or, by adopting a definition for abnormal SAP that includes more patients and a definition for mfERG that includes more patients as normal, one can influence the relative sensitivity of the two tests [83]. As a result, there are exceptions to any attempted generalization. For example, mfERG is generally abnormal before any fundus abnormality attributable to 4AQR is seen, yet counterexamples exist [16]. Nevertheless, it is worthwhile to sift through the sparse evidence that has been published on relative sensitivity and specificity of the ancillary tests for 4AQR. Table 8.17

Table 8.17 Published claims regarding the relative sensitivity and specificity of ancillary tests for detection of 4AQR

Study	Claimed most sensitive test	Claimed second most sensitive test	Claimed third most sensitive test	Claimed fourth most sensitive test
Farrell [16]	10-2 VF	mfERG	FAF	SD-OCT
Kellner [138, 139]	SD-OCT ONL thinning	mfERG	SAP, FAF	Color vision, global ERG
Neubauer [209]	mfERG	SAP	Color vision	Global ERG
Maturi [83]	SAP	mfERG	Global ERG	
Missner [23]	mfERG	SAP	Funduscopy, color vision changes	
So [77]	mfERG	SAP		
Moschos [110]	mfERG	SAP		
Tzekov [195]	mfERG	SAP		
Elder [49]	SAP	VA, color vision, funduscopy		
Anderson [78]	SAP	Funduscopy		
Michaelides [44]	mfERG	SD-OCT		
Lyons [52]	mfERG=SAP	VA, funduscopy		
Adam [47]	SAP	mfERG		
Chen [50]	SAP	mfERG	FAF	Funduscopy
Cruess [22]	Color fundus photography	FA		
Marmor [146]	mfERG=SD-OCT=SAP	FAF		
Rodriguez-Padilla [159]	mfERG=SD-OCT	SAP		

Table 8.18 Relative sensitivity and specificity of ancillary tests for 4AQR

Ancillary test	Sensitivity (%)	Specificity (%)
10-2 VF	85.7	92.5
mfERG	92.9	86.9
SD-OCT	78.6	98.1
10-2 VF + mfERG	100	82.2
10-2 VF + SD-OCT	85.7	92.5
mfERG + SD-OCT	100	86.0

Data from Browning and Lee [42]

gathers published claims on relative sensitivity and specificity of ancillary testing for 4AQR. No clear ordering is apparent from these informal observations.

One systematic investigation of the relative sensitivity and specificity of ancillary tests has been presented (Table 8.18) [42]. In this study 121 patients were screened for 4AQR using three of the four recommended ancillary tests (10-2 VF, mfERG, and SD-OCT). FAF was not used because clinicians seldom choose to use it despite recommendations that it is as valuable as the other tests [27]. Fourteen of the patients had 4AQR defined by the fact that the ophthalmologist and prescribing physician discontinued the 4AQR. They did so because retinopathy was considered to be present based on all the clinical evidence. One hundred and seven patients did not have 4AQR [42].

Visual field testing was done with the 10-2 program of the Humphrey Visual Field Analyzer. Visual fields with a III, white and III, red test object were pooled. The mfERGs were performed using the Espion system (Diagnosys LLC, Lowell, MA) running under version 6+ software. DTL fiber electrodes were used. The definition of an abnormal mfERG was that one or more of the following was true: R_1, R_2, or R_3 amplitudes less than the lower limit of normal determined in 32 normal volunteers tested on the same system or an R_1/R_2 ratio greater than 2.6. SD-OCTs were obtained with either the Cirrus or Spectralis systems. Loss of the perifoveal IS/OS junction and discontinuity of the RPE layer were used as the definition of an abnormal SD-OCT test [42].

The sensitivities of 10-2 VF, mfERG, and SD-OCT in detecting retinopathy were 85.7 %, 92.9 %, and 78.6 %, respectively. The specificities were 92.5 %, 86.9 %, and 98.1 %, respectively. The clinical message is that these tests rarely misclassify a patient who truly has hydroxychloroquine retinopathy as healthy, but can misclassify healthy persons as having hydroxychloroquine retinopathy. Moreover, the slight differences in the operating characteristics of the ancillary tests are swamped by the effect of prior probability of toxicity in analyzing a particular case using Bayesian logic. That is, it is imprudent to get too caught up in comparing relative performance characteristics of the ancillary tests. The appropriate clinical response is to make sure that the patient's sole modifiable risk factor, the adjusted daily dose, lies in a range of higher safety, to use more than one test to assess suspicious cases, and to evaluate the patient longitudinally with shortened follow-up intervals in suspicious cases.

8.17 Challenges

In the literature of ancillary testing of 4AQR, it is common for some tests to be called subjective and others objective [12, 26, 50, 89, 204]. The use of these value-laden terms should be discouraged, because all of the tests have a subjective aspect. With SAP there is considerable subjectivity injected by the patient and the interpreting physician [23]. Depending on whether the patient is alert or somnolent, bright or dim-witted, and intent on complying with test instructions or perverse, the results may be confounded and not reflect the true state of the macula. The subjectivity of mfERG enters less through the patient and more through the interpreting physician. Depending on the physician's choice of definitions of abnormal, the bar for defining disease may be set lower or higher. Similar comments apply to interpretations of SD-OCTs and FAF [79, 210]. Moreover, different physicians have different opinions about what is relatively more subjective. Marmor, Lee, and Chen label SAP as subjective, but Spalton calls SAP "the most objective technique for documenting visual field loss" as compared to the Amsler grid [89]. The challenge in screening for 4AQR is not to find more sensitive tests, but to raise the level of interpretation of tests that we use now to make them more reproducible. A prospective study examining the relative sensitivity and specificity of the ancillary tests used to detect 4AQR would be welcome. It would be useful to have standardized definitions that could be practically employed in the clinical arena.

Historically, more ancillary testing has been introduced over time. The impression has been that patients have been detected at earlier stages than earlier as a result [211]. This should not overshadow the practical fact that most 4AQR arises from iatrogenic overdosing of patients, not failures of ancillary testing. The screening ophthalmologist should focus first on making sure that dosing is correct based on IBW. Ancillary testing is the appropriate secondary concern.

8.18   Summary of Key Points

- The most important function of screening patients for 4AQR is to detect overdosing, which can be corrected.
- A subsidiary function is to detect the rare occurrence of retinopathy among properly dosed patients. For this, ancillary testing is needed because the clinical examination is insensitive.
- More than 10 ancillary tests have been proposed and discarded because they are too variable, not standardized, too insensitive, too sensitive, nonspecific, or not reimbursed.
- SAP with the 10-2 VF is widely available and understood as a screening test for 4AQR, but is hampered by variability and subjectivity in data acquisition and clinical interpretation.
- The mfERG is a sensitive test for 4AQR but has high variability and is fraught with pitfalls in technical application and interpretation.
- FAF is too subjective to have high value as a widely used ancillary test, but it can be helpful in certain cases.
- SD-OCT has the lowest variability of all the ancillary tests, is the most objective, is almost as sensitive as mfERG and 10-2 VF, and is more specific. It is almost as widely available

as the 10-2VF. Of the three recently introduced tests (mfERG, SD-OCT, and FAF), it is the most useful.

References

1. Albert DA, Debois LKL, Lu KF. Antimalarial ocular toxicity, a critical appraisal. J Clin Rheumatol. 1998;4:57–62.
2. Okun E, Gouras P, Bernstein H, von Sallmann L. Chloroquine retinopathy—a report of eight cases with ERG and Dark-Adaptation findings. Arch Ophthalmol. 1963;63:93–105.
3. Marks JS. Chloroquine retinopathy: is there a safe daily dose? Ann Rheum Dis. 1982;41:52–8.
4. Bienfang D, Coblyn JS, Liang MH, Corzillius M. Hydroxychloroquine retinopathy despite regular ophthalmologic evaluation: a consecutive series. J Rheumatol. 2000;27:2703–6.
5. Percival SPB, Behrman J. Ophthalmological safety of chloroquine. Br J Ophthalmol. 1969;53:101–9.
6. Easterbrook M. The ocular safety of hydroxychloroquine. Semin Arthritis Rheum. 1993;23:62–7.
7. Henkind P, Carr RE, Siegel IM. Early chloroquine retinopathy: clinical and functional findings. Arch Ophthalmol. 1964;71:157–65.
8. Kolb H. Electro-oculogram findings in patients treated with antimalarial drugs. Br J Ophthalmol. 1965;49:573–90.
9. Graniewski-Wijnands HS, Van Lith GHM, Vijfvinkel-Bruinenga S. Ophthalmological examination of patients taking chloroquine. Doc Ophthalmol. 1979;48:231–4.
10. Spalton DJ, Roe GMV, Hughes GRV. Hydroxychloroquine, dosage parameters and retinopathy. Lupus. 1993;2:355–8.
11. Dubois EL. Antimalarials in the management of discoid and systemic lupus erythematosus. Semin Arthritis Rheum. 1978;8:33–51.
12. Lee AG. Hydroxychloroquine screening. Who needs it, when, how, and why? Br J Ophthalmol. 2005;89:521–2.
13. Bishara SA, Matamoros N. Evaluation of several tests in screening for chloroquine maculopathy. Eye. 1989;3:777–82.
14. Maksymowych W, Russell AS. Antimalarials in rheumatology: efficacy and safety. Semin Arthritis Rheum. 1987;16:206–21.
15. Gouras P, Gunkel RD. The EOG in chloroquine and other retinopathies. Arch Ophthalmol. 1963;70:629–39.
16. Farrell DF. Retinal toxicity to antimalarial drugs: chloroquine and hydroxychloroquine: a neurophysiologic study. Clin Ophthalmol. 2012;6:377–83.
17. Almony A, Garg S, Peters RK, Mamet R, Tsong J, Shibuya B, Kitridou R, Sadun AA. Threshold amsler grid as a screening tool for asymptomatic patients on

hydroxychloroquine therapy. Br J Ophthalmol. 2005;89:569–74.

18. Easterbrook M. The use of Amsler grids in early chloroquine retinopathy. Ophthalmology. 1984;91: 1368–72.

19. Flach AJ. Amsler grids for chloroquine toxicity. Ophthalmology. 2011;118:2099.

20. Heravian J, Saghafi M, Shoeibi N, Hassanzadeh S, Shakeri MT, Sharepoor M. A comparative study of the usefulness of color vision, photostress recovery time, and visual evoked potential tests in the early detection of ocular toxicity from hydroxychloroquine. Int Ophthalmol. 2011;31:283–9.

21. Grierson DJ. Hydroxychloroquine and visual screening in a rheumatology outpatient clinic. Ann Rheum Dis. 1997;56:188–90.

22. Cruess AF, Schachat AP, Nicholl J, Augsburger JJ. Chloroquine retinopathy—is fluorescein angiography necessary? Ophthalmology. 1985;92:1127–9.

23. Missner S, Kellner U. Comparison of different screening methods for chloroquine/hydroxychloroquine retinopathy: multifocal electroretinography, color vision, perimetry, ophthalmoscopy, and fluorescein angiography. Graefe's Arch Clin Exp Ophthalmol. 2012;250:319–25.

24. Banks CN. Melanin: blackguard or red herring? Another look at chloroquine retinopathy. Aust N Z J Ophthalmol. 1987;15:365–70.

25. Marmor MF, Carr RE, Easterbrook M, et al. Recommendations on screening for chloroquine and hydroxychloroquine retinopathy. Ophthalmology. 2002;109:1377–82.

26. Marmor MF, Kellner U, Lai TYY, Lyons JS, Mieler WF. Revised recommendations on screening for chloroquine and hydroxychloroquine retinopathy. Ophthalmology. 2011;118:415–22.

27. Browning DJ. Impact of the revised American Academy of Ophthalmology guidelines regarding hydroxychloroquine screening on actual practice. Am J Ophthalmol. 2013;155:418–28.

28. Browning DJ. Diabetic retinopathy: evidence based management. New York: Springer; 2010. p. 1–454.

29. Bartel PR, Roux P, Robinson E, Anderson IF, Brighton SW, Van der Hoven HJ, Becker PJ. Visual function and long-term chloroquine treatment. S Afr Med J. 1994;84:32–4.

30. Lyons JS, Severns ML. Using multifocal ERG ring ratios to detect and follow Plaquenil retinal toxicity: a review. Doc Ophthalmol. 2009;118:29–36.

31. Garway-Heath DF, Friedman DS. How should results from clinical tests be integrated into the diagnostic process? Ophthalmology. 2006;113:1479–80.

32. Kellner S, Weinitz S, Kellner U. Spectral domain optical coherence tomography detects early stages of chloroquine retinopathy similar to multifocal electroretinography, fundus autofluorescence and near-infrared autofluorescence. Br J Ophthalmol. 2009;93:1444–7.

33. Jekel JF, Elmore JG, Katz DL. Epidemiology, biostatistics, and preventive medicine. Philadelphia: WB Saunders; 1996. p. 216–7.

34. Neubauer AS, Samari-Kermani K, Schaller U, Welge-Luben U, Rudolph G, Berninger T. Detecting chloroquine retinopathy: electro-oculogram versus color vision. Br J Ophthalmol. 2003;87:902–8.

35. Lai TYY, Chan WM, Li H, Lai RYK, Lam DSC. Multifocal electroretinographic changes in patients receiving hydroxychloroquine therapy. Am J Ophthalmol. 2005;140:794–807.

36. Marmor MF. The dilemma of hydroxychloroquine screening: new information from the multifocal ERG. Am J Ophthalmol. 2005;140:894–5.

37. Easterbrook M. Hydroxychloroquine retinopathy. Ophthalmology. 2001;108:2158–9.

38. Bonanomi MT, Dantas NC, Medeiros FA. Retinal nerve fiber layer thickness measurements in patients using chloroquine. Clin Experiment Ophthalmol. 2006;34:130–6.

39. Tanga L, Centofanti M, Oddone F, Parravano M, Parisi V, Ziccardi L, Kroegler B, Perricone R, Manni G. Retinal functional changes measured by frequency-doubling technology in patients treated with hydroxychloroquine. Graefe's Arch Clin Exp Ophthalmol. 2011;249:715–21.

40. Xiaoyun MA, Dongyi HE, Linping HE. Assessing chloroquine toxicity in RA patients using retinal nerve fiber layer thickness, multifocal electroretinography and visual field test. Br J Ophthalmol. 2010;94:1632–6.

41. Hayreh SS, Klugman MR, Beri M, Kimura AE, Podhajsky P. Differentiation of ischemic from non-ischemic central retinal vein occlusion during the early phase. Graefe's Arch Clin Exp Ophthalmol. 1990;228:201–17.

42. Browning DJ, Lee C. The relative sensitivity and specificity of 10-2 visual fields, multifocal electroretinography, and spectral domain OCT in detecting hydroxychloroquine retinopathy. Scientific poster 484. Presented at: American Academy of Ophthalmology 2013 Annual Meeting, 14–19 Nov 2013, New Orleans.

43. Mavrikakis I, Sfikakis PP, Mavrikakis E, Rougas K, Nikolaou A, Kostopoulos C, Mavrikakis M. The incidence of irreversible retinal toxicity in patients treated with hydroxychloroquine—a reappraisal. Ophthalmology. 2003;110:1321–6.

44. Michaelides M, Stover NB, Francis PJ, Weleber RG. Retinal toxicity associated with hydroxychloroquine and chloroquine: risk factors, screening, and progression despite cessation of therapy. Arch Ophthalmol. 2011;129:30–9.

45. Fleck BW, Bell AL, Mitchell JD, Thomson BJ, Hurst NP, Nuki G. Screening for antimalarial maculopathy in rheumatology clinics. Br Med J. 1985; 291:782–5.

46. Easterbrook M. Ocular effects and safety of antimalarial agents. Am J Med. 1988;85:23–9.

47. Adam MK, Covert DJ, Stepien KE, Han DP. Quantitative assessment of the 103 hexagon multifocal electroretinogram in detection of hydroxychloroquine retinal toxicity. Br J Ophthalmol. 2012; 96:723–9.

48. Easterbrook M. Detection of early hydroxychloroquine retinal toxicity enhanced by ring ratio analysis of multifocal electroretinography. Evid Based ophthalmol. 2008;9:50–1.

49. Elder M, Rahman AMA. Early paracentral visual field loss in patients taking hydroxychloroquine. Arch Ophthalmol. 2006;124:1729–33.

50. Chen E, Brown DM, Benz MS, Fish RH, Wong TP, Kim RY, Major JC. Spectral domain optical coherence tomography as an effective screening test for hydroxychloroquine retinopathy (the "flying saucer" sign). Clin Ophthalmol. 2010;4:1151–8.

51. Anderson C, Pahk P, Blaha GR, Spindel GP, Alster Y, Rafaeli O, Marx J. Preferential hyperacuity perimetry to detect hydroxychloroquine retinal toxicity. Retina. 2009;29:1188–92.

52. Lyons JS, Severns ML. Detection of early hydroxychloroquine retinal toxicity enhanced by ring ratio analysis of multifocal electroretinography. Am J Ophthalmol. 2007;143:801–9.

53. Vu BLL, Easterbrook M, Hovis JK. Detection of color vision defects in chloroquine retinopathy. Ophthalmology. 1999;106:1799–804.

54. Browning DJ. Reply to impact of the revised American Academy of Ophthalmology guidelines regarding hydroxychloroquine screening on actual practice. Am J Ophthalmol. 2013;156:410–1.

55. Hanley JA, Lippman-Hand A. If nothing goes wrong, is everything alright? JAMA. 1983;259:1743–5.

56. Schachat AP, Chambers WA, Liesegang TJ, Albert DA. Safe and effective. Ophthalmology. 2003;110:2073–4.

57. Bland JM, Altman DG. Statistical methods for assessing agreement between two methods of clinical measurement. Lancet. 1986;327:307–10.

58. Rynes RI. Ophthalmologic safety of long-term hydroxychloroquine sulfate treatment. Am J Med. 1983;75:35–9.

59. Massin P, Vicaut E, Haouchine B, Erginay A, Paques M, Gaudric A. Reproducibility of retinal mapping using optical coherence tomography. Arch Ophthalmol. 2001;119:1135–42.

60. Antonisamy B, Christopher S, Samuel PP. Biostatistics: principles and practice. New Delhi: Tata McGraw Hill; 2010. p. 227–40.

61. Parks S, Keating D, Williamson TH, Evans AL, Elliott AT, Jay JL. Functional imaging of the retina using the multifocal electroretinograph: a control study. Br J Ophthalmol. 1996;80:831–4.

62. Forooghian F, Cukras C, Meyerle CB, Chew EY, Wong WT. Evaluation of time domain and spectral domain optical coherence tomography in the measurement of diabetic macular edema. Invest Ophthalmol Vis Sci. 2008;49:4290–6.

63. Wolf-Schnurrbusch UEK, Ceklic L, Brinkmann CK, Iliev ME, Frey M, et al. Macular thickness measurements in healthy eyes using six different optical coherence tomography instruments. Invest Ophthalmol Vis Sci. 2009;50:3432–7.

64. Severin SL, Tour RL, Kershaw RH. Macular function and the photostress test 1. Arch Ophthalmol. 1967;77:2–7.

65. Altemir I, Pueyo V, Elia N, Polo V, Larrosa JM, Oros D. Reproducibility of optical coherence tomography measurements in children. Am J Ophthalmol. 2013;155:171–6.

66. Feuer WJ. Intraclass correlation analysis may alter conclusions. Invest Ophthalmol Vis Sci. 2007;48:1156–63.

67. Thomas JW. Visual fields: examination and interpretation. San Francisco: American Academy of Ophthalmology; 1996.

68. Stone JV. Bayes' rule: a tutorial introduction to Bayesian analysis. England: Sebtel Press; 2013.

69. Zarbin MA. Personalized medicine. Bayesian inference as applied to the measurement of glaucomatous visual field loss. JAMA Ophthalmol. 2013;131:837–8.

70. Newman DH. Hippocrates' shadow. Secrets from the House of Medicine. New York: Simon and Schuster; 2008.

71. Heijl A, Lindgren G, Olsson J, Asman P. Visual field interpretation with empiric probability maps. Arch Ophthalmol. 1989;107:204–8.

72. Lai TYY, Ngai JWS, Chan WM, Lam DSC. Visual field and multifocal electroretinography and their correlations in patients on hydroxychloroquine therapy. Doc Ophthalmol. 2006;112:177–87.

73. Mary JH. The field analyzer primer. San Leandro, CA; 1987.

74. Easterbrook M, Tullo A. Value of Humprey perimetry in the detection of early chloroquine retinopathy. Lens Eye Toxic Res. 1989;6:255–68.

75. Marmor MF, Chien FY, Johnson MW. Value of red targets and pattern deviation pots in visual field screening for hydroxychloroquine retinopathy. JAMA Ophthalmol. 2013;131:476–80.

76. Alward W. Glaucoma the requisites in ophthalmology. St. Louis: Mosby; 2000. p. 67–70.

77. So SC, Hedges TR, Schuman JS, Quireza MLA. Evaluation of hydroxychloroquine retinopathy with multifocal electroretinography. Ophthalmic Surg Lasers Imaging. 2003;34:251–8.

78. Anderson C, Blaha GR, Marx JL. Humphrey visual field findings in hydroxychloroquine toxicity. Eye. 2011;25:1535–45.

79. Browning DJ. Hydroxychloroquine and chloroquine retinopathy: screening for drug toxicity. Am J Ophthalmol. 2002;133:649–56.

80. Vavvas D, Huynh N, Pasquale L, Berson E. Progressive hydroxychloroquine toxicity mimicking low-tension glaucoma after discontinuation of the drug. Acta Ophthalmol. 2010;88:156–7.

81. Heijl A, Lindgren G, Olsson J. Normal variability of static perimetric threshold values across the central visual field. Arch Ophthalmol. 1987;105:1544–9.

82. Flammer J, Drance SM, Augustiny L, Funkhouse A. Quantification of glaucomatous visual field defects with automated perimetry. Invest Ophthalmol Vis Sci. 1985;26:176–81.

83. Maturi RK, Yu M, Weleber RG. Multifocal electro-retinographic evaluation of long-term hydroxychloroquine users. Arch Ophthalmol. 2004;122:973–81.

84. Hoskins HD, Magee SD, Drake MV, Kidd MN. Confidence intervals for change in automated visual fields. Br J Ophthalmol. 1988;72:591–7.

85. Blomquist PH, Chundru RK. Screening for hydroxychloroquine toxicity by Texas ophthalmologists. J Rheumatol. 2002;29:1665–70.

86. Heijl A, Asman P. A clinical study of perimetric probability maps. Arch Ophthalmol. 1989;107:199–203.

87. Johnson MW, Vine AK. Hydroxychloroquine therapy in massive total doses without retinal toxicity. Am J Ophthalmol. 1987;104:139–44.

88. Mititelu M, Wong BJ, Brenner M, Bryar PJ, Jampol LM, Fawzi AA. Progression of hydroxychloroquine toxic effects after drug therapy cessation. New evidence from multimodal imaging. Arch Ophthalmol. 2013;131:1187–97.

89. Spalton DJ. Retinopathy and antimalarial drugs—the British experience. Lupus. 1996;5:S70–2.

90. Wolfensberger TJ. Toxicology of the retinal pigment epithelium. In: Marmor MF, Wolfensberger TJ, editors. The retinal pigment epithelium. New York: Oxford University Press; 1998. p. 621–47.

91. Weisinger HS, Pesudovs K, Collin HB. Management of patients undergoing hydroxychloroquine (Plaquenil) therapy. Clin Exp Optom. 2000;83:32–6.

92. Weiner A, Sandberg MA, Gaudio AR, Kini MM, Berson EL. Hydroxychloroquine retinopathy. Am J Ophthalmol. 1991;112:528–34.

93. Hart WM, Burde RM, Johnston GP, Drews RC. Static perimetry in chloroquine retinopathy—perifoveal patterns of visual field depression. Arch Ophthalmol. 1984;102:377–80.

94. Akman F, Cerman E, Yenice O, Kazokoglu H. Two cases with chloroquine and hydroxychloroquine maculopathy. Marmara Med J. 2011;24:68–72.

95. Salu P, Uvijls A, van den Brande P, Leroy BP. Normalization of generalized retinal function and progression of maculopathy after cessation of therapy in a case of severe hydroxychloroquine retinopathy with 19 years follow-up. Doc Ophthalmol. 2010;120:251–64.

96. Schwartz SG, Mieler WF. Retinal and choroidal manifestations of systemic medications. In: Arevalo JF, editor. Retinal and choroidal manifestations of selected systemic diseases. New York: Springer; 2013. p. 479–92.

97. Razeghinejad MR, Torkaman F, Amini H. Blue-yellow perimetry can be an early detector of hydroxychloroquine and chloroquine retinopathy. Med Hypotheses. 2005;65:629–30.

98. Angi M, Romano V, Valldeperas X, Romano F, Romano M. Macular sensitivity changes for detection of chloroquine toxicity in asymptomatic patient. Int Ophthalmol. 2010;30:195–7.

99. Carr RE, Gouras P, Gunkel RD. Chloroquine retinopathy. Early detection by retinal threshold test. Arch Ophthalmol. 1966;75:171–8.

100. Bernstein H. Ocular safety of hydroxychloroquine sulfate (Plaquenil). South Med J. 1992;85:274–9.

101. Sutter EE, Tran D. The field topography of ERG components in man-I. The photopic luminance response. Vision Res. 1992;32:433–46.

102. Lai TYY, Chan WM, Lai RYK, Ngai JWS, Li H, Lam DSC. The clinical applications of multifocal electroretinography: a systematic review. Surv Ophthalmol. 2007;52:61–96.

103. Marmor MF, Hood DC, Keating D, Kondo M, Seeliger MW, Miyake Y. Guidelines for basic multifocal electroretinography (mfERG). Doc Ophthalmol. 2003;106:105–15.

104. Nebbioso M, Grenga R, Karavitas P. Early detection of macular changes with multifocal ERG in patients on antimalarial drug therapy. J Ocul Pharmacol Ther. 2009;25:249–58.

105. Ng J, Bearse Jr MA, Schneck ME, Barez S, Adams AJ. Local diabetic retinopathy prediction by multifocal ERG delays over 3 years. Invest Ophthalmol Vis Sci. 2008;49:1622–8.

106. Yoshii M, Yanashima K, Matsuno K, Wakaguri T, Kikuchi Y, Okisaka S. Relationship between visual field defect and multifocal electroretinogram. Jpn J Ophthalmol. 1998;42:136–41.

107. Schimitek T, Bach M. The effect of luminance on the multifocal ERG. Doc Ophthalmol. 2006;113:187–92.

108. Hood DC. Assessing retinal function with the multifocal technique. Prog Retin Eye Res. 2000;19:607–46.

109. Tzekov RT, Gerth C, Werner JS. Senescence of human multifocal electroretinogram components: a localized approach. Graefe's Arch Clin Exp Ophthalmol. 2004;242:549–60.

110. Moschos MN, Moschos MM, Apostopoulos M, Mallias JA, Bouros C, Theodossiadis GP. Assessing hydroxychloroquine toxicity by the multifocal ERG. Doc Ophthalmol. 2004;108:47–53.

111. Meigen T, Friedrich A. Zur reproduzierbarkeit von multifokalen ERG-Ableitungen. Ophthalmologe. 2002;99:713–8.

112. Keating D, Parks S, Evans A. Technical aspects of multifocal ERG recording. Doc Ophthalmol. 2000;100:77–98.

113. Seiple W, Vajaranant TS, Szlyk JP, Clemens C, Holopigian K, Paliga J, Badawi D, Carr RE. Multifocal electroretinography as a function of age: the importance of normative values for older adults. Invest Ophthalmol Vis Sci. 2003;44:1783–92.

114. Gundogan FC, Sobaci G, Bayraktar MZ. Intra-sessional and inter-sessional variability of multifocal electroretinogram. Doc Ophthalmol. 2008;117:175–83.

115. Tam A, Chan H, Brown B, Yap M. The effects of forward light scattering on the multifocal electroretinogram. Curr Eye Res. 2004;28:63–72.

116. Tzekov R. Ocular toxicity due to chloroquine and hydroxychloroquine: electrophysiological and visual function correlates. Doc Ophthalmol. 2005;110:111–20.

117. Teoh SC-B, Lim J, Koh A, Lim T, Fu E. Abnormalities on the multifocal electroretinogram may precede clinical signs of hydroxychloroquine retinotoxicity. Eye. 2006;20:129–32.

118. Harrison WW, Bearse Jr MA, Ng JS, Barez S, Schneck ME, Adams AJ. Reproducibility of the mfERG between instruments. Doc Ophthalmol. 2009;119:67–78.

119. Chang WH, Katz BJ, Warner JE, Vitale AT, Creel D, Digre KB. A novel method for screening the multifocal electroretinogram in patients using hydroxychloroquine. Retina. 2008;28:1478–86.

120. Bearse Jr MA, Adams AJ, Han Y, Schneck ME, Ng J, Bronson-Castain K, Barez S. A multifocal electroretinogram model predicting the development of diabetic retinopathy. Prog Retin Eye Res. 2006;25:425–48.

121. Yoshii M, Yanashima K, Wakaguri T, Sakemi F, Kikuchi Y, Suzuki S, Okisaka S. A basic investigation of multifocal electroretinogram: reproducibility and effect of luminance. Jpn J Ophthalmol. 2000;44:122–7.

122. Kondo M, Miyake Y, Horiguchi M, Suzuki S, Tanikawa A. Clinical evaluation of the multifocal electroretinogram. Invest Ophthalmol Vis Sci. 1995; 36:2146–50.

123. Parks S, Keating D, Evans A, Williamson TH, Lay JL, Elliott AT. Comparison of repeatability of the multifocal electroretinogram and Humphrey perimeter. Doc Ophthalmol. 1997;92:281–9.

124. Mendonca RHF, Maia Jr OO, Yukihiko Takahashi W. Electrophysiologic findings in chloroquine maculopathy. Doc Ophthalmol. 2007;115:117–9.

125. Gonzalez P, Parks S, Dolan F, Keating D. The effects of pupil size on the multifocal electroretinogram. Doc Ophthalmol. 2004;109:67–72.

126. Keating D, Parks S, Malloch C, Evans A. A comparison of CRT and digital stimulus delivery methods in the multifocal ERG. Doc Ophthalmol. 2001; 102:95–114.

127. Otto T, Bach M. Retest variability and diurnal effects in the pattern electroretinogram. Doc Ophthalmol. 1997;92:311–23.

128. Han Y, Bearse Jr MA, Schneck ME, Barez S, Jacobsen CH, Adams AJ. Multifocal electroretinogram delays predict sites of subsequent diabetic retinopathy. Invest Ophthalmol Vis Sci. 2004;45:948–54.

129. Chappelow AV, Marmor MF. Effects of pre-adaptation conditions and ambient room lighting on the multifocal ERG. Doc Ophthalmol. 2002;105:23–31.

130. Chen JC, Brown B, Schmid KL. Changes in implicit time of the multifocal electroretinogram response following contrast adaptation. Curr Eye Res. 2006; 31:549–56.

131. Chan HL, Siu AW. Effect of optical defocus on multifocal erg responses. Clin Exp Optom. 2003;86:317–22.

132. Bultmann S, Rohrschneider K. Reproducibility of multifocal ERG using the scanning laser ophthalmoscope. Graefe's Arch Clin Exp Ophthalmol. 2002;240:841–5.

133. Seeliger MW, Narfstrom K, Reinhard J, Zrenner E, Sutter E. Continuous monitoring of the stimulated area in multifocal ERG. Doc Ophthalmol. 2000;100: 167–84.

134. Seiple W, Greenstein VC, Holopigian K, Carr RE, Hood DC. A method for comparing psychophysical and multifocal electroretinographic increment thresholds. Vision Res. 2002;42:257–69.

135. Kretschmann U, Bock M, Gockeln R, Zrenner E. Clinical applications of multifocal electroretinography. Doc Ophthalmol. 2000;100:99–113.

136. Janaky M, Palffy A, Deak A, Szilagyi M, Benedek G. Multifocal ERG reveals several patterns of cone degeneration in retinitis pigmentosa with concentric narrowing of the visual field. Invest Ophthalmol Vis Sci. 2007;48:383–9.

137. Mohidin N, Yap MK, Jacobs RJ. The repeatability and variability of the multifocal electroretinogram for four different electrode types. Ophthalmic Physiol Opt. 1997;17:530–5.

138. Kellner U, Renner AB, Tillack H. Fundus autofluorescence and mfERG for early detection of retinal alterations in patients using chloroquine/hydroxychloroquine. Invest Ophthalmol Vis Sci. 2006; 47:3531–8.

139. Kellner U, Kraus H, Foerster MH. Multifocal ERG in chloroquine retinopathy: regional variance in retinal dysfunction. Graefe's Arch Clin Exp Ophthalmol. 2000;238:94–7.

140. Kretschmann U, Seeliger MW, Ruether K, Usui T, Apfelstedt-Sylla E, Zrenner E. Multifocal electroretinography in patients with Stargardt's macular dystrophy. Br J Ophthalmol. 1998;82:267–75.

141. Browning DJ, Lee C. The coefficient of repeatability for multifocal electroretinography measurements in normal volunteers and patients taking hydroxychloroquine. Scientific poster 483. Presented at American Academy of Ophthalmology 2013 Annual Meeting, 14–19 Nov 2013, New Orleans.

142. Penrose PJ, Tzekov RT, Sutter EE, Fu AD, Allen Jr AW, Fung WE, Oxford KW. Multifocal electroretinography evaluation for early detection of retinal dysfunction in patients taking hydroxychloroquine. Retina. 2003;23:503–12.

143. Aoyagi K, Kimura Y, Isono H, Akigawa H, Sugawara T. Reproducibility and wave analysis of multifocal electroretinography. Nihon Ganka Gakkai Zasshi. 1998;102:340–7.

144. Kondo M, Miyake T, Horiguchi M, Suzuki S, Ho Y, Tanikawa A. Normal values of retinal response densities in multifocal electroretinogram. Nihon Ganka Gakkai Zasshi. 1996;100:810–6.

145. Bergholz R, Schroeter J, Ruther K. Evaluation of risk factors for retinal damage due to chloroquine and hydroxychloroquine. Br J Ophthalmol. 2010; 94:1637–42.

146. Marmor MF. Comparison of screening procedures in hydroxychloroquine toxicity. Arch Ophthalmol. 2012;130:461–9.

147. Gilbert ME, Savino PJ. Missing the Bull's Eye. Surv Ophthalmol. 2007;52:440–2.

148. Maturi RK, Folk JC, Nichols B, Oetting TT, Kardon RH. Hydroxychloroquine retinopathy. Arch Ophthalmol. 1999;117:1262–3.

149. Marmor MF. Author reply. Ophthalmology. 2011;118:2099–100.

150. Garcia-Martin E, Pinilla I, Idoipe M, Fuertes I, Pueyo V. Intra and interoperator reproducibility of retinal nerve fibre and macular thickness measurements using Cirrus Fourier-domain OCT. Acta Ophthalmol. 2011;89:e23–9.

151. Menke M, Daov S, Knecht P, Sturm V. Reproducibility of retinal thickness measurements in healthy subjects using spectralis optical coherence tomography. Am J Ophthalmol. 2009;147:467–72.

152. Diabetic Retinopathy Clinical Research Network. Reproducibility of macular thickness and volume using Zeiss optical coherence tomography in patients with diabetic macular edema. Ophthalmology. 2007;114:1520–5.

153. Menke MN, Knecht P, Sturm V, Dabov S, Funk J. Reproducibility of nerve fiber layer thickness measurements using 3D fourier-domain OCT. Invest Ophthalmol Vis Sci. 2008;49:5386–91.

154. Pasadhika S, Fishman GA. Effects of chronic exposure to hydroxychloroquine or chloroquine on inner retinal structures. Eye. 2009;24:340–6.

155. Pasadhika S, Fishman GA, Choi D, Shahidi M. Selective thinning of the perifoveal inner retina as an early sign of hydroxychloroquine retinal toxicity. Eye. 2010;24:756–63.

156. Kellner U, Kellner S, Weinitz S. Chloroquine retinopathy: lipofuscin- and melanin-related fundus autofluorescence, optical coherence tomography and multifocal electroretinography. Doc Ophthalmol. 2008;116:119–27.

157. Stepien KE, Han DP, Schell J, Godara P, Rha J, Carroll J. Spectral-domain optical coherence tomography and adaptive optics may detect hydroxychloroquine retinal toxicity before symptomatic vision loss. Trans Am Ophthalmol Soc. 2009;107:28–34.

158. Fung AE. Patient complains of central shimmering lights, subtle OCT changes with hydroxychloroquine use. Ocul Surg News. 2013;31:25–6.

159. Rodriguez-Padilla JA, Hedges III TR, Monson B, Srinivasan V, Wojtkowski M, Reichel E, Duker JS, Schuman JS, Fujimoto JG. High-speed ultra-high-resolution optical coherence tomography findings in hydroxychloroquine retinopathy. Arch Ophthalmol. 2007;125:775–80.

160. Easterbrook M. Spectral domain optical coherence tomography detects early stages of chloroquine retinopathy similar to multifocal electroretinography, fundus autofluorescence and near-infrared autofluorescence. Evid-Based Ophthalmol. 2010;11:162–3.

161. Fung AE, Samy CN, Rosenfeld PJ. Optical coherence tomography findings in hydroxychloroquine and chloroquine-associated maculopathy. Retin Cases Brief Rep. 2007;1:128–30.

162. Fontaine F, Rougier MB, Korobelnik JF. Optical coherence tomography in hydroxychloroquine retinopathy: two observational case reports. Retin Cases Brief Rep. 2007;1:131–3.

163. Feeney L. Lipofuscin and melanin of human retinal pigment epithelium. Fluorescence, enzyme cytochemical, and ultrastructural studies. Invest Ophthalmol Vis Sci. 1978;17:583–600.

164. Kelmenson AT, Brar VS, Murthy RK, Chalam KV. Fundus autofluorescence and spectral domain optical coherence tomography in early detection of Plaquenil maculopathy. Eur J Ophthalmol. 2010;20:785–8.

165. Neville HE, Maundry-Sewry CA, McDougall J, Sewell JR, Dubowitz V. Chloroquine-induced cytosomes with curvilinear profiles in muscle. Muscle Nerve. 1979;2:376–81.

166. Labriola LT, Jeng D, Fawzi AA. Retinal toxicity of systemic medications. Int Ophthalmol Clin. 2012;52:149–66.

167. Gorovoy I, Gorovoy JB. Advances in ophthalmic monitoring for hydroxychloroquine toxicity. J Clin Rheumatol. 2013;19:46–7.

168. Kearns TP, Hollenhorst RW. Chloroquine retinopathy. Arch Ophthalmol. 1966;76:378–84.

169. Shearer RV, Dubois EL. Ocular changes induced by long-term hydroxychloroquine (Plaquenil) therapy. Am J Ophthalmol. 1967;64:245–52.

170. Tehrani R, Ostrowski RA, Hariman R, Jay WM. Ocular toxicity of hydroxychloroquine. Semin Ophthalmol. 2008;23:201–9.

171. Lozier JR, Friedlander MH. Complications of antimalarial therapy. Int Ophthalmol Clin. 1989;29:172–8.

172. American Academy of Optometry. Monitoring ocular toxicity of selected medications. www.aoa.org/optometrists/education-and-training/clinical-care/monitoring-ocular-toxicity-of-selected-medications. Accessed 5 July 2013.

173. Easterbrook M. Screening for antimalarial toxicity. Can J Ophthalmol. 1993;28:51–2.

174. Ormrod JN. Two cases of chloroquine-inducted retinal damage. Br Med J. 1962;1:918–9.

175. Easterbrook M. Comparison of threshold and standard Amsler grid testing in patients with established antimalarial retinopathy. Can J Ophthalmol. 1992;27:240–2.

176. Easterbrook M. The sensitivity of Amsler grid testing in early chloroquine retinopathy. Trans Ophthalmol Soc UK. 1985;104:204–7.

177. Morin JD. Discussion. Ophthalmology. 1984;91:1372.

178. Blomquist PH. Screening for hydroxychloroquine toxicity. Comp Ophthalmol Update. 2000;1:245–50.

179. Schuchard RA. Validity and interpretation of Amsler grid reports. Arch Ophthalmol. 1993;111:776–80.

180. Flach AJ. Improving the risk-benefit relationship and informed consent for patients treated with hydroxychloroquine. Trans Am Ophthalmol Soc. 2007;105:191–7.

181. Brown M, Marmor M, Vaegan, Zrenner E, Brigell M, Bach M. ISCEV standard for clinical electrooculography (EOG). Doc Ophthalmol. 2006;113:205–12.

182. Arden GB, Barrada A. Analysis of the electro-oculograms of a series of normal subjects. Br J Ophthalmol. 1962;46:468–82.

183. Reijmer CN, Tijssen JGP, Kok GA, Van Lith GHM. Interpretation of the electro-oculogram of patients taking chloroquine. Doc Ophthalmol. 1979;48:273–6.

184. Arden GB, Kolb H. Antimalarial therapy and early retinal changes in patients with rheumatoid arthritis. Br Med J. 1966;1:270–3.

185. Pinckers A, Broekhnyse RM. The EOG in rheumatoid arthritis. Acta Ophthalmol. 1983;61:831–7.

186. Butler I. Retinopathy following the use of chloroquine and allied substances. Ophthalmologica. 1965;149:204–8.

187. Carr RE, Henkind P, Rothfield N, Siegel IM. Ocular toxicity of antimalarial drugs-long-term follow-up. Am J Ophthalmol. 1968;66:738–44.

188. Wachtmeister L. Oscillatory potentials in the retina: what do they reveal? Prog Retin Eye Res. 1998;17:485–521.

189. Birch DG, Hood DC, Locke KG, Hoffman DR, Tzekov RT. Quantitative electroretinogram measures of phototransduction in cone and rod photoreceptors. Normal aging, progression with disease, and test-retest variability. Arch Ophthalmol. 2002;120:1045–51.

190. Rosenthal AR, Kolb H, Bergsma D, Huxsoll D, Hopkins JL. Chloroquine retinopathy in the rhesus monkey. Invest Ophthalmol Vis Sci. 1978;17:1158–75.

191. McConnell DG, Wachtel J, Havener WH. Observations on experimental chloroquine retinopathy. Arch Ophthalmol. 1964;71:552–3.

192. Ivanina TA, Zueva MV, Lebedeva MN, Bogoslovsky AI, Bunin AJ. Ultrastructural alterations in rat and cat retina and pigment epithelium induced by chloroquine. Graefe's Arch Clin Exp Ophthalmol. 1983;220:32–8.

193. Giorgi D, Rosati C, Verrastro G, Grandinetti F. What's the right patient management for early diagnosis of hydroxychloroquine retinal toxicity? Recenti Prog Med. 1996;87:308.

194. Schmidt B, Muller-Limmroth W. Electroretinographic examinations following application of chloroquine. Acta Ophthalmol Supp. 1962;70:245–51.

195. Tzekov RT, Serrato A, Marmor MF. ERG findings in patients using hydroxychloroquine. Doc Ophthalmol. 2004;108:87–97.

196. Grutzner P. Acquired color vision defects secondary to retinal drug toxicity. Ophthalmologica. 1969;158:592–604.

197. Easterbrook M. Clinical characteristics of hydroxychloroquine retinopathy. Evid Based Ophthalmol. 2011;12:132–3.

198. Warner AE. Early hydroxychloroquine macular toxicity. Arthritis Rheum. 2001;44:1959–61.

199. Nozik RA, Weinstock FJ, Vignos PJ. Ocular complications of chloroquine: series and case presentation with simple method for early detection of retinopathy. Am J Ophthalmol. 1964;58:774–8.

200. Nylander U. Ocular damage in chloroquine therapy. Acta Ophthalmol. 1966;44:335–8.

201. Payne JF, Hubbard III GB, Aaberg Sr TM, Yan J. Clinical characteristics of hydroxychloroquine retinopathy. Br J Ophthalmol. 2010;95:245–50.

202. Yam JCS, Kwok AKH. Ocular toxicity of hydroxychloroquine. Hong Kong Med J. 2006;12:294–304.

203. Morsman CDG, Livesey SJ, Richards IM, Jessop JD, Mills PV. Screening for hydroxychloroquine retinal toxicity: is it necessary? Eye. 1990;4:572–6.

204. Pulido JS, Barkmeier AJ, Leavitt JA. Screening for hydroxychloroquine toxicity. Ophthalmology. 2012;119:207.

205. Gonasun LM, Potts AM. In vitro inhibition of protein synthesis in the retinal pigment epithelium by chloroquine. Invest Ophthalmol Vis Sci. 1974;13:107–15.

206. Chader GJ, Pepperberg DR, Crouch R, Wiggert B. Retinoids and the retinal pigment epithelium. In: Marmor MF, Wolfensberger TJ, editors. The retinal pigment epithelium. New York: Oxford University Press; 1998. p. 135–51.

207. Khamis ARA, Easterbrook M. Critical flicker fusion frequency in early chloroquine retinopathy. Can J Ophthalmol. 1983;18:217–9.

208. Marmor MF, Kellner U, Lai TYY, Lyons JS, Mieler WF. Author response. Ophthalmology. 2012;119:207–8.

209. Neubauer AS, Stiefelmeyer S, Berninger T, Arden GB, Rudolph G. The multifocal pattern electroretinogram in chloroquine retinopathy. Ophthalmic Res. 2004;36:106–13.

210. Thorne JE, Maguire AM. Retinopathy after long term, standard doses of hydroxychloroquine. Br J Ophthalmol. 1999;83:1201–2.

211. Easterbrook M. Long-term course of antimalarial maculopathy after cessation of treatment. Can J Ophthalmol. 1992;27:237–9.

212. Ibrahim MA, Sepah YJ, Symons RCA, Channa R, Hatef E, Khwaja A, Bittencourt M, Heo J, Do DV, Nguyen M. Spectral - and time-domain optical coherence tomography measurements of macular thickness in normal eyes and in diabetic macular edema. Eye. 2012;26:454–62.

213. Hirasawa H, Araie M, Tomidokoro A, Saito H, Iwase A, Ohkubo S, et al. Reproducibility of thickness measurements of macular inner retinal layers using SD-OCT with or without correction of ocular rotation. Invest Ophthalmol Vis Sci. 2013;54:2562–70.

214. Leung CK, Cheung CY, Weinreb RN, Lee G, Lin D, Pang CP, Lam DSC. Comparison of macular thickness measurements between time domain and spectral domain optical coherence tomography. Invest Ophthalmol Vis Sci. 2008;49:4893–7.

Screening for Hydroxychloroquine and Chloroquine Retinopathy

9

Abbreviations

4AQR	4-Aminoquinoline retinopathy
4AQs	4-Aminoquinolines (chloroquine and hydroxychloroquine)
ABW	Actual body weight
AG	Amsler grid
C	Chloroquine
HC	Hydroxychloroquine
IBW	Ideal body weight
RA	Rheumatoid arthritis
RPE	Retinal pigment epithelium
SLE	Systemic lupus erythematosus

Screening guidelines for the detection of 4-aminoquinoline retinopathy (4AQR) retinopathy vary across countries [1–4]. One can infer that the superiority of one set of guidelines over another is not clear, and that the evidence to support screening is ambiguous. This chapter reviews the relevant studies on screening and attempts to clarify why different conclusions have been drawn from the same set of data.

Screening inevitably involves value judgments. For example, some argue that screening is justified when the prevalence of retinopathy reaches 1 % [5, 6]. However, this judgment depends on the wealth of the parties addressing the issue of screening and the competing interests for allocation of resources. Therefore, part of the variation in screening guidelines may reflect socioeconomic disparities across countries rather than disputes over the proper interpretation of the medical literature.

The efficacy of screening has not been studied in a valid manner [7]. Although for over 20 years the United States and the United Kingdom have had opposed guidelines on the need for 4AQR screening, it is unknown whether the prevalence of 4AQR is higher in the United Kingdom, where screening is discouraged, or in the United States, where it is standard practice.

Screening for retinopathy caused by the 4-aminoquinolines (4AQs) raises multiple issues, among them:

- Is screening warranted?
- If so, for what should one screen—toxic dosing or early retinopathy?
- If so, who should be screened?
- If so, how often should screening be performed?
- If so, what ancillary tests should be used [6, 8–10]?
- Where screening is advocated, how well is it done?
- Where screening is advocated, what explains the gap between the goals of screening and the practice of screening?

The considerations that influence a decision to screen include an assessment of the loss of sight if screening were omitted; the incidence of retinopathy in properly dosed and overdosed patients; the cost of screening; the consequences if these drugs are no longer used to treat systemic lupus erythematosus (SLE) or rheumatoid arthritis (RA); and medicolegal issues [3]. Potential

D.J. Browning, *Hydroxychloroquine and Chloroquine Retinopathy*,
DOI 10.1007/978-1-4939-0597-3_9, © Springer Science+Business Media New York 2014

legal risk arises from the gap between guidelines and adherence to them that exists in every country in which the matter has been investigated [1, 11–14]. Clinicians need to be cognizant of the guidelines that are advocated by the governing bodies of the geographical area in which they practice. These are the relevant guidelines in lawsuits to which they may become parties [11, 14].

Commonly used abbreviations in this chapter are collected in "Abbreviations" for reference. Each term will be first used in its full form, along with its abbreviation.

9.1   Indications for Screening

The indications for screening are generally accepted [15].

- A candidate disease for screening should be neither too common (else regular care is the goal—e.g., dental caries) nor too rare (else resources are wasted—e.g., population-wide screening for Tay–Sachs disease)
- The consequences of missing disease are serious
- There is effective treatment

However, a controversy arises over the interpretation of these guidelines. Part of the controversy has to do with what is the intent of screening. If the primary intent is to detect toxic dosing, as has been a theme of this book, then the first criterion is met, because at least 12.8 % of patients taking 4AQs are overdosed (see Chap. 7) [12, 16]. But if the primary intent is to detect retinopathy at an early stage, then it may not be satisfied, because the prevalence of 4AQR has not been established and some estimates of its prevalence are far less than 1 % (see Chap. 5). The best estimate for prevalence of 4AQR probably lies in the range from 0.1 to 5 % depending on drug (higher for chloroquine) and context. If it is close to 0.1 %, then the first criterion has probably not been satisfied. If it lies closer to 5 %, then it probably has been satisfied. Where the decision swings from probably not justified to probably justified is a matter of opinion and resources.

The second criterion is noncontroversial—all agree that advanced 4AQR is serious. The third is controversial, and depends again on the intent of screening. If it is to detect toxic dosing, then there is effective treatment, namely to correct dosing based on ideal body weight (IBW). If it is to detect early retinopathy, then the matter is unclear, because there is inconsistent evidence that retinopathy is reversible (see Chap. 6) [17].

In the debate on the intent of screening, one side holds that the main purpose is to detect retinopathy at an early stage and prevent its progression to a more advanced stage [18–21]. This point of view emphasizes that preventing retinopathy may not be possible [6, 20, 22]. The other view contends that prevention of retinopathy is the goal, which requires a shift in emphasis to the detection of toxic dosing [10, 12, 23–26]. The author's view is that not enough attention has been given to daily dosing. For example, in 2013 Schwartz and Mieler wrote that "Earlier recommendations emphasized dosing by weight," as though this point of view is now antiquated. However, such recommendations are forward-looking, because overdosing is common [12, 27, 28]. By reframing the purpose of screening as primarily detection of toxic dosing, with a subsidiary goal of detecting subclinical retinopathy, the tenor of the discussion about screening changes [4, 10, 29, 30].

Although detection of toxic dosing is the most important goal of screening, the lesser goal of detecting retinopathy early does deserve attention. Because 4AQR routinely develops before symptoms are noticed, it follows that screening asymptomatic subjects taking 4AQs will be necessary to detect most cases of retinopathy [31]. Because there is no evidence that retinopathy is reversible to a clinically important extent once it has advanced to the stage of funduscopic changes, a pertinent question is whether detection of retinopathy at the stage of premaculopathy is effective at preventing retinopathy. In Bernstein review of 1992, there were no cases in which premaculopathy had been followed and evolved into more advanced retinopathy [32]. However, in Chap. 6 a well-documented case was presented (Fig. 6.5), showing that such progression can occur.

The evidence is also strong that progression to advanced retinopathy occurs less frequently if retinopathy is detected early and the drug is stopped (see Chap. 6). Cessation of the drug at the premaculopathy stage is associated with a good prognosis [33].

There are other, less important, reasons to screen and reasons that offer incentives to screening. These include a desire to limit medicolegal liability, to respond to patient insistence, to remind patients of the possibility of toxicity so that the drug may be considered for discontinuation if not needed any longer, and to garner remuneration associated with screening [7, 12, 34–36]. These purposes deserve notice, because even if an analysis of the evidence leads to a conclusion at odds with screening, there is a probability that a culture of screening will continue [7].

9.2 Baseline Screening

The ophthalmic literature is inconsistent on the value of baseline screening [4, 13, 34, 37, 38]. For example, Marmor argues for uniformly obtaining baseline visual fields in one place and in another states, "I often omit baseline visual fields" [6, 22]. The rationale for baseline screening is that preexisting maculopathy is a risk factor for 4AQR and therefore needs to be established. Moreover, establishing the presence of a normal baseline makes subsequent determination of maculopathy more significant [39, 40].

When to perform baseline screening is an issue. Bernstein has recommended that it be performed within 4–8 weeks of initiating therapy, but there is no data to suggest that another window might not be acceptable. Others have recommended that the baseline examination be done after 6–12 months of treatment [14, 32]. Although one might argue for a baseline examination before beginning therapy, a practice of doing it within 4–8 weeks has the advantage of not screening those patients who will be intolerant of 4AQs due to gastrointestinal upset or another problem (see Chap. 3). Table 9.1 captures the spectrum of published recommendations on baseline screening for 4AQR.

9.3 Follow-up Screening Visits

As with recommendations regarding the need for a baseline screening visit, those for follow-up screenings are inconsistent (Table 9.1). The American Academy of Ophthalmology guidelines of 2011 and others suggest a second screening visit after 4–6 years, assuming that no risk factors for retinopathy are present [6, 14, 62, 67]. Despite these recommendations, in practice few clinicians adhere to the advice, because of fears that patients will be lost to follow-up during the prolonged gap [12, 34]. Instead, the prevailing practice is to screen at least yearly [12, 34]. Despite the lack of evidence supporting it, screening every 6 months is also widespread [12, 68].

A rational approach to the frequency of screening should include addressing the question of how fast a patient can go from no damage to visually disabling damage. The answer is not known and perhaps is unknowable since it will depend on the perspicacity of the screener. For example, the patient shown in Fig. 8.13 received recommended annual 10-2 VFs, but developed 4AQR because the ophthalmologist did not recognize the characteristic paracentral scotoma of the condition.

9.4 Who Should Screen and What Tests Should Be Used?

Many authors place a screening responsibility on the treating physician [4, 32, 39]. There is no objective way to measure the effectiveness of these admonitions, but the continuing occurrence of retinopathy and overdosed patients suggests that previous efforts have not been effective. Some treating physicians are adamant that ophthalmologic screening is needed rather than screening by the treating physician [25]. This appeals to common sense. Imagining the shoe on the other foot, the author shudders to think of ophthalmologists screening for heart murmurs. On the other hand, some rheumatologists view a requirement to involve ophthalmologists in

Table 9.1 Recommendations on screening for 4-aminoquinoline retinopathy

Study or report	Year	Screener	Baseline screening	When to do baseline?	Recommended elements of screening examination	Time of second screening examination for low-risk patients	Time of second screening examination for high-risk patients	Frequency of subsequent screening examinations
Percival [37]	1968	Ophthalmologist	Yes	NG	CE, VF, CV, FP	4 months	4 months	NG
Mackenzie [41]	1970	Ophthalmologist			CE	1 year	More frequently	NG
Dubois [42]	1978	Ophthalmologist	Yes	NG	VA, CE	4 months	4 months	4 months
Graniewski-Wijnands [43]	1979	Ophthalmologist	Yes	NG	NG	After cumulative dose of chloroquine of 75 g	After cumulative dose of chloroquine of 75 g	NG
Tobin [44]	1982	Ophthalmologist	Yes	NG	NG	6 months	6 months	NG
Scherbel [45]	1983	NG	NG	NG	NG	NG	NG	Every 3 to 6 months
Fleck [39]	1985	Treating Physician	Yes	NG	VA check, dilated funduscopy; if VA is subnormal or maculopathy detected refer to ophthalmologist	6 months	6 months	NG
Banks [13]	1987	Ophthalmologist	Yes	NG	VA, refraction, SLE, color VA, VF, CP, FA, AG	3 years	3 years	NG
Terrell [46]	1988	Ophthalmologist	Yes	NG	Funduscopy, SAP or tangent screen	6 months	6 months	NG
Lozier [47]	1989	Ophthalmologist	Yes	NG	NG	6 months	6 months	6 monthly
Bernstein [32, 48]	1991, 1992	Ophthalmologist	Yes	Within 4 weeks of starting drug	Ophthalmic examination, record height and weight and calculated ideal body weight for determining overdosage, Ishihara Plates, Amsler grid, SAP or GVF	1 year	1 year	1 year if low risk; q 4–6 months if high risk

Easterbrook [49–51]	1993	Ophthalmologist	Yes	NG	VA, SLE, fundus examination, AG, H, W	Yearly if AG reliable; 6 monthly if AG is unreliable	Yearly if AG reliable; 6 monthly if AG is unreliable	Yearly if AG reliable; 6 monthly if AG is unreliable
Spalton [52]	1993	Ophthalmologist	Yes	NG	VA, funduscopy	5 years	5 years	Yearly after 5 years of therapy
Grierson [53], Morsman [54], Morand [92]	1990–1997	NA	Screening only for indications	NA	NA	NA	NA	NA
American College of Rheumatology [55]	1996	Ophthalmologist	If patient ≥40 or if risk factors then do BL screen	6 months after starting drug	NG	12–18 months	Not specified, but consider more often	NG
Spalton [24]	1996	Ophthalmologist	Yes	NG	NG	3 years	3 years	NG
Rynes [56]	1997	Ophthalmologist	Yes	NG	Focused history, F, VF with red test object; if VF abnormal, check VF with white test object	6 months	6 months	6 months
Levy [57]	1997	Ophthalmologist	None if daily dose 6.5 mg/kg/day and normal renal function and duration <10 years	NG	NG	None	1 year if >10 years use, ≥6.5 mg/kg/day, or renal insufficiency	1 year if >10 years use, ≥6.5 mg/kg/day, or renal insufficiency
Canadian Rheumatology Association [58]	1998	Ophthalmologist	Yes	NG	NG	NG	NG	NG

(continued)

Table 9.1 (continued)

Study or report	Year	Screener	Baseline screening	When to do baseline?	Recommended elements of screening examination	Time of second screening examination for low-risk patients	Time of second screening examination for high-risk patients	Frequency of subsequent screening examinations
Royal College of Ophthalmologists and the British Society of Rheumatology [4, 8]	1998	Treating Physician	Yes	If symptoms are present or visual acuity is subnormal, refer to an optometrist; ophthalmologist sees patient if problem is nonrefractive	Determine baseline renal and liver function, ask about visual symptoms and check near visual acuity	Yearly	Yearly	Yearly
Block [14]	1998	Ophthalmologist	Yes	Wait until tolerance to the drug is established (6–12 months)	NG	5 years	Not stated, but before 5 years	NG
Albert [59]	1998	NG	No reason to screen unless daily dose by IBW is >6.5 mg/kg/day and cumulative dose >1,000 g	NA	NG	NA	NA	NA
May [60]	1998	Ophthalmologist	If preexistng maculopathy, renal or liver disease, age > 60, daily dose >6.5 mg/kg/day by ABW, or cumulative dose >500 g HC	NG	VA, SAP, funduscopy, fundus photographs	Not needed	1 year	Yearly, only if risk factors

Bray [61]	1998	Ophthalmologist	If patient ≥60 years or if a history of ocular pathology before starting 4AQ	NG	VA, red Amsler grid, color vision testing, slit lamp, and fundus examination	6 months	6 months	6 months
Jones [4]	1999	Treating physician	Yes	NG	Determine baseline renal and liver function, ask about visual symptoms and check near visual acuity; refer to ophthalmologist if problems detected	Perhaps after 5 years	Perhaps after 5 years	NG
Warner [3]	2001	Ophthalmologist	Yes	NG	VA, CE, SAP, CV	1 year	1 year	Yearly for 5 years, then 6 monthly
American Academy of Ophthalmology [18]	2002	Ophthalmologist	Yes	NG	H, W, CE, 10-2, AG	5 years	1 year	1 year
Mavrikakis [62]	2003	Ophthalmologist	Yes		VA, CE, Ishihara Plates, SAP, W	6 years	1 year	1 year for low-risk patients; more frequently for high-risk patients
Fielder	2004	Rheumatologist	Yes	Refer to ophthalmologist if any abnormality	Questions about visual symptoms and check BCVA	1 year	1 year	1 year
Elder [9]	2006	Ophthalmologist	Yes	NG	VA, CE, CV, SAP	2 year	2 year	Yearly after second year

(continued)

Table 9.1 (continued)

Study or report	Year	Screener	Baseline screening	When to do baseline?	Recommended elements of screening examination	Time of second screening examination for low-risk patients	Time of second screening examination for high-risk patients	Frequency of subsequent screening examinations
Payne [28]	2010	Ophthalmologist	Yes	NG	NG	Based on risk	Based on risk	Based on risk
Bergholz [63]	2010	Ophthalmologist	Yes	NG	VA, CE, SAP, mf ERG	Based on risk	Based on risk	Based on risk
European League Against Rheumatism	2010	Ophthalmologist	Yes	NG	H, W, CE, SAP	5 years	1 year	If low risk, yearly after 5 years of therapy; if high-risk yearly from start
American Academy of Ophthalmology [6]	2011	Ophthalmologist	Yes	NG	CE, 10-2 VF, and mf ERG, FAF, or SD-OCT if available	5 years	1 year	Based on risk
Farrrell [64]	2012	Ophthalmologist	Only if age >40 or >5 years drug usage	NG	NG	NG	NG	NG
American Optometric Association [65, 66]	2013	Optometrist	Yes	NG	CE, central threshold VF, AG, color vision testing (blue-yellow), CFP	6 months	6 months	6 months

CE clinical examination, *CFP* color fundus photographs, *FA* fluorescein angiography, *VA* visual acuity, *SLE* slit lamp examination, *NA* not applicable, *NG* not given, *DF* dilated funduscopy, *CV* color vision testing, *W* weight. Low risk means none of the following: age greater than 60, preexisting maculopathy, adjusted daily dosing above thresholds for increased toxicity, renal disease, or liver disease. High risk means presence of one or more of these risk factors

screening as a burden. If this need removed, that use of 4AQs might increase [39].

The screening methods recommended by authors have changed over the years, generally in the direction of more recommended tests in addition to clinical examination (Table 9.1). For example, in 1978 Dubois stated that screening should include clinical examination only and that routine use of visual fields, color vision testing, or any other ancillary modality was unnecessary. In 1992, visual field testing was still considered unnecessary for routine screening [69]. By 2002 standard automated perimetry (SAP) became a universally recommended screening modality [18]. In 2011 at least one of mfERG, SD-OCT, and fundus autofluorescence (FAF) was added to the list of routinely recommended ancillary tests, when these modalities were available [6].

Although governing bodies have issued guidelines [6], there remains no internationally accepted method of screening, any consensus as to which test is most useful, or in what order tests should be obtained [70, 71]. Experts have changed their opinions over time. For example, Easterbrook opined in 1993 that 10-2 VF testing was not indicated on a routine basis in patients taking hydroxychloroquine, but only to confirm a positive Amsler grid test [49, 50]. However, in 2002 he wrote that 10-2 VF testing should be routinely obtained in such patients [18]. In 2002, Marmor wrote that mf ERG should be optional, but by 2011 he changed his mind and wrote that it (or SD-OCT or FAF) should be obtained routinely if available [6]. He changed his mind again in 2013, stating "I often omit baseline fields and almost never order baseline mf ERG testing…I add mf ERG at some point between 5 and 10 years and usually order it only every few years or when something is suspicious on other tests" [22]. No level 1 evidence exists to address issues regarding 4AQR screening.

The single most important component of the clinical examination is the determination of the patient's height and IBW (see Chap. 7) [10]. This allows the clinician to detect the presence of toxic dosing and to correct it. The remainder of the clinical examination is not sufficiently sensitive to be of great value. It is universally agreed that

fundus changes of 4AQR are late (see Chap. 6), and therefore unhelpful for detecting retinopathy at a time when intervention can prevent damage. For this reason, ancillary testing has always been employed (see Chap. 8). The characteristics of the ancillary tests become important in choosing which tests to use. The ideal test should be both sensitive and specific. Unfortunately, in clinical practice, the more sensitive a test is, the less specific it is, and vice versa.

In the application of ancillary tests, the pretest probability of 4AQR is more important than the performance characteristics of the test [72, 73]. The clinician needs a sense of how likely disease is in any given patient before applying the test. For example, if the patient is a man who is 6 ft 4 in. tall, weighs 180 lb, has been taking hydroxychloroquine 400 mg/day for rheumatoid arthritis for 1 year, has normal renal and liver function, and no preexisting maculopathy, then the pretest probability of hydroxychloroquine retinopathy might be 0.001 % (with a range, perhaps, of 0.0001–0.01 %). Why is this important? Because, the clinical profile would be so atypical for 4AQR that regardless of the results of ancillary testing, one would not be swayed to think that retinopathy was present. Chapter 8 covers in detail the principles of Bayesian reasoning as applied to screening for 4AQR [73, 74].

In the interval between 2002 and 2011, the most commonly used screening test was the 10-2 VF, which was used in 35–98 % of cases [12, 34, 75]. Despite its inferiority to 10-2 VF testing in sensitivity, up to 28.2 % of ophthalmologists use 30° SAP as a screening visual field [34]. Nine percent of ophthalmologists screened with Amsler grid testing alone as a test of the central visual field. [34] Color vision testing (73 %), fundus photography (28 %), fluorescein angiography (3 %), and electroretinography (3 %) were used less commonly, but more than the evidence indicates is optimal [34, 75].

Some have recommended the use of a combination of ancillary tests because none is completely sensitive [6, 27, 50, 64, 76–78]. When these recommendations involve expensive office-based instruments they generally ignore cost considerations and are impractical in situations of relative economic constraint. In other cases, however, the use of more than one test is not expensive. For example, many authors recommend that the patient self-test using an Amsler grid (AG) [13, 14, 32, 56, 61, 65], and some then add the more expensive 10-2 VF for situations where the AG is abnormal [50]. Aside from anecdotal reports, there is no evidence that this strategy is an effective way to screen for 4AQR. It is not harmful, may detect some cases, may have educational value, and is inexpensive. When combination testing is employed, the number of tests to do and the interpretation of the various permutations of combined test results becomes complex and without clear guidelines (see Chap. 8). For example, Maturi recommended adding mfERG when the results of 10-2 VF testing alone were too noisy or when one wanted to verify that the presence of a pericentral scotoma on 10-2 VF testing arose from retinal abnormality [79].

9.5 Number Needed to Screen

In judging the efficacy of a treatment, a useful concept is the number needed to treat (NNT) [80]. This gives the number of patients who must be treated to change the outcome from negative to positive in one person [72]. An analogous concept in the setting of screening is the number needed to screen (NNS) [80]. This tells the number of persons who would have to be screened to detect one person destined to develop 4AQR. In this case we wish to prevent clinical 4AQR by detecting subclinical 4AQR—that is, in the vocabulary laid out in Chap. 6, we seek to find patients with premaculopathy.

At this point, the concept of NNS using plausible data for hydroxychloroquine is developed. No incontrovertible data exist, but these numbers are not likely to be far off, and in any event, once the analysis is completed, sensitivity testing regarding the assumptions will be done to see where more caution is needed in drawing inferences. The number of people taking hydroxychloroquine in the United States is not known, but one published estimate that is commonly used is 150,000 [57]. This number, first used in

Table 9.2 Patients taking hydroxychloroquine according to their retinopathy and 10-2 visual field status

	Patients with HC retinopathy	Patients without HC retinopathy
Patients with an abnormal 10-2 VF	707	11,188
Patients with a normal 10-2 VF	118	137,987

1997, is probably an underestimate in 2014, but it will be used for the purposes of the discussion. The median duration of hydroxychloroquine use in the author's sample of 285 patients taking hydroxychloroquine for whom duration of therapy is known is 5.9 years, IQR (2.5–10.6 years), range (0.1–37.3 years). A reasonable assumption for the prevalence of retinopathy in those with duration of therapy less than 5.9 years is 0.1 % [5]. Likewise, a reasonable assumption for the prevalence of retinopathy in those with duration of 5.9 years or more is 1 % [5]. With these assumptions, we can calculate that there are $0.001 \times 75{,}000$ or 75 cases of 4AQR among the patients taking hydroxychloroquine for less than 5.9 years and $0.01 \times 75{,}000$ or 750 cases among patients taking hydroxychloroquine for 5.9 years or more. Therefore, in the population there would be 825 patients with 4AQR and 149,175 patients without 4AQR.

The goal of hydroxychloroquine screening is to detect the 825 patients before they get clinical retinopathy so that their drug can be stopped and the disease prevented. Until 2011, the main method used was 10-2 visual field testing. The best data on the performance characteristics of this test suggest that a reasonable estimate is sensitivity = 85.7 % and specificity = 92.5 % [81]. We can therefore construct the following 2×2 table (Table 9.2).

If screening were not the standard of medical care, as is the case in Great Britain, the number of cases of 4AQR expected would be 825. The percentage of HC users developing retinopathy would be 825/150,000 or 0.55 %. With screening, under our assumptions, the number of cases would be 118. The percentage of hydroxychloroquine users developing retinopathy in the screening environment would be 118/150,000 or

Table 9.3 Sensitivity of 4-aminoquinoline screening outcomes to assumptions regarding prevalence and screening regimens

Assumption on test characteristics	Assumption on prevalence of retinopathy	Risk of HCR if unscreened (%)	Risk of HCR if screened (%)	Relative reduction in risk (%)	Absolute reduction in risk (%)	Number needed to screen
Sensitivity of 10-2 VF = 85.7 % and specificity = 92.5 %	0.1 % for duration <5.9 years; 1 % for duration ≥5.9 years	0.55	0.079	86	0.471	212
Sensitivity of 10-2 VF = 85.7 % and specificity = 92.5 %	1 % for duration <5.9 years; 10 % for duration ≥5.9 years	5.5	0.79	86	4.71	21
Sensitivity of 10-2 VF + SD-OCT + mf ERG = 100 % and specificity = 92.5 %	0.1 % for duration <5.9 years; 1 % for duration ≥5.9 years	0.55	0	100	0.55	182

0.079 %. Thus the reduction in rate of development of HC retinopathy experienced in a screening environment is 0.471 %. The number of patients who would need to be screened to detect a case of reversible retinopathy would be 1/0.00471 = 212.

We can test the sensitivity of the analysis to the assumptions by inspecting Table 9.2. Raising the assumption of prevalence of retinopathy from 0.1 to 1 % for the group on hydroxychloroquine for fewer than 5.9 years and from 1 to 10 % for the group on hydroxychloroquine for 5.9 years or greater changes the number needed to be screened to 21 (Table 9.3).

If we suppose that we institute a new ancillary testing regimen involving mfERG and SD-OCT (but not FAF because of evidence that clinicians shun this test [12]) in addition to 10-2 VF, as proposed in the 2011 American Academy of Ophthalmology guidelines, and assume that these tests improve sensitivity to 100 % and specificity to 92.5 % [79], the NNS is 182 (Table 9.3). Put in terms of direct medical expenses, to detect each case of 4AQR using the 2002 guidelines cost $40,962 and using the 2011 guidelines $67,924. To determine whether this allocation of money is worthwhile, one would have to put a cost on having an annular scotoma bilaterally. This has not been done.

9.6   Actual Screening Practice

The gap between recommended and actual screening practice has been frequently noted [1, 13, 82]. Reasons for the gap include access to physicians competent to screen for 4AQR, disagreement with guidelines, lack of required specialized equipment (e.g., mf ERG), and cost [13, 83].

Nonadherence to guidelines works in both directions. In Great Britain, many ophthalmologists, dermatologists, and rheumatologists screen even though they are guided not to do so [83]. In one survey of dermatologists in the United Kingdom, 56 % responded that they did screen patients for 4AQR even though their professional society guidelines recommend against doing so [83]. For rheumatologists, less than half adhered to any of the clinical guidelines published by the British rheumatological societies [11]. Approximately one quarter delegated all screening functions to ophthalmologists [11]. Sixty-one percent screened more frequently than recommended [11]. In the United States, the reverse is true. In addition, personal experience with individual cases of 4AQR makes many prescribers of 4AQs reluctant to forego screening no matter what governing bodies recommend. In a survey of rheumatologists in the United States, 75 %

responded that they would not forego screening even if the American College of Rheumatology changed its guidelines and recommended not to screen [7].

In the United States, where screening for 4AQR has been the standard of care for decades, many patients taking 4AQs do not receive screening. In Veterans Affairs Medical Centers, different case series estimate the proportion of unscreened at 34–40 % of all patients taking hydroxychloroquine [82, 84].

Possible reasons for the principle-practice gap include:

- Doubts by clinicians regarding validity of guidelines.
- Recognition by clinicians that some guidelines may be fallacious or impractical [75]. An example would be the enduring failure of practicing clinicians to adopt the recommendation that screening in low-risk patients be omitted between baseline and 5 years of drug use [12, 34].
- Lack of awareness by clinicians of guidelines. For example, knowledge of the risk factors for 4AQR by screening clinicians is poor. Incorrect responses for daily dosing, duration, and age were given by greater than 70 % of respondents in one survey [75].
- Hostility of clinicians toward oversight.
- Obstacles in the work environment (e.g., lack of resources or impracticality of patient flow) [11].

Ramifications of the principles-practice gap include medicolegal liability [11]. Clinical guidelines may have weight in setting a legal standard against which an individual practitioner might be measured in the case of a lawsuit [11].

Guidelines ought not to be overly rigid, but should recognize the possibly overriding importance of the clinical situation. For example, some patients taking 4AQs cannot be screened in the recommended manner secondary to dementia, or physical limitations. In such cases, departures from guidelines cannot be considered delinquent [11].

Auditing is a necessary practice for attempting to close the principles-practice gap. Monitoring needs to be continued over the long term to close gaps and prevent their reopening [11].

9.7 Responses to Positive Results of Screening

Regardless of the results of the screening examination, communication between the ophthalmologist or optometrist and the physician prescribing the 4AQ is critical to avert 4AQR [10, 12, 85]. It is rare for the prescribing physician and screening ophthalmologist to disagree on whether to discontinue 4AQs when both have the evidence. In the remarkable instance in which they disagree on stopping the medication, a reasonable secondary plan is 4AQ dosage reduction with monitoring of the patient [12].

The eye care provider can respond in five ways to clinical situations regarding 4AQ use:

- Continued monitoring as before
- Shorten the interval of follow-up, using the same screening regimen
- Add other ancillary tests
- Recommend a reduction in the daily dose of the 4AQ
- Recommend cessation of 4AQs

Inexplicably, writers on 4AQR have sometimes made dogmatic statements suggesting that the only option is cessation of drug [86, 87]. Because chloroquine and hydroxychloroquine are beneficial to patients who take these medications for autoimmune disease, and because cessation of the drugs increases the risk of disease flare-ups [88], action to stop the drugs should not be initiated lightly. In addition, the drugs other than 4AQs used to treat autoimmune diseases are generally more toxic [86]. One must weigh the probability that the observed changes are from the 4AQ and not from a masquerade syndrome [60]. One must be sure enough that retinopathy is present that the harm from retinopathy outweighs the harm from possible autoimmune disease reactivation. Therefore, the opinions of the ophthalmologist, the patient, and the treating rheumatologist must all be considered to resolve difficult trade-offs [60]. If a relative scotoma is present but the rheumatologist thinks that the 4AQ is the best treatment and the patient is willing to risk some visual loss to maintain autoimmune disease control, then dosage reduction might be a reasonable response rather than cessation of the 4AQ [51].

Because one is often not certain that toxicity is present and because toxicity often is not present, a more nuanced response to various scenarios encountered during screening is warranted. If toxic dosing is recognized, a good response is to reduce dosing to a nontoxic level based on IBW [12]. Even if no suspicion of 4AQR exists, if a patient has had a good therapeutic response to a dose of 4AQ, it is reasonable to consider whether the response could be maintained at a lower risk of retinopathy by decreasing the daily dose or by taking a drug holiday for several months of the year [82, 89]. However, if progression of a relative scotoma on SAP is apparent after reduction of dosage, the only alternative is to discontinue the medication [51]. Dosage reductions of 4AQs can be associated with disease flare-ups, which become more common when serum concentrations of HC drop below 10^{-6} M/L [90].

If there is a suspicion of 4AQR, but the probability seems too low to stop the drug, the interval of follow-up can be shortened and other ancillary tests can be employed. By applying Bayesian analysis sequentially to the results of selected tests in a patient with an informed pre-test probability of 4AQR, a conclusion can be reached about the need for stopping the drug (see Chap. 8). Patients can take 4AQs for decades, during which time mild macular pigmentary changes can naturally develop due to age. Therefore, development of mild macular pigmentary changes not present at baseline is not a reason to stop 4AQs but simply indicates that a heightened suspicion and more vigilant follow-up may be warranted.

9.8 Cost-Effectiveness of Screening for 4-Aminoquinoline Retinopathy

The cost of screening for 4AQ retinopathy has long been mentioned as a problem and is a factor in the policies of some countries and health care organizations not to screen [4, 5, 8, 77, 91].

The cost-effectiveness of screening for 4AQR has been questioned on many levels. Some question the value relative to cost in anyone [8, 52, 54, 92]. More forcibly, the cost-effectiveness of screening low-risk patients has been questioned [8, 24, 62, 93].

The cost-effectiveness of using certain expensive ancillary tests routinely has been questioned. For example, the universal use of 10-2 visual field testing was questioned in 1998 [94]. More recently, the revised recommendations of 2011 to universally screen patients with mf ERG, SD-OCT, or FAF, if available, were questioned [12, 94].

If the expense of screening is to be advocated selectively rather than universally, the threshold for its use becomes debatable. Both Bernstein and Mavrikakis advocated screening when the daily dose of hydroxychloroquine exceeds 6.5 mg/kg/day based on IBW [48, 62]. Mavrikakis advocates screening once the duration threshold of therapy exceeds 6 years [62]. Others consider screening cost-effective for all patients taking 4AQs [6].

If one accepts the view that universal screening is warranted, then the subsidiary issue of the cost-effectiveness of different screening strategies arises. In the United States the 10-2 VF became the gold standard ancillary test for 4AQR after the 2002 AAO guidelines [18], but was never shown to add clinical benefit over simpler screening using the Amsler grid [82]. Likewise, the revised guidelines of 2011 were made without evidence that they add value to screening over the former gold standard of the 10-2 VF [6]. In fact, there is evidence that they have added not value, but cost [12]. Although historically 10-2 VFs have been the most commonly employed ancillary test used for screening, more recently Pulido has suggested that SD-OCT or FAF be used as the entry test with 10-2 VF reserved for patients with symptoms or in the case of controversy [95]. The markedly low variability of SD-OCT relative to 10-2 VF, FAF, and mfERG together with similar sensitivity and specificity and lower cost elevates the significance of this test relative to the others (see Chap. 8).

Another aspect to the cost-effectiveness of screening relates to nonadherence of ophthalmologists to screening guidelines. For example, diverse evidence suggests that clinicians screen more frequently than recommended guidelines for both low-risk and high-risk patients [12, 75]. An estimated $44 million in excess medical expenses was incurred in one study of the first 5 years of hydroxychloroquine therapy by excessive screening of low-risk patients in the United States based on an estimated population of hydroxychloroquine users of 150,000 [75]. The addition of mfERG and SD-OCT to 10-2 VF testing was expected to increase the cost of screening by a factor of 1.93 [12]. In actual practice, the use of these tests increased the cost of screening by a factor of 1.4 [12].

9.9   Medicolegal Aspects of Screening

Screening recommendations must be weighed against cost and medicolegal considerations, which are judgments to be made by individual physicians, health plans, and patients [18]. Nevertheless, national bodies promulgate guidelines that differ dramatically. In the United States, screening is the standard of care [6]. In the United Kingdom, screening is not recommended [8]. As long as the professional governing organizations take a position on screening for 4AQR, there will be some medicolegal risk for an individual practitioner to hold an opposing view.

Some observers have stated that an important reason to screen is to protect against a lawsuit [52, 96]. Even those who advocate screening for medical reasons acknowledge the medicolegal risk involved in caring for patients taking 4AQs. At the outset of screening, it is important to inform the patient of the risks of hydroxychloroquine and chloroquine and the purpose of screening—to reduce the probability of retinopathy and detect it early should it occur [18]. The patient should be informed that it is possible to develop retinopathy despite all appropriate screening efforts although the risk is very low. These discussions need to be documented in the medical record. Some physicians think that written consent forms should be used, but others advise against them as they frighten patients unnecessarily and lead to nonuse of drugs that are valuable in treating rheumatologic disease [24].

Especially in early cases of retinopathy, there is frequently a disagreement regarding whether retinopathy is present [12, 22]. Moreover, predicting whether a case of retinopathy will regress, remain stable, or progress is unreliable. Therefore, patients must be made aware of the limitations of ophthalmic screening [82]. Screening can help to detect retinopathy earlier than if no screening were done, but retinopathy often develops even in a screening environment, and retinal damage may continue even if drug is stopped [10].

Not Screening Patients in a Screening Environment

Even in the United States, or another country where screening for 4AQR is the standard, there are cases in which a decision not to screen is rational and defensible. As an example from the author's practice, consider the case of a 79-year-old woman with SLE who had been treated with hydroxychloroquine for 2 years at a dosage of 200 mg/day. She was 63 in. tall and weighed 125 lb. She had suffered acute retinal necrosis of the left eye previously leaving her with hand motion's vision. In the right eye she had 20/25 visual acuity and a normal macula. She was confined to a recliner and could not sit up to cooperate with either visual field testing, SD-OCT imaging, or mf ERG testing. In this case, no ancillary testing was done either at baseline or follow-up. Her dosing and duration of therapy placed her at an extremely low risk for toxicity. The low risk of retinopathy was far overbalanced by the benefit that she obtained from hydroxychloroquine in the control of her SLE.

9.10 Patient Education and Home Medical Records

The importance of inquiring about visual symptoms has been stressed by some [32]. Unless specific inquiries are made by the ophthalmologist and education given about their importance, patients may overlook them. In a failure analysis of patients who developed 4AQR, Bergholz found that the median time between the onset of symptoms referable to 4AQR and cessation of drug was 12 months [97]. Because daily dosage, cumulative dosage, height, weight, and duration of therapy are all important variables in determining risk of 4AQR, patients should keep records of their 4AQ use and bring them to ophthalmologist visits [13]. These records need to include:

- Name of drug
- Diagnosis for which the drug was prescribed
- All dates of use and discontinuation
- All dosing
- Height
- Weight, including changes
- Renal disease
- Liver disease

Patient education can be enhanced by handouts of printed material to supplement the physician–patient encounter. An example of such a handout follows, written at the fifth-grade level (Fig 9.1) [6, 82].

Hydroxychloroquine Fact Sheet for Patients

You have an increased risk of eye damage from hydroxychloroquine if:

- You are older than 60

- You are shorter than 5 feet 3 inches

- You weigh less than 135 pounds

- You have taken the medicine for more than 5 years

- You have liver or kidney disease

- You have certain eye diseases before you begin the medicine

Eye exams are intended to see if you have any of these risks and to detect eye damage as early as possible, but they are not foolproof. You could get eye damage even if you receive screening. If you get eye disease, the damage could get worse even if you stop taking the medicine. If you stop taking your medicine for another reason, you could get eye damage that begins years later, although that is rare.

If hydroxychloroquine has reduced the symptoms of your disease, you can reduce your risk of later developing eye damage by lowering the amount of drug you take daily. You can ask your doctor if your daily dose can be reduced, but you should not lower the dose without permission from your doctor.

Fig. 9.1 Hydroxychloroquine fact sheet that can be given to patients at the time of screening. Using language aimed at the fifth-grade level, it educates, raises consciousness of risk, forms part of informed consent, and may help to protect the physician from medicolegal risk. Adapted from Flach [82]

9.11   Screening After Cessation of Chloroquine of Hydroxychloroquine

Because of the delayed occurrence of 4AQR after cessation of the drug, the question of whether patients who stop 4AQs should be screened arises. Based on the principles of screening laid out at the beginning of the chapter, there seems to be little rationale for this. Delayed development of retinopathy after cessation of 4AQs is even rarer than 4AQR in patients who are on the drug. There is already a controversy regarding the justification of screening in the latter group. It seems even less rational to screen the former group, especially as there is no treatment that can help. Nevertheless, there are contrary published recommendations [18]. One group recommended a follow-up evaluation 3 months after a diagnosis of definite 4AQR is made, and then annually [18]. Another has recommended that periodic visual fields or other functional test be administered to anyone taking a cumulative dose of chloroquine greater than 300 g who stops the drug [98].

9.12   Challenges

There is no foolproof method of preventing 4AQR, but the risk can be reduced by safe dosing and early detection of damage by monitoring of ocular functions [4, 25, 99]. The main public health problem with respect to use of 4AQs is overdosing. The focus of screening should be to detect and correct overdosing, and if the national policy recommends it, to detect the rare occurrence of retinopathy in those properly dosed. It is a challenge to write guidelines that are practical for the clinician who will actually do the screening that are consistent with the economic context and reflect the medical evidence. The author's attempt follows.

- Encourage prescribing physicians to adopt a policy not to prescribe a dose higher than 3.0 mg/kg/day for chloroquine and 6.5 mg/kg/day for hydroxychloroquine based on the lower of actual body weight (ABW) and IBW and to intentionally check renal and liver function before prescribing.
- In a screening culture, have eye care providers:
  - Check for overdosing based on the lesser of IBW and ABW and confirm normality of renal and liver function.
  - Check for preexisting maculopathy at a baseline examination that includes 10-2 VF and SD-OCT testing.
  - Recheck patients yearly with examinations that include alternating 10-2 VF or SD-OCT, but not both.
  - Restrict mfERG and FAF use to difficult cases.

9.13   Summary of Key Points

- Screening guidelines for 4AQR differ between the United States (pro) and the United Kingdom (con).
- The decision whether to screen depends on the prevalence of 4AQR, which is unknown, and for which estimates vary widely.
- At least 12.8 % of patients taking 4AQs are overdosed. Screening for overdosage is inexpensive and worthwhile.
- The prevalence of 4AQR in properly dosed patients is much less than 1 %. Screening to detect retinopathy in this population wastes money.
- Screening in the United States is likely to persist for historical reasons. If screening for 4AQR is retained in properly dosed patients, a reasonable approach is to obtain a baseline examination with 10-2 VF or SD-OCT followed by annual follow-up with one or the other, but not both. The 5-year gap recommended between baseline and a second screening should be abandoned as impractical. The use of mfERG and FAF should be less common. These tests are highly variable, less available, and less familiar to screening clinicians, but may add value in unclear cases.

References

1. Bernatsky S, Pinaeu CA, Gans M, Clarke A. Adherence to guidelines for monitoring of antimalarial-related retinal toxicity. Rheumatology. 2004;43:1058–9.
2. Samanta A, Goh L, Bawendi A. Guidelines for the monitoring of hydroxychloroquine: reply. Rheumatology. 2004;43:1059.
3. Warner AE. Early hydroxychloroquine macular toxicity. Arthritis Rheum. 2001;44:1959–61.
4. Jones SK. Ocular toxicity and hydroxychloroquine: guidelines for screening. Br J Dermatol. 1999; 140:3–7.
5. Wolfe F, Marmor MF. Rates and predictors of hydroxychloroquine retinal toxicity in patients with rheumatoid arthritis and systemic lupus erythematosus. Arthritis Care Res. 2010;62:775–84.
6. Marmor MF, Kellner U, Lai TYY, Lyons JS, Mieler WF. Revised recommendations on screening for chloroquine and hydroxychloroquine retinopathy. Ophthalmology. 2011;118:415–22.
7. Fraenkel L, Felson DT. Rheumatologists' attitudes toward routine screening for hydroxychloroquine retinopathy. J Rheumatol. 2001;28:1218–21.
8. Fielder A, Graham E, Jones S, Silman A, Tullo A. Royal college of ophthalmologists guidelines: ocular toxicity and hydroxychloroquine. Eye. 1998;12: 907–9.
9. Elder M, Rahman AMA. Early paracentral visual field loss in patients taking hydroxychloroquine. Arch Ophthalmol. 2006;124:1729–33.
10. Browning DJ. Hydroxychloroquine and chloroquine retinopathy: screening for drug toxicity. Am J Ophthalmol. 2002;133:649–56.
11. Samanta A, Goh L, Bawendi A. Are evidence-based guidelines being followed for the monitoring of ocular toxicity of hydroxychloroquine? A nationwide survey of practice amongst consultant rheumatologists and implications for clinical governance. Rheumatology. 2004;43:346–8.
12. Browning DJ. Impact of the revised American Academy of Ophthalmology guidelines regarding hydroxychloroquine screening on actual practice. Am J Ophthalmol. 2013;155:418–28.
13. Banks CN. Melanin: blackguard or red herring? Another look at chloroquine retinopathy. Aust N Z J Ophthalmol. 1987;15:365–70.
14. Block JA. Hydroxychloroquine and retinal safety. Lancet. 1998;351:771.
15. Jekel JF, Elmore JG, Katz DL. Epidemiology, biostatistics, and preventive medicine. Philadelphia: WB Saunders; 1996. p. 216–7.
16. Walvick MD, Walvick MP, Tongson E, Ngo CH. Hydroxychloroquine: lean body weight dosing. Ophthalmology. 2011;118:2100.
17. Michaelides M, Stover NB, Francis PJ, Weleber RG. Retinal toxicity associated with hydroxychloroquine and chloroquine: risk factors, screening, and progression despite cessation of therapy. Arch Ophthalmol. 2011;129:30–9.
18. Marmor MF, Carr RE, Easterbrook M, et al. Recommendations on screening for chloroquine and hydroxychloroquine retinopathy. Ophthalmology. 2002;109:1377–82.
19. Heravian J, Saghafi M, Shoeibi N, Hassanzadeh S, Shakeri MT, Sharepoor M. A comparative study of the usefulness of color vision, photostress recovery time, and visual evoked potential tests in the early detection of ocular toxicity from hydroxychloroquine. Int Ophthalmol. 2011;31:283–9.
20. Schwartz SG, Mieler WF. Retinal and choroidal manifestations of systemic medications. In: Arevalo JF, editor. Retinal and choroidal manifestations of selected systemic diseases. New York: Springer; 2013. p. 479–92.
21. Razeghinejad MR, Torkaman F, Amini H. Blue-yellow perimetry can be an early detector of hydroxychloroquine and chloroquine retinopathy. Med Hypotheses. 2005;65:629–30.
22. Marmor MF. Efficient and effective screening for hydroxychloroquine toxicity. Am J Ophthalmol. 2013;155:413–4.
23. Mackenzie AH. Dose refinements in long-term therapy of rheumatoid arthritis with antimalarials. Am J Med. 1983;75:40–5.
24. Spalton DJ. Retinopathy and antimalarial drugs-the British experience. Lupus. 1996;5:S70–2.
25. Mackenzie AH. Antimalarial drugs for rheumatoid arthritis. Am J Med. 1983;75:48–58.
26. Percival SPB, Behrman J. Ophthalmological safety of chloroquine. Br J Ophthalmol. 1969;53:101–9.
27. Marmor MF. Comparison of screening procedures in hydroxychloroquine toxicity. Arch Ophthalmol. 2012;130:461–9.
28. Payne JF, Hubbard III GB, Aaberg Sr TM, Yan J. Clinical characteristics of hydroxychloroquine retinopathy. Br J Ophthalmol. 2010;95:245–50.
29. Falcone PM, Paolini L, Lou PL. Hydroxychloroquine toxicity despite normal dose therapy. Ann Ophthalmol. 1993;25:385–8.
30. Bienfang D, Coblyn JS, Liang MH, Corzillius M. Hydroxychloroquine retinopathy despite regular ophthalmologic evaluation: a consecutive series. J Rheumatol. 2000;27:2703–6.
31. Henkind P, Rothfield NF. Ocular abnormalities in patients treated with synthetic antimalarial drugs. N Engl J Med. 1963;269:434–9.
32. Bernstein H. Ocular safety of hydroxychlotoquine sulfate (Plaquenil). South Med J. 1992;85:274–9.
33. Easterbrook M. Long-term course of antimalarial maculopathy after cessation of treatment. Can J Ophthalmol. 1992;27:237–9.
34. Blomquist PH, Chundru RK. Screening for hydroxychloroquine toxicity by Texas ophthalmologists. J Rheumatol. 2002;29:1665–70.
35. Bunch TW, O'Duffy JD. Disease modifying drugs for progressive rheumatoid arthritis. Mayo Clin Proc. 1980;55:161–79.

36. Maksymowych W, Russell AS. Antimalarials in rheumatology: efficacy and safety. Semin Arthritis Rheum. 1987;16:206–21.

37. Percival SPB, Meanock I. Chloroquine: ophthalmological safety and clinical assessment in rheumatoid arthritis. Br Med J. 1968;3:579–84.

38. Blyth C, Lane C. Hydroxychloroquine retinopathy: is screening necessary? Intensive screening is not necessary at normal doses. Br Med J. 1998;316:716–7.

39. Fleck BW, Bell AL, Mitchell JD, Thomson BJ, Hurst NP, Nuki G. Screening for antimalarial maculopathy in rheumatology clinics. Br Med J. 1985;291:782–5.

40. Rebello JA. Ocular reactions to antimalarial drugs. Arch Dermatol. 1961;83:123–7.

41. Mackenzie AH. An appraisal of chloroquine. Arthritis Rheum. 1970;13:280–91.

42. Dubois EL. Antimalarials in the management of discoid and systemic lupus erythematosus. Semin Arthritis Rheum. 1978;8:33–51.

43. Graniewski-Wijnands HS, Van Lith GHM, Vijfvinkel-Bruinenga S. Ophthalmological examination of patients taking chloroquine. Doc Ophthalmol. 1979;48:231–4.

44. Tobin DR, Krohel G, Rynes RI. Hydroxychloroquine-seven-year experience. Arch Ophthalmol. 1982;100:81–3.

45. Scherbel AL. Use of synthetic antimalarial drugs and other agents for rheumatoid arthritis: historic and therapeutic perspectives. Am J Med. 1983;75:1–4.

46. Terrell III WL, Haik KG, Haik Jr GM. Hydroxychloroquine sulfate and retinopathy. South Med J. 1988;81:1327–8.

47. Lozier JR, Friedlander MH. Complications of antimalarial therapy. Int Ophthalmol Clin. 1989;29:172–8.

48. Bernstein HN. Ocular safety of hydroxychloroquine. Ann Ophthalmol. 1991;23:292–6.

49. Easterbrook M. Screening for antimalarial toxicity. Can J Ophthalmol. 1993;28:51–2.

50. Easterbrook M. The ocular safety of hydroxychloroquine. Semin Arthritis Rheum. 1993;23:62–7.

51. Easterbrook M. Ocular effects and safety of antimalarial agents. Am J Med. 1988;85:23–9.

52. Spalton DJ, Roe GMV, Hughes GRV. Hydroxychloroquine, dosage parameters and retinopathy. Lupus. 1993;2:355–8.

53. Grierson DJ. Hydroxychloroquine and visual screening in a rheumatology outpatient clinic. Ann Rheum Dis. 1997;56:188–90.

54. Morsman CDG, Livesey SJ, Richards IM, Jessop JD, Mills PV. Screening for hydroxychloroquine retinal toxicity: is it necessary? Eye. 1990;4:572–6.

55. American College of Rheumatology Ad Hoc Committee on Clinical Guidelines. Guidelines for monitoring drug therapy in rheumatoid arthritis. Arthritis Rheum. 1996;39:723–31.

56. Rynes RI. Antimalarial drugs in the treatment of rheumatological diseases. Br J Rheumatol. 1997;36:799–805.

57. Levy GD, Munz SJ, Paschal J, Cohen HB, Prince KJ, Peterson T. Incidence of hydroxychloroquine retinopathy in 1,207 patients in a large multicenter outpatient practice. Arthritis Rheum. 1997;40:1482–6.

58. Esdaile JM. Canadian consensus conference on hydroxychloroquine. J Rheumatol. 2000;27:2919–21.

59. Albert DA, Debois LKL, Lu KF. Antimalarial ocular toxicity, a critical appraisal. J Clin Rheumatol. 1998;4:57–62.

60. May K, Metcalf T, Gough A. Screening for hydroxychloroquine retinopathy. Br Med J. 1998;317:1388–9.

61. Bray VJ, Enzenauer RJ, Enzenauer RW, West SG. Antimalarial toxicity in rheumatic disease. J Clin Rheumatol. 1998;4:168–9.

62. Mavrikakis I, Sfikakis PP, Mavrikakis E, Rougas K, Nikolaou A, Kostopoulos C, Mavrikakis M. The incidence of irreversible retinal toxicity in patients treated with hydroxychloroquine—a reappraisal. Ophthalmology. 2003;110:1321–6.

63. Bergholz R, Schroeter J, Ruther K. Evaluation of risk factors for retinal damage due to chloroquine and hydroxychloroquine. Br J Ophthalmol. 2010;94: 1637–42.

64. Farrell DF. Retinal toxicity to antimalarial drugs: chloroquine and hydroxychloroquine: a neurophysiologic study. Clin Ophthalmol. 2012;6:377–83.

65. American Academy of Optometry. Monitoring ocular toxicity of selected medications. 2013. www.aoa.org/optometrists/education-and-training/clinical-care/monitoring-ocular-toxicity-of-selected-medications. Accessed 5 July 2013.

66. Hanna B, Holdeman NR, Tang RA, Schiffman JS. Retinal toxicity secondary to Plaquenil therapy. Optometry. 2008;79:90–4.

67. Alarcon GS. How frequently and how soon should we screen our patients for the presence of antimalarial retinopathy? Arthritis Rheum. 2002;46:561.

68. Shinjo SK, Junior OOM, Tizziani VAP, Morita C, Kochen JAL, Takahashi WY, Laurindo IMM. Chloroquine-induced bull's eye maculopathy in rheumatoid arthritis: related to disease duration? Clin Rheumatol. 2007;26:1248–53.

69. Easterbrook M. Comparison of threshold and standard Amsler grid testing in patients with established antimalarial retinopathy. Can J Ophthalmol. 1992;27:240–2.

70. Marmor MF. The dilemma of hydroxychloroquine screening: new information from the multifocal ERG. Am J Ophthalmol. 2005;140:894–5.

71. Chen E, Brown DM, Benz MS, Fish RH, Wong TP, Kim RY, Major JC. Spectral domain optical coherence tomography as an effective screening test for hydroxychloroquine retinopathy (the "flying saucer" sign). Clin Ophthalmol. 2010;4:1151–8.

72. Newman DH. Hippocrates' shadow. Secrets from the house of medicine. New York: Simon and Schuster; 2008.

73. Newman DH. Hippocrates' shadow. Secrets from the house of medicine. New York: Scribner; 2008. p. 101–2.

74. Stone JV. Bayes' rule: a tutorial introduction to Bayesian analysis. Lexington: Sebtel Press; 2013.

75. Semmer AE, Lee MS, Harrison AR, Olsen TW. Hydroxychloroquine retinopathy screening. Br J Ophthalmol. 2008;92:1653–5.

76. Marmor MF, Kellner U, Lai TYY, Lyons JS, Mieler WF. Author response. Ophthalmology. 2012;119:207–8.

77. Kellner S, Weinitz S, Kellner U. Spectral domain optical coherence tomography detects early stages of chloroquine retinopathy similar to multifocal electroretinography, fundus autofluorescence and near-infrared autofluorescence. Br J Ophthalmol. 2009;93:1444–7.

78. Rodriguez-Hurtado FJ, Saez-Moreno JA, Rodriguez-Ferrer JM. Maculopathy in patient with systemic lupus erythematosus treated with hydroxychloroquine. Reumatol Clin. 2012;8:280–3.

79. Maturi RK, Yu M, Weleber RG. Multifocal electroretinographic evaluation of long-term hydroxychloroquine users. Arch Ophthalmol. 2004;122:973–81.

80. Barratt A, Irwig L, Glasziou P, Cumming R, Raffle A, Hicks N, Gray JAM, Guyatt G, Lijmer J. Moving from evidence to action. Recommendations about screening. In: Guyatt G, Rennie D, editors. User's guide to the medical literature. A manual for evidence-based practice (JAMA and Archives Journals). Chicago: AMA; 2002. p. 583–97.

81. Browning DJ, Lee C. The relative sensitivity and specificity of 10-2 visual fields, multifocal electroretinography, and spectral domain OCT in detecting hydroxychloroquine retinopathy. Scientific poster 484. Presented at: American Academy of Ophthalmology 2013 Annual Meeting, New Orleans; 14–19 Nov 2013.

82. Flach AJ. Improving the risk-benefit relationship and informed consent for patients treated with hydroxychloroquine. Trans Am Ophthalmol Soc. 2007;105:191–7.

83. Cox NH, Paterson WD. Ocular toxicity of antimalarials in dermatology: a survey of current practice. Br J Dermat. 1994;131:878–82.

84. Gupta G, Greenberg PB, Tsiaras WG. The prevalence of high-risk factors and adherence to screening guidelines for hydroxychloroquine retinopathy in a cohort of US veterans. Scientific poster 461. Presented at: American Academy of Ophthalmology 2005 Annual Meeting, Chicago; 17–18 Oct 2005.

85. Fung AE, Samy CN, Rosenfeld PJ. Optical coherence tomography findings in hydroxychloroquine and chloroquine-associated maculopathy. Retinal Cases Brief Rep. 2007;1:128–30.

86. Yam JCS, Kwok AKH. Ocular toxicity of hydroxychloroquine. Hong Kong Med J. 2006;12:294–304.

87. Lyons JS. Impact of the revised American Academy of Ophthalmology guidelines regarding hydroxychloroquine screening on actual practice. Am J Ophthalmol. 2013;156:410.

88. The Canadian Hydroxychloroquine Study Group. A randomized study of the effect of withdrawing hydroxychloroquine sulfate in systemic lupus erythematosus. N Engl J Med. 1991;324:150–4.

89. Elman A, Gullberg R, Nillson E, Rendahl I, Wachtmeister L. Choroquine retinopathy in patients with rheumatoid arthritis. Scand J Rheumatol. 1976;5:161–6.

90. Lafyatis R, York M, Marshak-Rothstein A. Antimalarial agents: closing the gate on toll-like receptors? Arthritis Rheum. 2006;54:3068–70.

91. Lai TYY, Ngai JWS, Chan WM, Lam DSC. Visual field and multifocal electroretinography and their correlations in patients on hydroxychloroquine therapy. Doc Ophthalmol. 2006;112:177–87.

92. Morand EF, McCloud PI, Littlejohn GO. Continuation of long term treatment with hydroxychloroquine in systemic lupus erythematosus and rheumatoid arthritis. Ann Rheum Dis. 1992;51:1318–21.

93. Lee AG. Hydroxychloroquine screening. Who needs it, when, how, and why? Br J Ophthalmol. 2005;89:521–2.

94. Easterbrook M. Current concepts in monitoring patients on antimalarials. Aust N Z J Ophthalmol. 1998;26:101–3.

95. Pulido JS, Barkmeier AJ, Leavitt JA. Screening for hydroxychloroquine toxicity. Ophthalmology. 2012;119:207.

96. Coyle E. Hydroxychloroquine retinopathy [letter]. Ophthalmology. 2001;108:243–4.

97. Bergholz R, Ruther K, Tillack H, Joussen AM, Schroeter J. Ophthalmologic screening history and vision-targeted health status of patients suffering from chloroquine maculopathy. Ophthalmologe. 2012. doi:10.1007/s00347-012-2657-1.

98. Ehrenfeld M, Nesher R, Merin S. Delayed-onset chloroquine retinopathy. Br J Ophthalmol. 1986;70:281–3.

99. McChesney EQ, Fitch CD. 4-Aminoquinolines. In: Peters W, Richards WHG, editors. Antimalarial drugs II. Current antimalarials and new drug developments. Berlin: Springer; 1984. p. 3–60.

Abbreviations

4AQR	4-Aminoquinoline retinopathy
4AQs	4-Aminoquinolines (chloroquine and hydroxychloroquine)
AAO	American Academy of Ophthalmology
ABW	Actual body weight
AG	Amsler grid
C	Chloroquine
HC	Hydroxychloroquine
IBW	Ideal body weight
RA	Rheumatoid arthritis
RPE	Retinal pigment epithelium
SLE	Systemic lupus erythematosus

The first nine chapters of this book were thematic. This chapter takes a topical approach, presenting clinical examples that illustrate the principles developed in the earlier chapters. In many cases, the details of the clinical scenario modify a straightforward extrapolation of a theoretical assertion from an earlier chapter. By reviewing many cases, the clinician can learn to assess the risk of retinopathy and detect it early in patients who take 4-aminoquinolines (4AQs). The format in the chapter will be case reports with ancillary test images followed by an analysis of the case, and when available, a description of the outcome and follow-up.

The overriding message of the cases to be presented is how often patients are overdosed, and how the problems entailed are potentially avoidable if the principle of dosing based on the lesser of ideal body weight (IBW) and actual body weight (ABW) is followed (see Chap. 7) [1]. When both hydroxchloroquine and chloroquine are under discussion, they will be termed 4-aminoquinolines and their retinopathies will be termed 4-aminoquinoline retinopathy (4AQR). Commonly used abbreviations in this chapter are collected in "Abbreviations" for reference. Each term will be first used in its full form, along with its abbreviation.

10.1 A Case of Prolonged Toxic Dosing with Evidence of Premaculopathy

A 48-year-old woman with systemic lupus erythematosus (SLE) had been taking hydroxychloroquine for 20 years at 400 mg/day. She was 5 ft 3 in. tall and weighed 167 lb. She had no renal or liver disease, nor any preexisting macular abnormalities on funduscopy. She had annual 10-2 visual fields (10-2 VFs), which were normal (Fig. 10.1). When the American Academy of Ophthalmology (AAO) guidelines were revised in 2011 to add multifocal electroretinography (mf ERG) and spectral domain optical coherence tomography (SD-OCT), where available, these were also obtained. Three consecutive 10-2 mf ERGs showed progressive decrease in N1P1 amplitude for rings R_1 to R_3 in both eyes and progressive increase in the R_1/R_2 ratio (Fig. 10.1). By the third study, these variables were all in the

D.J. Browning, *Hydroxychloroquine and Chloroquine Retinopathy*,
DOI 10.1007/978-1-4939-0597-3_10, © Springer Science+Business Media New York 2014

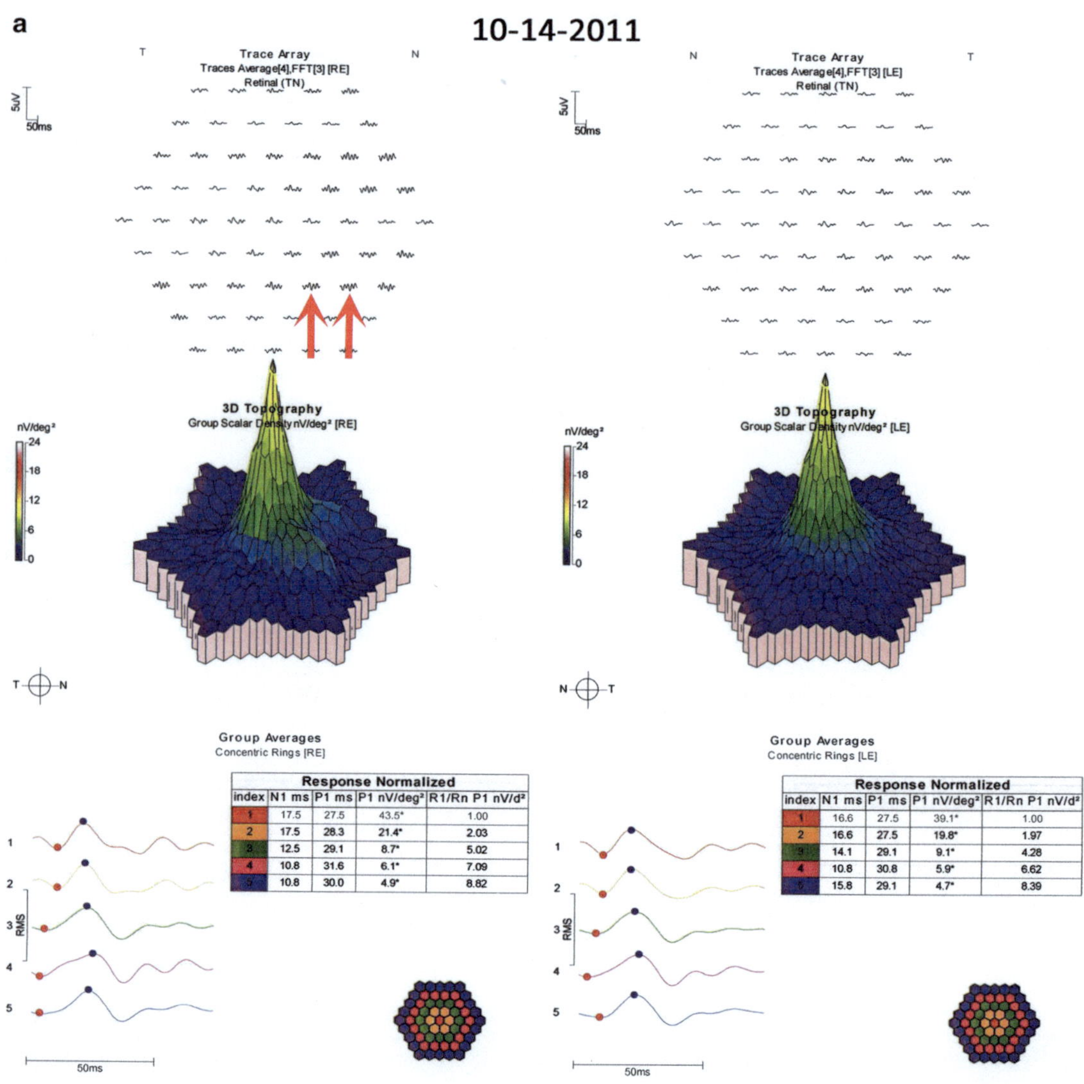

Fig. 10.1 Ancillary testing in a patient on toxic dosing of hydroxychloroquine for 20 years. (**a**) The initial multifocal electroretinogram (mf ERG) from 10/14/2011. There is some 60 cycle noise evident in some of the hexagonal recordings (*red arrows*). The amplitudes and R_1/R_2 ratio for both eyes are normal. (**b**) The second mf ERG from 10-19-2012 is technically better than that of (**a**). The N1P1 amplitudes are decreased in comparison to those in (**a**). (**c**) The third mf ERG from 10-18-2013 is of good quality and shows a further trend in decreasing N1P1 amplitudes compared to those of (**a**, **b**). (**d**) Plots of the N1P1 amplitudes and the R_1/R_2 ratios for the three mf ERGs shown in (**a**–**c**). The *green horizontal bars* identify the lower limits of normal for the ring

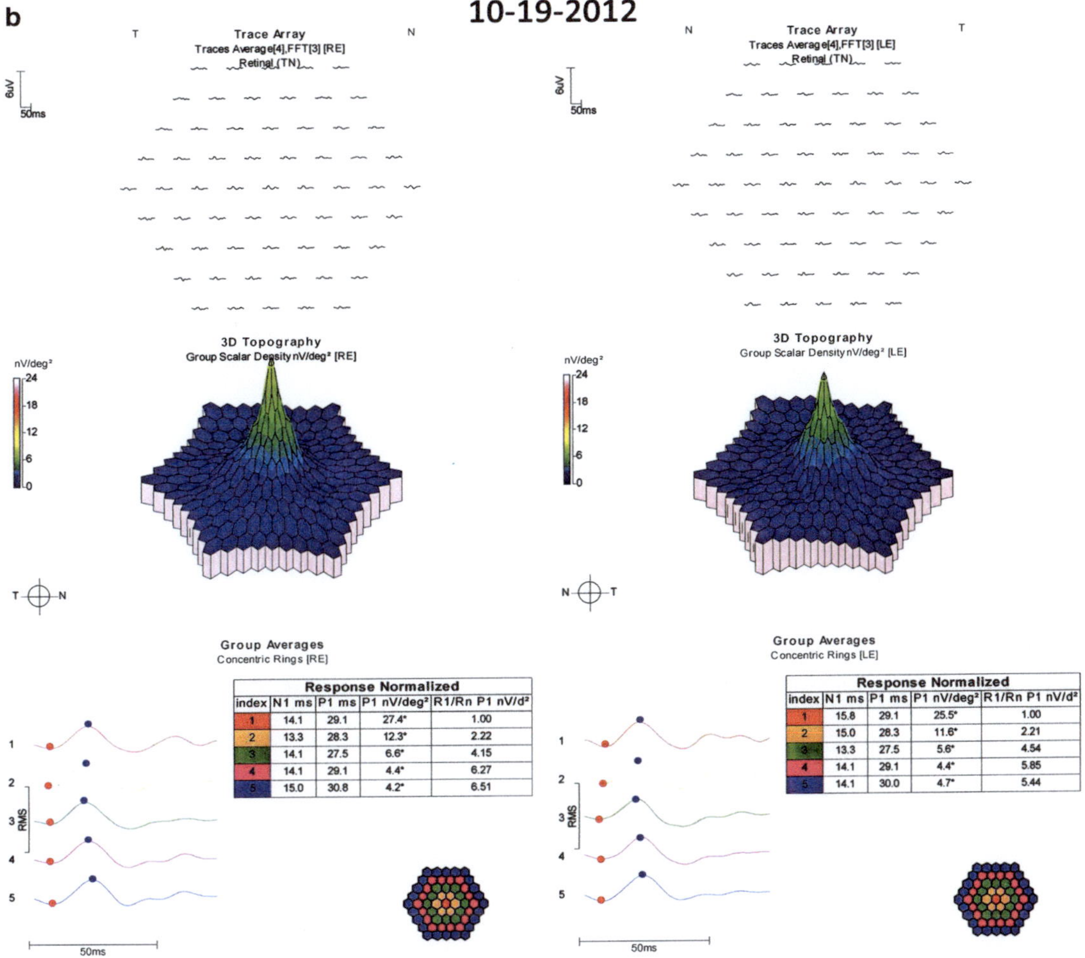

	Response Normalized			
index	N1 ms	P1 ms	P1 nV/deg²	R1/Rn P1 nV/d²
1	14.1	29.1	27.4*	1.00
2	13.3	28.3	12.3*	2.22
3	14.1	27.5	6.6*	4.15
4	14.1	29.1	4.4*	6.27
5	15.0	30.8	4.2*	6.51

	Response Normalized			
index	N1 ms	P1 ms	P1 nV/deg²	R1/Rn P1 nV/d²
1	15.8	29.1	25.5*	1.00
2	15.0	28.3	11.6*	2.21
3	13.3	27.5	5.6*	4.54
4	14.1	29.1	4.4*	5.85
5	14.1	30.0	4.7*	5.44

Fig. 10.1 (continued) amplitudes and the upper limit of normal for the R_1/R_2 ratio. There is a three-study trend toward increasing abnormality consistent with hydroxychloroquine toxicity. (**e**) The false color maps of macular thickness from spectral domain optical coherence tomography (SD-OCT) show parafoveal thinning bilaterally (*red arrows*), which is most severe temporally in the right eye. (**f**) SD-OCT line scans showing normal inner segment/outer segment junction morphology (*yellow arrows*) at a time when parafoveal thinning was present. (**g**) 10-2 visual fields from 2005 through 2013 are normal

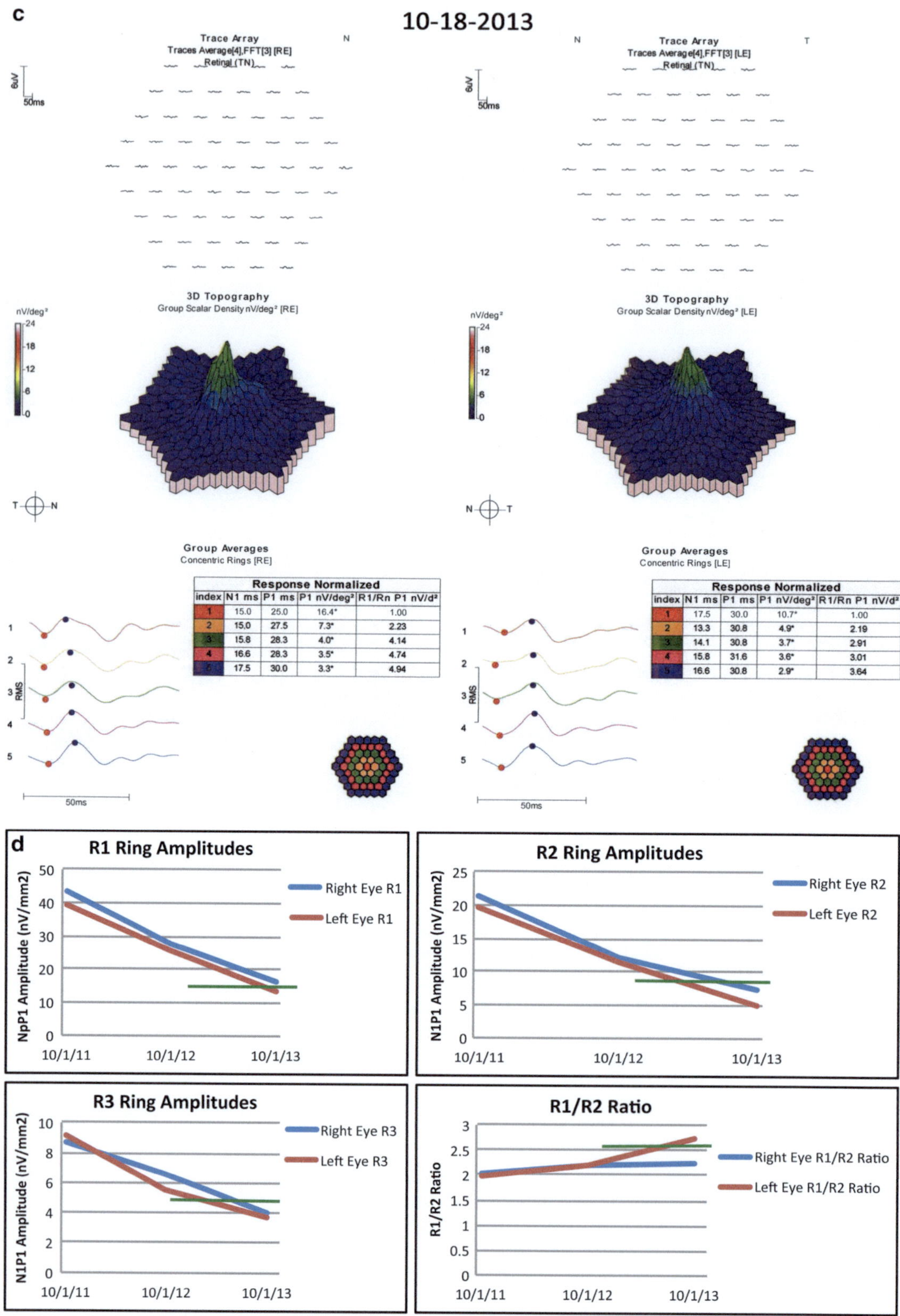

Fig. 10.1 (continued)

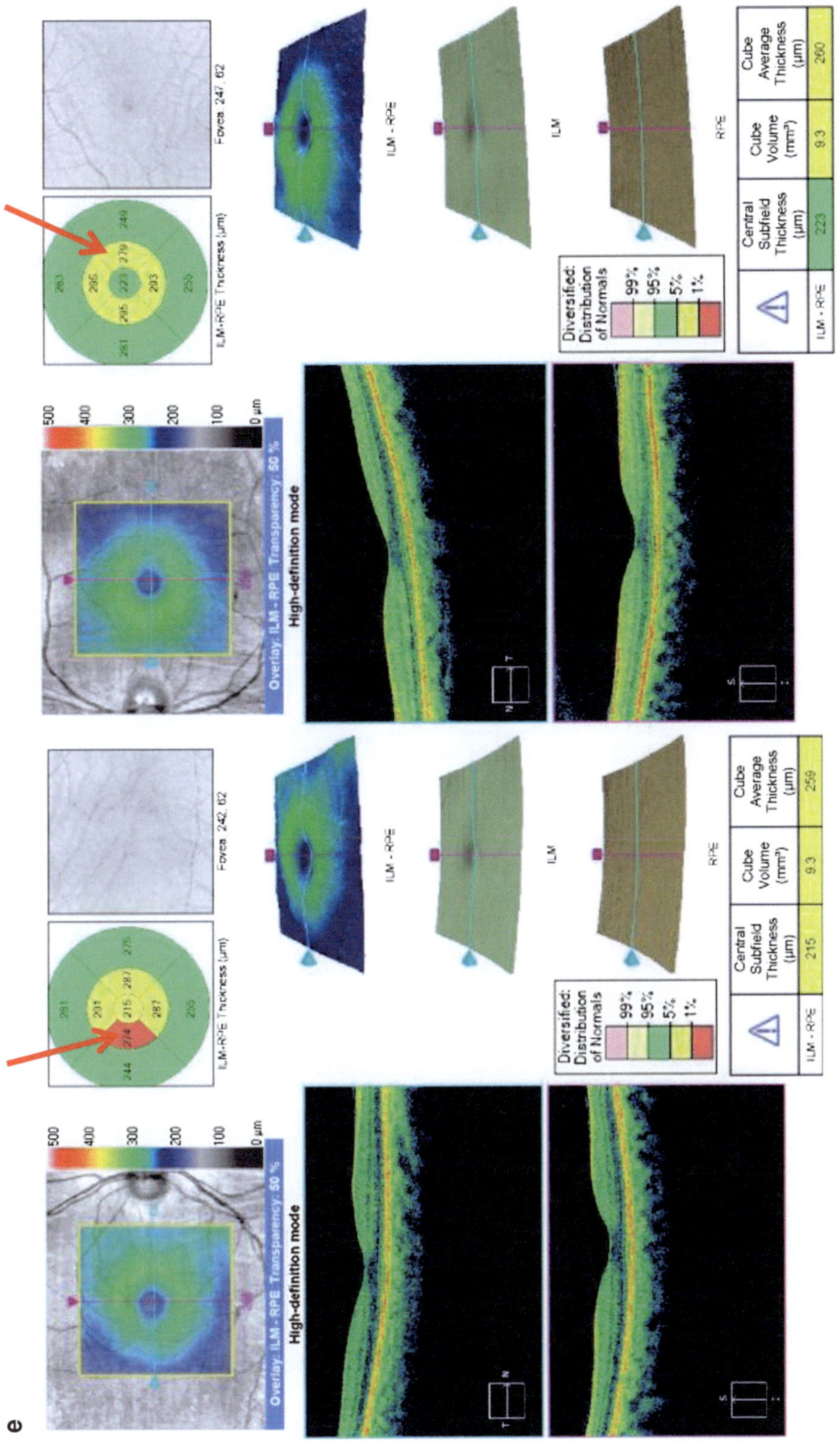

Fig. 10.1 (continued)

f

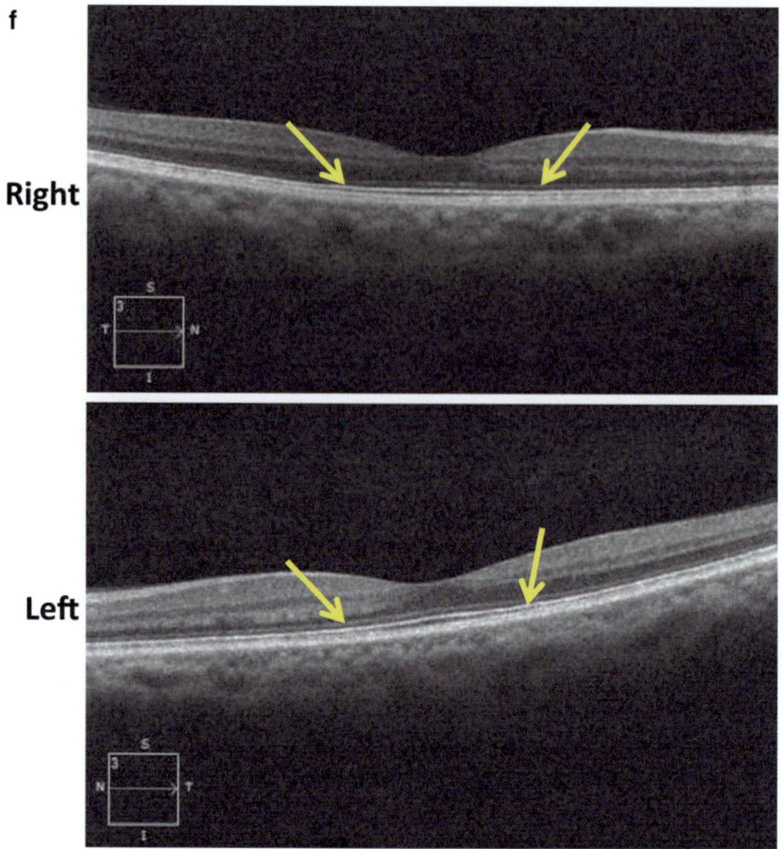

g

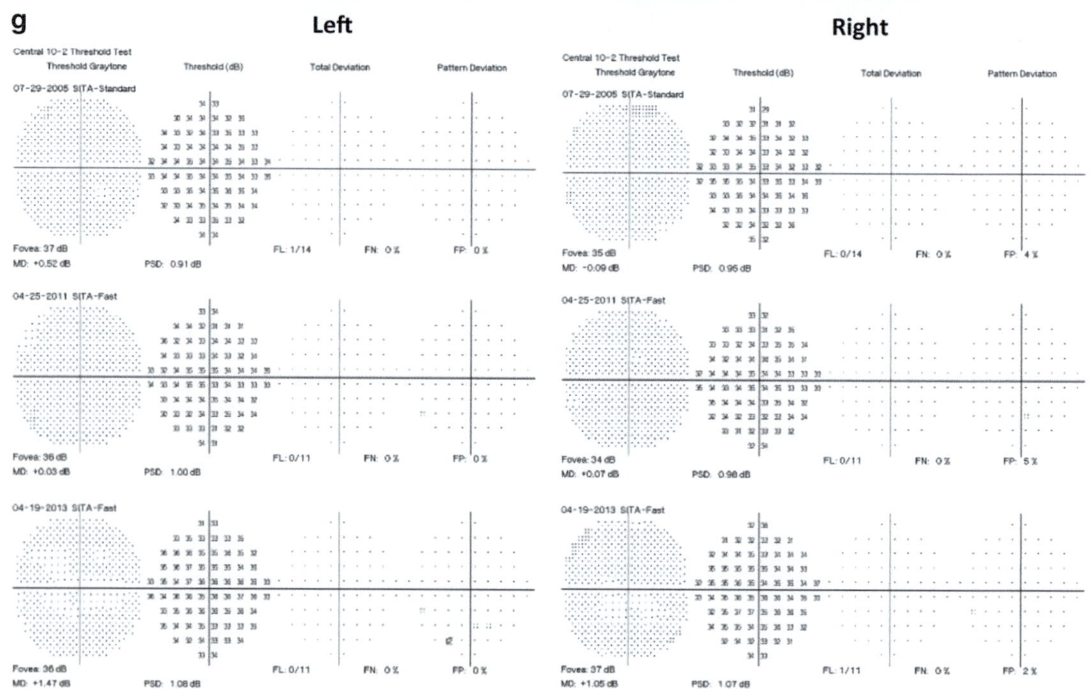

Fig. 10.1 (continued)

abnormal range in both eyes except for the R_1/R_2 ratio for the right eye (Fig. 10.1). Nevertheless, the 10-2 VFs were normal for both eyes. The SD-OCT showed paracentral thinning temporally in the right eye, but no abnormality of the inner segment/outer segment junction (IS/OS junction) (Fig. 10.1). How would you manage this patient?

In this case, the trend in mfERG indices carried more weight than any single abnormal study. The SD-OCT documentation of parafoveal thinning despite normal outer retinal morphology was also compelling for toxicity. The 10-2 VFs in this case were technically excellent and were less sensitive than the other tests. The patient was taking a toxic dose of hydroxychloroquine. The lesser of IBW and ABW in this case was 135 lb using the National Heart Lung and Blood Institute table [2], implying that she had been on 6.52 mg/kg/day for 20 years, receiving a cumulative dose of 2,920 g. Reasonable options in this case would include reduction of dosage or cessation of drug. After discussion with the patient and the rheumatologist, it was decided to reduce dosing to 300 mg/day (4.89 mg/kg/day) and to recheck her ancillary tests in 3 months. The suspicion of 4AQR was high with a pretest probability of retinopathy estimated to be 60 %. At the 3 month follow-up, any further evidence of retinopathy (e.g., further parafoveal thinning on SD-OCT or a new paracentral scotoma on 10-2 VF) would raise the posttest probability of retinopathy into a range (e.g., greater than 85 %) compatible with cessation of drug. This follow-up had not occurred by the time of publication of this book.

205 lb. He had normal renal and liver function. There was no preexisting maculopathy. Visual acuity was 20/20 in each eye. The ancillary tests chosen were the mfERG and the 10-2 VF. There were abnormalities of each test. In the case of the 10-2 VF, there were paracentral scotomas bilaterally (Fig. 10.2). The mfERG had low N1P1 amplitudes for ring R_1 in the right eye and rings R_1 and R_2 in the left eye, but the R_1/R_2 ratios were normal in both eyes. How would you manage this case?

The patient is properly dosed based on IBW at 5.05 mg/kg/day (see Chap. 7), and has only been on a 4AQR for 8 months. The pretest probability of 4AQR is on the order of 0.01 % or less (see Chap. 8). With the performance characteristics of 10-2 VF and mfERG, the posttest probability of 4AQR is no greater than 1 %. The clinician properly would not consider stopping the hydroxychloroquine or reducing the dose. Further testing with SD-OCT would be worthwhile. A normal SD-OCT would be associated with a negative predictive value (NPV) of close to 100 %, and reassure the clinician that follow-up in 1 year would be reasonable.

This case makes the point that the clinical situation is crucial in the correct interpretation of ancillary testing. Ancillary tests do not diagnose 4AQ. Clinicians considering a collection of evidence do. All ancillary tests have false positives, including 10-2 VF and SD-OCT. Based on the data reported in Chap. 8, the clinician should expect that 7.5 % of 10-2 VFs and 13.1 % of mf ERGs will have false positive results.

10.2   The Importance of the Clinical Estimation of Pretest Probability of 4-Aminoquinoline Retinopathy for Proper Interpretation of Ancillary Tests

A 50-year-old man underwent a baseline screening for hydroxychloroquine retinopathy 8 months after beginning the drug at 400 mg/day for rheumatoid arthritis. He was 6 ft tall and weighed

10.3   Hydroxychloroquine Retinopathy Due to Long-Term Overdosing, Misinterpretation of 10-2 Visual Fields, and an Internist's Unresponsiveness to a Recommendation to Stop Medication

A 79-year-old woman had been treated for rheumatoid arthritis for 15 years with hydroxychloroquine at 400 mg/day. She was 5 ft 5 in. tall and

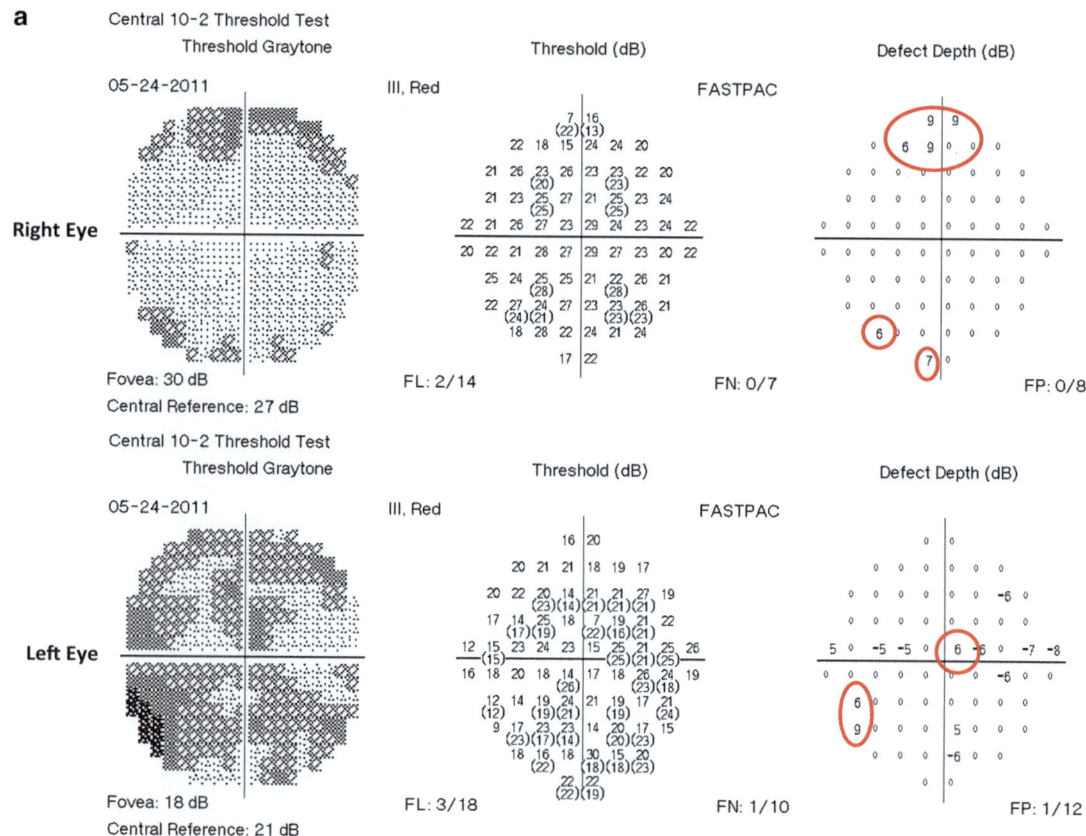

Fig. 10.2 Ancillary test images obtained at baseline in a 50-year-old man taking hydroxychloroquine for rheumatoid arthritis. (**a**) The 10-2 visual fields obtained with a III, red target have paracentral scotomas (*circled* in *red*) but the reliability indices are not excellent with 14 % and 17 % fixation losses in the right and left eyes, respectively, and one suspects a learning curve effect. (**b**) Based on N1P1 amplitude criteria, these mf ERGs are abnormal, but are not abnormal based on R_1/R_2 ratio criteria

weighed 100 lb. She had no renal or liver disease, nor any preexisting maculopathy. She complained of blurred vision in 2012 and had best corrected visual acuity of 20/20 right eye, 20/25 left eye. She was screened yearly with 10-2 VF testing using the III, red target and was declared free of retinopathy by the screening ophthalmologist each year. The author, in reviewing the charts of patients taking hydroxychloroquine in the practice during 2012, noted the typical presence of annular scotomata in each eye (Fig. 10.3) and suggested to the screening ophthalmologist that discontinuation of the hydroxychloroquine be recommended, which was done.

The prescribing internist reduced the dosing to 200 mg/day, but did not discontinue the medication. In 2013, the annular scotoma was worse and the visual acuity in the left eye had decreased to 20/30. How would you manage this case?

This case illustrates another overdosed patient. The weight to use in calculating adjusted daily dosing in this patient's case is the ABW, not the IBW, because her ABW was less than her IBW. One should use the lesser of ABW and IBW (see Chap. 7) [1]. Using ABW, her daily dosing was 8.8 mg/kg/day. Her cumulative dosage was 2,190 g. The case also shows that obtaining a 10-2 VF on a regular basis does not ensure

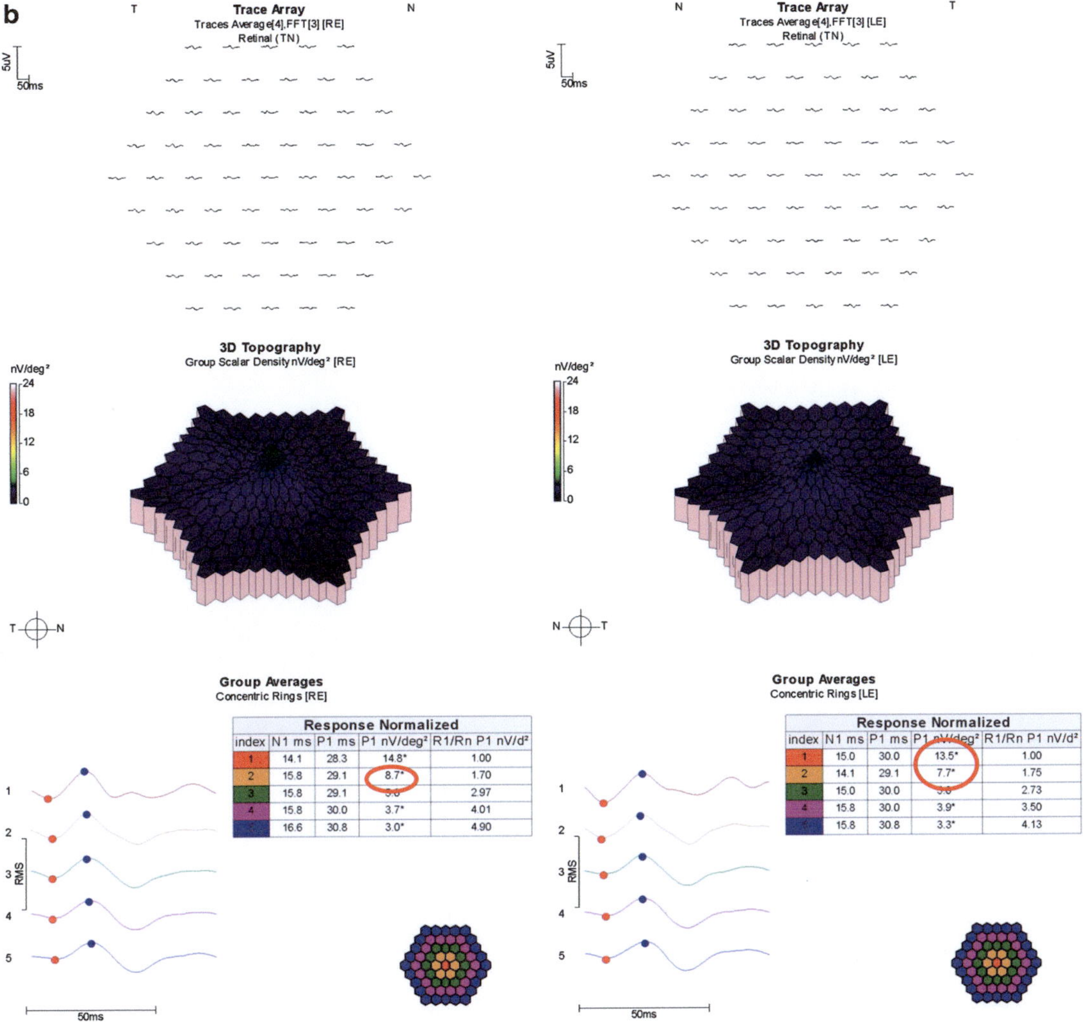

Group Averages
Concentric Rings [RE]

index	N1 ms	P1 ms	P1 nV/deg²	R1/Rn P1 nV/d²
1	14.1	28.3	14.8*	1.00
2	15.8	29.1	8.7*	1.70
3	15.8	29.1	5.0	2.97
4	15.8	30.0	3.7*	4.01
5	16.6	30.8	3.0*	4.90

Group Averages
Concentric Rings [LE]

index	N1 ms	P1 ms	P1 nV/deg²	R1/Rn P1 nV/d²
1	15.0	30.0	13.5*	1.00
2	14.1	29.1	7.7*	1.75
3	15.0	30.0	5.0	2.73
4	15.8	30.0	3.9*	3.50
5	15.8	30.8	3.3*	4.13

Fig. 10.2   (continued)

detection of 4AQR if the result is misinterpreted. The diagnosis was delayed at least 3 years because of visual field misinterpretation. Note that the graytone display was more useful than the defect depth display for showing the scotoma when the 10-2 VF with the III, red target and FASTPAC display is used. Finally, the proper response was cessation of drug, not reduction of dosage. Reduction of dosage is a proper response when there is doubt about the diagnosis. In this case, a convincing series of progressively abnormal 10-2 VFs makes the diagnosis incontrovertible and the drug needed to be stopped. Ancillary testing with SD-OCT would have been useful to confirm the findings indicated by 10-2 VFs. If drug cessation had been stopped at 4-25-2013, it is probable that continued field loss and acuity loss would have occurred anyway, as the best corrected visual acuity had already dropped to 20/30 (see Chap. 6).

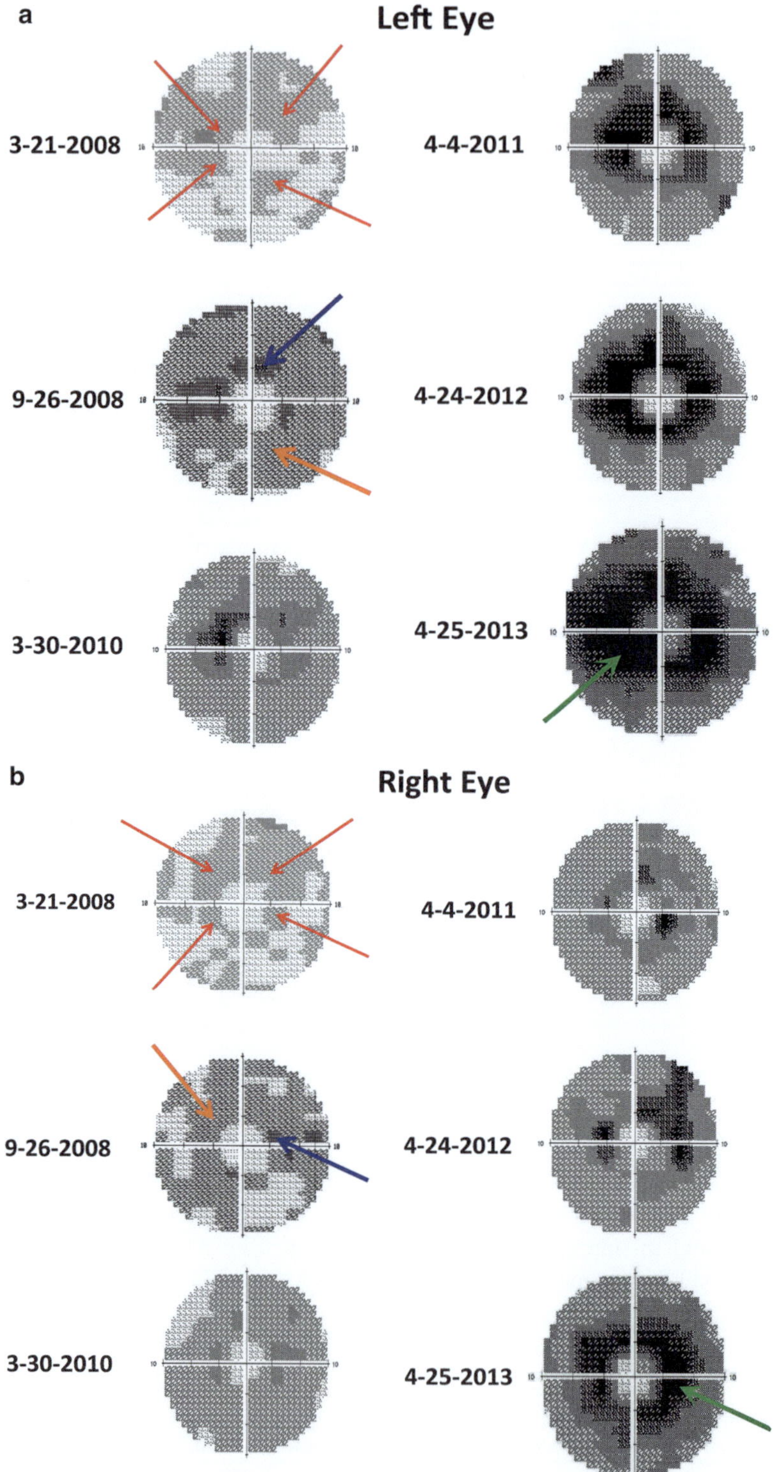

Fig. 10.3 10-2 visual fields (10-2 VFs) from a chronically overdosed patient on hydroxychloroquine. (**a**, **b**) Graytone displays of the left and right eyes, respectively. A suspicious annular scotoma is present on the first 10-2 VF from 2008 (*red arrows*), which progressively worsens for the next four fields. All of these 10-2 VFs were misinterpreted as normal. *Red arrows* show a shallow relative scotoma. The *blue arrow* shows a deeper relative scotoma.

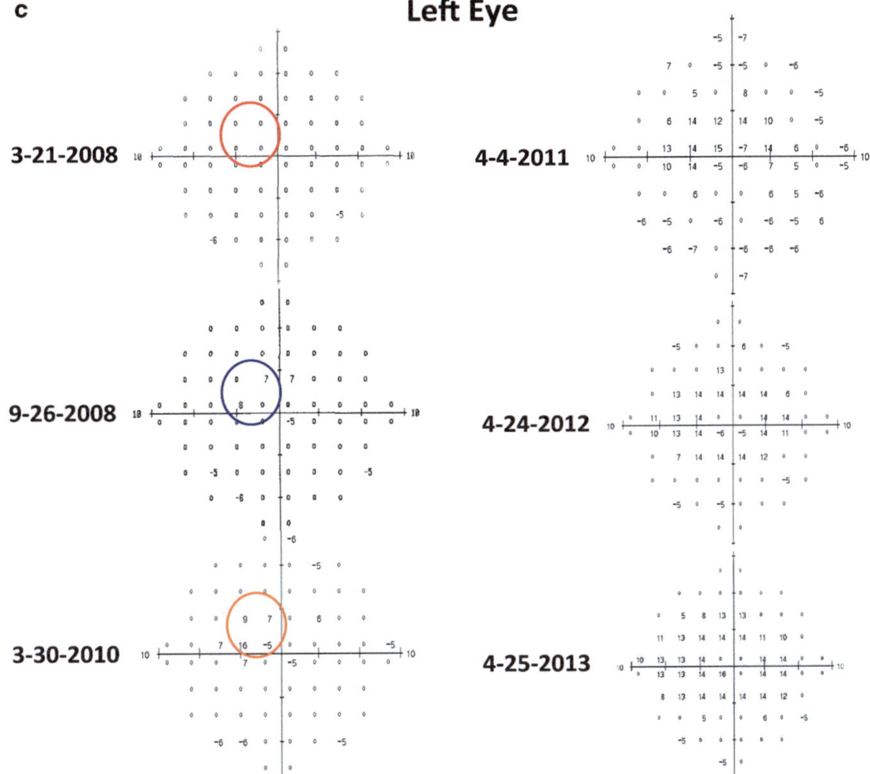

Fig. 10.3 (continued) The *orange arrow* shows a broadening of a shallow relative scotoma. The *green arrow* shows an absolute scotoma. At 4-24-2012 the dosing was reduced to 200 mg/day but the annular scotoma worsened anyway over the next year. (**c**) Defect display of the left eye. This display is less sensitive than the graytone display. In 3-21-2008 the red circled points are within normal sensitivity ranges. By 9-26-2008 two of the same points have developed elevated thresholds (*blue-circled area*). By 3-30-2010 three of the four points have elevated thresholds and the two points already abnormal on 9-26-2008 study have even higher thresholds than on that date (*orange-circled area*). (**d**) Defect display of the right eye. This display is less sensitive than the graytone display. In 3-21-2008 the *red-circled* points are within normal sensitivity ranges. By 4-4-2011 one of the same points has developed an elevated threshold (*blue-circled area*). By 4-25-2013 three of the four points have elevated thresholds and the point already abnormal on the 4-4-2011 study has an even higher threshold than on that date (*orange-circled area*)

10.4   A Case of Hydroxychloroquine Retinopathy in an Overdosed, Regularly Monitored Patient in Whom the Fundus Changes Were Atypically Mild and in Which Progression of Damage Occurred Despite Cessation of Drug

A 68-year-old woman with SLE had been on hydroxychloroquine at a dosage of 400 mg/day for 8 years. Her height was 5 ft 3 in. and her weight was 135 lb. She had no renal or liver disease, nor any preexisting maculopathy. She was screened yearly by her optometrist, but the fields done from year to year were inconsistent with a mixture of 10-2 and 24-2 VFs. At the eighth year visual field scotomata were suspected but her fundi were considered to be normal. She was referred to an ophthalmologist who diagnosed retinopathy and recommended cessation of hydroxychloroquine. She was followed for an additional 18 months and despite cessation of drug had progression of retinopathy (Fig. 10.4). How would you analyze this case?

This case illustrates many pitfalls. The most egregious was that the patient was overdosed by the prescribing rheumatologist and the screening optometrist did not recognize it nor recommend

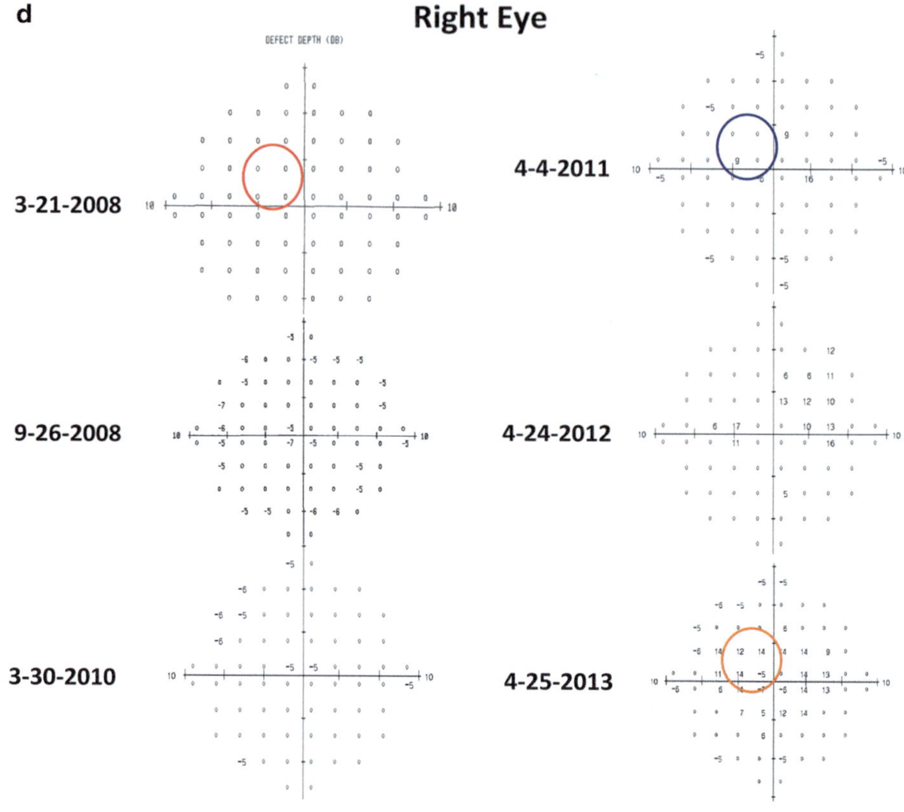

Fig. 10.3 (continued)

reduction of dosing [3, 4]. The case also illustrates the dangers of mixing visual field types in screening. The 10-2 VF is better for screening than the 24-2 or 30-2 VF [5]. In 2009 a 24-2 VF was used rather than a 10-2 VF. Had a 10-2 VF been used, comparison with the fields obtained before and after would have been easier. Also illustrated is the difference in 10-2 VFs obtained with red and white test objects. The 10-2 VF obtained with the red test object is more sensitive but less specific than the 10-2 VF obtained with the white test object (see Chap. 8). Scotomas obtained with the red test object are broader and deeper than those obtained with the white test object. There is no clearly preferable option as long as the 10-2 VF is used (see Chap. 8).

Unfortunately, the case further illustrates that no matter how sensitive the 10-2 VF is, the interpreting clinician must be able to recognize a relevant abnormality [3]. In this case, recognition was delayed. The 10-2 VFs of 5/29/2011 showed worrisome characteristics, but action was not taken until the absolute scotomata of 5/29/2011 were recorded. The mfERG and SD-OCT confirmed advanced 4AQR when they were obtained. It is speculative whether routine use of these extra tests all along would have led to earlier diagnosis of retinopathy.

10.5 Hydroxychloroquine Overdosage in a Patient with Renal Failure

A 65-year-old woman with SLE and renal failure requiring dialysis was placed on hydroxychloroquine in 2007. She was initially on 200 mg/day but after 1 year had her dose increased to 400 mg/day. After 1 year at this dosage, her daily dosage was reduced to 300 mg. She was 5 ft 3 in. tall and

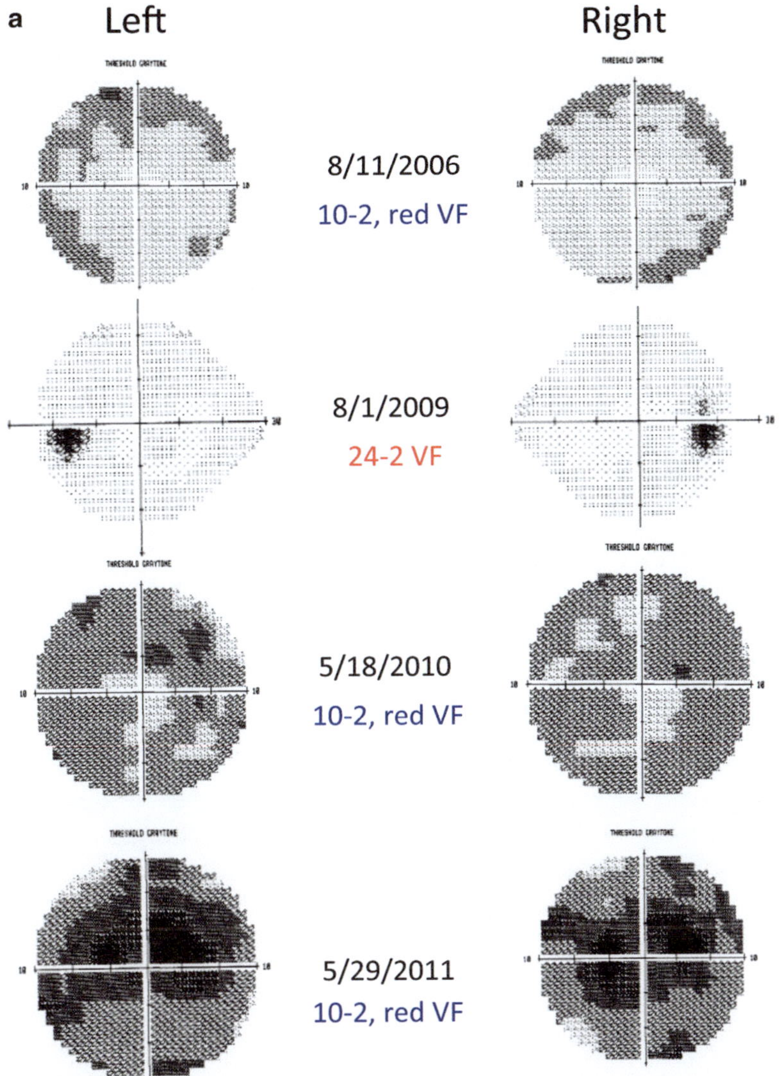

Fig. 10.4 Ancillary test images from a 68-year-old woman overdosed with hydroxychloroquine for 8 years who developed retinopathy. (**a**) A series of visual fields of the left and right eyes. In 2006, 2010, and 2011 the chosen test was the 10-2 VF with the III, red test object, but in 2009 a 24-2 VF with the III, white test object was used. This may have obscured the development of bilateral paracentral scotomas. The 10-2 VFs from 5/18/2010 were abnormal, but this was not recognized. In 5/29/2011 it was recognized by the screening optometrist that the 10-2 VFs were abnormal and the patient was referred to an ophthalmologist with suspected retinopathy. By this time, the retinopathy was advanced, with absolute paracentral scotomas. (**b**) The ophthalmologist who consulted on the patient obtained a 10-2 VF with the III, white test object. The scotomas with this test are not so broad as with the III, red test object (compare to (**a**)). (**c**) Color fundus photographs of the patient at the time that retinopathy was diagnosed. The optometrist and the ophthalmologist considered the fundi normal, but there are subtle retinal pigment epithelial (RPE) changes present (*white arrows*). (**d**) Frames from the fluorescein angiogram show a faint window defect temporally (*white arrows*) and an early hint of the same inferonasally in the left eye (*yellow arrow*). (**e**) Multifocal electroretinography (mfERG) at this time shows flat waveforms (*green-circled areas*). The ring averaged waveforms for R_1 are so small that the machine-placed cursors are artifactiously placed erroneously (*red arrows*). (**f**) SD-OCT retinal thickness maps show macular thinning bilaterally.

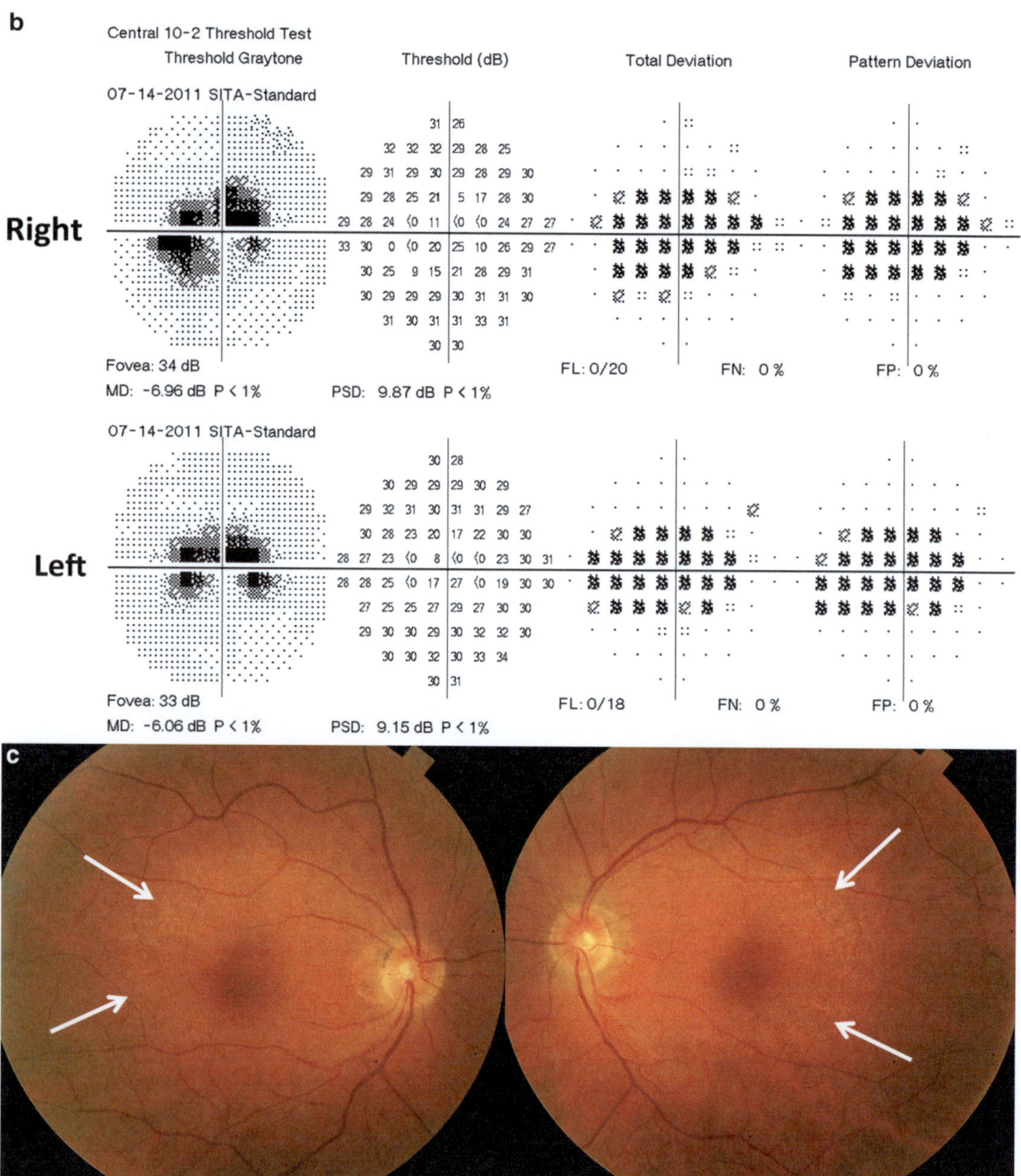

Fig. 10.4 (continued) (**g**) SD-OCT line scans show foveal retention of the inner segment/outer segment (IS/OS) junction (*blue arrows*) but loss parafoveally. Both the IS/OS junction and the RPE are lost at the *orange arrows*, but the RPE begins to be present more eccentrically at the *yellow arrows*, although the IS/OS junction is missing at this paracentral location. (**h**) 10-2 VFs of the right eye at the time of drug cessation and 18 months later shows progression of damage with deterioration of foveal sensitivity (*red-* and *blue-circled areas*). (**i**) 10-2 VFs of the left eye at the time of drug cessation and 18 months later shows progression of damage with deterioration of foveal sensitivity (*red-* and *blue-circled areas*)

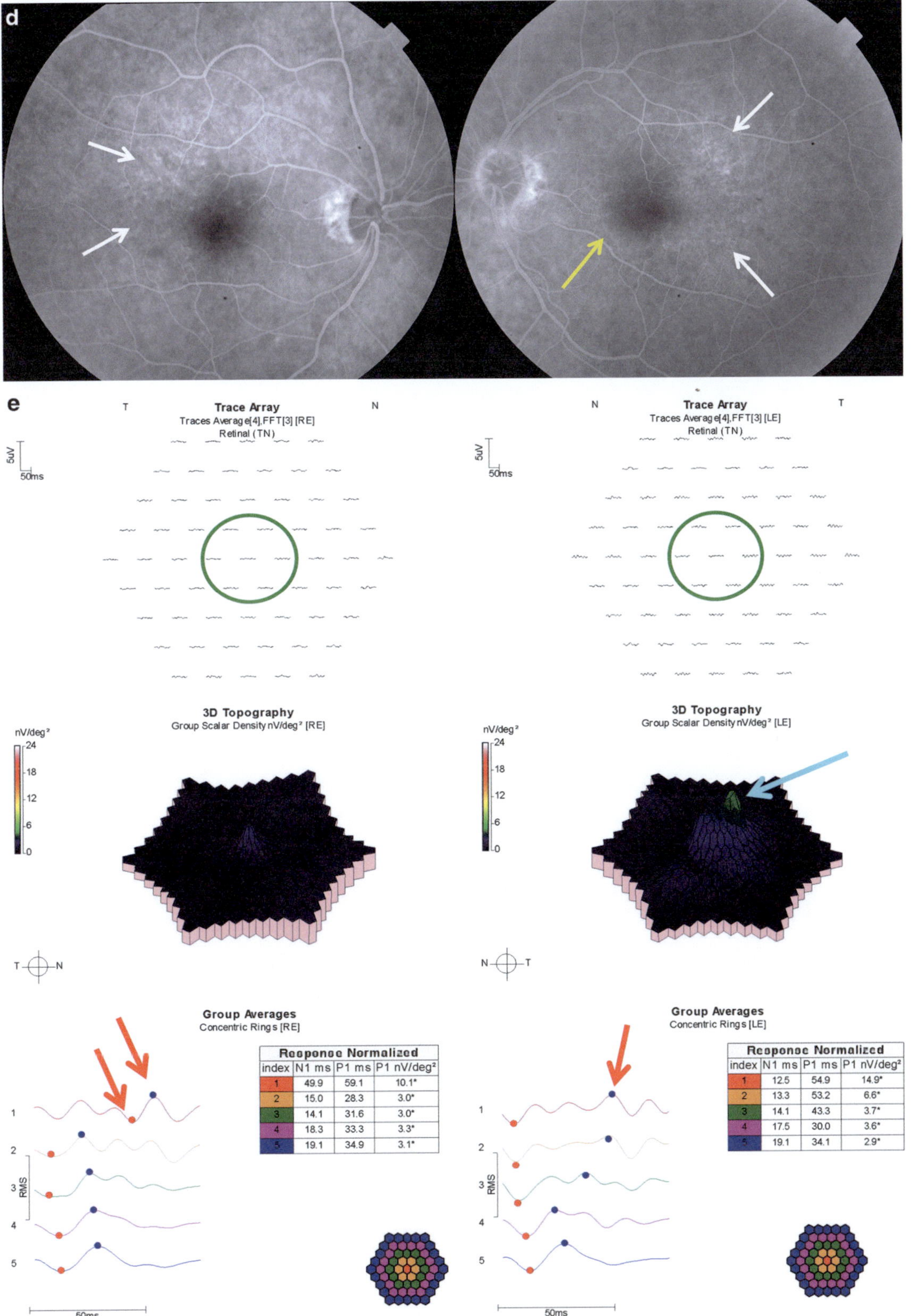

Fig. 10.4   (continued)

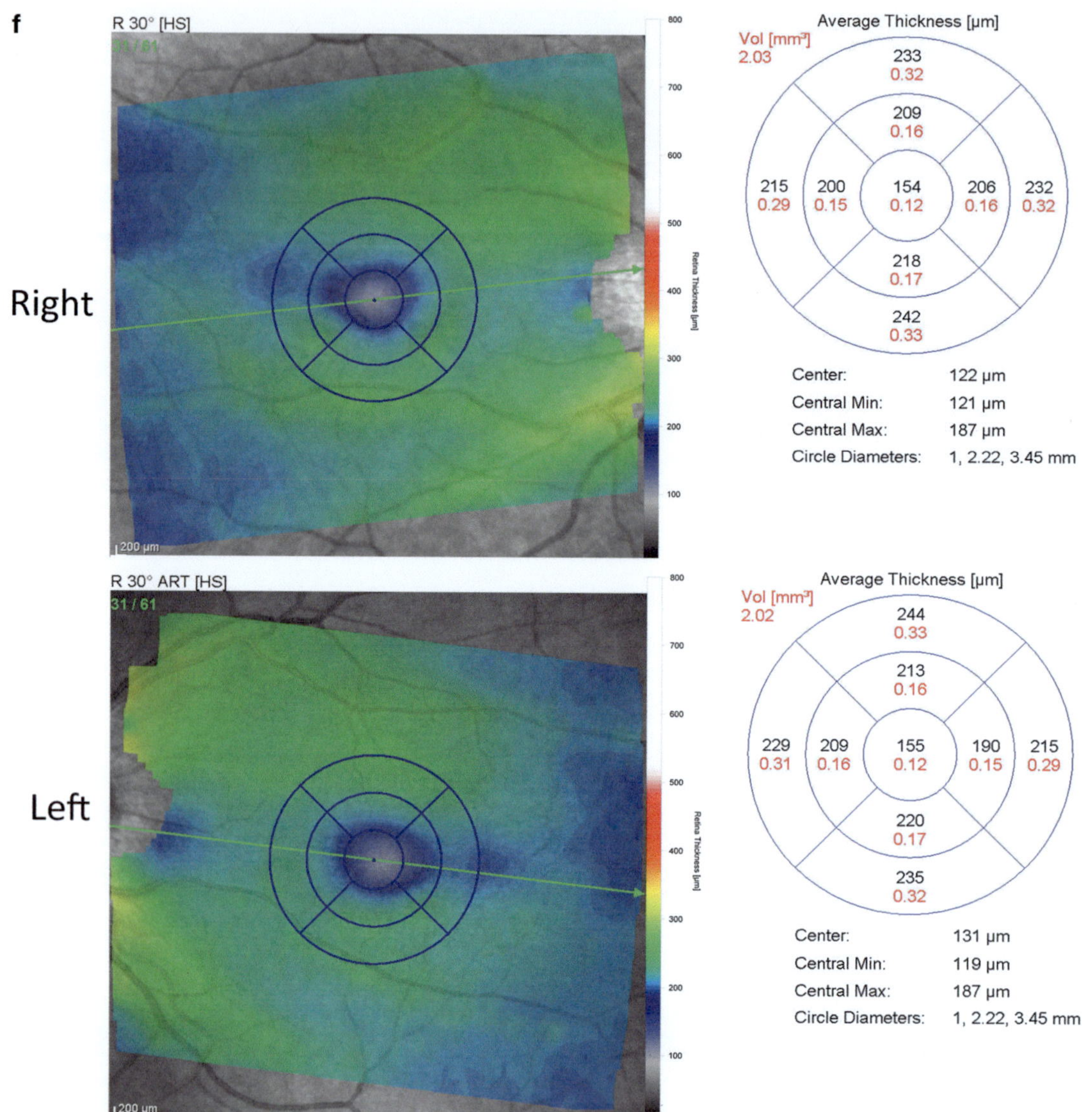

Fig. 10.4 (continued)

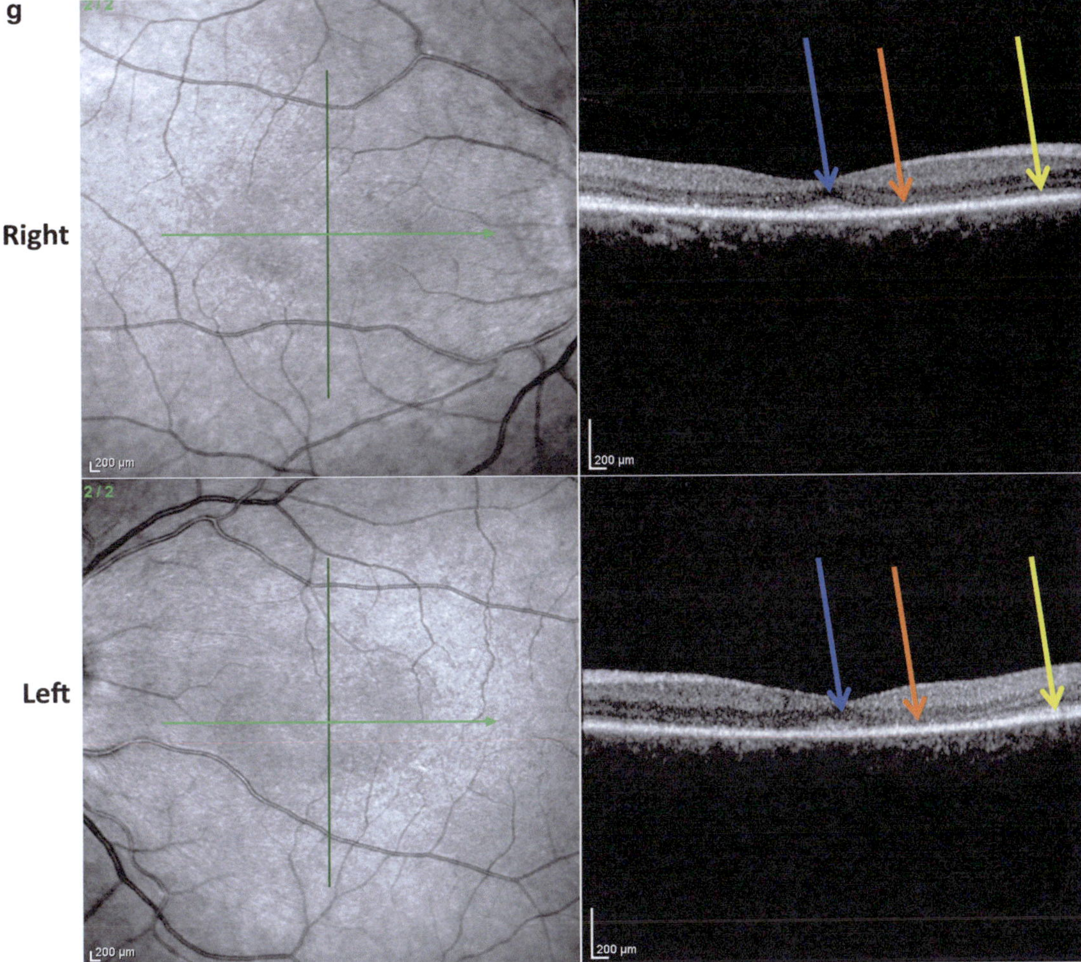

Fig. 10.4   (continued)

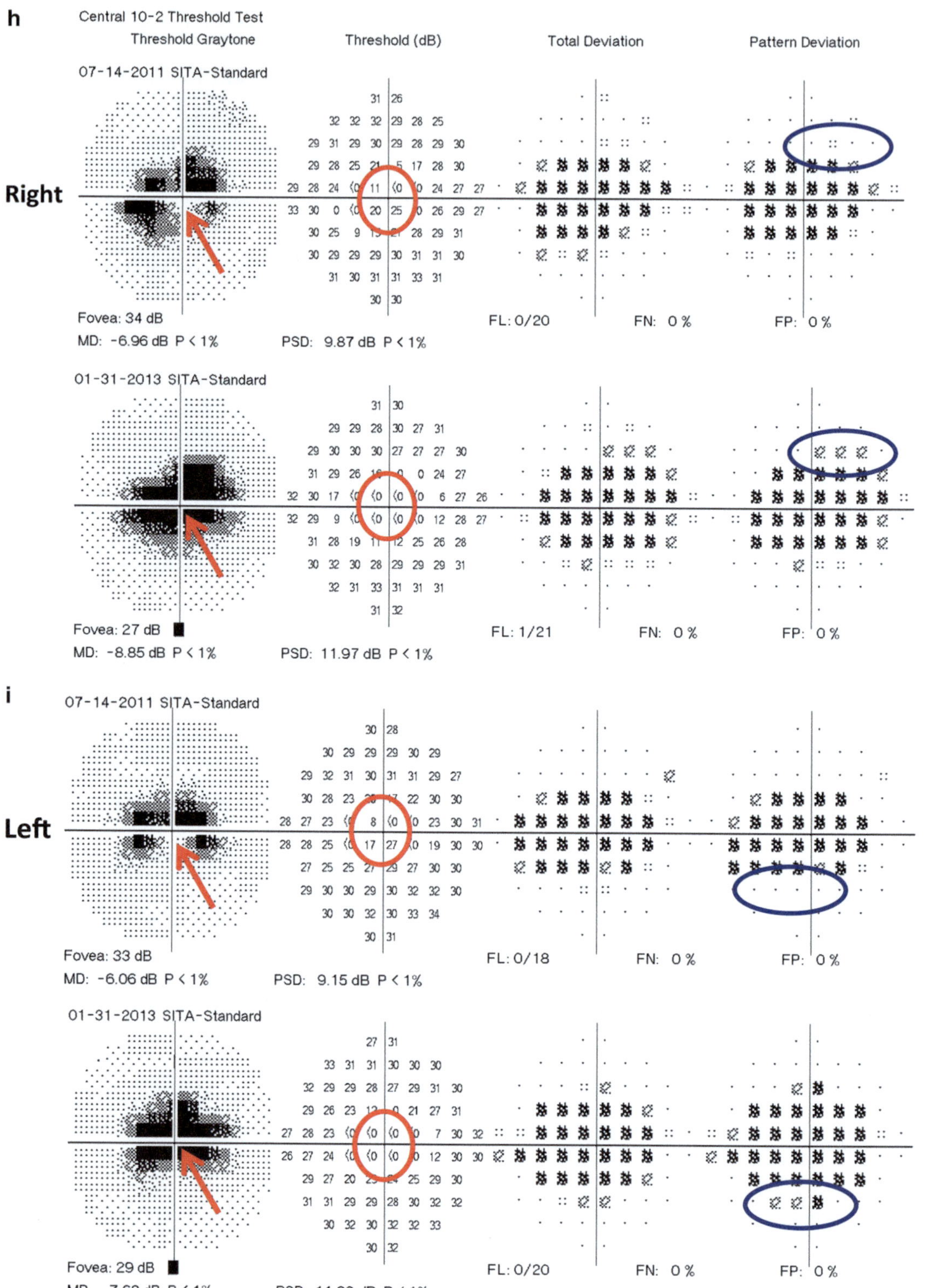

Fig. 10.4   (continued)

weighed 105 lb. She had no preexisting macular abnormalities, nor any liver disease. Her best corrected visual acuity was 20/30 in the right eye and 20/63 in the left eye. She was pseudophakic in the right eye and had a cataract consistent with her visual acuity in the left eye. Her ophthalmologist noted paracentral scotomas that were variable on serial 10-2 VFs. SD-OCT showed diffuse macular thinning but no disruption of outer retinal morphology (Fig. 10.5). How would you manage this case?

In analyzing this case, the most important fact to note is that the patient is overdosed. The weight to use to determine dosing is her ABW, which is lower than her IBW. When she was on 400 mg/day, she was overdosed based on this weight even if she had normal renal function. As she is on renal dialysis, the degree of overdosage is more severe. Inquiry regarding renal and liver dysfunction is often overlooked, and can be avoided by using a checklist of important risk factors for 4AQR (see Chap. 7) [1]. There are no good studies that allow one to rationally determine a correction factor for dosing in the situation of renal failure, although a rule of thumb to reduce dosing by 50 % has been espoused [6]. It was recommended that her dosage be reduced to 100 mg/day. There is no good evidence that the patient has hydroxychloroquine retinopathy. The variability of her 10-2 VFs makes the significance of her paracentral scotomata suspect. The paramacular thinning of the SD-OCT is concerning, but the intact IS/OS junction allows one to continue to monitor this patient taking a reduced dosage. Investigation with fundus autofluorescence and mf ERG if these modalities were available would be helpful. A follow-up interval of 3–6 months would be reasonable.

10.6 Unexpected Location of Retinopathy with Misinterpretation of the SD-OCT in a Chronically Overdosed Patient Taking Hydroxychloroquine

A 58-year-old woman with SLE had been taking 400 mg/day of hydroxychloroquine for 16 years. She was 5 ft 2 in. tall and weighed 150 lb.

Her IBW was 131 lb and her adjusted daily dosage based on the lesser of IBW and ABW was 6.72 mg/kg/day. Her cumulative dose of hydroxychloroquine was 2,336 g. She had no renal or liver disease and no preexisting maculopathy. She had been receiving annual 10-2 VFs with the III, red test object and in 2011 also received her first SD-OCT examination, concomitant with the revised AAO screening guidelines. Both 10-2 VF and SD-OCT were interpreted as normal. She was later sent for an mf ERG test as well, which was interpreted by a retina specialist. Her ancillary studies are shown in Fig. 10.6. How would you manage this patient?

The primary problem in this case was 16 years of overdosing. A second problem was misinterpretation of ancillary testing. The scotomata to 10-2 VF testing occurred more peripherally than expected (see Chap. 6 for the expected location closer to the fovea), as did the SD-OCT changes and ring of RPE atrophy. The take-home message is that the spectrum of 4AQR is broader than the classical picture illustrated in reviews over the decades. The clinician will only see what he expects to see. This case broadens that expectation.

The various ways that the clinician could respond to abnormalities detected on screening were reviewed in Chap. 7. The clinician in this case recommended reduction in dosing to 300 mg/day, because he thought the ancillary tests were normal. The proper response would have been to stop the drug, which did occur 1 year later upon consultation with a retinal specialist and understanding that all three ancillary tests (10-2 VF, SD-OCT, and mf ERG) were abnormal, not normal. Progression of retinopathy was evident on the SD-OCT and 10-2 VF during the year of reduced dosage of hydroxychloroquine.

10.7 Hydroxychloroquine Monitoring in the Setting of Preexisting Maculopathy

A 53-year-old woman with Sjogren's syndrome started hydroxychloroquine 400 mg/day in 2003 and had her dosage reduced to 200 mg/day in

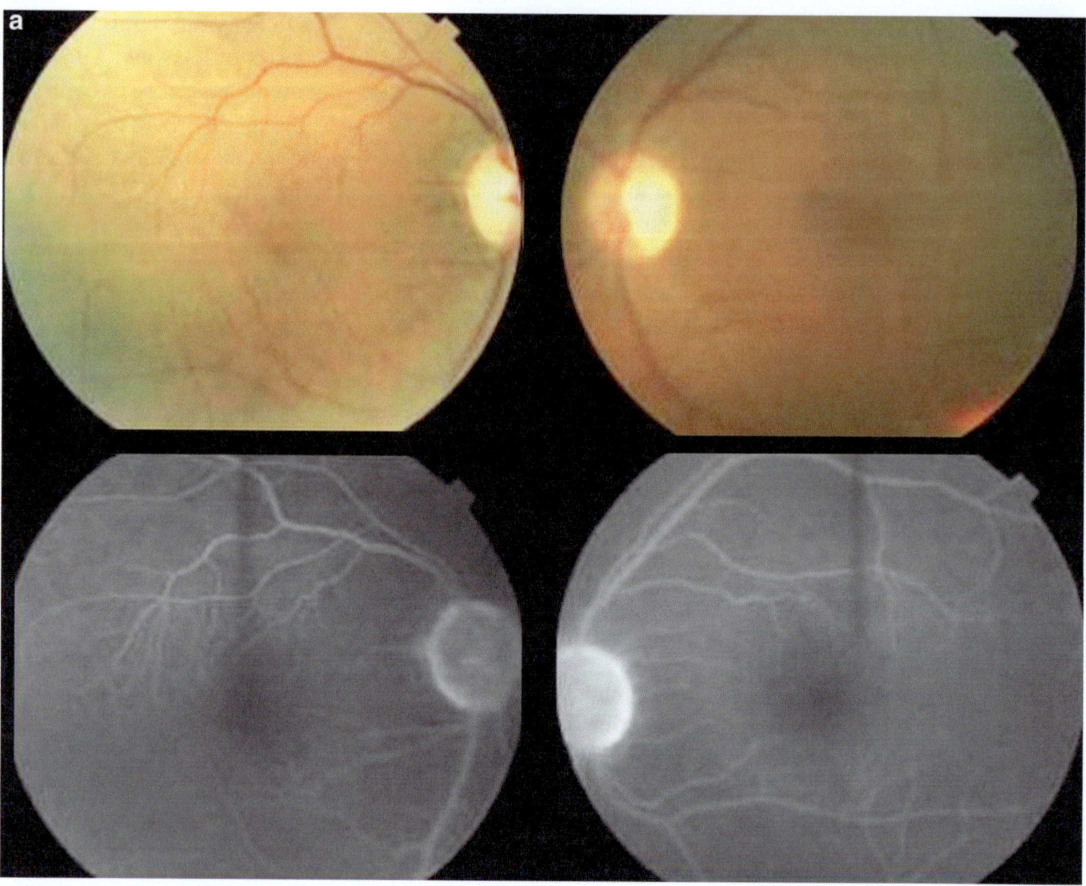

Fig. 10.5 Images from ancillary studies of a 65-year-old patient with renal failure overdosed with hydroxychloroquine. (**a**) Color fundus photographs and frames from a fluorescein angiogram taken of both eyes. The fundus photographs have some mild, nonspecific mottling of the retinal pigment epithelium (RPE) that is not diagnostic of hydroxychloroquine retinopathy. The fluorescein angiogram is normal bilaterally. (**b**) 10-2 visual fields (10-2 VFs) of both eyes show inconsistent paracentral scotomas. The *red-circled* scotomata are not reproducible from one field to the next. However, the *blue-circled* scotomata are reproducible. (**c**) SD-OCT of both eyes shows diffuse macular thinning (*red arrows*). For example, the paracentral subfields of the right and left eyes have thicknesses of approximately 250–270 µm, whereas normal thickness of these subfields is $318 \pm SD14$ µm for the Cirrus SD-OCT instrument (see Chap. 1). (**d**) SD-OCT line scans of the right and left eyes showing normal outer retinal morphology

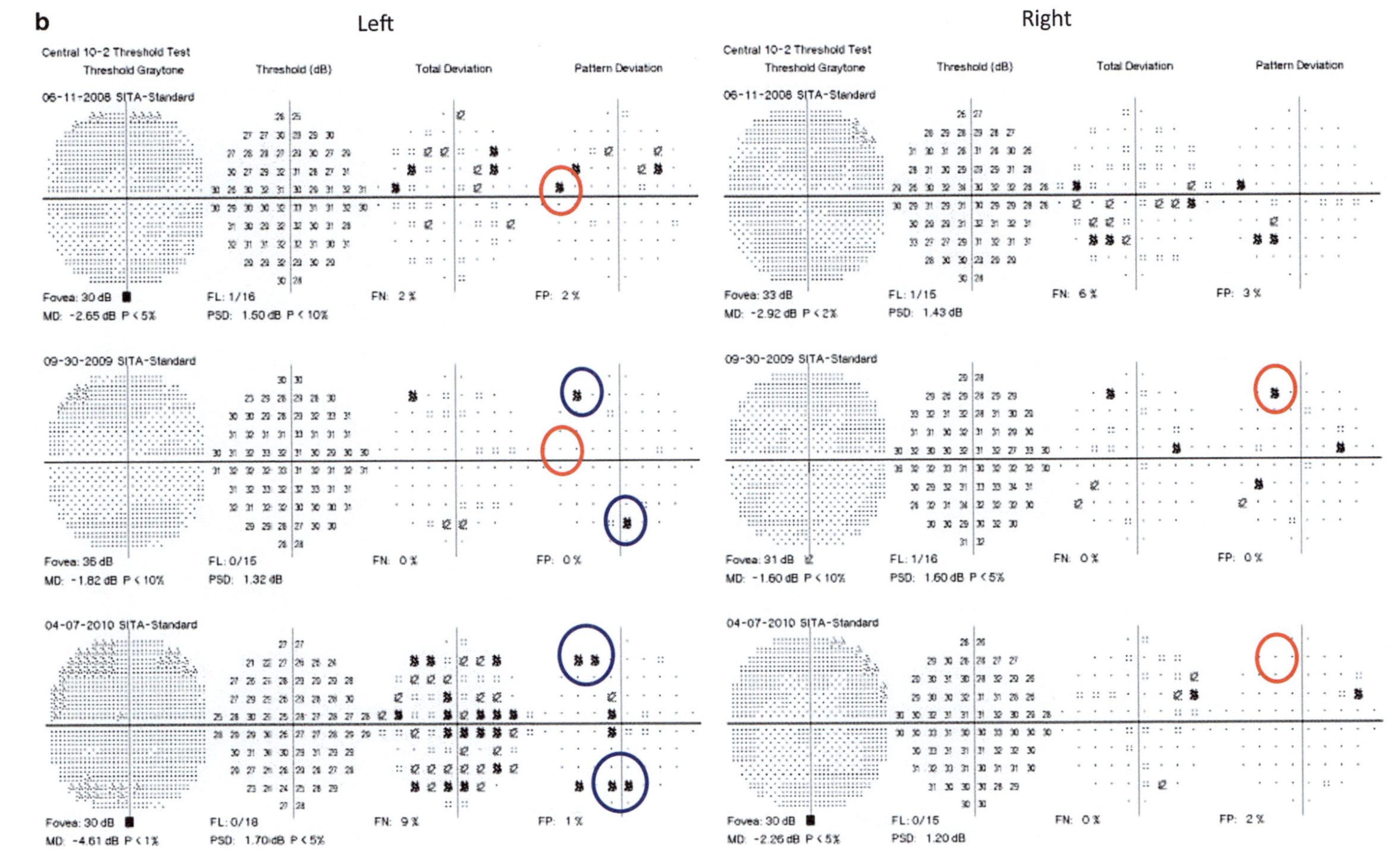

Fig. 10.5 (continued)

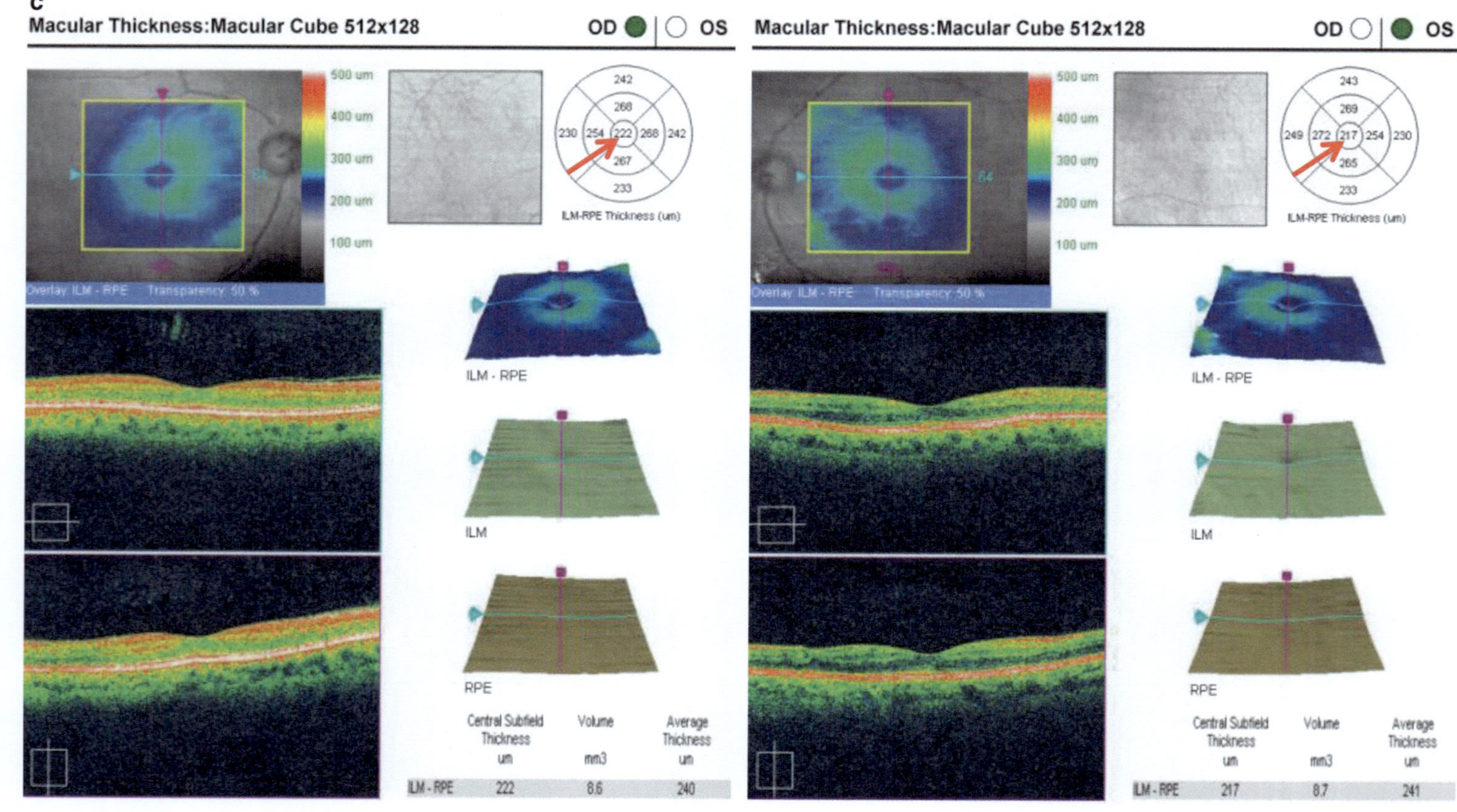

Fig. 10.5 (continued)

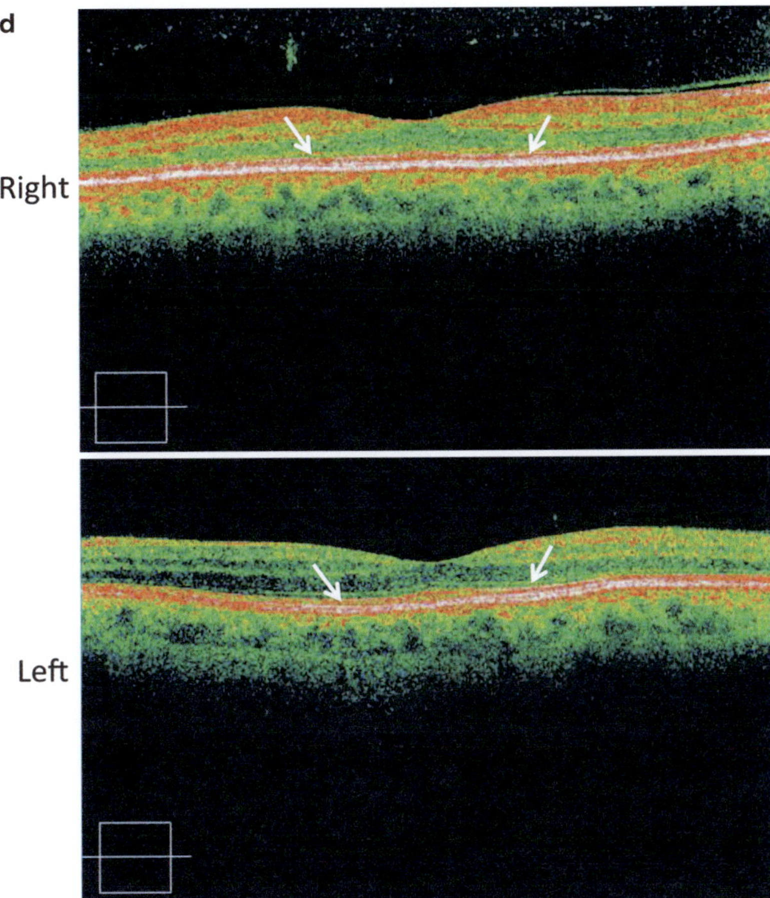

Fig. 10.5 (continued)

2010. She was 5 ft 7 in. tall and weighed 134 lb. She had no renal or liver disease. In 2004 she had an ischemic central retinal vein occlusion of the right eye that reduced her visual acuity to 20/200 and left her with a macular scar. The left eye had a normal macula and visual acuity of 20/20. Her ophthalmologist monitored her with yearly 10-2 visual fields (10-2 VFs) and after the revised AAO guidelines were published in 2011 with SD-OCT and mfERG as well, which are shown in Fig. 10.7. How would you manage this case?

The patient's ABW is less than her IBW, thus the ABW should be used in the calculation of the adjusted daily dose (see Chap. 7). Her adjusted daily dose was toxic from 2003 to 2010 at 6.57 mg/kg/day. After 2010 her dosing was in a safer range at 3.28 mg/kg/day. There is no evidence that the macular scarring induced by the chronic macular edema secondary to the central retinal vein occlusion renders the right macula more susceptible to 4AQR. The problem with the preexisting maculopathy is that it makes the job of detecting retinopathy in the right eye more difficult. All the tests—10-2 VF, SD-OCT, and mfERG—are confounded for the right eye. In a case like this, screening is based on the healthy left macula. There is no evidence of any toxicity in the 10-2 VF, SD-OCT, or mfERG of the left eye. The patient was advised that continued use of hydroxychloroquine at 200 mg/day was safe and that she should be rechecked in 1 year. In cases with bilateral preexisting maculopathy this approach will

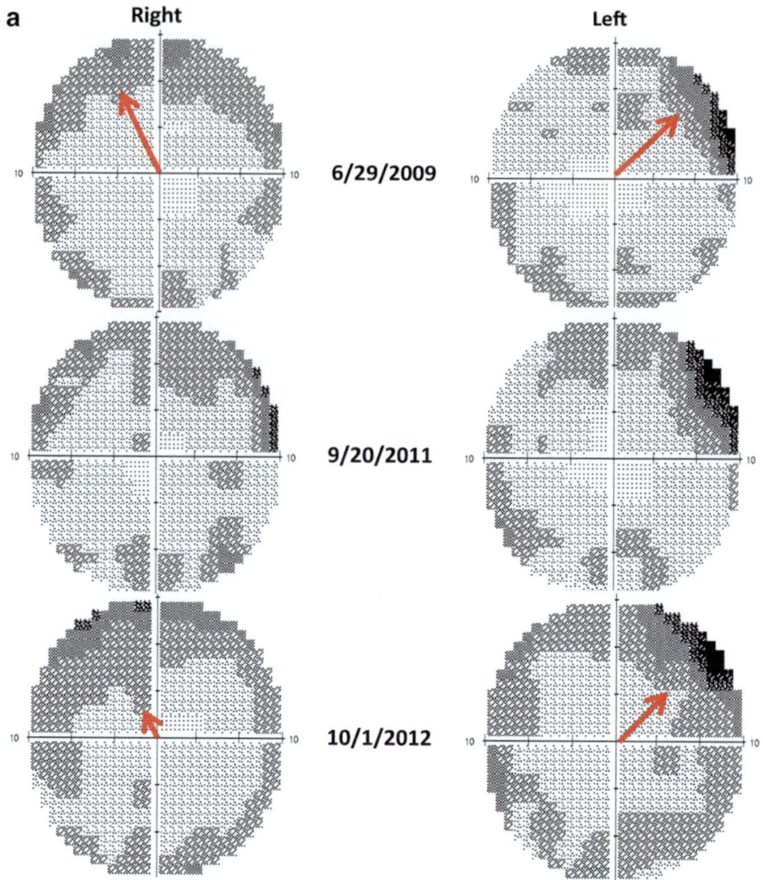

Fig. 10.6 Ancillary test images of a patient chronically overdosed with hydroxychloroquine who developed retinopathy more eccentrically than is classically described. (**a**) Three sequential 10-2 visual fields (10-2 VFs) obtained with the III, red test object. The annular scotoma is outside the typically described region of hydroxychloroquine involvement (2–8° from fixation). Over time the scotoma spreads centrally (compare *red arrows*). (**b**) SD-OCT line scans from right and left eyes. Although the ophthalmologist read these as normal, they are not. Note that the inner segment/outer segment (IS/OS) junction is lost at the *yellow arrows*, a more peripheral location for this sign of hydroxychloroquine damage than typically described. (**c**) SD-OCT line scans separated by 1 year in the right eye. Note that the IS/OS junction loss has moved centrally (compare *yellow* to *orange arrows*). (**d**) SD-OCT line scans separated by 1 year in the left eye. Note that the IS/ OS junction loss has moved centrally (compare *yellow* to *orange arrows*). (**e**) Abnormal mf ERG showing flat hexagonal waveforms (*green-circled areas*). The R_1/R_2 ratios are not abnormal because the R_1 amplitude is decreased as well as the R_2 amplitude. The machine drawn cursor is erroneously positioned because the ring averaged waveform for R_1 has no signal, but only noise (*red arrow*). (**f**) The fundi were interpreted as normal by the screening ophthalmologist, but they are not. Subtle RPE atrophy is seen (*white arrows*) with greater visibility of the choroidal vascular pattern compared to the more perifoveal macula. (**g**) The fluorescein angiogram shows window hyperfluorescence more peripheral and less sharply demarcated than classical examples of hydroxychloroquine retinopathy. (**h**) Fundus autofluorescence images show hyperautofluorescence (*red arrows*) and in the left eye a more peripheral zone of hypoautofluorescence (*blue arrow*)

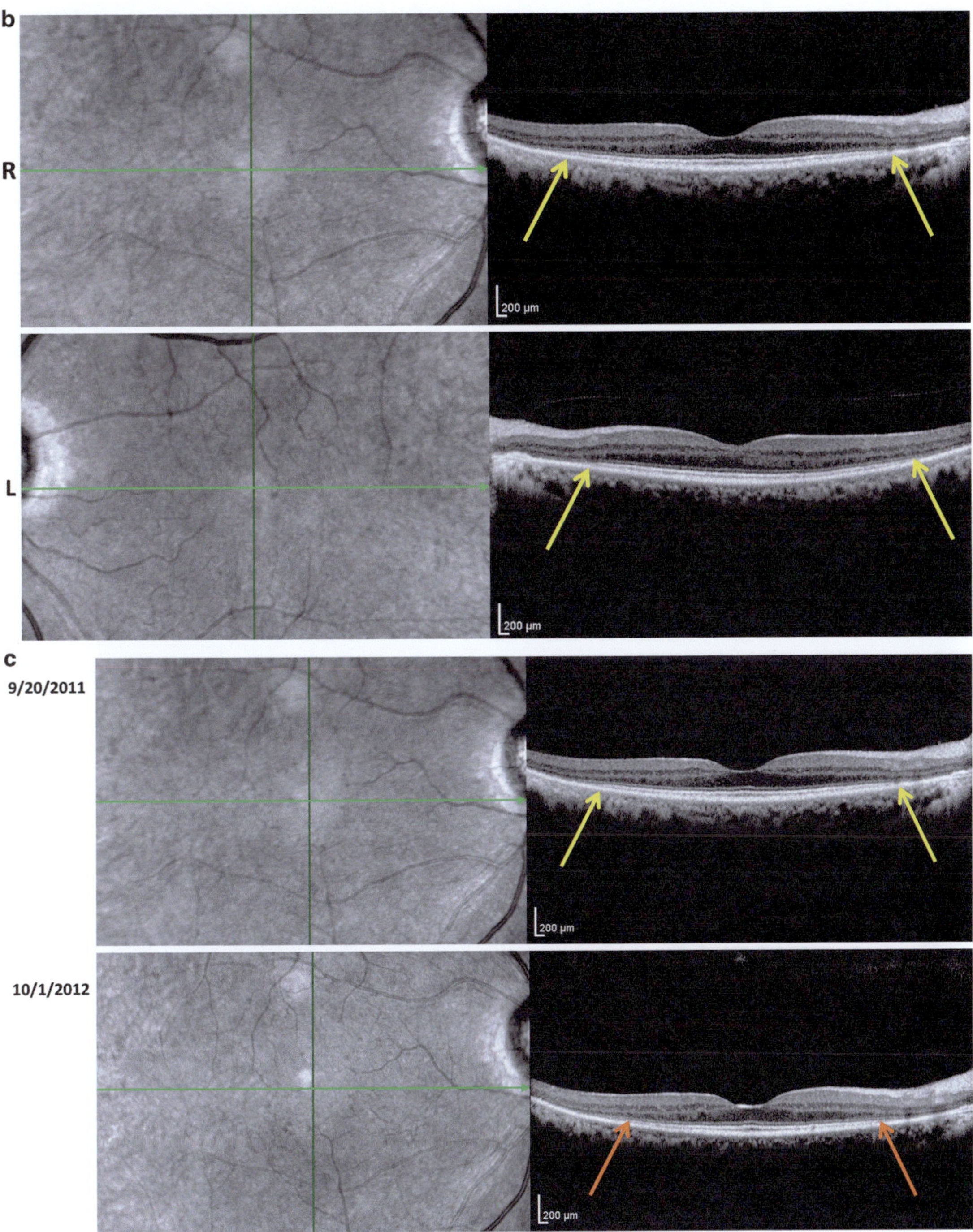

Fig. 10.6 (continued)

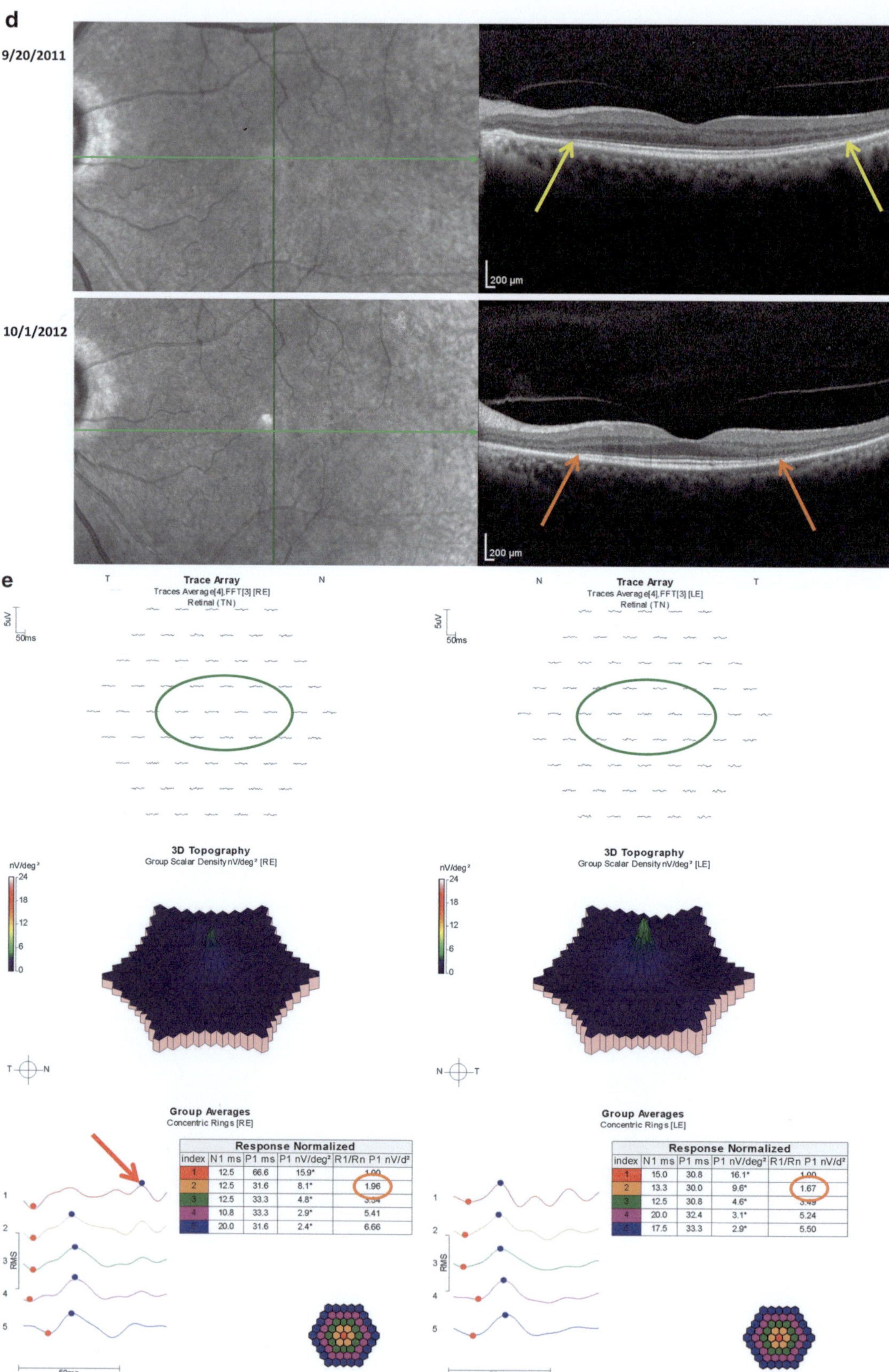

Group Averages — Concentric Rings [RE]

		Response Normalized		
index	N1 ms	P1 ms	P1 nV/deg²	R1/Rn P1 nV/d²
1	12.5	66.6	15.9*	1.00
2	12.5	31.6	8.1*	1.96
3	12.5	33.3	4.8*	3.34
4	10.8	33.3	2.9*	5.41
5	20.0	31.6	2.4*	6.66

Group Averages — Concentric Rings [LE]

		Response Normalized		
index	N1 ms	P1 ms	P1 nV/deg²	R1/Rn P1 nV/d²
1	15.0	30.8	16.1*	1.00
2	13.3	30.0	9.6*	1.67
3	12.5	30.8	4.6*	3.49
4	20.0	32.4	3.1*	5.24
5	17.5	33.3	2.9*	5.50

Fig. 10.6 (continued)

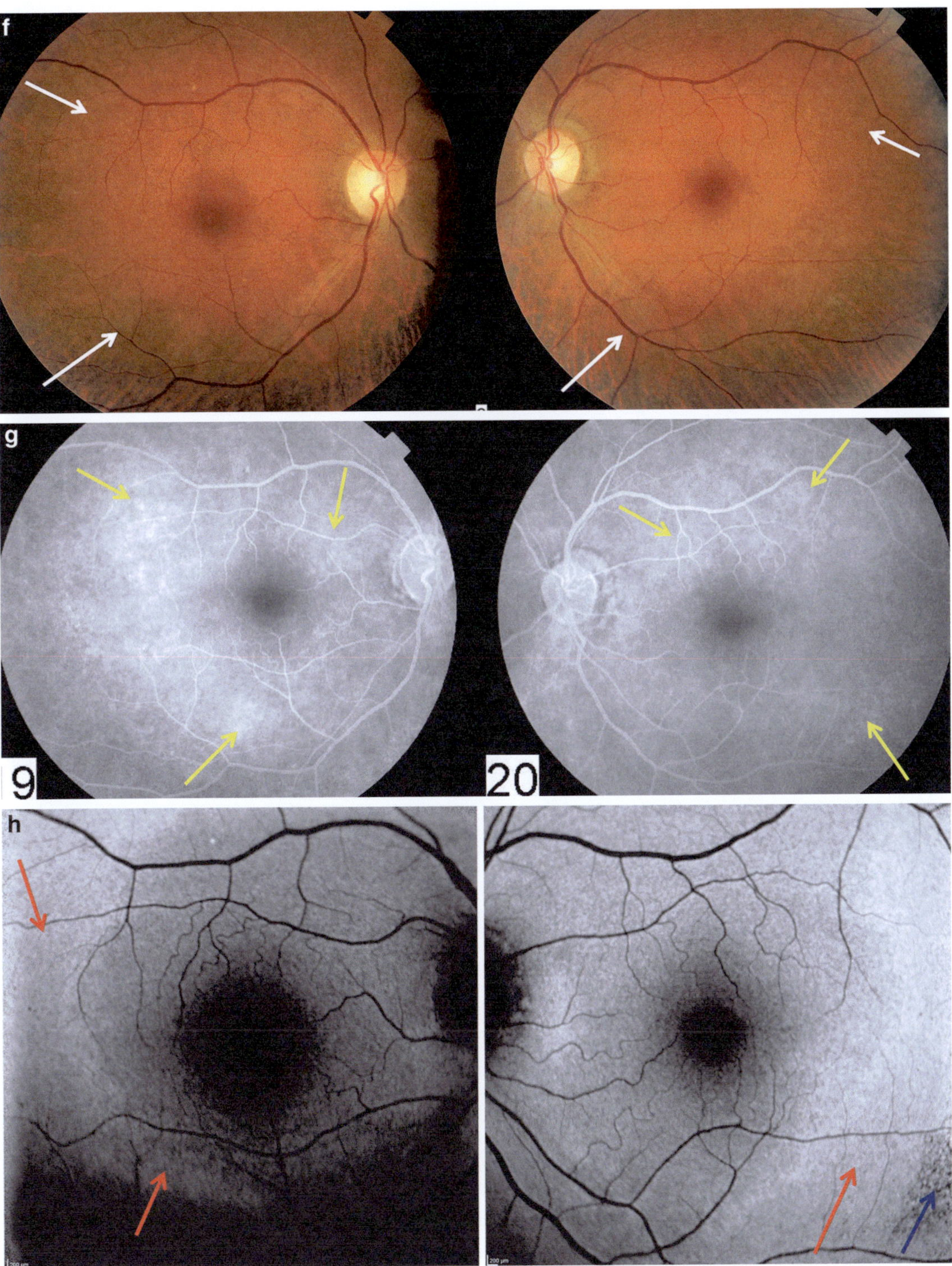

Fig. 10.6 (continued)

not work. Instead, more weight is placed on modifiable risk factor optimization (i.e., safer daily dosing based on the lesser of ideal and ABW).

10.8   Asymmetric Hydroxychloroquine Retinopathy in an Appropriately Dosed Patient with Progression of Retinopathy After Cessation of the Drug

A 73-year-old woman with rheumatoid arthritis was treated with hydroxychloroquine 400 mg/day from 1992 through 2010 for a cumulative dose of 2,628 g. She was 5 ft 5 in. tall and weighed 145 lb. Her IBW and ABW were the same, thus her adjusted daily dosage was 6.1 mg/kg/day. She had no renal or liver disease. She had been screened for 18 years by her optometrist, but was referred by her rheumatologist to an ophthalmologist because of complaints of photophobia. Her best corrected visual acuity was 20/40 right eye and 20/60 left eye. She was noted to have a bull's-eye maculopathy of the right eye and pigmentary mottling of the left eye (Fig. 10.8). Her 10-2 VFs showed a paracentral annular scotoma more pronounced on the right than the left. Time domain OCT showed paracentral thinning of the macula and loss of paracentral IS/OS junction. How would you manage this case?

In contrast to many of the cases shown in this chapter, this patient was properly dosed, yet she still developed retinopathy. Her risk factors were age greater than 60 and high cumulative dose (Chap. 7). We do not have records from the screening by her optometrist, and cannot analyze the failure to detect retinopathy at that level of care. Her rheumatologist responded admirably to her new symptom of photophobia. Symptoms are an insensitive index of 4AQR, but when present, are helpful and should lead to redoubled efforts to discern retinopathy (Chap. 6). The asymmetry in retinopathy is not typical but is not rare (see another case in Chap. 6). The local factors that rendered the right eye more susceptible to retinopathy than the left eye are unknown. Progression of retinopathy once bull's-eye changes have developed is common (see Chap. 6). The line scans on TD-OCT

are less useful than the false color maps of macular thickness which show the parafoveal distribution of thinning in striking manner. Line scans are much more useful for SD-OCT than for the less sensitive TD-OCT. Yearly follow-up of this patient would be suitable with 10-2 VF testing to give some indication regarding the functional progression of her damage.

10.9   Screening for Hydroxychloroquine Retinopathy in a Setting of Confounding Glaucomatous Visual Field Defects and Preexisting Maculopathy from Resolved Central Retinal Vein Occlusion and Macular Epiretinal Membrane

A 58-year-old woman with SLE and a secondary antiphospholipid antibody syndrome had taken hydroxychloroquine 200 mg/day for 15 years. She was 5 ft tall and weighed 95 lb. She had no renal or liver disease. She had keratoconus, previous bilateral nonischemic central retinal vein occlusions that had resolved, and primary open angle glaucoma. Her best corrected visual acuity was 20/30 in the right eye and 20/20 in the left eye. Fundus examination was notable for glaucomatous optic disc cupping of both eyes and a macular epiretinal membrane of the right eye (Fig. 10.9). Images from fundus photography, 10-2 VF testing, and SD-OCT are shown in Fig. 10.9. How would you manage this case?

The most important fact to note in this case is that dosing is in an acceptably safe range at 4.63 mg/kg/day using her ABW, which is lower than her IBW (see Chap. 7). Her main risk factor for 4AQR is a large cumulative dose of hydroxychloroquine at 1,095 g. This case illustrates the importance of several ancillary testing modalities in cases of multiple ocular comorbidities. Glaucoma is common in patients taking 4AQs, and the visual field defects from glaucoma must be separated from those possibly arising from 4AQs. This is best done by obtaining separate fields for the glaucoma and the 4AQR screening. It is not easy to detect 4AQR using 24-2 or 30-2 VFs (see

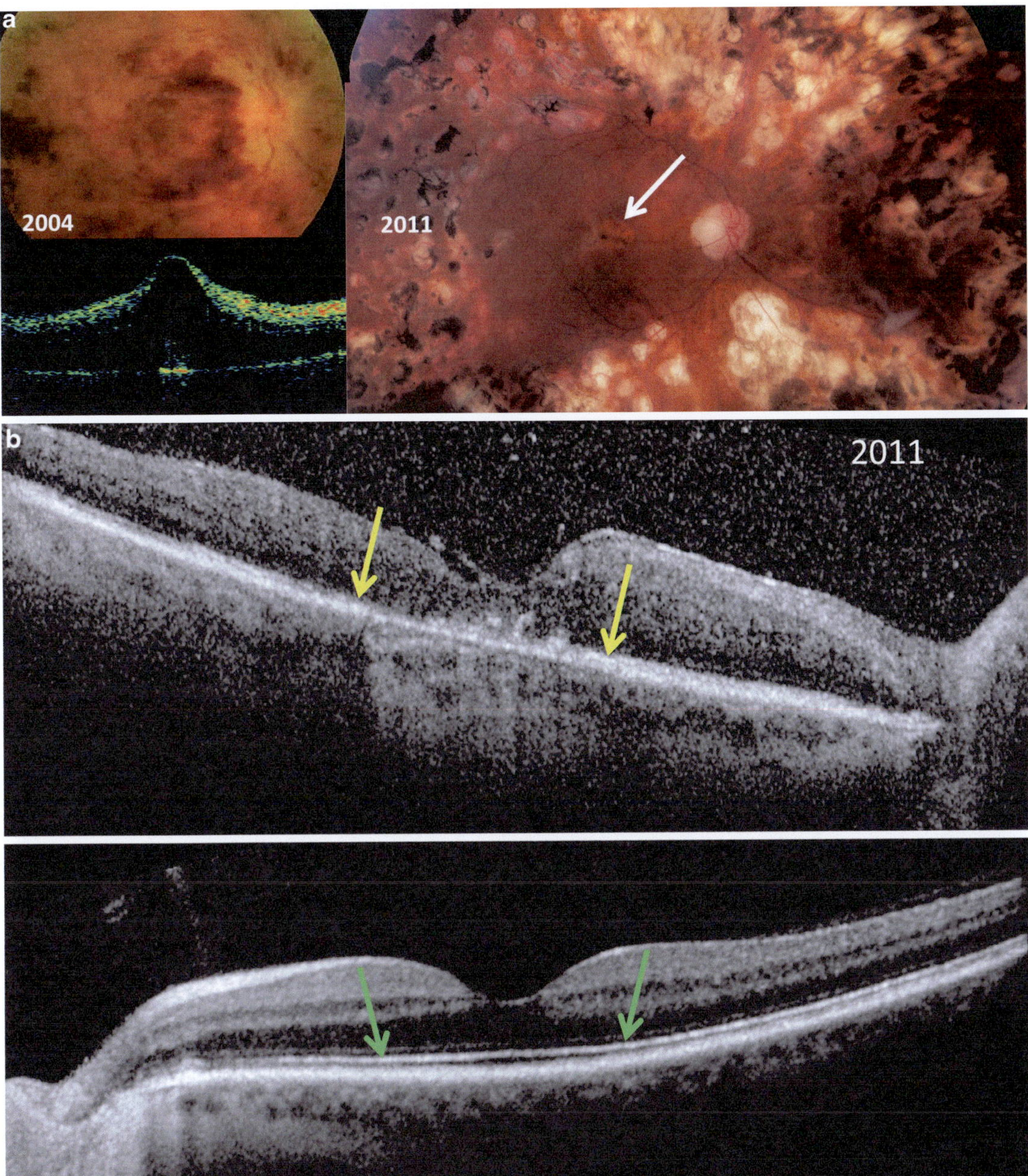

Fig. 10.7 Images from ancillary testing of a 53-year-old woman on hydroxychloroquine therapy for Sjogren's syndrome who had a preexisting maculopathy of the right eye. (**a**) The *upper left panel* shows the appearance of her acute central retinal vein occlusion (CRVO) of the right eye in 2004. The *bottom left panel* shows the marked macular edema as imaged by time domain OCT. The *right panel* shows the macular scarring that resulted from the chronic macular edema (*white arrow*). She has had extensive panretinal photocoagulation as a response to iris neovascularization that followed the CRVO. (**b**) SD-OCT line scans of the right eye (*top panel*) and left eye (*bottom panel*). The macular scarring of the right eye has disrupted the inner segment/outer segment (IS/OS) junction (space between the *yellow arrows*). The IS/OS junction is normal in the left eye (space between the *green arrows*). (**c**) Serial 10-2 VFs of the right and left eyes. The right eye has a stable central scotoma best seen on the pattern deviation display. The fields from the left eye are consistently normal with nonreproducible point scotomas that vary from study to study. (**d**) mf ERG of the right and left eyes. The central hexagonal waveforms are nearly flat in the right eye (compare *red-circled area* to *green-circled area*). The ring averaged waveform for R_1 is also nearly flat, such that the machine is unable to properly place the cursors (*blue-circled area*). The R_1 amplitude (*orange-circled area*) cannot be taken at face value because the cursors are erroneously placed

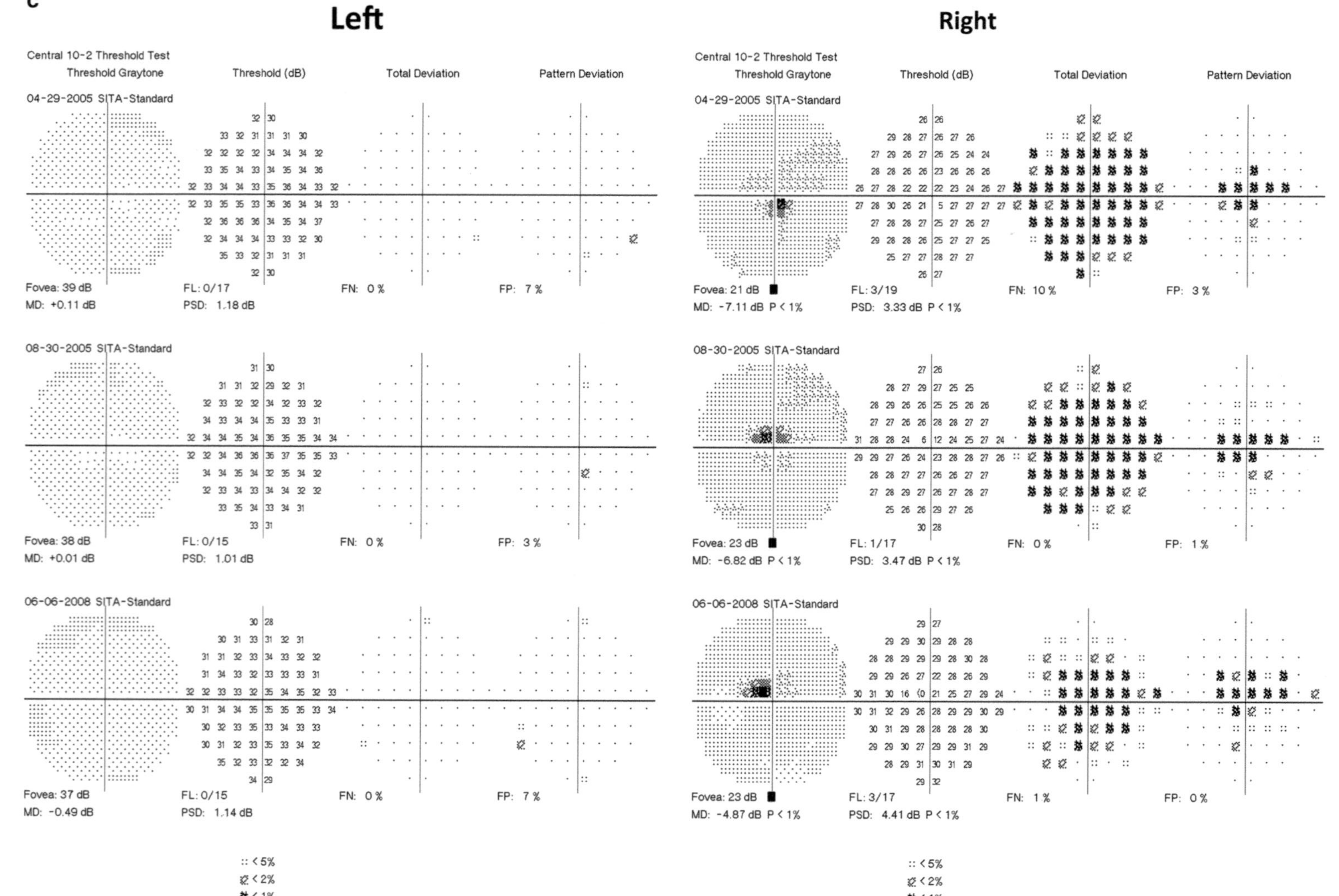

Fig. 10.7 (continued)

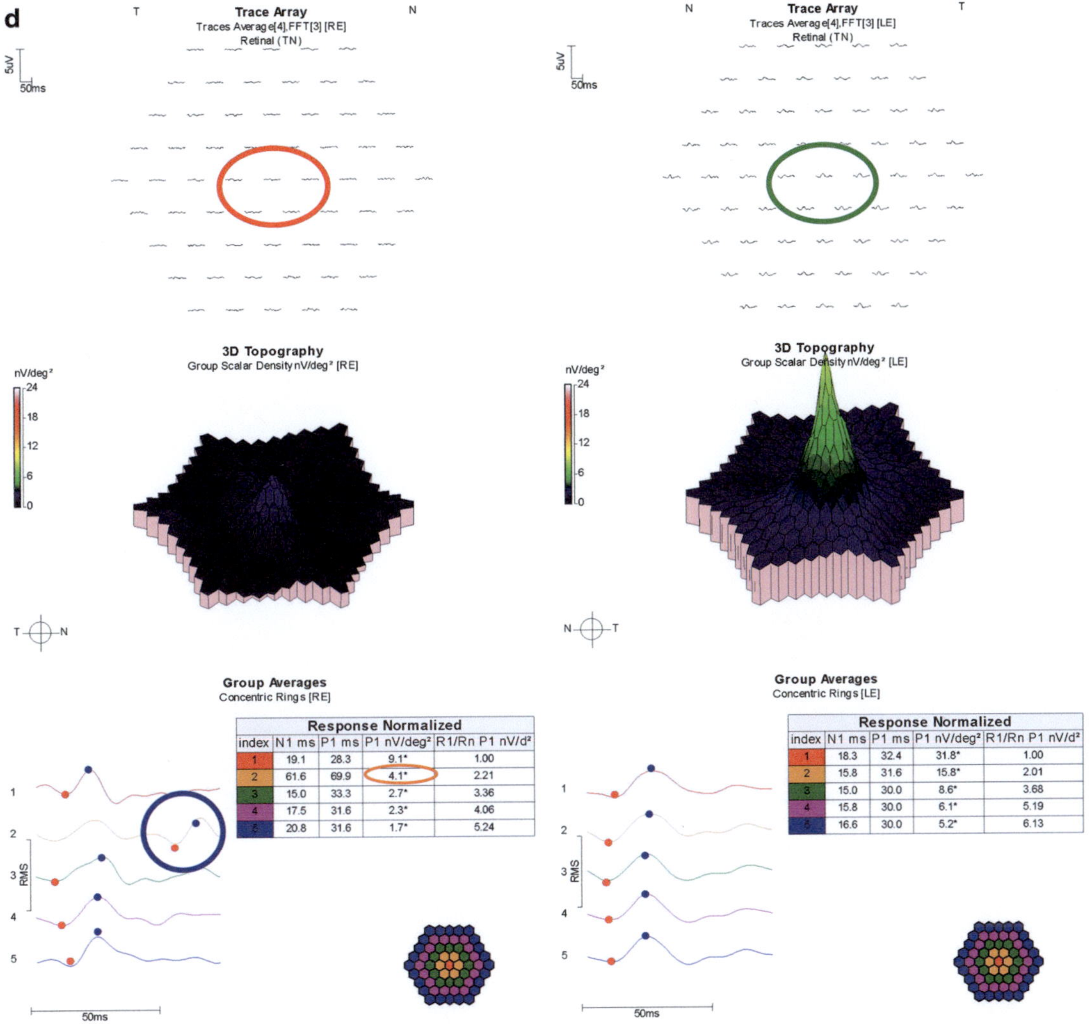

Group Averages
Concentric Rings [RE]

	Response Normalized			
index	N1 ms	P1 ms	P1 nV/deg²	R1/Rn P1 nV/d²
1	19.1	28.3	9.1*	1.00
2	61.6	69.9	4.1*	2.21
3	15.0	33.3	2.7*	3.36
4	17.5	31.6	2.3*	4.06
5	20.8	31.6	1.7*	5.24

Group Averages
Concentric Rings [LE]

	Response Normalized			
index	N1 ms	P1 ms	P1 nV/deg²	R1/Rn P1 nV/d²
1	18.3	32.4	31.8*	1.00
2	15.8	31.6	15.8*	2.01
3	15.0	30.0	8.6*	3.68
4	15.8	30.0	6.1*	5.19
5	16.6	30.0	5.2*	6.13

Fig. 10.7 (continued)

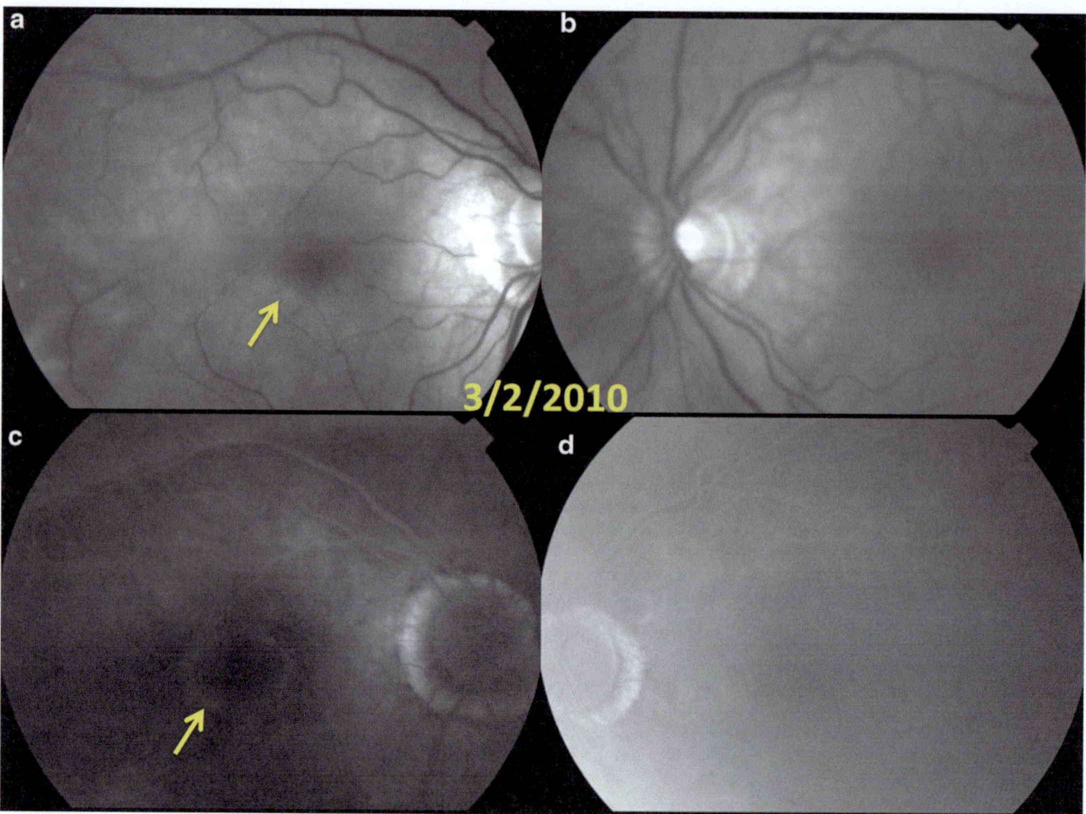

Fig. 10.8 Images from ancillary testing of a 73-year-old woman receiving appropriate dosing of hydroxychloroquine who developed retinopathy anyway. Red-free photographs of the right and left eyes are shown in (**a**) and (**b**), respectively. Frames from the fluorescein angiogram of the right and left eyes are shown in (**c**) and (**d**), respectively. A bull's-eye lesion is evident in the right eye (*yellow arrows*), but not the left eye. Red-free photographs of the right and left eyes 18 months after cessation of hydroxychloroquine are shown in (**e**) and (**f**), respectively. Frames from the fluorescein angiogram of the right and left eyes 18 months after cessation of hydroxychloroquine are shown in (**g**) and (**h**), respectively. The bull's-eye lesion has progressed in the right eye, and now an inferior partial bull's-eye lesion has developed in the left eye (*yellow arrow* (**h**)). 10-2 VFs obtained with the III, white test object of the right and left eyes from 2010 at the time that retinopathy was diagnosed and 2012, 18 months after cessation of the drug are shown in (**i**). The pattern deviation plots show best that paracentral scotomas deepened and broadened in both eyes despite cessation of the drug. Asymmetry in degree of involvement of the two eyes persists. The right eye has more advanced damage. (**j**) Time domain optical coherence tomography (TD-OCT) line scans of the right and left eyes show loss of inner segment/outer (IS/OS) segment junction parafoveally (*purple arrows*). The IS/OS junction at the fovea remains (*white arrow*). (**k**) False color maps of TD-OCT measured macular thickness at diagnosis showing paracentral thinning (*red sectors*). (**l**) False color maps of TD-OCT measured macular thickness at 18 month follow-up showing further paracentral thinning (*red sectors*)

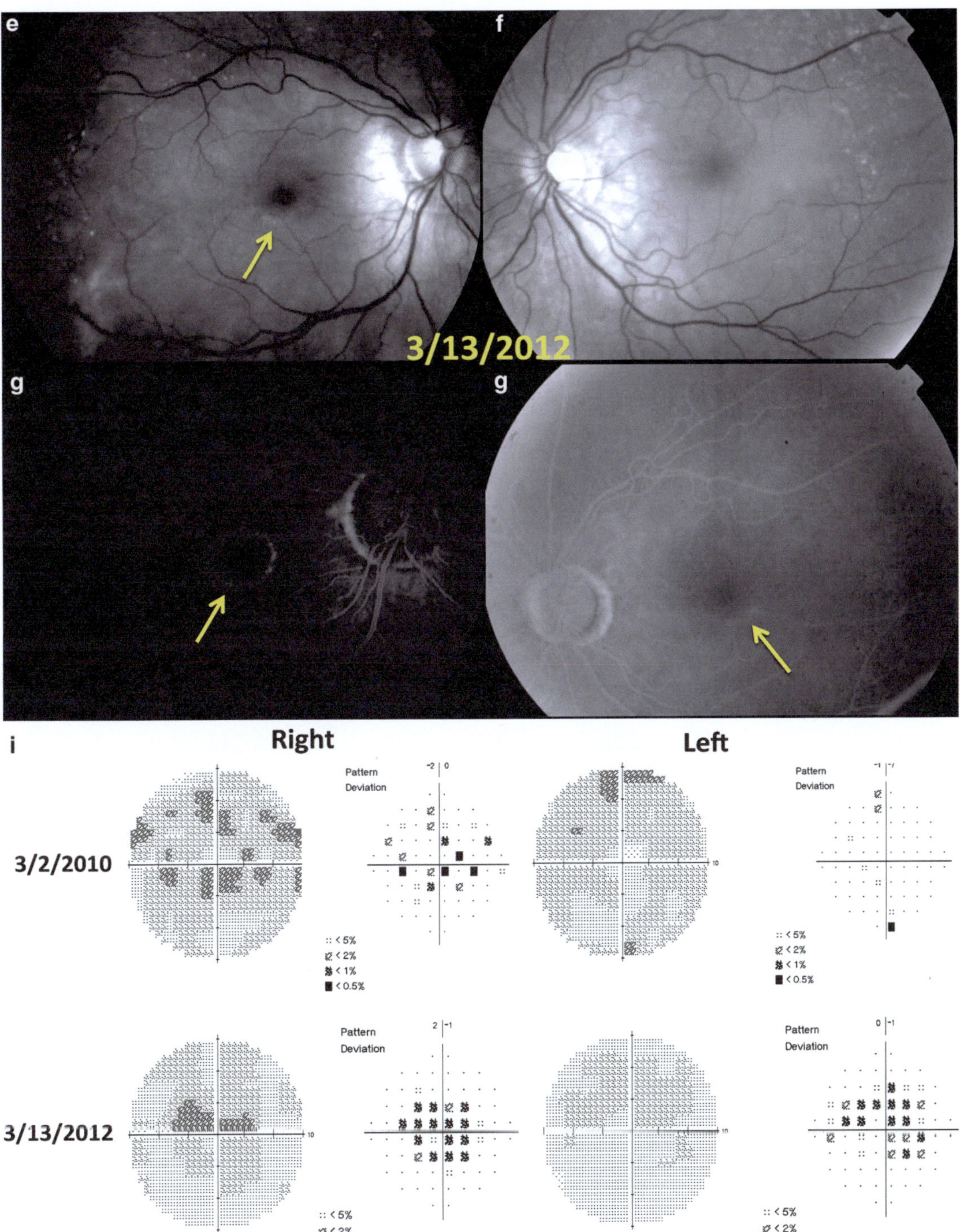

Fig. 10.8 (continued)

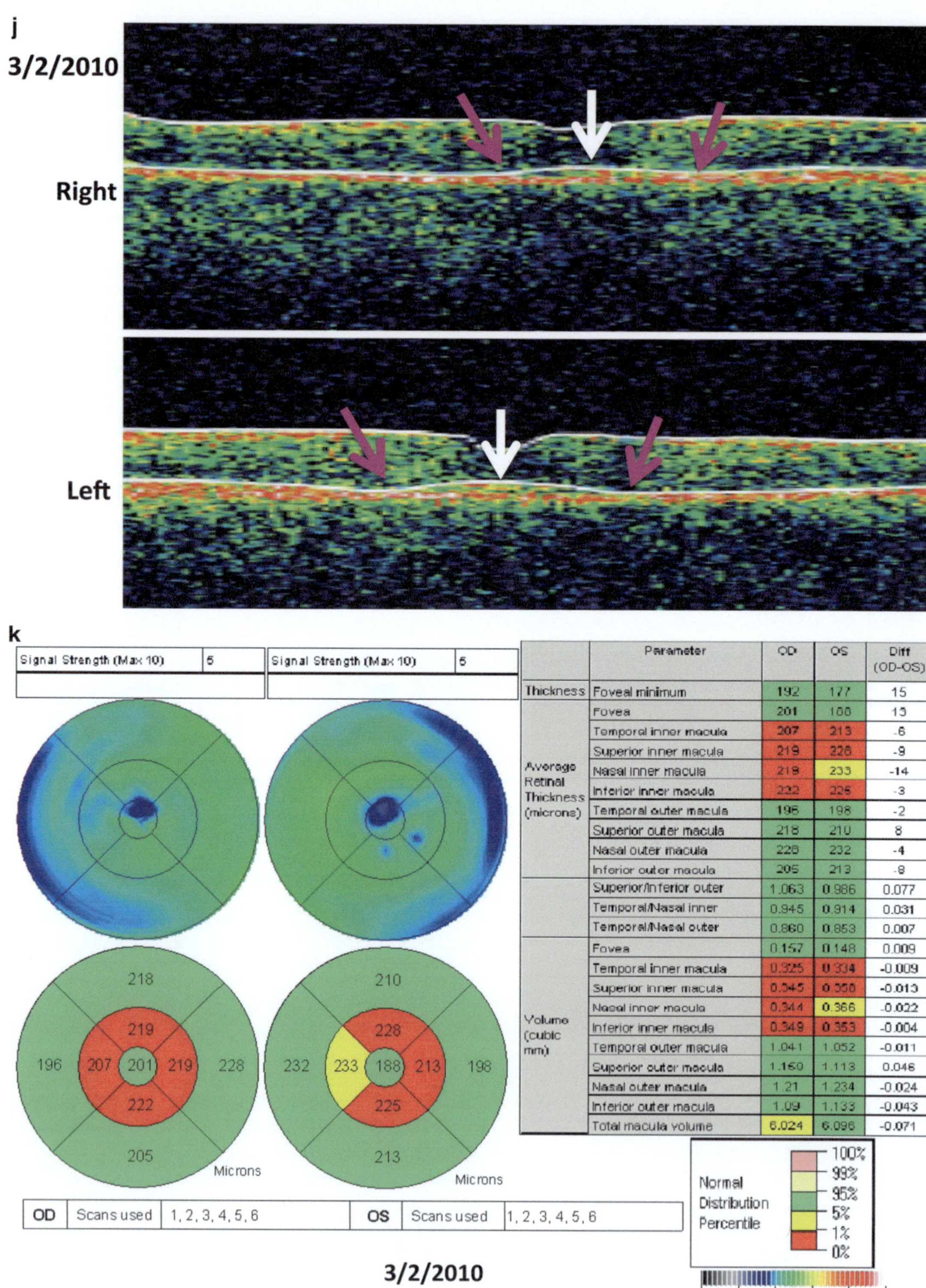

	Parameter	OD	OS	Diff (OD-OS)
Thickness	Foveal minimum	192	177	15
Average Retinal Thickness (microns)	Fovea	201	188	13
	Temporal inner macula	207	213	-6
	Superior inner macula	219	228	-9
	Nasal inner macula	219	233	-14
	Inferior inner macula	222	225	-3
	Temporal outer macula	196	198	-2
	Superior outer macula	218	210	8
	Nasal outer macula	228	232	-4
	Inferior outer macula	205	213	-8
	Superior/Inferior outer	1.063	0.986	0.077
	Temporal/Nasal inner	0.945	0.914	0.031
	Temporal/Nasal outer	0.860	0.853	0.007
Volume (cubic mm)	Fovea	0.157	0.148	0.009
	Temporal inner macula	0.325	0.334	-0.009
	Superior inner macula	0.345	0.358	-0.013
	Nasal inner macula	0.344	0.366	-0.022
	Inferior inner macula	0.349	0.353	-0.004
	Temporal outer macula	1.041	1.052	-0.011
	Superior outer macula	1.160	1.113	0.046
	Nasal outer macula	1.21	1.234	-0.024
	Inferior outer macula	1.09	1.133	-0.043
	Total macula volume	6.024	6.096	-0.071

Fig. 10.8 (continued)

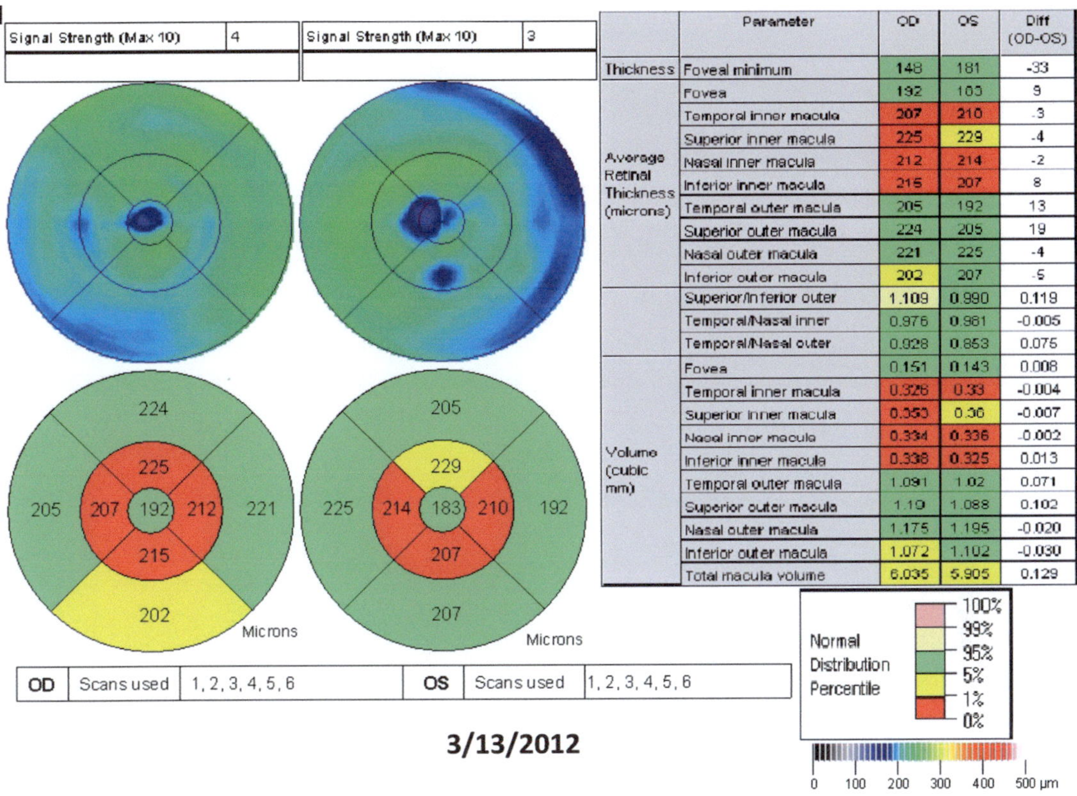

	Parameter	OD	OS	Diff (OD-OS)
Thickness	Foveal minimum	148	181	-33
Average Retinal Thickness (microns)	Fovea	192	183	9
	Temporal inner macula	207	210	-3
	Superior inner macula	225	229	-4
	Nasal inner macula	212	214	-2
	Inferior inner macula	215	207	8
	Temporal outer macula	205	192	13
	Superior outer macula	224	205	19
	Nasal outer macula	221	225	-4
	Inferior outer macula	202	207	-5
	Superior/Inferior outer	1.109	0.990	0.119
	Temporal/Nasal inner	0.976	0.981	-0.005
	Temporal/Nasal outer	0.928	0.853	0.075
Volume (cubic mm)	Fovea	0.151	0.143	0.008
	Temporal inner macula	0.326	0.33	-0.004
	Superior inner macula	0.353	0.36	-0.007
	Nasal inner macula	0.334	0.336	-0.002
	Inferior inner macula	0.338	0.325	0.013
	Temporal outer macula	1.091	1.02	0.071
	Superior outer macula	1.19	1.088	0.102
	Nasal outer macula	1.175	1.195	-0.020
	Inferior outer macula	1.072	1.102	-0.030
	Total macula volume	6.035	5.905	0.129

Fig. 10.8   (continued)

Chap. 8) [3, 5]. The SD-OCT is the most reliable ancillary test and has comparable sensitivity to the 10-2 VF and is unaffected by glaucoma. Therefore, it makes a suitable complementary test to 10-2 VF testing in this situation. Reasonable advice in this case is approval of continued hydroxychloroquine therapy with follow-up in 1 year.

10.10   Interpreting an Abnormal 10-2 Visual Field in a Patient with a Low Pretest Probability of Having Hydroxychloroquine Retinopathy

A 61-year-old woman with Sjogren's syndrome was started on hydroxychloroquine 200 mg/day in 2006. She was 5 ft 3 in. tall and weighed 183 lb. She had no renal or liver disease and no preexist-

ing macular abnormalities. She underwent annual screening for retinopathy with 10-2 VFs (Fig. 10.10). In 2011, paracentral scotomata in the left eye led her screening optometrist to obtain an mf ERG (Fig. 10.10). Is there evidence of retinopathy? How would you have managed this case?

Ancillary testing should be interpreted within the context of a pretest probability of retinopathy. In this case the pretest probability was low because the adjusted daily dose was in a safer range (3.26 mg/kg/day using the IBW of 135 lb for her height), her cumulative dose was low (365 g in 2011), and she had no renal or liver disease. A reasonable estimate of her pretest probability of 4AQR would be 0.1 %. No single 10-2 VF can modify this extremely low clinical suspicion to the point of stopping the medication. Moreover, her 10-2 VFs show high variability over the years, thus the particularly bad appearing study for the right eye in 2011 should not be alarming, especially

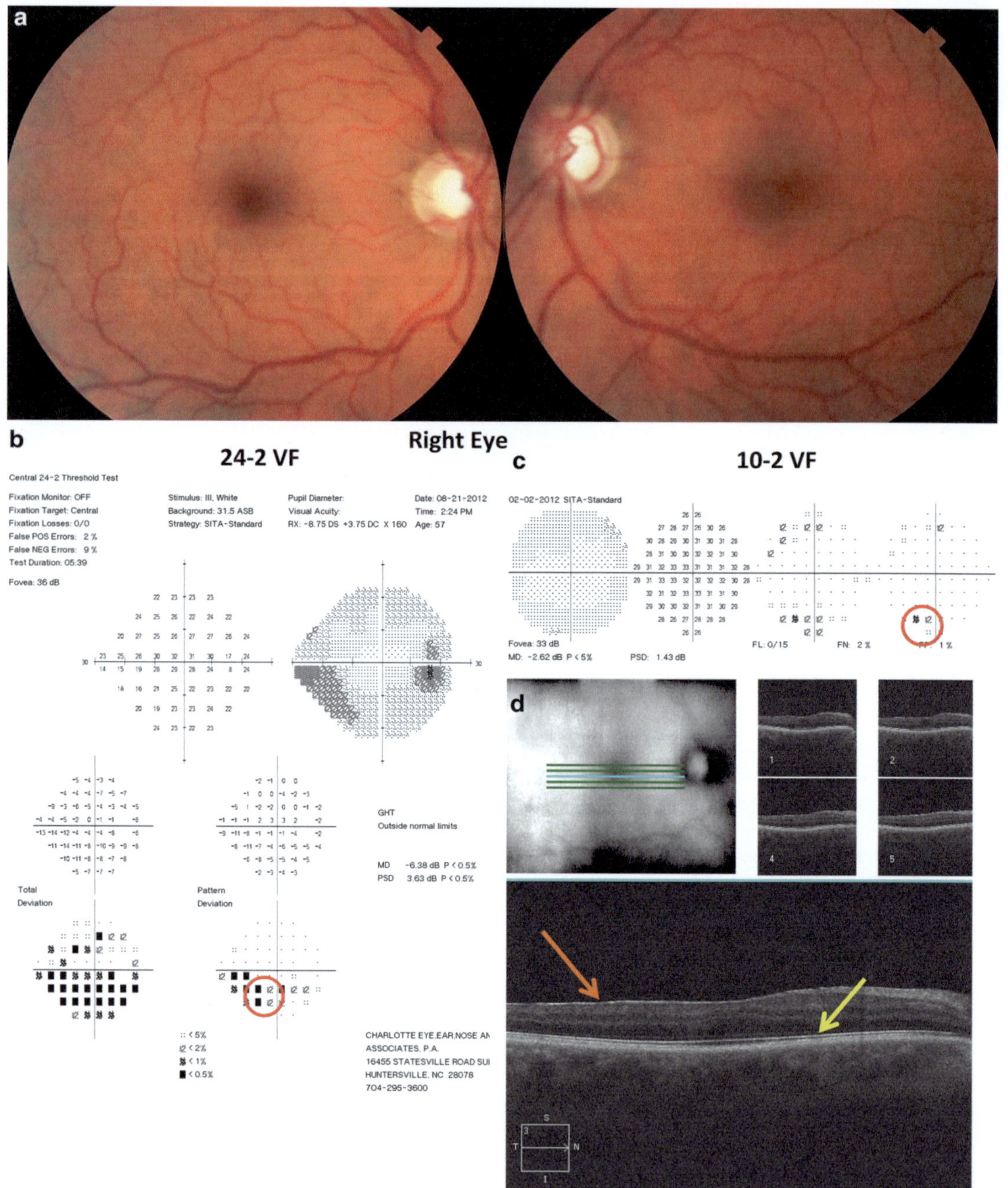

Fig. 10.9 Images from ancillary testing of a 58-year-old woman on appropriately dosed hydroxychloroquine therapy who had ocular comorbidities. (**a**) Color fundus photographs show enlarged optic disc cups left greater than right. She had primary open angle glaucoma. She also had keratoconus which degraded the quality of the photographs slightly. An epiretinal membrane was present on the right but cannot be appreciated in this photograph. (**b**) 24-2 VF testing of the right eye shows a Bjerrum scotoma with a nasal step (*red-circled area*). (**c**) 10-2 VF testing of the right eye shows a paracentral scotoma that might be interpreted as an effect of hydroxychloroquine retinopathy, but in view of the glaucomatous field defect shown in (**b**) more likely represents a 10-2 VF manifestation of her glaucoma. (**d**) SD-OCT line scans of the right eye show the epiretinal membrane (*orange arrow*) and an intact inner segment/outer segment (IS/OS) junction parafoveally (*yellow arrow*). (**e**) 24-2 VF testing of the left eye shows upper and lower arcuate scotomas that represent a combination of damage from glaucoma and her previous CRVO. (**f**) 10-2 VF testing shows a paracentral scotoma that might be interpreted as an effect of hydroxychloroquine retinopathy, but in view of the field defect shown in (**e**) more likely represents a 10-2 VF manifestation of her glaucoma and former CRVO. (**g**) SD-OCT line scans of the left eye show an intact inner segment/outer segment (IS/OS) junction parafoveally (*yellow arrow*)

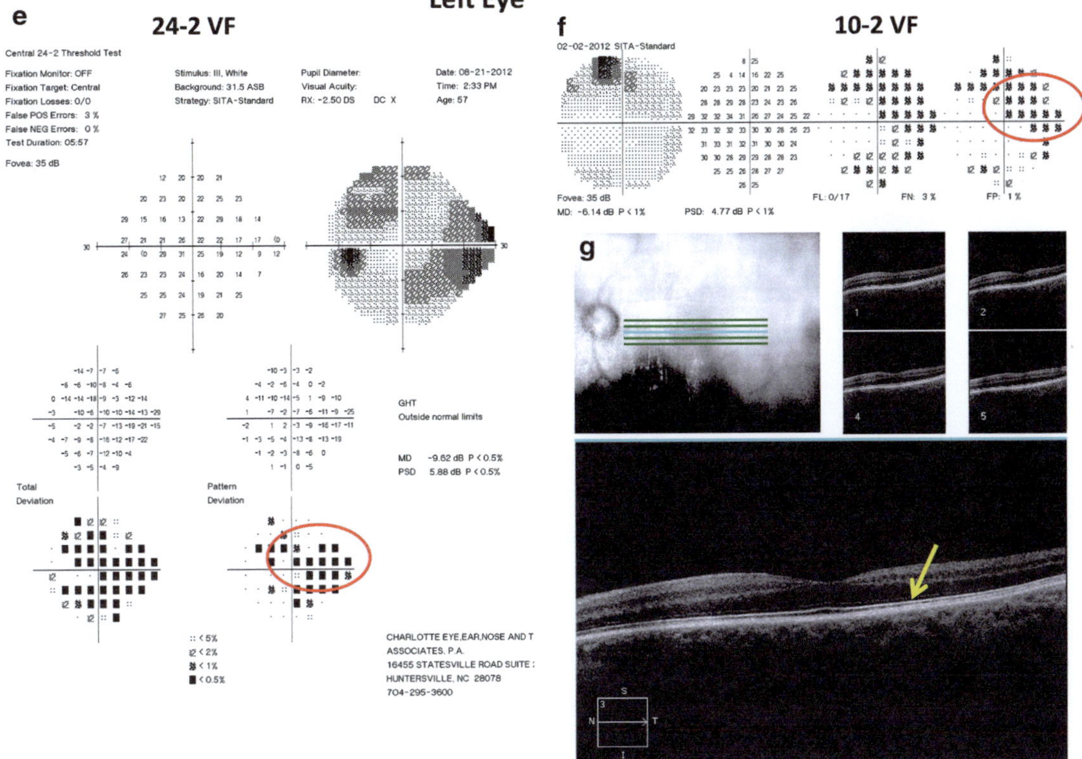

Fig. 10.9 (continued)

as the left eye study was not similarly bad. The appropriate response was to check other ancillary testing not sharing the variability of the 10-2 VFs. The mf ERG and SD-OCT studies were normal, reassuring the clinician that the 10-2 VF of 2011 was a false positive study. The patient was told to continue hydroxychloroquine at the same dosage and to return in 1 year for follow-up.

10.11 Summary of Key Points

- The most important function in screening for 4AQR is to detect and correct overdosing. This single action will have the greatest impact on the incidence of this largely preventable condition.
- The clinician can estimate the pretest probability of 4AQR from the patient's height, weight, daily dosage, duration of therapy, and the presence of renal and liver disease. An estimate of the pretest probability of 4AQR is a necessary prerequisite for proper interpretation of ancillary tests.
- A trend in progressive abnormality of an ancillary test over time carries greater weight than a single abnormal test.
- Mild suspicion of 4AQR should prompt shortening of follow-up screening interval and addition of complementary ancillary tests.
- Moderate suspicion of 4AQR should prompt reduction of dosage with shortened follow-up and multimodal ancillary tests.
- An estimated probability of 4AQR above 80–90 % should prompt cessation of the 4AQ unless other clinical factors are more important (e.g., transplant rejection or high risk of reactivated autoimmune disease).
- Continuing work by clinicians to refine their skills in interpreting ancillary tests is worthwhile. This includes understanding variability and reproducibility of the different tests. Obtaining the correct test but misinterpreting it is a common problem.
- A checklist of risk factors can help the clinician avoid overlooking important infor-

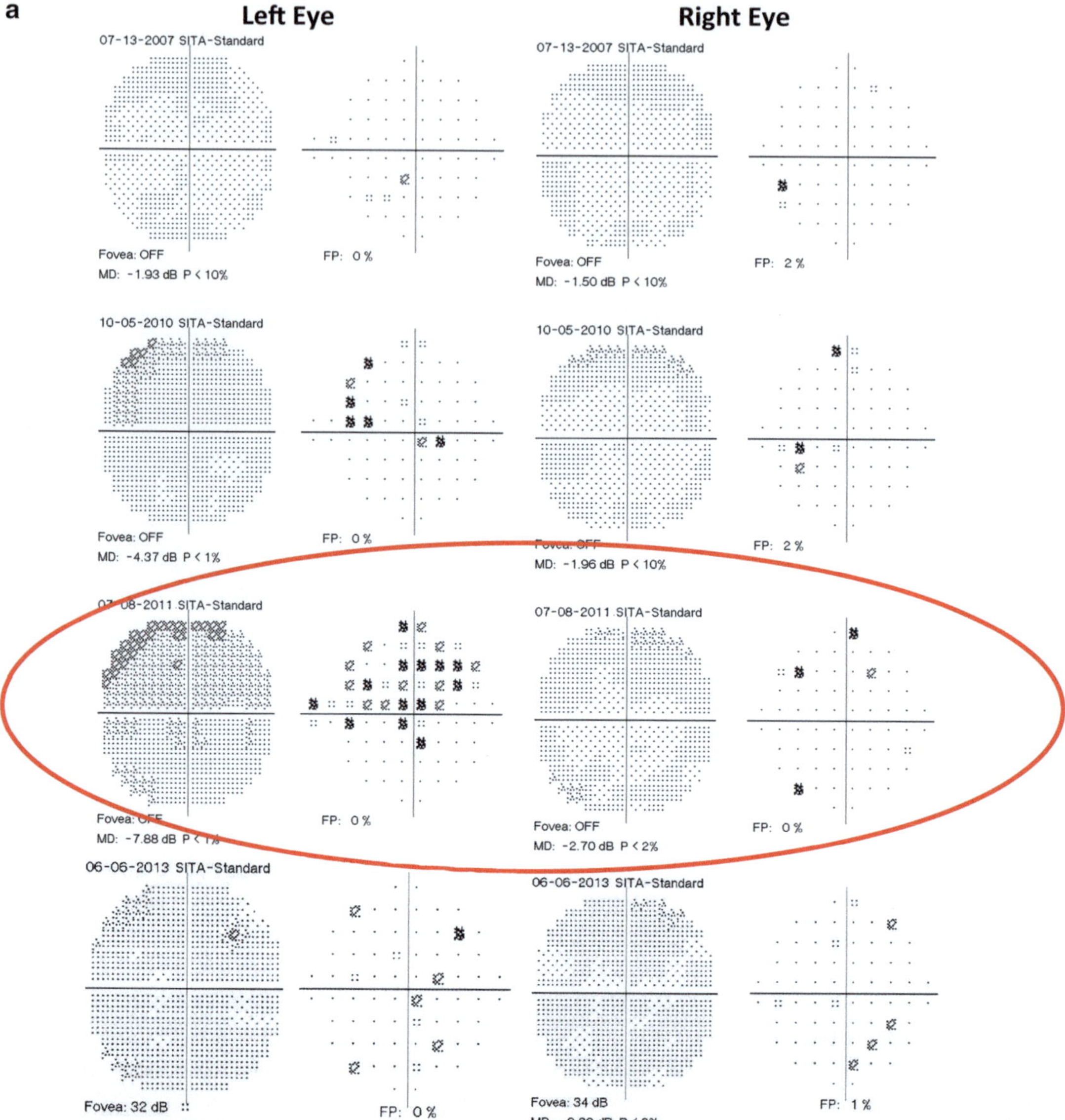

Fig. 10.10 Images from ancillary testing of a 61-year-old woman taking 200 mg/day of hydroxychloroquine for Sjogren's syndrome. (**a**) 10-2 VFs from four serial screening visits. Paracentral scotomas are present in both eyes but they are not reproducible and change in location, breadth, and depth over time. The scotomas appeared worse in 2011 (*red-circled* studies) prompting the optometrist to obtain the mf ERG. However, at the next 10-2 VF in 2013 the apparently worsened scotomata in the right eye had largely resolved. The theme in this sequence of studies is high variability of 10-2 VF testing in this patient. (**b**) mf ERG testing is normal in both eyes using both N1P1 amplitudes and R_1/R_2 ratios. The indices are closer to abnormal in the right eye. (**c**) SD-OCT line scans of both eyes show normal inner segment/outer segment morphology bilaterally

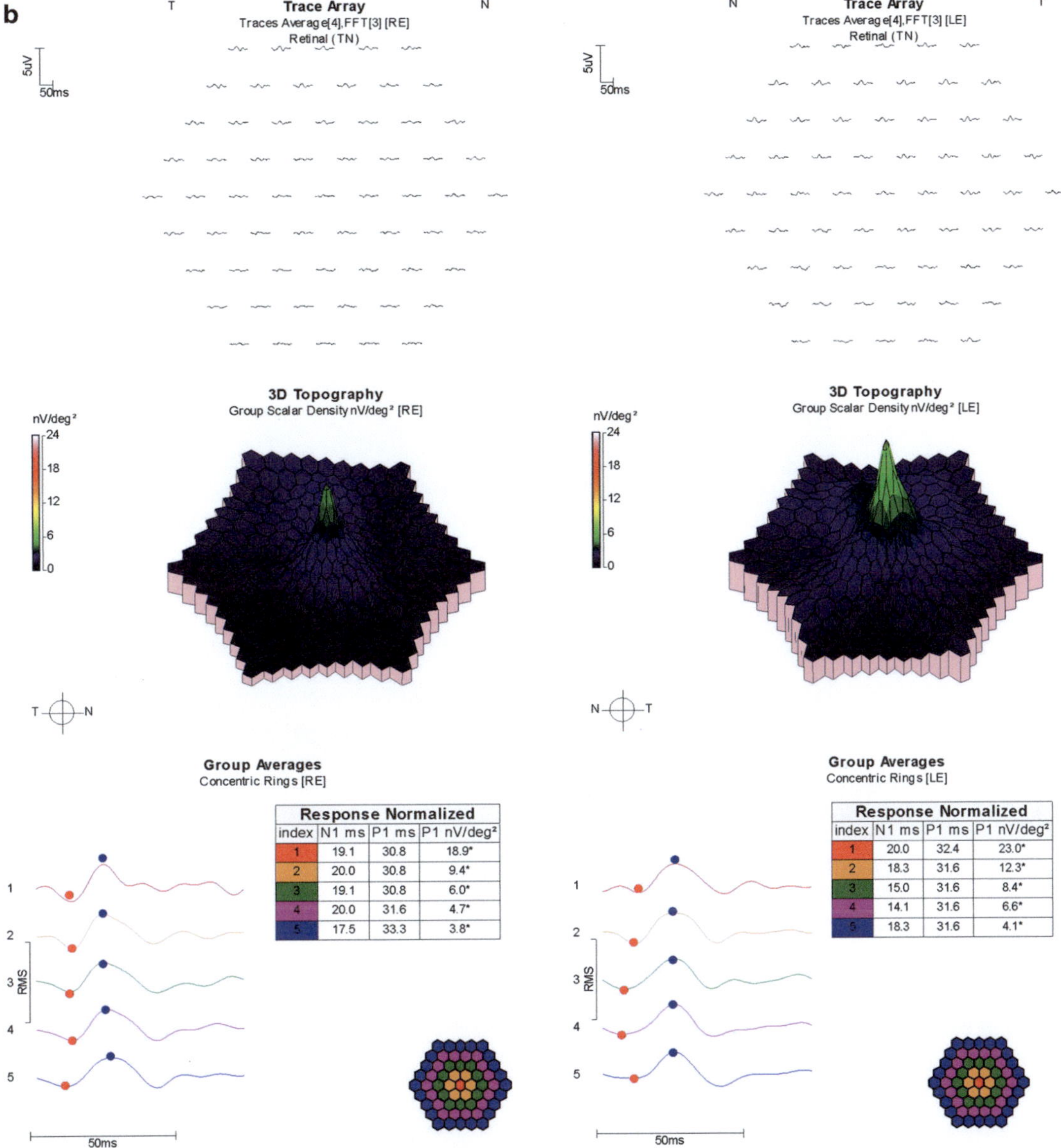

Group Averages — Concentric Rings [RE]

| Response Normalized | | |
index	N1 ms	P1 ms	P1 nV/deg²
1	19.1	30.8	18.9*
2	20.0	30.8	9.4*
3	19.1	30.8	6.0*
4	20.0	31.6	4.7*
5	17.5	33.3	3.8*

Group Averages — Concentric Rings [LE]

| Response Normalized | | |
index	N1 ms	P1 ms	P1 nV/deg²
1	20.0	32.4	23.0*
2	18.3	31.6	12.3*
3	15.0	31.6	8.4*
4	14.1	31.6	6.6*
5	18.3	31.6	4.1*

Fig. 10.10 (continued)

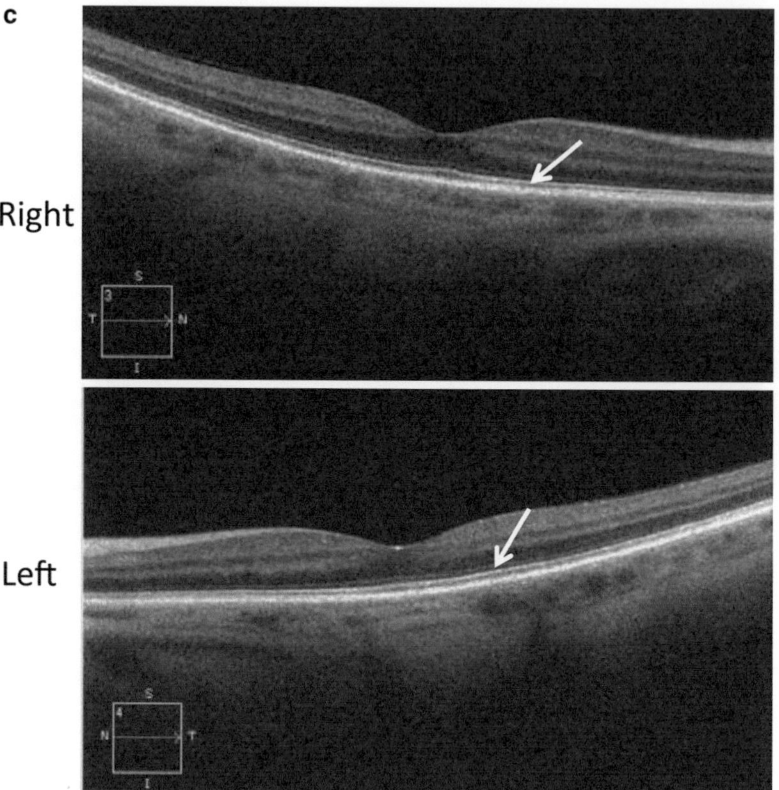

Fig. 10.10 (continued)

mation (e.g., renal dysfunction) affecting the probability of retinopathy.

- In screening patients with unilateral preexisting maculopathy, the uninvolved eye is scrutinized for evidence of retinopathy.
- In cases with bilateral preexisting maculopathy, more weight must be placed on modifiable risk factor optimization (i.e., safer daily dosing based on the lesser of ideal and ABW). Although rare, cases of 4AQR do occur in properly dosed patients, especially if the cumulative dose is high.
- Avoid screening for 4AQR with the 24-2 or 30-2 visual field; use the 10-2 VF. In patients with glaucoma who take 4AQs, use both the 10-2 VF and one of the broader visual field tests according to the reason for testing.

References

1. Browning DJ. Impact of the revised American Academy of Ophthalmology guidelines regarding hydroxychloroquine screening on actual practice. Am J Ophthalmol. 2013;155:418–28.
2. Browning DJ. Reply to defining ideal body weight. Am J Ophthalmol. 2002;134:935–6.
3. Browning DJ. Hydroxychloroquine and chloroquine retinopathy: screening for drug toxicity. Am J Ophthalmol. 2002;133:649–56.
4. Mackenzie AH. Dose refinements in long-term therapy of rheumatoid arthritis with antimalarials. Am J Med. 1983;75:40–5.
5. Anderson C, Blaha GR, Marx JL. Humphrey visual field findings in hydroxychloroquine toxicity. Eye. 2011;25:1535–45.
6. Aronoff GR, Brier M. Prescribing drugs in renal disease. In: Brenner BM, editor. Brenner and Rector's the kidney. Philadelphia: Saunders; 2004. p. 2850–70.

Index

D.J. Browning, *Hydroxychloroquine and Chloroquine Retinopathy*,
DOI 10.1007/978-1-4939-0597-3, © Springer Science+Business Media New York 2014